DATE DUE

Integrating Complementary Medicine into Health Systems

Edited by

Nancy Faass, MSW, MPH
Writer
San Francisco, California

AN ASPEN PUBLICATION®
Aspen Publishers, Inc.
Gaithersburg, Maryland
2001

This publication is designed to provide accurate and authoritative information in regard to the Subject Matter covered. It is sold with the understanding that the publisher is not engaged in rendering legal, accounting, or other professional service. If legal advice or other expert assistance is required, the service of a competent professional person should be sought. (From a Declaration of Principles jointly adopted by a Committee of the American Bar Association and a Committee of Publishers and Associations.)

The author has made every effort to ensure the accuracy of the information herein. However, appropriate information sources should be consulted, especially for new or unfamiliar procedures. It is the responsibility of every practitioner to evaluate the appropriateness of a particular opinion in the context of actual clinical situations and with due considerations to new developments. The author, editors, and the publisher cannot be held responsible for any typographical or other errors found in this book.

Library of Congress Cataloging-in-Publication Data

Integrating complementary medicine into health systems / edited by Nancy J. Faass.
p.; cm.
Includes index.
ISBN 0-8342-1216-1
1. Alternative medicine. 2. Integrated delivery of health care. I. Faass, Nancy.
[DNLM: 1. Alternative Medicine—organization & administration. 2. Delivery of Health
Care, Integrated. WB 890 I6065 2001]
R733 .I57 2001
362.1—dc21
00-069523

Aspen Publishers, Inc., grants permission for photocopying for limited personal or internal use. This consent does not extend to other kinds of copying, such as copying for general distribution, for advertising or promotional purposes, for creating new collective works, or for resale. For information, address Aspen Publishers, Inc., Permissions Department, 200 Orchard Ridge Drive, Suite 200, Gaithersburg, Maryland 20878.

Orders: (800) 638-8437
Customer Service: (800) 234-1660

About Aspen Publishers • For more than 40 years, Aspen has been a leading professional publisher in a variety of disciplines. Aspen's vast information resources are available in both print and electronic formats. We are committed to providing the highest quality information available in the most appropriate format for our customers. Visit Aspen's Internet site for more information resources, directories, articles, and a searchable version of Aspen's full catalog, including the most recent publications: **www.aspenpublishers.com**
Aspen Publishers, Inc. • The hallmark of quality in publishing
Member of the worldwide Wolters Kluwer group.

Editorial Services: Ruth Bloom
Library of Congress Catalog Card Number: 00-069523
ISBN: 0-8342-1216-1

Printed in the United States of America

1 2 3 4 5

_____

To my father

_____

Table of Contents

Acknowledgments and Contributors

Like good research, a resource typically reflects the concerted efforts of more than one person. This book would not be possible without the contributions of a number of people: Sandy Cannon, Ruth Bloom, and Tara Tomlinson at Aspen Publishers; Charles A. Simpson, medical director of Complementary Healthcare Plans, Portland, OR; Roger Jahnke, director of Health Action, Santa Barbara, CA; and John Weeks, founder-editor of *The Integrator*, Seattle, WA.

A number of people have kindly reviewed portions of the manuscript or provided additional resources. Many others have been generous with their time and consideration. I would also like to express my gratitude to David Kailin, Leah Kliger, Phil Herre, Robert Strub, MD, and Anita Armstrong for their advice on the manuscript; to Benjamin Druss, MD, Michael Menke, and Maria Van Rompay for their insight regarding the research; and to the research and production team: Karen, Esther, Norm, Dennis, and Joel. My most sincere appreciation goes to the contributing authors because their insight and understanding comprise the substance of the book.

Special Acknowledgments

The following individuals and organizations made significant contributions to this text:

Acupuncture and Oriental Medicine Alliance
Steven G. Aldana, PhD
American Massage Therapy Association
David Bearman, MD
Donald M. Berwick, MD
Clement Bezold, PhD
Lori L. Bielinski, LMP
Jeffrey S. Bland, PhD
Francis Brinker, ND
Claire M. Cassidy, PhD
The Center for Health Design
David Chapman-Smith, LLB
Michael H. Cohen, MBA, JD

Complementary Medicine Program, University of Maryland School of Medicine
Tiffany M. Field, PhD
David H. Freedman
Thomas A. Glass, PhD
Ron Z. Goetzel, PhD
Greta Golden
Deborah Grandinetti
Songping Han, PhD
Ji-sheng Han, MD
Daniel T. Hansen, DC
Maria Hill, MS, RN
Bert H. Jacobson, EdD

Lawrence H. Kushi, ScD
Jeffrey S. Levin, PhD, MPH
Allison R. McCutcheon, PhD
Judith McKinnon, CMT
Michael T. Murray, ND
National Cancer Institute
National Center for Complementary and Alternative Medicine
Ornish Preventive Medicine Research Institute
Amanda J. Owens, JD
The Picker Institute
Barbara Raley, LVN, OMA
Ralph F. Rashbaum, MD

Haya R. Rubin, MD, PhD
Len Saputo, MD
Paul Saunders, ND
Robyn Scherr
John R. Schuck, PhD
Thomas Snook

Lea Steele, PhD
Stephen E. Straus
John J. Triano, DC, PhD
Edward L. Trimble
George A. Ulett, MD, PhD
Kris Vardell, MS

Washington State, Office of the
    Insurance Commissioner
David O. Weber
John Weeks
Melvyn Werbach, MD
Leslie Yee, MD, MPH

Contributors

Sita Ananth, MHA
Associate Director of Education
Health Forum/AHA
San Francisco, California

William Mac Beckner
Director, Information Services
Complementary Medicine Program
University of Maryland School of Medicine
Trial Registry Coordinator
Cochrane Complementary Medicine Field
Baltimore, Maryland

Linda L. Bedell-Logan
President and CEO
Solutions in Integrative Medicine
Saco, Maine

Stephen Birch, PhD, LAc
Director
Stichting (Foundation) for the Study of
    Traditional East Asian Medicine
Amsterdam, The Netherlands

James Blair, LAc, Dipl Ac
Director
Seattle Acupuncture Associates
Co-Founder
Center for Comprehensive Care
Seattle, Washington

Brian Bouch, MD
Medical Director
Hillpark Clinic
    and
OneBody.com
Clinical Instructor
UCLA Medical Acupuncture for Physicians
Los Angeles, California

Richard A. Branson, DC
Director of Chiropractic
Institute of Athletic Medicine
Eagan, Minnesota

Richard D. Brinkley, MPA
President and CEO
Complementary Healthcare Plans, Inc.
Portland, Oregon

Carlo Calabrese, ND, MPH
Product Development Manager
Rexall Sundown
Boca Raton, Florida
Adjunct Senior Scientist
Bastyr University Research Institute
Kenmore, Washington

Debra Canfield
Operations Coordinator
Alternative Medicine Division
Department of Medicine
Hennepin County Medical Center
Minneapolis, Minnesota

Kim M. Carlson
Administrator
Seattle Cancer Treatment and Wellness Center
Seattle, Washington

Linda Chrisman, MA
Rosen Method Bodywork Practitioner
Continuum Movement Teacher
Oakland, California

Robert E. Christenson
Co-Founder and Senior Principal
CAM Consults
Minneapolis, Minnesota

Cliff K. Cisco
Senior Vice President
Hawaii Medical Service Association
Honolulu, Hawaii

James E. Connolly, MBA, CMCE
Assistant Vice President
Allied Products Department
Regence BlueCross BlueShield of Oregon
Portland, Oregon

Nancy Faass, MSW, MPH
Writer
San Francisco, California

Christopher Foley, MD
Director
Integrative Health, HealthEast
Clinical Assistant Professor
College of Pharmacy
University of Minnesota
St. Paul, Minnesota

Susan B. Frampton, PhD
Executive Director
Planetree, Inc.
Derby, Connecticut

Tracy W. Gaudet, MD
Associate Director
The Duke Center for Integrative Medicine
Assistant Professor
Clinical Obstetrics and Gynecology
Duke University
Durham, North Carolina
Former Director and Medical Director
Program in Integrative Medicine
University of Arizona College of Medicine
Tucson, Arizona

Melinna Giannini
Chief Executive Officer
Alternative Link, Inc.
Las Cruces, New Mexico

Richard Hammerschlag, PhD
Research Director
Oregon College of Oriental Medicine
Portland, Oregon

Lon Hatfield, MD, PhD
Founding Medical Director, Healing Arts
  Center
Co-Founder
Northeast Washington Medical Group
Colville, Washington

H. Phil Herre, MBA
Chief Executive Officer
East-West Health Centers
Greenwood Village, Colorado

Karen A. Hohenstein, MBA
Director and Consultant
Tiber Group
Chicago, Illinois

Tori Hudson, ND
Professor
National College of Naturopathic Medicine
Medical Director and Naturopathic Physician
A Women's Time
Portland, Oregon

Vickie S. Ina, MBA
Former Senior Vice President
Practitioner Product Development
Consensus Health dba OneBody.com
Emeryville, California

Roger Jahnke, PhD, OMD
Chief Executive Officer
Health Action
Santa Barbara, California

Wayne B. Jonas, MD
Associate Professor
Departments of Family Medicine and of
    Preventive Medicine/Biometrics
Uniformed Services University of the Health
    Sciences
Former Director
Office of Alternative Medicine
National Institutes of Health
Bethesda, Maryland

David C. Kailin, MPH, PhD Candidate
Chief Executive Officer
Convergent Medical Systems, Inc.
Corvallis, Oregon

Alan M. Kittner, MBA
Chief Executive Officer
Consensus Health dba OneBody.com
Emeryville, California

Leah Kliger, MHA, CH
Director
Program for Integrative Medicine
Evergreen Healthcare
Kirkland, Washington
Assistant Clinical Professor
University of Washington Graduate Program in
    Health Services Administration
Seattle, Washington
Principal
The Lakes Group
Kirkland, Washington

Tony Knox
Supervisor
Member Services
Consensus Health dba OneBody.com
Emeryville, California

Efrem Korngold, OMD, LAc
Co-Director
Chinese Medicine Works
Adjunct Faculty
American College of Traditional Chinese
    Medicine
San Francisco, California

Mary Jo Kreitzer, MA, PhD
Director
Center for Spirituality and Healing
University of Minnesota
Minneapolis, Minnesota

Patrick E. Linton, MHA
Consultant
Five Mountain Medical Community
Kamuela, Hawaii
Former Chief Executive Officer
North Hawaii Community Hospital
Waimea, Hawaii

Pamella J. Marchand, MBA
Vice President and Chief Operating Officer
Complementary Healthcare Plans, Inc.
Portland, Oregon

M. Caroline Martin, RN, MHA
President, Chief Executive Officer
Riverside Regional Medical Center
Executive Vice President
Riverside Health System
Newport News, Virginia

Lynn McDowell, RN, BS
Vice President
Medical Services
American WholeHealth Networks, Inc.
Hartland, Wisconsin

William C. Meeker, DC, MPH
Principal Investigator
Consortial Center for Chiropractic Research
Director of Research
Palmer Center for Chiropractic Research
Davenport, Iowa

J. Michael Menke, MA, DC
Consultant in Integrative Medicine
Chiropractic Clinician
Palo Alto, California
Technical Advisor
Program in Integrative Medicine
University of Arizona
Tucson, Arizona
Adjunct Faculty
Palmer Center for Chiropractic Research
Davenport, Iowa

Adrianne Mohr, CMT
Health Educator
Institute for Health and Healing
California Pacific Medical Center
San Francisco, California

Nancy S. Moore, RN, PhD
Vice President
Healing Health Services
St. Charles Medical Center

Robert D. Mootz, DC, FICC
Editor, *Topics in Clinical Chiropractic*
Associate Medical Director for Chiropractic
State of Washington, Department of Labor and
     Industries
Olympia, Washington

Dean Ornish, MD
Director and Founder
Preventive Medicine Research Institute
Sausalito, California
Clinical Professor of Medicine
University of California, San Francisco
San Francisco, California

Marla Jane Orth, MS, MPH
President and CEO
Dimensional Health Systems, Inc.
Dimensional Capital, Inc.
Corte Madera, California

Laura Patton, MD
Clinical Director
Alternative Services Program
Group Health Cooperative
Seattle, Washington
Associate Clinical Professor
University of Washington School of Medicine
Seattle, Washington

Glenn Perelson
Director of Network Development
Preventive Medicine Research Institute (Ornish
     Program)
Sausalito, California

Douglas Ribley, MS
Director
LifeStyles of Akron General Health System
Akron, Ohio

Malcolm Riley, DDS
Director
Associate Fellowship Program
Program in Integrative Medicine
University of Arizona
Tucson, Arizona

Lisa K. Rolfe, MBA
Vice President and Consultant
Tiber Group
Chicago, Illinois

Martin L. Rossman, MD
Co-Founder and Co-Director
Academy for Guided Imagery
Mill Valley, California

Richard Sheff, MD
Chairman of the Board
CommonWell
Boston, Massachusetts
Managing Director
The Greeley Company
Marblehead, Massachusetts

Charles A. Simpson, DC, DABCO
Chief Medical Director
Complementary Healthcare Plans, Inc.
Portland, Oregon
Private Practice
Cornelius Chiropractic Clinic
Cornelius, Oregon

Neil Sol, PhD
Vice President
Outpatient Services
Valley Care Health System
Pleasanton, California

William B. Stewart, MD
Medical Director
Institute for Health and Healing
California Pacific Medical Center
San Francisco, California

Cheryl E. Stone, MSPH
Senior Vice President
Rynne Marketing Group
Evanston, Illinois

Eileen Stretch, ND
Associate Medical Director
American WholeHealth Networks, Inc.
Naturopathic Physician
Institute of Complementary Medicine
Seattle, Washington

Karl J. Toubman, LAc, LMT
Adjunct Medical Provider
North Hawaii Community Hospital
Acupuncturist
Waimea Natural Health Center
Waimea, Hawaii

Thomas Trompeter, MPA
Executive Director
King County Community Health Centers
Kent, Washington

Jeffrey A. Weih, PA, LAc
Physician Assistant, Licensed Acupuncturist
Physiatry Department
Kaiser Permanente Northwest
Portland, Oregon

Andrew Weil, MD
Director
Program in Integrative Medicine
University of Arizona
School of Medicine
Tucson, Arizona

Jay Witter
Vice President of Government Relations
American Chiropractic Association
Arlington, Virginia

Simone B. Zappa, MBA, RN
Program Director/Administrator
Integrative Medicine Service
Memorial Sloan-Kettering Cancer Center
New York, New York

Foreword

The speed and magnitude of change in complementary and alternative medicine (CAM) in the United States today are compelling:

- Complementary health care disciplines are being studied by the National Institutes of Health. The White House Commission on Complementary and Alternative Medicine Policy is working to maximize the benefits of CAM for the general public. Conventional medical schools are integrating CAM topics into medical curricula. The United States Congress, after objectively proving its effectiveness and efficiency, has integrated one CAM discipline, chiropractic, into its military health care systems and has authorized two federal demonstration projects of the Ornish Program.
- CAM providers are emerging as an industry. CAM business leaders have met in an industry summit. CAM organizations are now meeting with each other in various forums to discuss, as professionals not competitors, issues confronting the integration of CAM: health care quality, evidenced-based practice, practitioner credentialing, utilization management, and health care contracting.
- For the first time, a CAM organization sits on the Board of the American Association of Preferred Provider Organizations (AAPPO) as an equal with major medical PPOs. In another example, a major Oregon health plan requested the participation of a CAM medical director on its credentialing committee, alongside allopathic physicians, an event that could not have occurred ten years ago.
- CAM health care benefit designs are now incorporated as "core" benefits in many health plans having evolved out of non-insured discount affinity benefits and carve-out rider insurance products. These products are now delivered by sophisticated CAM specialty PPOs that, in many instances, are licensed to carry insurance risk.
- CAM organizations, heretofore isolated and provincial, have recruited experienced health care executives to co-lead integration efforts with their clinical professionals, while simultaneously appointing outside directors to their boards to provide sophisticated policy and strategy insight.
- Experienced health care executives are being called upon to lead the integration of CAM services into their own traditional health systems.

Today's health care consumers expect performance at the highest level. Performance in complementary health care is measured by cost, quality, access, convenience, and innovation. Competition requires that health care executives and practitioners make the right decisions in order to leverage competitive advantages from CAM. They only can do so if they have accurate and timely information on which to ask the right questions and gather the right information. *Integrating Complementary Medicine into Health Systems* is this resource.

Knowledgeable health care executives and decision makers that quickly need to transition into CAM-savvy health care executives and decision makers will find this book invaluable. Conventional and CAM practitioners alike will also profit from these insights into the integration process as the continuum of health care expands. Students in the healing disciplines need to know what the future of truly integrated health care will be.

The structure of the book is planned around three major concepts:

- Administrative functions
- Organizational models
- Complementary health care disciplines

Readers may seek out information on one of these broad topics or on a specific subject area such as credentialing and staffing. Others may wish to peruse the perspective of experts such as Wayne Jonas, MD, Donald Berwick, MD, and other health care professionals and executives who have pioneered the integration of CAM into the mainstream of health care.

Health care executives may wish to focus on network organizational models or quality management programs, the challenges of credentialing CAM practitioners, and complementary health care or integrative disciplines. Clinicians may be more interested in seeking out chapters on clinical management strategies, clinical perspectives in risk management or review in-depth resources on other CAM disciplines.

Those unfamiliar with administrative or management functions within a health care organization may want to start with the Management Functions section. Whether a seasoned health care professional, experienced clinician, or newcomer to complementary health care, *Integrating Complementary Medicine into Health Systems* will provide a complete resource.

This book has been almost two years in the making with many of the authors directly competing against each other in the marketplace while indirectly cooperating with each other under Nancy Faass's editorial leadership in an endeavor surely to benefit all CAM organizations and professionals. To all the authors and Nancy Faass . . . my admiration for a job well done.

Richard D. Brinkley
President and CEO
Complementary Healthcare Plans, Inc.
Portland, Oregon

Preface

Recent studies have demonstrated the desire of patients for access to complementary and alternative medicine (CAM). Other studies have demonstrated the efficacy and beneficial nature of complementary and alternative approaches, particularly in wellness and in the management of certain chronic conditions. Many administrators and clinicians have responded to these data by referring patients to CAM practitioners and by developing programs and practices in which CAM practitioners and mainstream physicians work synergistically by using alternative therapies in conjunction with standard medical treatments. In integrative medicine centers, CAM professionals have enjoyed the benefits of working within a unified team of professionals in a collegial atmosphere. They also have realized the economic benefits of shared office space and reduced administrative responsibilities and paperwork. Mainstream physicians who become involved in integrative medicine come to value the expanded range of treatment options available to their patients. Their patients appreciate access to a physician who can guide them in all their treatment options, particularly for conditions that have not responded to traditional approaches. Patients are also increasingly interested in prevention, exercise, stress management, nutrition, and herbal therapies and are more likely to seek out physicians who have become knowledgeable in these areas.

Other health professionals have made the decision to integrate CAM into their hospital programs or practices, but want additional baseline information and data before they begin the process. They want to know more about the actual demand for CAM, the best way to introduce CAM to their patients, the most efficient way to identify capable CAM professionals in their community, and the data that support CAM efficacy. In this evolving field, who are the experts? What are the best sources of data?

Integrating Complementary Medicine into Health Systems is a compendium containing a wealth of information, including discussions of the latest research and thinking in integrative medicine and resources linked to realms of knowledge on many related topics. The book is a comprehensive resource that provides up-to-date information on this rapidly developing field. Health care administrators, physicians, and CAM practitioners will benefit from the fresh insights of the many expert contributors. Their varied contributions provide the perspectives of seasoned insiders, offering insight into the manifold pressing issues of this emerging field. Topics cover virtually every facet of integrative medicine from safety and efficacy data in the CAM disciplines to credentialing guidelines and referral protocols.

The overall organization of the book involves five domains:

1. The Emerging Field of Integrative Medicine—an overview of current trends and data
2. Management Functions—field reports on major aspects of CAM administration
3. Organizational Structures—case studies of model programs
4. Integrative Disciplines—descriptions, research, and resources for five major disci-

plines: acupuncture, chiropractic, therapeutic massage, clinical nutrition, and
herbal therapy
5. The Future—perspectives on potential
developments

The reader will find a variety of helpful elements within the chapters that make this book
a useful reference tool; these include case studies, field reports, model programs, and profiles;
perspectives and vantage point; checklists; bibliographies; and resources that contain indispensable lists of references, associations, Web sites,
and other materials for those wishing to explore
each topic further. The chapters in the section
on Integrative Disciplines also contain relevant
utilization data, clinical descriptions, and over-
views of each discipline.

PART I—INTRODUCTION

This initial section explores the major trends
in CAM including credentialing, medical education, insurance issues, employer interests, federal initiatives, and entrepreneurial endeavors; a
review of the best available data on CAM utilization, drawn from the most extensive research
studies of the past decade; trends in consumer
demand and demographics of CAM users from
the GI Generation to Generation X; and how
the epidemiology of disease will influence the
role of CAM in the future. Part I concludes with
considered discussions of two environments in
which complementary medicine is being integrated into the mainstream: the state of Washington and the program at the University of Arizona.

PART II—PRACTICAL STRATEGIC PLANNING

Health care administrators will find Part II of
value, particularly the discussions of the crucial
issues surrounding the development of integrative programming. The initial stages of planning, covered in Chapter 5, include evaluating

organizational readiness; adopting a plan that is
consistent with the organization's overall mission, vision, and organizational mandates; and
conducting a self-assessment of capabilities and
resources to determine the potential for success.
Chapter 6 discusses a strategy for phasing in the
implementation of a CAM program:

1. maximizing health promotion programming
2. expanding the capacity of the infrastructure
3. integrating complementary therapies

In Chapter 7, an overview of strategic planning looks at the entire range of developmental
activities from market analysis to facility design,
program implementation, and billing. Other
topics in this part include potential roles for integrative medicine programs in hospitals and the
possible benefits associated with establishing
such programs. The practical steps involved in
implementing a multisite program are examined
in a case study of the Ornish Program of the
Preventive Medicine Research Institute, including site evaluation, marketing, training, program
development, client motivation, and evaluation.
The section concludes with a model for integrating the administrative, practitioner-related, and
clinical aspects of CAM into mainstream health
care environments.

PART III—REIMBURSEMENT, MARKETING, AND POLICY

Considerations for successful reimbursement
are discussed in Chapter 11, including program
design based epidemiologic data and clinical
outcomes. As consultants, the authors of Chapter
12 share their insights on assessing the market
and developing a marketing campaign. The following chapters discuss insurance coverage, reimbursement, and benefits design from the perspective of the actuary, the insurer, the software
designer, and the underwriter. Federal and state
initiatives relating to CAM are discussed in
Chapters 15 and 16.

PART IV—CREDENTIALING AND STAFFING

Credentialing is covered in-depth, including credentialing rationale, protocol, guidelines, and resources. Chapter 17 also discusses the pros and cons of contracting out the credentialing function to an outside vendor or providing those services in-house. Specific information on state licensure for 22 medical specialties in all 50 states is included. Chapter 18 focuses on recruitment and staffing, organizational culture, compensation and benefits, training, and other aspects of the developing of a team in an integrative clinic.

PART V—REGULATIONS

Important legal issues that affect both practitioners and administrators are examined in Part V. Detailed discussions consider the variability in state laws regulating the practice of medicine (and therefore complementary medicine), as well as malpractice and informed consent and their implications for risk managers. The reader will find the representative statutes, cases, and references invaluable, providing the basis for additional research into this crucial area of health care practice.

PART VI—CLINICAL OPERATIONS

A variety of perspectives are introduced, relevant to the development of clinical education and training in integrative medicine. Chapter 22 showcases two leaders in this developing field: Wayne Jonas and Andrew Weil. Dr Jonas highlights the tremendous successes of technological medicine, which have literally changed patterns of health and disease in technological societies. He discusses the rationale for lifestyle medicine, its potential benefits, and the current limitations in implementing such programs. Dr Weil suggests the potential of integrative medicine to reduce health care costs through the management of chronic illness in the aging population and the provision of less expensive low-tech

treatment options. He also discusses the need for medical education that will provide physicians training in integrative medicine and describes the innovative Program in Integrative Medicine at the University of Arizona.

Nurses and case managers will particularly benefit from the review of care management in Chapter 23, which includes a conceptual framework and information on the management of complex cases. In Chapter 24, five respected clinicians discuss a variety of clinical strategies, including group models for the management of chronic illness and services in women's health. Two essays chronicle the evolution of an integrative practice and the development of mentoring and networking relationships in integrative medicine. The chapter closes with an excellent overview of interprofessional referral protocols describing the etiquette and administrative guidelines as the basis for cooperative patient co-management. Part VI concludes in Chapter 25 with a concise discussion of clinical risk management and its clear importance to CAM providers.

PART VII—ASSESSMENT AND RESEARCH

Chapter 26 is essentially a checklist health care administrators can use to evaluate the degree of integration within their organization, in the context of administration, practitioner-system interface, and clinical operations. In Chapter 27, a discussion of the relevance of technology assessment is provided as it relates to both mainstream medicine and CAM. The authors suggest that CAM therapies need to undergo the same type of assessment as mainstream therapies to determine efficacy, reliability, and cost for treatment and insurance purposes. A useful list of resources completes the chapter.

Chapter 28 outlines the major issues in CAM research today, summarizing the work of a panel from the National Institutes of Health. Some of the most stimulating thinking on the topic of research in the past decade is applied in this discussion of methodology and design. The range of research opportunities available to clinical centers is explored in the following section, which describes participation in research at the Hennepin County Clinic. A resource list is also included in this section on the eleven NIH-funded centers under the National Center for Complementary and Alternative Medicine, as well as a description of the work of the Cochrane Collaboration registry of CAM clinical trials. Chapter 29, based on an interview with Dr Wayne Jonas, provides his insightful perceptions of the current status of CAM research and funding.

PART VIII—NETWORKS

The role of networks in the administration of CAM is examined in Part VIII. Chapter 30 is a thorough overview of network structures and functions, describing the organization of discount (affinity) benefit programs, preferred provider organizations (PPOs), and independent practice associations, as well as financial risk, capitation, and barriers to financial integration. The chapter includes practical guidelines for evaluating networks. Discount or affinity services are the focus of Chapter 31. The section explores major considerations in the development of affinity services by Consensus Health aka OneBody.com, a leader in the field of affinity networks. The second provides the perspective of Hawaii Medical Service Association (HMSA) (BlueCross BlueShield), in a state with nearly universal health care coverage; and the third section profiles a model customer service program, developed through staff education, technical initiatives, and quality management. (Imagine if every businesses could respond to your phone calls in 2 to 20 seconds!). The authors of Chapter 32, from the leadership of Complementary Healthcare Plans based in Portland, present two important aspects of CAM in preferred provider networks: an open access model for CAM delivery in PPOs, as well as utilization and quality management in preferred pro-

vider networks. The final chapter in Part VIII, Chapter 33, looks at the development of utilization guidelines in Group Health Cooperative of Washington state and the quality assurance program of American Whole Health Networks, Inc.

PART IX—INTEGRATIVE MEDICINE CENTERS

Chapter 34 discusses design considerations in the development of integrative medicine centers. Topics range from on-site evaluations to staff training and patient protocols, including an economic profile of the Healing Arts Center in Washington state. Interviews with three free-standing integrative medicine centers are presented in Chapters 35: King County Community Clinics, the Center for Comprehensive Care, and Seattle Cancer Treatment and Wellness Center. Chapters 36 and 37 discuss operations management in a multispecialty group practice—East-West Health Centers in Denver—and in an alternative medicine clinic within a teaching hospital—Hennepin Clinic in Minneapolis. Chapter 38 provides insight into the clinical services of Texas Back Institute, integrating chiropractic into spine care. Two useful case studies provide the reader insight into the institute's methods and rationale. Chapter 39 concludes this part with a presentation of quality management in a hospital-based integrative medicine center—The Institute of Health and Healing at California Pacific Medical Center in San Francisco.

PART X—HOSPITAL-BASED PROGRAMS

Part X opens with a discussion of the role of integrative medicine in disease management and the enormous potential available to hospitals in this approach. A report from the Preventive Medicine Research Institute continues the discussion of disease management, summarizing the findings and data of the Multicenter Lifestyle Demonstration Project. The goal of this clinical research has been to determine whether patients with coronary conditions can avoid medical interventions by making low-cost lifestyle changes, without increasing cardiac morbidity or mortality.

Chapter 41 focuses on North Hawaii Community Hospital, which provides leading-edge medical technology and holistic healing services in a beautiful facility that maximizes the surrounding Hawaiian environment and culture. Memorial Sloan-Kettering Cancer Center is the focus of Chapter 42. Its Integrative Medicine Service provides inpatient and outpatient programs, including an integrative medicine center designed expressly for the program. The range of CAM therapies offered have been carefully selected, based on existing research, in order to support patients in healing and enhance their quality of life.

In this context, researchers from Johns Hopkins Medicine provide a metanalysis of the research literature on the physical environment of health care institutions and its effects on therapeutic outcomes. Their extensive review of more than 70,000 studies and their subsequent analysis has resulted in some significant conclusions well worth the reader's attention. In the second section of Chapter 43, the Picker Institute presents a synopsis of the results from a series of consumer focus groups concerning factors most important to patients in the health care environment. Health care workers will benefit from a better understanding of the patients' points of view after reading these findings. This same sensitivity to the patient's perspective underlies the transformation of Griffin Hospital in Connecticut, described in Chapter 44. The metamorphosis of this facility into a financially successful patient-centered institution over the last 15 years has resulted in an astounding 96% satisfaction rate. The chapter offers a succinct overview of the Planetree model of progressive health care. The section concludes with checklist for administrators, physicians, and nurses who are interested in implementing new programs.

PART XI—WELLNESS PROGRAMS

This section contains five chapters that all relate to health promotion. Chapter 45 provides an overview of CAM's potential role in the expansion of the continuum of care to include programs in health enhancement and prevention. Chapter 46 focuses on the Akron General Health and Wellness Center. The most financially stable unit within the Akron General Health System, the center was begun in 1996 and contains a diagnostic unit, outpatient surgery facilities, rehabilitation programs, and a state-of-the-art fitness center, LifeStyles. LifeStyles includes one of the few truly integrated rehabilitation units in the country, an important element of its success. The Relationship Focused Services of the St. Charles Medical Center in Bend, Oregon, reflects a decade of effort to maximize services for patients that has resulted in exceptionally high patient satisfaction rates and the development of award-winning programs. Chapter 48 explores the innovative programs of Riverside Health System of Virginia, a hospital system turned "health improvement company" that includes not only three acute care centers, but six fitness centers and one of the most extensive, multifaceted community outreach programs in the country. These programs, also recently acknowledged with a national award, serve essentially every major sector of the community, in a service delivery area that extends over hundreds of square miles. The final chapter in this part, Chapter 49, presents the results of a study that compared the medical care costs of employees who participated in a health promotion program with the costs of those who did not participate, reflecting a savings of more than $1.4 million in the third year of the program.

The fourth domain focuses on the integrative disciplines—acupuncture, chiropractic, massage, clinical nutrition, and herbal therapy, examined in detail in Parts XII through XVI. Discussion centers around utilization data, an overview of each discipline, research on efficacy and cost-effectiveness, resources, and extensive bibliography.

PART XII—ACUPUNCTURE

Chapter 50 provides an introduction to the discipline of acupuncture and contains utilization data on acupuncture's acceptance; an overview of clinical acupuncture; resources including national associations, books, references, journals, and Web sites; and a brief summary of the data regarding the cost-effectiveness of acupuncture treatment. The next chapter presents data from in-depth research conducted to survey acupuncture patients in the United States. Performed at six clinics, the study supplies interesting results that will provide insight for program planners in the field of integrative medicine. A seminal review of the literature concerning acupuncture efficacy is offered in Chapter 52. Two bibliographies of important research round out the chapter. In addition, two decades of research are reviewed, intended to document and explain the physiological mechanisms of analgesia induced by electroacupuncture (Chapter 53). Clinical applications of this form of acupuncture for pain, depression, addiction, cerebrovascular accidents, digestive disorders, and anxiety are also briefly discussed.

PART XIII—CHIROPRACTIC

Administrators as well as practitioners will benefit from the information in Part XIII, Chiropractic. Chapter 54 opens with a presentation on the utilization of chiropractic care and continues with an overview of legal scope of practice, epidemiology and treatment, safety and education, education and licensure, and reimbursement. The chapter closes with a list of valuable resources. Chapter 55 provides a review of all the major research on cost-effectiveness of chiropractic in the treatment of common musculoskeletal disorders. Readers will find the extensive reference list useful. Chapter 56 examines the literature on safety and effectiveness of

spinal manipulation for certain complaints. The topics in Chapter 57 include the barriers to the introduction of chiropractic into multidisciplinary practices, the differences between alternative and complementary chiropractors, and a comparison of chiropractic and physical therapy.

PART XIV—MASSAGE

Written by a number of experts, Chapter 58 is a thorough introduction to the discipline of massage therapy. Utilization data, a general overview, clinical applications and contraindications, and resources are included. Two brief essays provide exceptional insight into the role of massage therapy in mind-body medicine—one focusing on applications in psychotherapy, the other on trauma care. An exhaustive glossary that succinctly groups dozens of variations of massage into a few major categories provides readers a mental framework for organizing their thinking. Seminal research that laid the groundwork for the field of therapeutic massage is presented by the Touch Research Institutes (TRI), University of Miami, in an overview of the research on the effectiveness of massage and a bibliography of research conducted at TRI (Chapter 59).

PART XV—CLINICAL NUTRITION

Chapter 60 in Part XV, Clinical Nutrition, reviews the field of clinical nutrition through utilization and efficacy data and summaries of a number of major clinical trials on nutrition; resources include books, videotapes, monthly publications, audiotape series, Web sites, and databases, chosen with clinicians in mind who may wish to deepen their knowledge of this expanding field. Concepts in clinical nutrition from the perspective of functional medicine are offered in Chapter 1. The concept of biochemical individuality is described, which looks at the surprisingly wide range of variability from one individual to the next. Examples and data from clinical research and explanations are included. The multidisciplinary approach of functional medicine is also described.

PART XVI—HERBAL THERAPY

This rapidly expanding field is the theme of Part XVI, which consists of three chapters. Chapter 62 reviews the utilization data in the literature on herbal and homeopathic products. The chapter continues with a discussion of the rebirth of herbal medicine, the role herbs play in modern medicine, the advantages of herbal therapeutics, perspectives on the standardization of herbal medicines, and the processing of botanical products. The chapter closes with an excellent checklist that can be used in credentialing herbal suppliers and a reference list of the major resources in herbal medicine research. Chapter 63 is a crucial examination of the interactions of pharmaceuticals and botanicals—a frequently overlooked and poorly understood area relevant to lay persons and health professionals alike. Chapter 64, on naturopathic medicine, describes a multidisciplinary approach to the evaluation of research literature that could expand our understanding of naturopathy using the knowledge base already available in the peer-reviewed literature.

PART XVII—RESOURCES FOR CONTINUING EDUCATION IN INTEGRATIVE MEDICINE

Mainstream and alternative health practitioners who want to learn more will value the synopsis of continuing education in integrative medicine in Chapter 65. The Program in Integrative Medicine at the University of Arizona is discussed by the program's founder and executive director, including the new distributive learning program conducted over the Internet and through periodic seminars. Three levels of integrative practice and the training needed to achieve them are described. Finally, an annotated list of resources is provided for those wishing to pursue further training in integrative medicine, including a seminal overview of Internet resources.

PART XVIII—FUTURE PERSPECTIVES

This section considers the future of integrative medicine and its evolving niche in the health care system. The author of Chapter 66, a respected futurist, offers a series of forecasts regarding the potential of CAM. The book concludes with Chapter 67, The Total Customer Relationship in Health Care: Broadening the Bandwidth, by Donald Berwick. He closes with this, "When the patient enters our gates, all our encounters must begin with a single question, 'How can I help you?' All the investment of our time, our energies, and our dollars must move ever in the direction of the answers to that question." In part, the answer to that question is to expand the range of options in health care—from the most sophisticated diagnostics, surgery and trauma care, across the spectrum to also include complementary services, self-care resources, prevention, and wellness. This expanded continuum of care will reflect integrative medicine at its best.

Nancy Faass

THE EMERGING FIELD OF INTEGRATIVE MEDICINE

PART I Introduction

Introduction

CHAPTER 1

Major Trends in the Integration of Complementary and Alternative Medicine

John Weeks

Health care systems and managed care organizations across the country are charting their course in the flourishing integration of complementary medicine. For these explorers, the sublime questions posed by natural medicine's health-creating paradigm tend to quickly break into a number of operational challenges:

- Which complementary therapies work? Why do they work? Will they be cost effective?
- Shall we establish an integrative clinic? With which providers? How will we credential them?
- Should we add benefits to our health plan, or add a panel of complementary practitioners to our network?
- Is complementary medicine relevant to inpatient care? If so, which therapies and which providers?

- How do we work with our medical staff—both those who have expressed interest in alternative medicine and those who are adamantly opposed to even opening a conversation?
- How do we respond to the often conflicting wishes of our patients or members, our purchasers, payers, and mainstream providers?

The challenges may seem overwhelming, particularly given the continued wrestling with other forms of health care change already required of physicians and health care executives. Yet significant trends toward the greater integration of complementary and alternative medicine (CAM), presently visible among all of medicine's major stakeholders, suggest that grappling with this new set of issues is part and parcel of health care's core business, not a subplot.

EMERGING TRENDS

Complementary Professions Enhance Their Credentials

The distinctly licensed CAM professions—chiropractic, acupuncture, naturopathic medicine, and massage therapy—matured significantly in the past quarter century. Each of these four professions now offers standardized national exams. Chiropractors, naturopathic physicians, and acupuncturists have each successfully established an accrediting agency for their schools that has gained recognition from the U.S. Department of Education. Licensing for

John Weeks, Publisher-Editor of *THE INTEGRATOR for the Business of Alternative Medicine* <www.onemedicine.com>, is widely recognized as a national expert in the business of CAM integration into mainstream payment and delivery systems. Through his Seattle-based firm, Integration Strategies for Natural Healthcare, he has consulted on integration issues with all types of stakeholders, including hospitals, physician groups, HMOs, federal, state, and local government, employers, venture capital firms, and CAM professional organizations. Weeks, whose early professional work was in politics and journalism, worked from 1983 to 1993 in a variety of leadership positions in the maturation of the CAM movement.

Source: Reprinted from *Healthcare Forum Journal*, Vol. 41, No. 6, by permission, November/December 1998, Copyright 1998 by Health Forum, Inc.

one or more of these disciplines expands into new jurisdictions annually, except for chiropractic, which is licensed in all 50 states. Malpractice insurance is now available to practitioners with licenses. In short, in states where licensing exists, these CAM providers stand at the doorstep of the mainstream payment and delivery systems with their basic entrance credentials pretty well in order (ACA, 2000; NCCAOM, 2000; AANP, 2000; ABMP, 2000).

Current estimates suggest that the United States has approximately:

- 50,000 to 60,000 chiropractors
- 8,000 to 10,000 licensed acupuncturists (plus another 3,000 to 5,000 physicians licensed as acupuncturists)
- 1,500 licensed naturopaths
- Over 120,000 massage therapists and other bodyworkers.

A study that appeared in *Health Affairs* estimated that in 1994, 11% of the "direct care providers" in the United States were chiropractors, acupuncturists, or naturopathic physicians, with that percentage growing to 17% by 2010 (Cooper and Stoflet, 1996). Continuity of care concerns alone argue for expanded integration.

Increased Inclusion in Medical Education

In 1993, some 15 of the nation's 125 medical schools included some education in complementary medicine. Five years later, 75 schools included such courses or electives (Wetzel et al, 1998). Medical schools associated with the University of Pittsburgh, Albert Einstein College of Medicine, Stanford University, and Harvard University are among those developing integrative clinics. New CAM residencies and fellowships have been stimulated by the model offered in the 2-year program at the University of Arizona School of Medicine, directed by Andrew Weil, MD (Gaudet, 1998).

An expansion of CAM continuing education offerings is becoming available to physicians across the country, sponsored by dozens of medical schools. A growing number of publications and online resources allow physicians to receive recognized CME credits through readings on the scientific basis for CAM. These initiatives in medical education have sparked a debate inside the American Association of Medical Colleges and the Society of Teachers of Family Medicine over whether to expand programs from teaching about CAM to courses that promote the clinical use of complementary medicine.

An estimated 15,000 to 20,000 physicians have already crossed over into CAM use in their clinical practices (Eisenberg et al, 1998). Natural product manufacturers view the MD market as a significant growth area for sales of botanical medicines, vitamins, and minerals (Annual industry overview, 1999).

The "Bamboo Curtain" Splinters

Awareness of high consumer use has transformed CAM into a legitimate area of study. The NIH Center for Complementary and Alternative Medicine (NCCAM), originally funded in 1992 at $2 million through the leadership of US Senator Tom Harkin (D-IA), saw federal appropriations increase to $110 million for 2001 (NCCAM, 2000). An ambitious 5-year plan for the Center, developed under the leadership of NCCAM director Stephen Straus, MD, was publicly announced in mid-2000. Included is at least $3 million a year to explore integrated medicine—the real-world challenges in payment and delivery.

Federal support for research is essential for natural health care. Most CAM therapies involve natural agents and procedures that are part of the public domain and cannot be patented. This author views them as a kind of natural health care "Commons," which will only be understood and appropriately utilized in U.S. health care if we significantly expand public funding of CAM research well beyond current levels.

Researchers in the field of complementary medicine are also witnessing significant advances in publication opportunities. Peer-reviewed publications like *Alternative Therapies in Health and Medicine* (founded and edited by Larry Dossey, MD, a physician and researcher) took the lead and are now indexed and included among the journals that appear in the MEDLINE database of the National Library of Medicine.

A breakthrough in mainstream medical science publications came in late 1997 when an editorial in the *Journal of the American Medical Association* (December 17, 1997) called for papers for a special, historic CAM issue that was published November 11, 1998 (Fontanarosa and Lundberg, 1998a; 1998b). *JAMA*'s new direction was fostered by a startlingly rapid shift in interest in alternative medicine, discovered in two annual surveys by the editors of the American Medical Association's family of publications. In 1996, of 73 topics, CAM ranked close to last, 68th. Just 12 months later, a similar survey found that of 86 topics, CAM ranked second. What accounts for this rapid shift? *JAMA* editor George Lundberg, MD, used a cold-war metaphor to eloquently describe the change: "The bamboo curtain between conventional medicine and CAM is splintering."

Insurers and Managed Care Reevaluate CAM

A multiyear project led by Stanford's Kenneth Pelletier, PhD, MD, for the *American Journal of Health Promotion* offers the most definitive peer-reviewed data to date on the penetration of CAM into managed care offerings (Pelletier et al, 1997, 1999). A commercial survey by Sacramento-based Landmark Healthcare found that nearly two-thirds of HMOs offered some CAM coverage (National Market Measures, 1999). Chiropractic dominated, followed by acupuncture and massage. Yet the desired data points are difficult to pin down, because of the multiple meanings of both CAM and coverage.

What we know for certain is that most of the major national health plans either have a CAM product in place or a team working on CAM; this includes United, Kaiser, many local and multistate Blues plans like Anthem and Highmark, Aetna-U.S. Healthcare, and others. Re-

gional plans have also jumped into the field, including Providence Healthplan in Oregon, Oxford Health Plans in New York and Connecticut, Health Net in California, and Sloan's Lake in Colorado (Weeks, 1999a; 1999b; and others).

Chiropractic—if only for acute low-back pain—is a staple offering for a majority of plans, initially in conjunction with Worker's Compensation insurance, and generally as a rider unless mandated. Interest in acupuncture coverage was spurred by the positive report of the 1997 NIH Consensus Conference on acupuncture. The programs developed by Dean Ornish, MD, for reversing coronary artery disease are reported to be covered by 30 to 40 insurers (Ornish, 1998).

The dominant trend during 1998 to 2000, however, was a conservative move to offer CAM through discounted, value-added affinity programs. When plans actually cover CAM services, most do so as an added benefit contracted by employers or groups through insurance riders, with services provided at an added cost and through credentialed networks of practitioners. The current increase in insurer interest is seen as a positive trend primarily in the context of the extreme antagonism of the past. Still, for the average person, the likelihood of coverage for CAM services remains slim at present.

Employer Purchasers Become Involved

Employer purchasers were a relatively quiet stakeholder in the CAM integration process until 1998 when William Mercer became the first employer group to routinely include questions about CAM coverage in national employer surveys (William M. Mercer Inc, 1998). Chiropractic offerings were highest, at 55% to 65% of employers, with acupuncture found to be covered by roughly one-third. Interest was highest among large employers. A 1999 survey of employee benefits professionals by the International Foundation for Employee Benefits Plans presented not only a strong expectation of growing coverage but also of significant use by these decision makers. Nearly 50% personally used some CAM (IFEBP, 2000).

Another indication of purchaser behavior is the experience reported by Oxford Health Plans. Since their CAM benefit was first offered in January 1997, Oxford doubled the plan's projections for the sales of a rider covering chiropractic, acupuncture, and naturopathy.

The strong economic climate and tight labor market in the late 1990s are viewed as a key factor for most employers who have increased CAM offerings. An economic downturn could be expected to dampen employer and payer interest. However, a significant subset views CAM coverage as part of more fundamental efforts to enhance effective care. By 2000, rising base premiums increased the interest of some employer-oriented interests, such as the Institute for Health and Productivity Management, in exploring CAM's role in enhancing employee effectiveness and usefulness (IHPM, 2000).

Federal Interest Is Increasing and Diversifying

Numerous federal initiatives outside the NIH's NCCAM warrant mention (see Chapter 15). In late 1996, the CAM coverage issue officially appeared on the federal agenda when the United States Agency for Health Care Policy and Research linked with the NCCAM's predecessor, the Office of Alternative Medicine, to hold a 1-day workshop on coverage issues in CAM.

A year later, the Health Care Financing Administration (HCFA) began its first CAM exploration beyond chiropractic. A collaboration with the Preventive Medicine Research Institute, directed by Dean Ornish, MD, to investigate the efficacy of multifaceted lifestyle intervention in reversing coronary artery disease among the elderly led to a 1,800-person, multisite demonstration project formally kicked off 2 years later (see Chapter 15). HCFA officials are also reviewing the efficacy of acupuncture for Medicare recipients. In the Department of Veterans Affairs, a $200,000 contract was awarded in spring of 1998 to explore the application of CAM therapies inside the VA's diverse facilities nationwide. The Bureau of Primary Care is look-

ing into CAM's usefulness in serving the underserved (Bureau of Primary Care, 2000). Consumer use of herbs and vitamins is the subject of diverse examinations, with the NIH Office of Dietary Supplements in the point position.

The diversity of federal interest in CAM began to have a centralized focal point in July of 2000. A White House Commission on Complementary and Alternative Medicine Policy, enabled through the NCCAM legislation in late 1998, began its 2-year work plan. Many view this group as setting the course of federal CAM activity for the foreseeable future (see Chapter 15).

CAM Entrepreneurs

Health systems considering the inclusion of CAM have questions about credentialing, quality, utilization, outcomes, and cost. Answers for many of these questions are few and far between. A vice president of underwriting in an innovative managed care organization captured this status succinctly: "Our actuaries took a leap of faith."

However, the information gap is beginning to narrow, in part due to the rapid development of a CAM industry with a stake in providing both services and information. Many of the leaders in these businesses formerly held executive positions inside mainstream health care organizations. Their personal interest in CAM led to decisions to move into CAM professionally. These individuals are becoming culturally bilingual—learning the content and the values of both arenas—and are playing significant roles in the process of bringing CAM services into the mainstream.

Some of these new CAM businesses are sifting the available clinical information and making it readily available on CD-ROM, or in some cases, via Internet and intranet. These organizations include Portland, Oregon-based Healthnotes and Boston-based Integrative Medicine Communications, which owns the newsletter for which this author serves as publisher-editor, *THE INTEGRATOR for the Business of Alter-*

native Medicine. CAM work groups are also forming inside well-known health care publishers such as Aspen, Medical Economics, and the American Hospital Association.

Many of these ventures are working on the creation of clinical pathways and disease management plans that integrate CAM. Alternative Link, in Las Cruces, New Mexico, has developed a product that links a set of CAM procedure codes with attached relative value units (see Chapter 14). Sloan's Lake, a Colorado HMO that is part of Catholic Health Initiatives, is piloting the codes. These CAM information companies know that a part of their economic viability requires that they regularly update their data banks.

Many of these and other CAM entrepreneurs are promising outcomes data as part of the services they provide. Alternare, a CAM services organization in Washington state, is among the first to make good on the promise, reporting on a survey of CAM use to two of its clients, Group Health Cooperative of Puget Sound (see Chapter 33) and Premera Blue Cross of Washington and Alaska.

The findings of Alternare (based on the report of 291 patients) indicate that 92% of patients surveyed found CAM services to be helpful (Weeks and West, 1999). The insurers offer services in acupuncture, naturopathy, and massage:
- Found treatment extremely helpful—56%
- Very helpful—26%
- Helpful—10%
- Decreased use of mainstream medical services—55%
- Decreased use of prescription drugs—61%
- Those who would definitely (70%) or probably (15%) return to the same CAM provider with the same condition—70%
- Those who have had the condition for more than a year—76%

For some CAM entrepreneurs, venture capital is fueling business plans and the expansion of services and networks. One area of investment is integrated clinics. A significant boom in interest in 1995–1996 tapered off, however, amidst the health care industry's general awakening to the problematic marriage of venture capital and primary care, compounded by the struggles of pioneering integrated clinics. The most significant venture was an aggressive plan announced in 1996 by Reston, Virginia-based American WholeHealth to roll out a network of 50 to 100 branded physician-led integrative clinics in major markets within 4 years. By 2000 only 11 clinics were developed and they were not returning the value required by the firm's venture backers. The firm's clinic division was shut down in favor of the firm's Internet and CAM network arms.

The business of developing and offering credentialed networks of CAM providers is another area of significant CAM investment. Successful chiropractic management organizations began adding other CAM specialties. The national leaders here are San Diego-based American Specialty Health, Inc. and American WholeHealth's network division. Each has over 10,000 to 20,000 credentialed providers. Over four dozen regional and national networks of CAM providers now exist, spreading up and down much of both coasts and across many metropolitan areas. The principals of these networks are eager to partner with large health systems and HMOs.

Clearly, this field is in a time of significant growth, even as the first phase of active CAM integration has shown that the economic meeting of disparate paradigms is not easy. Network businesses have been hit by the minuscule revenues in leasing their networks to deliver discount benefits relative to the income and profit potential in managing covered benefits. Challenges in developing successful business models for integrative clinics, combined with the difficult economic climate for health systems post-Balanced Budget Act, have moved many system leaders into a wait-and-see attitude.

Consumers Lead the Way

Meanwhile, the engine for this activity—burgeoning consumer interest in CAM—continues to churn. To all accounts, CAM has gained the attention of leaders in mainstream medicine from the impetus of consumer interest.

The initial mainstream recognition developed from the publication in 1993 of David Eisenberg's study showing that in 1990, 34% of adult Americans were using some form of alternative medicine (1993). Eisenberg's survey update, from data collected in 1997, found use at 42% (1998). A survey in the same year by John Astin found that the percentage of users of alternative medicine had grown to 42% (1998). A survey in 1999, jointly sponsored by Stanford University, Health Net, and American Specialty Health (2000), found that 69% of the respondents had used some form of CAM in the previous year. While some of the increase is due to methodology, the trend among consumers was clearly up in 2000.

Significant areas of growth appear to be vitamin therapy, botanical/herbal medicine, massage, chiropractic, homeopathy, and, where the practitioners are licensed, the services of naturopathic physicians. The population group with the most significant use is baby boomers, particularly women, who tend to influence health care purchasing for their families. Overall, the numbers of individual visits are significant: Eisenberg estimated that 627 million visits were made to complementary practitioners in 1997, more than all visits to primary care physicians in the same year (1998).

FUTURE DIRECTIONS

The CAM movement, driven by consumers, is beginning to reshape the care that consumers receive from their mainstream organization. This represents a tremendous change, particularly when you consider that as late as 1990, these services were still widely denigrated as quackery, fraud, or placebo. By 2010, following these trends, we will see:

- A new generation of physicians less estranged from CAM, with many offering some CAM services or comfortably referring to neighborhood providers.
- Outcomes from explorations like the HCFA/Ornish demonstration project will have begun to shift routine care of chronic conditions to multifactorial mind-body interventions.
- A new scientific literature will expand the outcomes on which physicians and payers can build their decision-making processes.
- Economic and clinical outcomes will be available through various claims-based projects undertaken by the early adopting payers and providers.
- A new sort of care will emerge in some conventional delivery systems—a hybrid that is part conventional and part CAM.
- Consumers will have increased access to distinctly trained CAM professionals whose professional organizations will have become more skilled at distinguishing between their services and the CAM treatments that are minor appendages to conventional practice.

The integration and coverage process, with the increased scrutiny from payers and mainstream providers, will be humbling for some CAM advocates. We will learn that some CAM treatments don't live up to their reputation. Others may produce outcomes beyond the current expectations of the mainstream.

By 2010, consumer experience in the United States may be comparable to current CAM utilization in Germany, where acupuncture, botanical medicine (phytomedicine), and other natural therapies are already routinely covered services. In England, 75% of the population presently reports using homeopathy, herbs, or aromatherapy. The British Medical Association has called for formal and routine inclusion of acupuncture in that nation's National Health Services (Ernst, 1996).

The average consumer-patient in 2010 will be much more likely to have botanicals, vitamins, massage, chiropractic adjustments, and acupuncture treatments prescribed in regular, medical visits. More CAM will be covered.

A fundamental question is whether selected CAM therapies and treatments will be merely grafted onto the conventional experience as in, "take this botanical instead of this drug." Or will the use of these natural modalities become part of a significantly altered patient experience of the medical delivery system? In the health care of the future will CAM advocates become partners in a systemwide campaign to take on the challenge: How shall we create health?

The stand-alone CAM clinic is one of the starting points for integration. So is increased access to carved-out CAM benefits or discounted access. But in their own ways, neither brings CAM into the heart of the organization or mainstream health care delivery. The natural tendency in both is still an externalized grafting of CAM therapies onto the existing system and current paradigms.

We are also seeing indicators of the emergence of a deeper conversation on the role of CAM in health creation through a dialogue that values many voices. One hotbed is Washington state, which in 2000 was in its fifth year of a statewide integration fostered on a 1995 legislated mandate that required all insurers to include every category of licensed provider. For Washington, this meant chiropractors, acupuncturists, massage practitioners, naturopathic physicians, and licensed, direct-entry midwives.

The Washington mandate provoked significantly deepened conversation on optimal integration at all levels of public policy:

- The King County Council, in the Seattle area, sponsored a publicly funded integrative clinic, cosponsored by Bastyr University, a premier center for research and education in natural health care, and the Community Health Centers of King County (see Chapters 16 and 35).
- Bastyr linked with the leadership of Region X of the U.S. Public Health Service in 1997 to explore the potential for a joint mission

between CAM and public health. One product: co-creation of a daylong workshop on integrative diabetes care.
- Through the state Office of the Insurance Commissioner, a Clinician Workgroup on Integrative Care was created involving medical directors of seven health plans, four delivery systems, three CAM networks, seven CAM professional organizations, and four CAM educational institutions. The organizations jointly funded the work for 2 years.
- Harborview Hospital, a teaching hospital for the medical school at the University of Washington, and the Seattle-King County Board of Health each made history by bringing naturopathic physicians onto their boards.
- These breakthroughs were not only in the public sector. The Microsoft Corporation brought a CAM provider onto an advisory panel to help the employer think about optimal approaches to health and productivity.

Creating Relationships

As a Seattle-based participant in the national CAM integration process who has had working relationships on integration with diverse local stakeholders—HMOs, government agencies, CAM professions, and delivery organizations—this author personally had the opportunity to serve on some of the teams that created and evolved a number of these initiatives.

These opportunities allowed him to witness how the value of CAM integration deepens in these communitywide, cooperative environments. Bringing CAM experts into core strategic thinking about the direction of our organizations and essential strategies becomes a possibility once relationships of trust are established. With the creation of relationships, the conversation increasingly shifts from the mechanical, "how do we integrate?" to the more sublime, which lured many into the health care arena, "how do we create health in the populations we serve?"

When we engage this question, we find ourselves in an era beyond the polarization of alternative medicine and conventional medicine. In this context, the best CAM tools, clinical orientations, and service providers have an opportunity to become a seamless part of an integrated system that might rightfully be called, simply, *health care.*

REFERENCES

American Association of Naturopathic Physicians; www.aanp.org; accessed 6/00.

American Chiropractic Association; www.amerchiro.com; accessed 6/00.

American Specialty Health (ASH) and Stanford University. National consumer trends in complementary and alternative medicine. San Diego: ASH. 6/00.

Annual industry overview. *NBJ*. 1999; IV(6):1–5.

Associated Bodywork and Massage Professionals; www.abmp.com; accessed 6/00.

Astin J. Why patients use alternative medicine: results of a national study. *JAMA*. 1998;279(19):1548–1553.

Bureau of Primary Care; www.bphc.hrsa.gov; accessed 6/00.

Cooper RA, Stoflet SJ. Trends in the education and practice of alternative medicine clinicians. *Health Aff*. 1996;15(3):226–238.

Eisenberg D, Davis R, Ettner S, et al. Trends in alternative medicine use in the United States, 1990–1997: results of a follow-up national survey. *JAMA*. 1998; 280(18):1569–1575.

Eisenberg DM, Kessler RC, Foster C, et al. Unconventional medicine in the United States. *N Engl J Med*. 1993;328(4):246–252.

Ernst E. Regulating complementary medicine. Only 0.08% of funding for research in NHS goes to complementary medicine. *BMJ*. 1996;313(7061):882.

Fontanarosa PB, Lundberg GD. Alternative medicine meets science. *JAMA*. 1998a;280(18):1618–1619.

Fontanarosa PB, Lundberg GD. Complementary, alternative, unconventional, and integrative medicine. Call for papers for the annual coordinated theme issues of the AMA Journals. *Arch Gen Psychiatry*. 1998b;55(1):82–83.

Gaudet TW. Integrative medicine: the evolution of a new approach to medicine and to medical education. *Integr Med*. 1998;1:67–73.

IFEBP (International Federation of Employee Benefit Professionals). Census of employee benefit specialists. www.ifebp.org/recen99d.html; accessed 4/00.

IHPM (Institute for Health and Productivity Management); www.ihpm.org; accessed 6/00.

National Market Measures. *The Landmark Report II*. Sacramento, CA: Landmark Healthcare; 1999.

NCCAM (National Center for Complementary and Alternative Medicine). Spring 2000 CAM newsletter. http://nccam.nih.gov/nccam/ne/newsletter/spring200/index/html; accessed 7/00.

NCCAOM (National Council for the Certification of Acupuncture and Oriental Medicine); www.NCCAOM.org; accessed 8/00.

Ornish DM. Avoiding revascularization with lifestyle changes: The Multicenter Lifestyle Demonstration Project. *Am J Cardiol*. 1998;82(10B):72T–76T.

Pelletier KR, Astin JA, Haskell WL. Current trends in the integration and reimbursement of complementary and alternative medicine by managed care organizations (MCOs) and insurance providers: 1998 update and cohort analysis. *Am J Health Promot*. 1999;14(2):125–133.

Pelletier KR, Marie A, Krasner M, Haskell WL. Current trends in the integration and reimbursement of complementary and alternative medicine by managed care, insurance carriers, and hospital providers. *Am J Health Promot*. 1997;12(2):112–122. Review.

Weeks J. Sloan's Lake: spiritual care and CAM in core benefits. *The Integrator*. 1999a;3(11):1, 3.

Weeks J. A kind of blue: alternative medicine spreads in Blue Cross Blue Shield plans. *The Integrator*. 1999b;3(12):1, 3–5.

Weeks J, West P. Presentation on Washington's Clinician Workgroup on Integration of CAM. Healthcare Forum Best Practices meeting, Honolulu, HI, February 10–13, 1999.

Wetzel MS, Eisenberg DM, Kaptchuk TJ. Courses involving complementary and alternative medicine at US medical schools. *JAMA*. 1998;280(9):784–787.

William M. Mercer Inc. National Survey of Employer-Sponsored Health Plans. San Francisco: William M. Mercer, Inc. 1998.

CHAPTER 2

Utilization Data on Complementary and Alternative Medicine

Nancy Faass

SIZE OF THE MARKET

Research Data

In 1993, a seminal article in the *New England Journal of Medicine* changed the way in which we view American medicine. A research team affiliated with Harvard Medical School and led by Eisenberg et al (1993) estimated that, in 1990, Americans made 425 million visits to practitioners of alternative medicine. The researchers projected expenditures for alternative medicine in the United States at more than $13.6 billion. In that same year, out-of-pocket expenditures on hospitalization totaled $12.8 billion.

A second study done by Eisenberg et al (1998) found a 47.5% increase in the number of total visits to alternative medicine practitioners (629 million in 1997), with total expenditures in that year estimated as high as $47.5 billion (see Table 2–1).

The research has expanded our understanding of complementary and alternative medicine (CAM). Three of the surveys conducted in 1998–1999 are in approximate agreement that 40–42% of the general population used CAM in some form:

- Eisenberg et al (1998), in a national telephone survey, found 42% of respondents reporting CAM use
- Astin (1998), in a national mail survey, found 40% reported use
- InterActive Solutions for Landmark Healthcare (1998), in a national telephone survey, reported 42% use
- Druss and Rosenheck (1999), using a federal data set, found 8.2% CAM practitioner utilization
- The Consumers Union, conducting a written survey for *Consumer Reports* (2000), reported 35% CAM use
- Stanford University and American Specialty Health, in a 1998 survey (2000), reported 69% CAM use
- Gordon et al (1998), in a large health maintenance organization (HMO) population, found 50% total past use of CAM and 31% recent use
- Wooten and Sparber (1999), using meta-nalysis of condition-specific research on CAM utilization, found the range of CAM use to be 9–63%

Retail Data

Since these studies, the firmest data we have are sales figures from the natural foods industry. In 1998, consumer purchases in supplements, natural foods, and related products were indicated to be $25.4 billion, reflecting 11% growth from the previous year (Raterman, 1999; Annual Industry Overview, 1999). Sales in 1999 again reflected 11% overall growth, with total sales of $28.2 billion (Figure 2–1) (Traynor, 2000).

Nancy Faass, MSW, MPH, is a writer and editor in San Francisco who provides book and project development in integrative medicine and the social sciences. With an MPH from the University of California at Berkeley and an MSW from Catholic University, she has worked as a science editor at the University of California, San Francisco; as an archivist; and in scholarly publishing. Ms. Faass has also served as program coordinator in social services and education.

Table 2–1 Projections of National Expenditures for CAM in 1997 in Billions of Dollars (Eisenberg, 1998)

Source of Payment and Type of Expense	Conservative to Liberal Estimate	
	Estimated Range of Expenditures on CAM 1990	Estimated Range of Expenditures on CAM 1997
Reimbursed Expenditures—CAM Professional Services and Therapies*	7.4–11.6 B	9.0–13.1 B
Out-of-Pocket Expenditures—CAM Professional Services and Therapies*	7.2–11.0 B	12.2–19.6 B
Out-of-Pocket Spent on Self-Care—Megavitamins, Diet Products, Books, Herbs, Classes, Equipment*	—	14.8–14.8 B
Total CAM Expenditures	$14.6–22.6 B	$36.0–47.5 B

Source: Adapted with permission from D. Eisenberg et al, Trends in Alternative Medicine Use in the United States, 1990–1997: Results of a Follow-Up National Survey, *Journal of the American Medical Association*, Vol. 280, No. 18, p. 1574, © 1998, American Medical Association.

ALTERNATIVE OR COMPLEMENTARY MEDICINE?

The apparently extensive public interest in complementary and alternative medicine goods and services raises a series of questions. In the context of medical services, to what extent do patients use alternative therapies exclusively? Do they seek a combination of conventional and complementary care (often referred to as *integrative medicine*)? The data provide a clear indication that the vast majority of patients seek care in both systems. Of survey respondents who indicated they used CAM, the following percentages reported using both CAM and conventional medicine:

- Eisenberg et al (1998), respondents using both types of care—96%
- InterActive Solutions for Landmark Healthcare (1998), those using both in some combination—86%
- Druss and Rosenheck (1999), those using both—approximately 80%

A study by Astin (1998) at Stanford University specifically addressed the issue of whether people who use complementary medicine use conventional care, as well. The study also looked at the motivation for CAM use and inquired as to whether respondents were dissatisfied with conventional biomedical care. Only 9% of respondents indicated dissatisfaction with conventional care, and less than half of those used CAM. Astin found that, overall, only 4.4% relied primarily on CAM. "The vast majority of individuals appear to use alternative therapies in conjunction with, rather than instead of, more conventional treatment" (Astin, 1998).

Two considerations are suggested by these data. The very high use of conventional care among patients who also utilize CAM reflect broad appreciation of the value of biomedicine. It can be suggested that most patients are grateful for the benefits of Western medicine.

The other implication is that patients are not neglecting conventional care for alternative treatment. A primary concern has been that serious conditions might go undetected by CAM practitioners. The fact that the vast majority of CAM patients continue to use conventional services does not provide an automatic conclusion to this question of safety, but it at least indicates

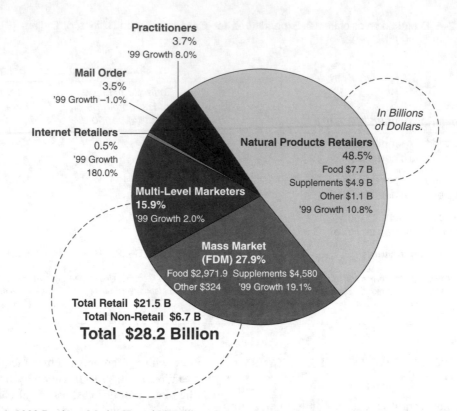

Figure 2–1 1999 Products Market Tops $28 Billion. *Source:* Reprinted with permission from *Products for the Natural and Organic Products Industry*, Vol. 21, No. 6, © 2000, New Hope Communications.

that patients continue to avail themselves of access to biomedical services.

DEMOGRAPHICS

What do we know about who uses complementary medicine? The studies of Eisenberg et al (1993, 1998) surveyed a population selected at random that essentially parallels the U.S. population. Overall, reported utilization of 42.1% reflected a measurable increase from the finding of 33.8% in 1990 (see Table 2–2). Among certain subsets of the population, Eisenberg and colleagues (1998) found that CAM utilization approached 50%, including:

- Respondents with some college—50.6%
- The age group 25–49 years old—50.1%

- Female respondents—48.9%
- Those with incomes above $50,000—48.1%

The Astin analysis (1998) was a written survey mailed to individuals randomly selected from a nationally representative panel. The overall projection was CAM utilization by approximately 40% of the population. Astin's survey identified respondents by demographics and by subculture (see Table 2–2). Groups reporting highest utilization included:

- "Cultural Creatives" (23% of the U.S. population)—55%
- Those with graduate degrees—50%
- Respondents who maintained a holistic philosophy—46%

Table 2–2 Demographics of Patients Who Use CAM, Projected Percentage U.S. Population (Eisenberg et al, 1998 and Astin, 1998)

	Percentage CAM Use in Each Category	
Demographic Characteristic	Eisenberg 1997 Data N = 2,055	Astin 1997 Data N = 1,035
Overall Utilization	42.1	40
Age		
18–24	(ages 18–34) 41.8	35
25–34		41
35–49	50.1	42
≥ 50	39.1	(older than 64 = 35%) 44
Gender		
Female	48.9	41
Male	37.8	39
Education		
High school or less	36.4	31
College graduate	(some college) 50.6	(college/higher) 45/50
Ethnicity		
White	(white/other races) 44.5	41
Black	33.1	29
Hispanic		40
Income		
Lower income	(≤ $50,000) 42.6	(< $40,000) 33
Higher income	(> $50,000) 48.1	(> $40,000) 44

Source: Data from D. Eisenberg et al, Trends in Alternative Medicine Use in the United States, 1990–1997: Results of a Follow-up National Survey, *Journal of the American Medical Association*, Vol. 280, No. 18, pp. 1569–1575, © 1998, American Medical Association and J. Astin, Why Patients Use Alternative Medicine: Results of a National Study, *Journal of the American Medical Association*, Vol. 279, No. 19, pp. 1548–1553, © 1998, American Medical Association.

- Respondents earning $40,000 or greater— 44%

It has been suggested that major expansion and shifts in CAM utilization would occur if complementary medicine were provided as a covered benefit by more insurers and/or employers. Currently, factors in utilization include the availability of disposable income, health insurance coverage, and circumstance (such as coverage under workers' compensation insurance or automobile accident coverage) (Eisenberg et al, 1998; Herre, 1999; Orth, 2000).

PHYSICIAN REFERRAL

For two decades, researchers have monitored physician perceptions of alternative medicine. A number of major studies conducted from 1995 to 2000 evaluated physician referral patterns regarding CAM. Several trends are almost universal in the research findings, and particularly evident in the metanalysis of Astin et al (1998):

- Among the physicians surveyed, more believe CAM therapies to provide therapeutic benefit than actually refer patients to their use.
- Until recently, acceptance of CAM has been greater in Europe and worldwide than in the United States.
- Referrals to CAM therapies by American physicians appear to be increasing steadily.

Astin's analysis (Astin et al, 1998) indicates that, in the majority of studies conducted since

1995, more than a third of physicians report referring patients to acupuncture and chiropractic. Berman et al (1998) found that, among 783 physicians trained in pediatrics, internal medicine, and general practice, more than 90% had used or would use diet, exercise, and stress reduction. The survey of Gordon et al (1998), conducted in a large managed care organization in northern California, found that the level of interest among physicians was significantly associated with clinicians' reports of how often patients mentioned using or considering alternative therapies. The study included 624 primary care clinicians—two-thirds of whom expressed at least moderate interest in the use of alternative therapies.

- Berman et al (1998) found use or referral to chiropractic to be 48.2% and use or referral to acupuncture, 60.4%

- Berman et al (1998) reported that 27% of physicians in general practice had training in chiropractic, and 23.8% had training in acupuncture
- Gordon et al (1998) found the percentage of primary care clinicians who used or recommended chiropractic to be 33.6% and those who used or recommended acupuncture to be 57.2%

REIMBURSEMENT

Given this level of interest on the part of consumers and physicians, what is the level of participation among insurers and employers? Utilization by managed care organizations is reflected in the *Landmark Report II* (National Market Measures, 1999), a telephone survey of senior HMO executives in 114 managed care organizations (25% of the 449 companies in the

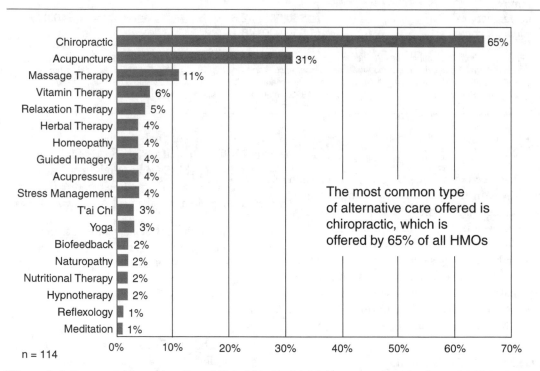

n = 114

Figure 2–2 Types of Alternative Care Offered by Health Maintenance Organizations (HMOs). *Source:* Reprinted with permission from *The Landmark Report II on HMOs and Alternative Care,* © 1999, Landmark Healthcare Inc.

United States at that time). Chiropractic was offered by 65% of the companies surveyed, acupuncture by 31%, and massage therapy by 11% (see Figure 2–2).

A survey by William M. Mercer, Inc. (1998) of different types of managed care organizations reflected variability in the offerings of various therapies but indicated trends similar to those in *Landmark Report II* (see Table 2–3). A survey by the International Association of Employee Benefit Specialists (IFEBP, 2000) reported that 89% of the responding employers offered chiro-

practic. In the IFEBP survey, a range of other CAM therapies was offered by approximately 19% of the companies participating.

UTILIZATION OF CAM THERAPIES

Use of Specific Therapies

Which therapies are most widely used? The research of Eisenberg et al (1998) indicates that five of the most popular CAM therapies involve the use of a practitioner. Of these, the most fre-

---

Interest in Complementary and Alternative Medicine Worldwide

CAM is widely used in other industrialized countries, according to a summary published in the *British Medical Journal* (1996). In Britain, one person in ten consults CAM practitioners each year, and the most popular therapies are acupuncture, chiropractic, osteopathy, homeopathy, herbal medicine, and hypnotherapy. In France, one-third of the population uses CAM, with homeopathy being the most popular treatment. In Norway, homeopathy is also the most popular CAM practice, followed by acupuncture and aromatherapy. Russia legalized alternative medicine in 1993; the officially recognized practices are reflexology, chiropractic, homeopathy, and a breathing method. In Australia, a third of the population regularly visits natural therapists, and two-thirds regularly take vitamins and use other "natural" treatments, the most popular being chiropractic, naturopathy, massage, herbal medicine, and homeopathy. In Japan, scientific Western medicine and CAM coexist. Two-thirds of the population in Tokyo report using CAM treatments. The most popular CAM therapies are herbal medicine, acupuncture, and acupressure (shiatsu), and more than 600 herbal medicines are available under the national health insurance system. In Germany and the United Kingdom, the national health payment system also covers many CAM practices.

Source: Reprinted with permission from *Enhancing the Accountability of Alternative Medicine*, p. 3, © 1998, Milbank Memorial Fund. Print copies of this report are available on request from the Fund at 645 Madison Avenue, New York, NY 10022; an electronic edition is available on the Fund's website: http://www.milbank.org

---

Table 2–3 Therapies Offered by Managed Care Organizations (MCOs) and by Employers

	Acupuncture	Chiropractic	Massage
Landmark (1999)—MCOs	31%	65%	11%
Mercer/Foster Higgins National Survey (1998)—MCOs	9%	45 to 65%	6 to 9%
Employee Benefit Specialists (2000)	14%	86%	8%

Sources: Data from *The Landmark Report II on HMOs and Alternative Care*, © 1999, Landmark Healthcare Inc., *Mercer/Foster Higgins National Survey of Employer-Sponsored Health Plans*, © 1999, William M. Mercer, Inc., and IFEBP (International Federation of Employee Benefit Professionals), CENSUS of employee benefit specialists, www.ifebp.org/recen99d.html.IFEBP; accessed 4/00.

quently utilized have been chiropractic and massage, accounting for approximately 70% of all CAM visits to practitioners (see Table 2–4). The research of Gordon and others at Kaiser Permanente (1998) also found highest utilization percentages for chiropractic (24.2%) and massage (15.1%).

MOTIVATION FOR USE

Why do people use complementary therapies? Both research and experience suggest that there are multiple markets for CAM (Eisenberg et al, 1993, 1998; Astin, 1998; Druss and Rosenheck, 1999; Consumers Union, 2000; Kittner, 1998; Jahnke, 1998).

Health Promotion

One major arena of consumer interest in CAM appears to be health promotion. The data of Eisenberg et al (1993, 1998), Gordon et al (1998), and others reflect major expenditures on various forms of self-help. In these studies, the greater majority of the responses reflects participation in CAM activities, practiced as self-

care (Jahnke, 1998). This utilization includes self-help activities such as:

- Exercise, including yoga and T'ai chi
- Stress reduction, meditation, and imagery
- Use of nutrition, vitamins, and herbal supplements
- Involvement in support groups and spiritual activities

In 1997, out-of-pocket expenditures on supplements, books, classes, and equipment were $14.8 billion. As mentioned, by 1999, expenditures on supplements, natural foods, and natural products totaled $28.2 billion (Traynor, 2000; Annual Industry Overview, 1999). The high level of interest expressed in health enhancement holds implications for both program design and marketing. It has been suggested that employers who offer CAM gain a competitive edge in attracting and retaining highly qualified workers (Sheff, 1999). Others in this field perceive a segment of the CAM market as proactive individuals who tend to use CAM for prevention and health enhancement (Ina, 1998). In the context of the future development of health care,

---

Table 2–4 Prevalence and Frequency of Use of Alternative Therapies in United States, 1997 (Eisenberg et al, 1998)

Therapy	Total Estimated Annual Visits (in Millions)	Number of Visits per Thousand Members of the U.S. Population	Mean Number of Visits per User Annually
Chiropractic	192 M	969.1	9.8
Massage	114 M	574.4	8.4
Self-help groups	80 M	402.8	18.9
Commercial diet	27 M	138.8	7.3
Imagery	22 M	114.3	11
Megavitamins	22 M	112.1	n.a.
Herbal medicine	10 M	53.0	2.9
Acupuncture	5 M	27.2	3.1
Hypnotherapy	4 M	21.1	1.6
Biofeedback	4 M	19.5	3.6

Source: Adapted with permission from D. Eisenberg et al., Trends in Alternative Medicine Use in the United States, 1990–1997: Results of a Follow-up National Survey, *Journal of the American Medical Association*, Vol. 280, No. 18, pp. 1574, © 1998, American Medical Association.

Table 2–5 Conditions Treated by CAM Therapies, Percentage of Use Reported by Respondents Experiencing Those Conditions

Condition	Eisenberg 1997 Data	Astin 1997 Data
Neck conditions	57.0	—
Back conditions	47.6	—
Chronic pain	—	37
Depression	40.9	31
Anxiety	42.7	31
Headaches	32.2	24
Arthritis/rheumatism	26.7	25
Sprains and strains	23.6	26
Addiction	—	25
Insomnia	26.4	—
Fatigue	27.0	—
Digestive disorders	27.3	—
Allergies	16.6	—

Source: Data from D. Eisenberg et al., Trends in Alternative Medicine Use in the United States, 1990–1997: Results of a Follow-up National Survey, *Journal of the American Medical Association*, Vol. 280, No. 18, pp. 1574, © 1998, American Medical Association.

self-help activities are predicted by many to play a greater role (see Chapter 45 on health enhancement and Chapter 66 on futures).

Use of CAM for Chronic Conditions

Researchers and planners have suggested that individuals with chronic illness make up a major market for CAM services (Eisenberg et al, 1993, 1998; Astin, 1998; Druss and Rosenheck, 1999; Kittner, 1999). The Astin survey (1998) found that the two most frequently endorsed benefits indicated "relief for symptoms" and "efficacy for a particular health problem." *Consumer Reports*, reflecting survey responses from more than 46,000 readers, reported, "Those who said they were in severe pain or stress were more likely to try alternatives" (Consumers Union, 2000).

The Astin (1998) and Eisenberg et al (1998) data are in general agreement in their findings

on the conditions for which respondents most often seek CAM therapies (see Table 2–5). Astin (1998) found higher use of CAM correlated with the presence of specific health conditions. For example:

- The likelihood of CAM use among respondents with back problems was found to be twice that of respondents not reporting back problems.
- The likelihood of CAM use among respondents with chronic pain was found to be twice that of respondents not reporting chronic pain.
- Respondents who reported anxiety were three times as likely as the average survey respondent to use CAM.

United States Prevalence of Chronic Conditions

In the context of potential CAM applications in the management of chronic illness, what is the size of this population? According to an analysis of disability in the United States by a team of Stanford researchers (Hoffman et al, 1996), approximately 44.5% of the ambulatory, noninstitutionalized adult population experienced one or more forms of chronic illness in 1989. Addressing the needs of this population holds relevance for the public health system, because more than three-fourths of all premature deaths were found to occur due to chronic conditions. According to this study, demographics of this population suggest that:

- The total number of persons in 1989 with one or more chronic conditions was 88.5 million.
- The total direct medical costs of these disabilities (in 1996 U.S. dollars) was $425 billion.
- Indirect costs totaled an additional $234 billion.
- Over 40% of direct health care costs for persons with chronic conditions were paid with public funds.

DISCUSSION

The research indicates that the public is willing to pay out of pocket to expand its medical options for care. High levels of satisfaction with CAM are reported in both preferred provider organizations and managed care networks (see Chapters 32 and 33). High levels of patient satisfaction with CAM are recorded in publicly funded programs (see Chapters 16 and 35). Improved health outcomes are reported for both acupuncture (Chapter 51) and chiropractic (Chapter 54). There is also a substantial body of research indicating cost-effectiveness for chiropractic (Chapter 55). These data suggest an expanded market if CAM coverage were to become more widely available.

Actuaries, insurers, and employers are awaiting the data to determine the economic feasibility of complementary medicine. Do CAM services represent additional health care costs or the replacement of current expenditures? To what extent would CAM drive up overall expenditures or offset the cost of other forms of treatment? Will reimbursement for programs offset the expense of providing them in more elaborate conventional environments? Will the attractiveness of these programs expand market share to an extent that makes them worth offering?

In the context of cost-effectiveness, will the inclusion of wellness programming and complementary medicine in health systems improve the overall health of clients? Will these therapies provide new tools for prevention and performance enhancement? Will they provide meaningful options for treatment? Will complementary medicine improve health outcomes?

The economics of CAM will eventually be defined in the marketplace. The question of effectiveness will play out in clinical environments, particularly those that employ effective methods of tracking outcomes. Currently, data suggest affordability and cost-effectiveness, but the health care community awaits further confirmation. This book is offered to provide a range of perspectives that continues the dialogue on these questions and offers additional insight.

REFERENCES

Annual industry overview. *Nutr Business J.* 1999;4(6):1–5.

American Specialty Health (ASH) and Stanford University. *National Consumer Trends in Complementary and Alternative Medicine.* San Diego, CA: ASH; 6/00.

Astin J. Why patients use alternative medicine: Results of a national study. *JAMA.* 1998;279(19):1548–1553.

Astin JA, Marie A, Pelletier KR, Hansen E, Haskell WL. A review of the incorporation of complementary and alternative medicine by mainstream physicians. *Arch Intern Med.* 1998;158:2303–2309.

Berman BM, Singh BB, Hartnol SM, et al. Primary care physicians and complementary-alternative medicine: Training, attitudes, and practice patterns. *J Am Board Fam Pract.* 1998;11:272–281.

British Medical Journal. Complementary medicine is booming worldwide (News). *Br Med J.* 1996;313:131–133.

Consumers Union. The mainstreaming of alternative medicine. *Consumer Reports.* May, 2000:17–25.

Druss B, Rosenheck R. Association between use of unconventional therapies and conventional medical services. *JAMA.* 1999;282(7):651–656.

Eisenberg D, Davis R, Ettner S, et al. Trends in alternative medicine use in the United States, 1990–1997: Results of a follow-up national survey. *JAMA.* 1998;280(18):1569–1575.

Eisenberg DM, Kessler RC, Foster C, et al. Unconventional medicine in the United States. *N Engl J Med.* 1993;328(4):246–252.

Gordon N, Sobel D, Tarazona E. Use of and interest in alternative therapies among adult primary care clinicians and adult members in a large health maintenance organization. *WJM.* 1998;169(3):153–161.

Herre HP, CEO, East-West Health Centers. Oral communication; 10/99.

Hoffman C, Rice D, Sung HY. Persons with chronic conditions: Their prevalence and costs. *JAMA.* 1996;276(18): 1473–1479.

IFEBP (International Federation of Employee Benefit Professionals). Census of employee benefit specialists. <http://www.ifebp.org/recen99d.html>. Accessed 4/00.

Ina V, vice president, Network Development, OneBody.com. Oral communication; 6/98.

InterActive Solutions. *Landmark Report I on Public Perceptions of Alternative Care.* Sacramento, CA: Landmark Healthcare; 1998.

Jahnke R, Director, Health Action Group. Written communication; 1/98.

Kittner A, CEO, OneBody.com. Oral communication; 3/98.

Milbank Memorial Fund. *Enhancing the Accountability of Alternative Medicine.* New York: Milbank Memorial Fund; 1998:3.

National Market Measures. *The Landmark Report II.* Sacramento, CA: Landmark Healthcare; 1999.

Orth MJ, President, Dimensional Health Systems. Oral communication; 6/00.

Raterman K. Change: The only constant in natural market. *Nat Foods Merchandiser.* 1999;20(6):1, 34–35.

Sheff R, Chairman of the Board, Commonwell. Oral communication; 8/99.

Traynor M. Natural products market tops $28 billion. *Nat Foods Merchandiser.* 2000;21(6):1, 21.

William M. Mercer, Inc. *National Survey of Employer-Sponsored Health Plans.* William M. Mercer; 1998.

Wooten JC, Sparber AG. Surveys of complementary and alternative medicine. In MS Micozzi, ed. *Current Review of Complementary Medicine.* Philadelphia: Current Medicine; 1999:139–153.

CHAPTER 3

Evolving Demands and Demographics in Health Care

Clement Bezold

Complementary and alternative approaches to health and medicine are among the fastest growing aspects of health care in the United States. In 1990, one-third of the U.S. population used some form of complementary therapy or wellness activity (Eisenberg et al, 1993). By 2010, at least two-thirds will be using one or more of the approaches now considered complementary or alternative.

In some cases, these treatments will be applied instead of current conventional approaches, and in others, will complement current treatments. These modalities also extend beyond treatment; they will be used for serious prevention and health promotion activities. Although

Clement Bezold, PhD, is the President of the Institute for Alternative Futures (IAF) and its for-profit subsidiary Alternative Futures Associates. He received his doctorate in political science from the University of Florida. He has authored or edited 11 books and numerous articles focused on the future of health, health care, and the health professions, as well as government and the justice system. He is a renowned speaker on the future for voluntary organizations, national and international corporations, and health care and education groups and has taught at the University of Florida, Antioch University, and American University.

The IAF is a nonprofit research and educational organization founded in 1977. IAF specializes in aiding organizations and individuals to more wisely choose and create their preferred futures. IAF and its profit subsidiary, AFA, are leading providers of training and services in scenario planning and vision development to large associations, governments, and corporations.

Courtesy of Clement Bezold, Institute for Alternative Futures, Alexandria, Virginia.

the current focus is on the use of complementary and alternative medicine (CAM) in health care, an important subtheme is that some of these alternative therapies and activities are now being pursued, not for treating illness, but for prevention or wellness. This parallel use of various complementary and alternative approaches is already a significant part of their demand and is likely to grow.

It is important to keep in mind the relative importance of medical care in health. Roughly 90% of the variance in premature death in modern society is related to factors other than the lack of health care. Currently, the vast majority of morbidity and mortality is associated with lifestyle, genetic, and environmental factors. Health care is moving from a focus on medical interventions to the factors affecting this 90%, particularly lifestyle. This new focus will increasingly favor prevention and treatment approaches with certain core components that are nutritional, physical, psychological, or spiritual. One reason for the growing interest in CAM is that it includes or reinforces these components of care.

CHANGING DEMOGRAPHICS

Diversity

By 2010, demographic shifts will trigger dramatic quantitative and qualitative changes in U.S. health care. The racial composition of society also will change markedly, with particularly high growth among Hispanic groups. Health care practitioners will see increasingly diverse populations of consumers, requiring even greater need for sensitivity to physical, social, mental, emotional, and economic distinctions among patients. As health care moves toward prevention and self-care, new customized health maintenance and treatment protocols will be devised for these diverse populations, rather than favoring one generalized treatment for most patients.

Complementary and alternative approaches to medicine are relevant to the health care needs of a diverse population. The World Health Organization has estimated that in 1990, the four most widely used medical therapeutics were acupuncture, homeopathy, herbal medicine, and conventional biomedicine (World Health Organization, 1993).

Aging Markets

Quantitatively, a generally lower birth rate and higher life expectancy will shift attention to the growing proportions of elderly and minority Americans, also expanded through immigration and higher birth rates in some minority populations. In 2011, the oldest members of the baby boomer generation will turn 65. Although a growing percentage of America's elderly will be healthy later in life, another large percentage will not.

Thus, aging markets mean that health care providers—both conventional and CAM—will need to target their services to retirees, many with limited incomes. They will address a broad spectrum of geriatric health problems, given the predomination of chronic conditions among older members of the population, with 50% experiencing at least one chronic condition by the age of 75 (Ostir et al, 1999). Consequently, CAM may see increasing application in the management of disease and chronic illness.

GENERATIONS

Qualitative population changes may be even more significant than demographics due to the passage of one dominant generational cohort and the rise of the next. Psychographic research has identified a set of generational personalities that characterize successive cohorts of Americans, with one type following the next in a continuous cycle, shaped in part by the milestone events of their time. Although there is certainly great diversity within a cohort, as a whole each tends to exhibit a primary behavior pattern (a core set of preferences) as the cohort passes through successive phases of life. Each of these generationwide personalities tends to react in characteristic ways to the opportunities and challenges of youth, middle age, and old age (Strauss and Howe, 1991).

The GI Generation

This is the cohort now entering its 70s and 80s. The GI generation has been one of the most assertive in American history. The strong civic spirit of its members led them to invent and strengthen large institutions and to look for support from these institutions in return. After winning World War II, the members of this generation were the leaders who consolidated medical authority and built and expanded hospitals, university medical centers, and research institutions such as the National Institutes of Health. Medicare is a legislated reflection of their vision, a funding structure designed to support successive generations in their old age.

The Silent Generation

The cohort currently in its 50s and 60s is sandwiched between two more powerful generational personalities. History shows that generations with these attributes typically have many great legislators, but few presidents. This group will continue to benefit from the tremendous resources institutionalized by the preceding generation. They may modify these institutions but will probably refrain from radical reconstruction.

The Baby Boomers

This 77-million-strong cohort now taking political power is characterized as idealist in its desire to place individuals over institutions.

Thus, it is no surprise that the first baby boomer president would seek to reform health care, or that his generation will drive continued change in health care. The trend is likely to lead to a weakening of institutional power since baby boomers tend to place a high value on autonomy and believe in greater personal responsibility for health and the costs of health care.

Generation X

This cohort has already experienced the weakening of institutions. These individuals were born into a time when the social institution of marriage was weakened by rising divorce rates, and public institutions such as schools were weakened by tax revolts. This cohort has come to expect that opportunities and benefits available to previous generations will not be open to them. Consequently, as a group they tend to be quite pragmatic; they look very realistically at issues such as career, Social Security, and Medicare, and are likely to accept reforms aimed at shifting resources (Strauss and Howe, 1997).

Given this ongoing dynamic between generational cohorts, the developing trends in health care are likely to include a series of reforms that decrease the role of institutions and strengthen individual freedoms and responsibilities. The powerful financing, research, and health care delivery organizations that dominated the second half of the 20th century will be subjected to increasing challenges. Public spending for the elderly may decline. These trends are all congruent with the emphasis on patient participation evident in many CAM disciplines. The health care paradigm emphasizing self-care, prevention, and wellness will join the current treatment-focused model and take its place in the continuum of care.

DEMOGRAPHICS AND THE USE OF CAM

David Eisenberg's (1993) landmark study on unconventional medicine found that the use of CAM was significantly more common among people who are 25 to 49 years old, are college-educated, have relatively higher incomes, and live in the West.

A study for the Institute of Noetic Sciences by Paul Ray (1996) had similar findings regarding values and interest in holistic health. Ray identifies three subsets of American culture that are influencing the demand for health services.

1. *Heartlanders* preserve traditional or rural values, tend to resist change, are somewhat isolationist, and are most often among middle- to lower-income populations. They currently represent 29% of the U.S. population, but by 2010 are predicted to represent 20%.
2. *Cultural moderns* are found in the mainstream, in all income categories. Currently 48% of the U.S. population; in 2010 they will probably maintain a similar niche at 45% of population.
3. *Cultural creatives* are most often found in upper income levels, tend to be leaders of cultural change, and see a desirable future. They are growing in numbers, and although they currently reflect 23% of the U.S. population, they are projected to be 35% by 2010. Cultural creatives have nontraditional values that require a different paradigm of health and they are willing to try a variety of approaches to health care. These consumers believe in holistic health through a unified approach to the body, mind, and spirit. Although this group tends to be fairly healthy, some members have been described as the "worried well." They are more prevention-oriented than the two other groups that make up the U.S. population.

As the size of the cultural creatives group increases and comes to the forefront in American culture, its members could push for increased coverage and reimbursement for CAM and increased availability of CAM therapies. They are also more likely to be willing and able to purchase complementary and alternative services as "wellness" expenditures, out of their own pockets, beyond the limits of health care cost reimbursements.

Ray found that 37% of Americans were using alternative health care at the time of his 1994 survey—a figure that is up 4% from the 33% cited by Eisenberg in his 1990 survey (Eisenberg et al, 1993). This survey by the Institute of Noetic Sciences reflected use of alternative health care by 52% of cultural creatives, 32% of cultural moderns, and 34% of heartlanders.

Nonusers of CAM

Information gathered from focus group participants in the Institute for Alternative Futures' (IAF) study (1998) on the future of CAM suggests that there is a fine line between users and nonusers of CAM. Most nonusers appear to be less aware of different alternative therapies but are not opposed to using them, particularly if they are scientifically proven. However, some nonusers had a strong bias against particular therapies. Other factors that may determine use of CAM include:

- the predominant locus of control for the particular therapy—a focus on expert opinion or on self-reliance
- cost-effectiveness and affordability—participants responded positively to a future in which CAM is supported by additional scientific evidence and is affordable
- lower-income persons are "as excluded from alternative health care as [they are] from regular health care: they can't afford it" (Ray, 1996)

EPIDEMIOLOGY OF NEED

Trends in Infectious Disease

Contagious disease has been a major factor in human history. The development of antibiotics provided a 50-year respite in industrialized nations from the threat of outbreaks and epidemics. However, a number of trends have been developing over the past 20 years that concern researchers at the Centers for Disease Control and Prevention (CDC) in Atlanta and the World Health Organization (WHO). For example, as this book goes to press, legislation has been submitted to the U.S. Congress to provide approximately $300 million to fight drug-resistant tuberculosis in the United States and abroad. Current changes in the epidemiology of infectious disease include:

- *Emerging infectious disease.* At least 30 new disease-causing agents have been identified over the past 20 years. They include the viruses that cause AIDS, Legionnaire's disease, Lyme disease, and hepatitis C and microspora (Iruka et al, 1998).
- *Reemerging infection.* Illnesses that were once thought to be under control have developed drug-resistant strains, increasing in prevalence. The most dangerous include resistant forms of tuberculosis, gonorrhea, malaria, and cholera. New strains occur naturally as microbes adapt to challenges in their environment and through mutation.
- *New links between infection and illness.* Recent research indicates a major role for microbial pathogens in the development of diseases not previously linked to infection, such as chlamydia in heart disease and aflatoxin molds in cancer. Human papilloma virus is considered a causal factor in cervical cancer in approximately 8 out of 10 cases (Cichocki, 2000; Myers et al, 2000). *Helicobacter pylori* is now known to be a major cause of gastric ulcers, and approximately 40% of people with *H. pylori* eventually develop gastric cancer (Konturek et al, 1999).
- *Drug-resistant microbes.* Resistant bacteria have been a growing problem for decades. In 1946, just 5 years after penicillin came into use, doctors discovered a strain of staphylococcal bacteria that had already become drug resistant. Penicillin-resistant streptococcus was documented in 1985,

and by 1995 more than 100 frequently used antibiotics had become ineffective against certain strains of bacteria (Garrett, 1994).

Viral diseases have taken an incredible toll in this century. The influenza epidemic of 1918 is reported to have caused the death of more than 40 million people (Kolata, 1999). In our time, AIDS continues to be a disease that is essentially untreatable. To date, AIDS has been the cause of more than 19 million deaths worldwide, and 5.8 million new cases develop each year (Forossa, 2000).

Antibiotic-resistant bacterial infection is also a major problem. Currently in the United States, the CDC estimates that 249,000 cases of drug-resistant infections occur yearly in hospitals, of which 70,000 to 90,000 are fatal (Yoffe, 2000). In Thailand, *Campylobacter* species, with its accompanying acute gastrointestinal symptoms, tested as drug resistant in 84% of samples reviewed in 1995, having been totally treatable with ciprofloxacin in 1991 (Hoge et al, 1998). In Iceland, the frequency of penicillin-resistant streptococcus increased by eight times in 3 years, from 2% in 1989 to 17% in 1992 (Soares et al, 1993). In Holland, the prevalence of drug-resistant *H. pylori* detected through laboratory testing increased fourfold from 7% in 1993 to 32% in 1996 (van der Wouden et al, 1997).

Super germs are strains of viruses and sometimes bacteria that can cause immediate, intense symptoms that are often fatal. Some experts believe that many are exotic rain forest viruses that are being unearthed in the process of tropical rain forest destruction (Zimmerman and Zimmerman, 1996). These pathogens include Ebola virus, Lassa fever virus, Hantavirus, and dengue hemorrhagic fever virus. Some super germs have migrated from animals to people. Lethal microorganisms that have recently adapted to human hosts include agents causing bovine spongiform encephalopathy (mad cow disease from prions) in cattle and the Hong Kong avian flu (a virus) (Zimmerman and Zimmerman, 1996).

The new paradigm of integrative medicine becomes highly relevant in the context of drug-resistant infection and emerging contagion. For example, medical research in the Third World on integrative protocols found greater reductions in mortality when antibiotics were used in combination with nutrients. Vitamin C used in conjunction with medication in the treatment of life-threatening tetanus in Bangladesh improved outcomes by 60% to 80% (Jahan et al, 1984). Problems of drug resistance also reinforce the importance of preventive and lifestyle measures such as improvements in hygiene, diet, and exercise. In mind-body medicine and the emerging field of psychoneuroimmunology, stress reduction has been clearly linked to enhanced immune system function (Pert, 1997; Pert et al, 1998).

Other Changes in Disease and Morbidity

The pattern of disease is changing in other areas as well. Data from the WHO cited in its report titled *Global Comparative Assessments in the Health Sector* describe the leading causes of morbidity in terms of disability-adjusted life years (DALYs) (Murray and Lopez, 1996). (See Table 3–1.) This is a measure that combines the losses from premature death (the difference between actual age of death and life expectancy at that age in a low-mortality population) and loss of healthy life resulting from disability. Diseases that disable or kill younger people generate higher resulting DALYs, compared with those that are short in duration. For example, in 1990 in established market countries (essentially the nations of North America and Western Europe as well as Japan and Australia), there were 9,362,000 DALYs lost to ischemic heart disease; heart disease was the leading cause of premature death and disability in those countries in that year.

Projected global trends of morbidity and mortality include:

- *The rising rate of injury globally.* This rising rate is due to both intentional and unintentional causes. By 2020, trauma may rival infectious diseases as a chief source of ill health.

Table 3–1 Projections of the World Health Organization on Morbidity in Industrialized Nations: Disability-Adjusted Life Years

1990		2020 Projection	
Cause	In Millions	Cause	In Millions
Ischemic heart disease	9.4	Ischemic heart disease	9.1
Cerebrovascular heart disease	4.9	Unipolar disorders/major depression	6.6
Dementia	4	Cerebrovascular heart disease	4.8
Traffic accidents	3.3	Tracheal and lung cancer	4.5
Tracheal and lung cancer	3	Alcohol abuse	4.3
Alcohol abuse	2.8	Dementia	4.3
Congenital abnormalities	2.4	Osteoarthritis	3.4
Osteoarthritis	2.2	Traffic accidents	3.3
Unipolar disorders/major depression	2.1	Bacterial meningitis	2.3
Self-inflicted injuries	1.9	Self-inflicted injuries	2.2

Source: Reprinted with permission from the World Health Organization website www.who.ch

- *Tobacco-related deaths.* Tobacco is anticipated to cause more premature deaths and disability than any other single risk factor; it may cause as much as 9% of the adult disease burden by 2020 (Murray and Lopez, 1996).
- *Psychosocial disorders.* Disorders such as depression are among the fastest growing forms of morbidity. Although depression has genetic, biochemical, and physiological

components, the exacerbations that result from an unsatisfactory social context and loss of personal meaning are major factors. These aspects of dysfunction are anticipated to intensify as world society becomes almost entirely concentrated in crowded, yet often isolating urban enclaves, with a greater majority of the world's populations living in megacities with populations that range from 4 to 20 million. (See Table 3–2

Table 3–2 Global Disease Burden Measured in Disability-Adjusted Life Years (DALYs)

	Estimate 1990			Projection 2020	
Rank	Cause	% Total	Rank	Cause	% Total
1	Lower respiratory infections	8.2	1	Ischemic heart disease	5.9
2	Diarrheal disease	7.2	2	Unipolar major depression	5.7
3	Perinatal conditions	6.7	3	Road traffic accidents	5.1
4	Unipolar major depression	3.7	4	Cerebrovascular disease	4.4
5	Ischemic heart disease	3.4	5	Chronic pulmonary disease	4.2
6	Cerebrovascular disease	2.8	6	Lower respiratory infections	3.1
7	Tuberculosis	2.8	7	Tuberculosis	3.0
8	Measles	2.7	8	War	3.0
9	Road traffic accidents	2.5	9	Diarrheal diseases	2.7
10	Congenital abnormalities	2.4	10	HIV	2.6

Source: Reprinted with permission from the World Health Organization website www.who.ch

for projected shifts in the burden of disease.)

The challenge for CAM providers and risk reduction programs is to identify patients whose "crisis of meaning" can be prevented or ameliorated through clinical intervention. It is also important to identify and diagnose physiological conditions that produce symptoms of depression so that the underlying disorder can be treated. Many complementary approaches offer useful tools and a range of interventions to improve general physical and emotional well-being; address issues that relate to the mind, body, and spirit; provide early intervention; and correct underlying imbalances in physiological function. Other complementary approaches focus on family, community, and societal arenas in which individuals can enhance their sense of personal meaning and coherence.

These trends may provide a leadership role for some CAM practitioners within their communities. As recognition of the growth and causes of depression and diseases of meaning becomes more prevalent, health care providers will be looked to for their expertise and interventions.

Prevalence of Chronic Illness

Chronic illness may be considered a silent epidemic in the United States. According to 1987 data published in *JAMA* (Hoffman et al, 1996), more than 45% of noninstitutionalized Americans (90 million people) had one or more chronic conditions in that year. Their direct health care costs in 1987 accounted for three-fourths of U.S. health care expenditures. The total associated costs for chronic conditions projected to 1990 amounted to $659 billion—$425 billion in direct health care costs and $234 billion in indirect costs, such as lost productivity.

Hoffman and colleagues point out that the majority of people with chronic conditions are not totally disabled, but lead relatively normal lives. However, they live with the threat of recurrent episodes of illness, higher personal health care costs, more days lost from work, and the risk of long-term limitations and disabilities. They are reported to be at greater risk for being underinsured. This study also found that the per capita costs of those with chronic conditions were typically three times higher than those of others in the population, and that people with two or more chronic disorders incurred costs more than twice those of people with one chronic condition.

It is estimated that in the context of 1995 data, the prevalence of chronic illness was likely to involve at least 100 million people. This population is likely to continue to increase, given declining mortality rates across the entire life span, advances in medical technology, and higher survival rates associated with life-threatening conditions. The Hoffman study points out that our health care delivery system is still essentially designed to provide acute care. These researchers suggest that the level of need among those with chronic illness is approaching critical mass and may ultimately provide the impetus for major changes within the health care system.

Poverty

Poverty is increasingly recognized as the largest risk factor for ill health in the United States. Poor living conditions, high-stress lifestyle and environments, violence, poor nutrition, and limited access to preventive health care all increase the risk of disease and disability. For example, the health status of residents in parts of Washington, DC, is as compromised as that in Haiti. Rates of infant mortality among poorer populations in cities like Washington are worse than those in most developing countries (Brown and Goldstein, 1997). In 1960, 22% of the U.S. population was at or below the poverty line. Following the Great Society legislation, by the end of the 1970s, poverty had fallen to 11.4%. However, this trend is shifting, and in 1998, the level of poverty had risen to 12.7 percent, and among American children it had risen to 22% (Census Bureau, 1998).

The impact of poverty on health will become increasingly apparent as outcomes data continue to build. Populations in need include not only the poor, but disabled children and adults, the elderly with chronic and disabling conditions, and those institutionalized. In response to the challenges of service provision for these populations—overuse of emergency department care, rising costs, lack of preventive care, and poor health outcomes—many states have moved their Medicaid populations into managed care systems, often with mixed results. Yet these managed care programs offer environments in which the greatest wisdom of CAM could be applied to serve those most in need. One outstanding example is the King County Community Health Center in Kent, Washington, where poor and uninsured people can receive integrated conventional and CAM services (see Chapters 16 and 35).

Environmental Issues

Over the past decade, the environment has emerged as a major concern in health care. Water quality, for example, has become a health issue in some parts of the United States and is a critical health issue in developing nations throughout Asia and elsewhere. In 2000, for example, outbreaks of cholera in Madagascar resulted from flooding due to monsoons (WHO, 2000).

Environmental threats to health are increasing on a global scale, despite significant progress in certain areas. Even in the richest nations, poor areas often bear heavy burdens of pollution and toxic waste exposure. Deforestation and habitat destruction in the tropics are major factors in the emergence of new diseases, particularly those caused by the exotic viruses classified as super germs. Depletion of the stratospheric ozone layer is believed to be causing a rise in the incidence of skin cancers worldwide, but particularly in parts of the Southern Hemisphere.

Also of importance is the possible role of endocrine-disrupting chemicals linked with breast cancer, testicular cancer, endometriosis, and developmental problems in exposed children (Dumanoski and Myers, 1996). Endocrine-disrupting chemicals have been associated with the

drop in sperm count of various species of male animals in different regions of the world, and by extrapolation are believed to play a role in the decrease of human sperm counts in industrial nations over the past 50 years.

Shifts in global weather could have enormous impact on human health. Global warming threatens to bring tropical diseases into northern latitudes and may cause more weather extremes. This warming trend is also likely to enlarge the "hot zones" that produce new strains of disease. Worsening problems of soil erosion, water scarcity, and overfishing could undermine the nutritional status of hundreds of millions of people in the decades ahead. Environmental problems, such as the shortage of water for agriculture or eventually for cities, can also contribute to economic problems and outbreaks of conflict, which in turn pose threats to human health.

As wellness increasingly becomes the focus of health care, health care providers (mainstream, complementary, and alternative) will of necessity deal with the repercussions of these broader issues and will ultimately have their work judged in relation to them. Many will seek to discover and invent ways in which they have an impact on environmental issues.

NEW DIRECTIONS

Much of Disease Is Preventable

Of current health care expenses, 70% result from preventable illnesses, according to the U.S. Department of Health and Human Services (1991). According to Dr. Everett Koop, former U.S. surgeon general, and Dr. James Fries of Stanford University, eight of every nine diseases have preventable causes (Fries et al, 1993). The concepts of health and disease have become reconceptualized to some degree, particularly over the last decade. As a result, the trend toward risk reduction and health promotion has become more visible. Although health promotion has been a foundation of public health programming since the 1980s, the essence of new preventive initiatives is currently being redefined in leading-edge institutions throughout the health care system. This expanded vision involves the creation of a continuum of care ranging from acute care to prevention. Activities that focus on prevention and wellness are relevant to most of the major CAM therapies. Yet, as with conventional health care providers, CAM practitioners could easily fall prey to financial incentives and health care practices that ignore prevention because it takes more of the provider's time, requires additional effort on the part of the patient, or is not paid for by insurers or many patients.

Changing the Disease Curve: Compressing Morbidity

Within the range of complementary and alternative approaches, it is prevention rather than the therapies that offers the greatest prospect of lowering morbidity, particularly for the elderly. James Fries, professor of medicine at Stanford University Medical School, has developed the theory of compression of morbidity (Fries, 1996). He suggests that appropriate lifestyle changes can sustain health and delay the onset of disease in late life, ideally compressing disabling morbidity into the last year or last few months of life, rather than having it dominate the last several years.

Fries forecasts that health care costs can actually be reduced by 20% just by using currently available and proven demand management and health promotion techniques (Fries, 1996). His work stands in striking contrast to the forecasts that show an aging population pushing morbidity and health care costs skyward. As health care embraces the new paradigm of forecasting, preventing, and managing disease, the potential is generated to manage chronic disorders such as arthritis, back pain, and other degenerative conditions.

IMAGES OF THE FUTURE

Within a decade, we predict that health care will likely operate within a new paradigm—one oriented to prevention, self-care, and holism. It will be capable of addressing an individual's unique status from the microscopic (genotype) to the macroscopic (environment). Treatment options will be far more numerous, but resolving a health problem could also extend to social and environmental interventions aimed at uprooting problems at their source. Much health care will be self-care, with the services of health care professionals applied more strategically and even more effectively.

Pessimistic images exist as well. Any of a variety of wildcards could intrude and redirect U.S. health care into less-desirable channels—environmental, economic, or social dislocations; slowdown or reversal of health care's movement toward monitoring outcomes and accountability; or the failure to ensure greater health equality in terms of both access and outcomes.

Outcomes increasingly will drive better prevention and therapeutics, including the integration of complementary and alternative approaches into standard health care. Individuals will experience a greater range of options with regard to their health, with a range of supporting tools and resources available for managing personal health. Society will also be faced with choices about how healthy we want society to be and how accessible health care should be. If we make the right choices, 2010 will be far healthier.

REFERENCES

Brown D, Goldstein A. Long and short of life. *Washington Post.* December 4, 1997:A1.

Census Bureau. Poverty 1998. U.S. Census Web site. Available at: http:///www.census.gov/hhes/poverty/poverty98/table5.html. Accessed March 15, 2000.

Cichocki, M. Papilloma: papilloma protection. About.com Web site. Available at: http://www.aids.about.com/library/weekly/aa031500.htm. Accessed March 15, 2000.

Dumanoski D, Myers JP. *Our Stolen Future.* London: Abacus; 1996.

Eisenberg D, Kessler RC, Foster C, et al. Unconventional medicine in the United States: prevalence, cost and patterns of use. *N Engl J Med.* 1993;328(4):246–283.

Forossa U. AIDS in Africa: bleak future. *San Francisco Examiner.* 6/27/00: A1, A12.

Fries JF. Aging, society, and health. In: *Future care: responding to the demand for change.* Bezold C, Mayer E., eds. *Aging, Society and Health.* New York: Faulkner & Gray; 1996.

Fries JF, Koop CE, Beadle CE, et al. Reducing health care costs by reducing the need and demand for medical services: the Health Project Consortium. *N Engl J Med.* 1993;329:321–325.

Garrett L. *The Coming Plague: Newly Emerging Diseases in a World Out of Balance.* New York: Penguin USA; 1994.

Hoffman C, Rice D, Sung HY. Persons with chronic conditions: their prevalence and costs. *JAMA.* 1996;276: 1473–1479.

Hoge CW, Gambel JM, Srijan A, Pitarangsi C, Echeverria P. Trends in antibiotic resistance among diarrheal pathogens isolated in Thailand over 15 years. *Clin Infect Dis.* 1998;26:341–345.

Institute for Alternative Futures. *The Future of Complementary and Alternative Approaches (CAAs) in US Health Care.* Alexandria, VA: NCMIC Insurance Company; 1998.

Iruka NO, Adebayo L, Edelman R. Socioeconomic and behavioral factors leading to acquired bacterial resistance to antibiotics in developing countries. *Perspectives. Emerging Infectious Diseases.* 1998. National Center for Infectious Diseases, Centers for Disease Control and Prevention Web site. Available at: http://www.cdc.gov. Accessed March 15, 2000.

Jahan K, Ahmad K, Ali MA. Effect of ascorbic acid in the treatment of tetanus. *Med Res Counc Bull.* 1984;10(1):24–28.

Kolata G. *Flu: The Story of the Great Influenza Pandemic of 1918 and the Search for the Virus That Caused It.* New York: Farrar, Straus, & Giroux; 1999.

Konturek PC, Konturek SJ, Bielanski W, et al. Role of gastrin in gastric cancerogenesis in *Helicobacter pylori* infected humans. *J Physiol Pharmacol.* 1999;50(5):857–873.

Murray C, Lopez AD, eds. The global burden of disease. In: *The Global Burden of Disease and Injury Series*, vol 1. Cambridge, MA: Harvard University School of Public Health;1996: 990–994.

Myers ER, McCrory DC, Nanda K, Bastian L, Matchar DB. Mathematical model for the natural hisory of human papillomavirus infection and cervical carcinogenesis. *Am J Epidemiol.* 2000;151(12):1158–1171.

Ostir GV, Carlson JE, Black SA, Rudkin L, Goodwin JS, Markides KS. Disability in older adults: 1. prevalence, causes, and consequences. *Behav Med.* 1999;24(4): 147–156.

Pert CB. *Molecules of Emotion.* New York: Touchstone Books; 1997.

Pert CB, Dreher HE, Ruff MR. The psychosomatic network foundations of mind-body medicine. *Alt Ther.* 1998;4(4):30–41.

Ray P. *The Integral Culture Survey: A Study of the Emergence of Transformational Values in America.* Sausalito, CA: Institute of Noetic Sciences; 1996. Research Report 96-A.

Soares S, Kristinsson KG, Musser JM, Tomsz A. Evidence for the introduction of a multiresistant clone of serotype 6B *Streptococcus pneumoniae* from Spain to Iceland in the late 1980s. *J Infect Dis.* 1993;168:158–163.

Strauss W, Howe N. *Generations.* New York: William Morrow and Company; 1991.

Strauss W, Howe N. *The Fourth Turning.* New York: Broadway Books; 1997.

U.S. Department of Health and Human Services. *Healthy People 2000: National Health Promotion and Disease Prevention Objectives.* Washington, DC: U.S. Department of Health and Human Services, Public Health Service; 1991.

van der Wouden EJ, van Zwet AA, Vosmaer GD, Oom JA, de Jong A, Kleibeuker JH. Rapid increase in the prevalence of metronidazole-resistant *Helicobacter pylori* in the Netherlands. *Emerging Infect Dis.* 1997;3:385–389.

WHO reports cholera deaths in Madagascar. Geneva: Reuters News Service; March 10, 2000.

World Health Organization. *Bulletin of WHO Collaborating Centres for Traditional Medicine.* Geneva, Switzerland: World Health Organization; March 1993.

Yoffe E. Doctors are reminded "wash up." *New York Times.* February 9, 2000: Health and Fitness section.

Zimmerman BE, Zimmerman DJ. *Killer Germs: Microbes and Diseases That Threaten Humanity.* Chicago: Contemporary Books; 1996.

CHAPTER 4

New Perspectives

4.1   The Evolution of Integrative Medicine in Washington State

Eileen Stretch with Nancy Faass

The broad-based integration of complementary medicine began in Washington state in 1996, in response to an insurance commission ruling to expand insurance coverage for complementary and alternative forms of treatment. In order to facilitate the integrative process, a forum was convened by the Office of the Insurance Commissioner, which became identified as the Clinician Workgroup on the Integration of Complementary and Alternative Medicine. The group initially consisted of medical directors from various health plans and practitioners who are representative of CAM professions, such as naturopathy, acupuncture, chiropractic, midwifery, clinical nutrition, and others. Representatives from various networks of CAM providers also took part in the group; the author partici-

pated as medical director for American Whole-Health Networks in Washington state and as a naturopathic physician. In 1999, additional representatives joined the group from various CAM educational institutions and became active participants. At this time, the group has fulfilled its charter, has disbanded, and has produced a report summarizing its activities. The report can be accessed on the World Wide Web at <www.insurance.wa.gov> or through the Office of the Insurance Commissioner of Washington State. The report's Executive Summary is reproduced in Chapter 16.

THE GROWTH OF INTEGRATIVE MEDICINE

When the group began in 1997, there was some serious skepticism on the part of all the participants. The medical directors were involved primarily because their companies had requested that they take part. There was also mistrust on the part of CAM practitioners: we were concerned that insurance companies might not be willing to work with us or address us as peers. However, communication improved dramatically as participants came to know one another—not just as people, but as professionals of our disciplines.

Eileen Stretch, ND, is Associate Medical Director for American WholeHealth Networks, Inc (AWHN), which assists health plans integrate CAM by providing networks nationwide. She leads their credentialing activities and has also been instrumental in developing AWHN's clinical quality and utilization management system for CAM services. Dr. Stretch is a partner in the Institute of Complementary Medicine, Seattle, where she practices naturopathic medicine in an integrated setting. She served on the Clinician Workgroup for the Integration of CAM and is on the adjunct faculty of Bastyr University in the Department of Naturopathic Medicine.

Development of Practice Guidelines

When the group first convened, few of the CAM professions participating had developed both practice and treatment guidelines, with the exception of dietitians, midwives, and chiropractors. There was a great deal of hesitation and resistance to the use of guidelines. Practitioners did not want to be pinned down. However, at the time of this writing, every one of the CAM participant groups has developed some form of practice and treatment guidelines. In the discipline of naturopathic medicine, this has provided the impetus to the national organization to begin the process of treatment guideline development.

Increased Interest in Integrative Medicine

The medical directors have become increasingly interested in integration and in finding ways to foster integration. The insurance companies represented in the group have made great strides in discussing and evaluating strategies and implementation plans for the integration of CAM into their health plans. The HMOs and the primary care groups that are involved are also taking active steps to move the integration forward. Naturopathic physicians are now included as primary care providers with a major health plan in Washington state, and the experience has been positive for the practitioners, patients, and the health plan. Other insurers are following suit.

Expanded Communication

When people sit down together, they have the opportunity to exchange meaningful information. They have access to the facts. They are no longer just making assumptions. When insurers and health plans open the dialogue with alternative practitioners, the next steps become clearer.

Open communication provides the basis for trust, and when trust develops, people begin to overcome the obstacles. They begin to identify problems not as obstacles, but as opportunities.

The collegial relationships that have developed in the group provide the basis for professional networking. Now, when the health plans need information or referrals, they have associates in various complementary fields they can contact as resources.

Although it will probably take some time to achieve true integration of CAM into conventional medicine, this type of experience will lay the groundwork. Open dialogue is one of the most important initial steps in the successful application of CAM in mainstream medical environments. In Washington state, people have become so interested in integrative medicine and so highly motivated, the greatest problem has become finding the resources (the time, people, and energy) to actually implement all the ideas that have come out of the group.

Increased Referrals

Currently, the author receives requests for referrals from providers who in the past have been hostile toward CAM. To some degree, the impetus for these referrals has grown out of the increasing number of requests by health plan members for CAM services (from patients with chronic illness, for example). Now, however, interest from primary care providers and specialists is also motivating these referrals, out of desire to provide the best of both worlds to their patients.

The number of interdisciplinary referrals has increased dramatically. More medical doctors and specialists are referring their patients to CAM providers. If that trend could be tracked, the percentage of increase would be in the thousands. Earlier, referrals were relatively rare. At this point, as a provider, this author receives referrals from physicians every single day. Many other providers receive daily referrals as well.

In naturopathic medicine, the appropriate use of referral is part of the training. Naturopathic physicians are well schooled in the scope of practice since they do not perform surgery or prescribe certain medications. Consequently, they refer patients back to medical doctors and other allopathic providers as appropriate. Now, the referral process has become more reciprocal.

The current transition is occurring as an extension of the development of trust and increased information dissemination. As practitioners in the mainstream gain an in-depth understanding of the alternative disciplines and their potential, they become more interested in the possibility of collaboration.

THE PROCESS OF INTEGRATION

The Expanding Knowledge Base

The process of integration definitely entails a learning curve. CAM is very multifaceted. Many of the disciplines encompass an immense aggregate of knowledge and practical wisdom. There is also a sizeable body of information involved in credentialing CAM providers. A genuine effort to implement integrative medicine will always involve a stage of self-education. The important first step is to explore options with an open mind.

Reframing the Options

Health plans are beginning to recognize the value of these services. Physicians and specialists such as oncologists are reporting that patients who include complementary therapies in their treatment do better. Although this is anecdotal, impressions are important because they are based on observation by professionals who have extensive experience with the usual course of disease. When practitioners observe a positive difference in the long-term outcomes of patients using integrative approaches, they begin to reframe their opinion of complementary therapies. As more patients seem to do better or are able to manage their diseases better, practitioners have become more interested in the research that supports these clinical observations.

Those physicians are expressing the desire for expanded options with which to treat chronic ill-ness. They want new tools. Here in Washington state, many physicians are very excited about the prospect of having additional clinical resources available. They are also attracted by the practice style of CAM—they, too, would like to be able to spend 30 or 60 minutes with a patient in an office visit.

The Expansion of Integrative Practice

When the integration of CAM began, it was exceptionally rare to find conventional physicians who were providing integrative medicine in conjunction with alternative care practitioners. In a few cases, acupuncturists were in the same building with physicians, but not in the same group practice. Now it is very common for conventional physicians to seek out CAM providers to work in their offices. An endocrinologist may look for a naturopathic physician to provide nutrition counseling for diabetic patients. The rheumatologist may be looking for a naturopathic physician or acupuncturist. There are also integrative pain clinics that did not exist 2 or 3 years ago. This trend is accelerating in Oregon as well. In Portland, an integrative clinic is being developed for women with breast cancer, in affiliation with a major hospital and a medical school. The National College of Naturopathic Medicine has an integrative medicine residency program, and there is also a residency exchange program with Oregon Health Sciences University and Providence Hospital. Children's Hospital in Seattle is providing an integrative program in conjunction with Bastyr University clinicians.

The State of Research

The question of "Where is the proof?" is beginning to be answered. Research studies and data are becoming more widely available. Now conventional providers can read about CAM in their own journals. For example, University of Washington researchers are working with clinical researchers at Bastyr University to look at the efficacy of phytoestrogens, herbs, and natural hormones, compared to conventional hormone replacement therapy. The Fred Hutchinson Cancer Research Center in Seattle is evaluating 900 women with breast cancer in a case-control study to determine if the use of synthetic and/or natural hormones increases the risk of breast cancer.

A PERSONAL PERSPECTIVE

I have always said that if I get into a serious accident, take me directly to the hospital emergency department. Do *not* take me to a naturopathic physician. However, once they stop the hemorrhaging, I want the hospital to call my naturopathic doctor, because then I want to integrate. I want the best of both medicines.

4.2 Developing an Integrative Medicine Program: The University of Arizona Experience

Tracy W. Gaudet with Nancy Faass

Integrative medicine is based on the best of mainstream and complementary therapies. This approach is committed to the practice of good medicine founded in good science, whether its origins are biomedical or complementary. At its most effective, this perspective is inquiry-driven and open to new paradigms, neither rejecting mainstream medicine nor uncritically accepting alternative practices.

Tracy W. Gaudet, MD, is recognized as a leader in the emerging field of integrative medicine. She has served as executive director and medical director of the University of Arizona Program in Integrative Medicine and led the Program in the design of the country's first comprehensive curriculum in the new field of integrative medicine. Dr. Gaudet is also assistant professor of clinical medicine in the Departments of Medicine and Obstetrics and Gynecology at University of Arizona and has taught at the University of Texas, San Antonio, as assistant professor in the Maternal-Fetal Medical Division. Her work has been featured in the national media; she has presented at conferences throughout the United States, and is an invitational member of the National Health Council's Integrated Patient-Centered Care Initiative Advisory Committee.

Source: A portion of this chapter has been adapted from *Integrative Medicine*, Vol. 1, No. 2, Integrative Medicine: The Evolution of a New Approach to Medicine and to Medical Education, Tracy Gaudet, pp. 67–73, Copyright 1998, with permission from Elsevier Science.

THE ISSUES WITHIN MEDICINE

A large percentage of the American population is reported to be using alternative methods about which, by definition, their physicians have not been formally educated. Recent studies found that 40% to 42% of Americans had used alternative medicine within the previous year (Eisenberg et al, 1998; Astin, 1998). Consequently, physicians and health systems are realizing that they must begin to address the issues surrounding the use of alternative therapies by their patients. This ultimately involves research, regulation, and education.

The majority of patients are not informing their doctors about these choices (Eisenberg et al, 1998). Given that the practice of good medicine is based on the physician's working knowledge of the treatments in which patients are engaged and their potential effects, this is a potentially dangerous set of circumstances. Physicians clearly need to have a working knowledge of alternative methods. They need to know which practices are potentially harmful, could cause dangerous interactions, or are unlikely to be of benefit, thereby delaying timely treatment. This knowledge is also necessary to help patients avoid spending what can be substantial financial resources.

If the objective is to practice the best medicine possible, physicians want to be aware of which alternative modalities can be of greatest benefit to patients when selectively and intelligently integrated into health care. At present, there is little formalized academic training to support integrative practice and no certification process covering these areas. With the lack of information in these domains, this newly evolving medicine is left extremely vulnerable to those who may be more motivated by market share and profit than by regard for the highest medical and academic standards.

The Patients' Perspective

Why do patients want to be seen in an integrative environment? The Program in Integrative Medicine of the University of Arizona informally surveyed their waiting list to determine why patients wanted to be seen here. By far the most important reason was that people wanted to be advised by a well-informed physician who would advise them on all of their treatment options, including alternative medicine. They did not want to go to their own conventional doctor only to have all alternative therapies dismissed and then go to their alternative practitioner to be told the opposite.

Patients recognize that they do not have the in-depth knowledge of a physician. They want to be seen by someone medically trained, a physician who will work with them collaboratively to guide them through the maze of alternative options. They want a health care provider who involves them in designing a treatment plan focused on their whole person, on their health as well as their disease, integrating the best of conventional medicine with the best of alternative therapies.

The Practitioners' Perspective

What are the issues from the perspective of alternative providers? Through case conferences held with the multidisciplinary team, we have learned that alternative providers are no more accustomed to the integrative process than mainstream physicians. A Chinese medicine practitioner knows how to practice Chinese medicine. Most have never had any conversations about whether or how to integrate with conventional medicine or with another alternative system. These conversations have not occurred on either side.

The Patients' Dilemma

Patients often feel caught in the middle, and they tend to be the ones who suffer. The greatest struggle is seen in cancer patients. They feel their lives are on the line, and often they are. They may ask their oncologist for advice, but many oncologists have not explored CAM in great depth. From an oncologist's perspective, the safest solution is not to use any alternative treatments since there are many unknowns involved, such as possible side effects from herbs or potential interactions between nutrients and chemotherapy.

When patients talk to their friends, their Internet contacts, and alternative providers, everyone gives them different advice. They come to feel as if they are totally alone, singularly responsible for medical decisions for which there seem to be no answers. They are not medically trained, they may have a potentially fatal condition, and they have no idea how to make these decisions. They are looking for someone they can trust who is medically trained and who can help them through the medical maze. We as health care providers have a responsibility to these patients. If we are committed to good health care, we must look at these issues.

Patients are hungry to be able to have a conversation with someone who is genuinely knowledgeable about the range of treatment options. To some degree, the question of integration is as much about openness and willingness to consider alternatives as it is about being thoroughly expert. In that context, the issue of retraining becomes greatly simplified.

CONTINUING EDUCATION IN INTEGRATIVE MEDICINE

Physicians who are interested in integrative practice may find themselves wondering if they will have to drop everything and take part in an intensive training program for 2 years. Most doctors are relieved to learn that they can begin where they are in their own communities and their own organizations. Options include the following:

- *Participating in an interest group.* This can be an effective way to begin.
- *Case conferences.* Informal seminars could involve bringing in alternative providers to discuss complex cases.
- *A journal club or a steering committee.* A review of the literature is another option. Even meeting once a month can be meaningful because the goal is to raise awareness and involve people in dialogue.
- *Experiencing the treatment.* It can also be highly useful for doctors to be seen as patients by skilled alternative practitioners in their own communities so that they can develop an experiential sense of various disciplines.
- *Observing a practitioner.* Another option is to visit practitioners and observe them working with patients. The opportunity to observe the therapy, the treatment process, and the outcome is what is meaningful.
- *Conferences.* This is another useful way to become involved in integrative medicine, to learn, and to network.

The Program at the University of Arizona sponsors a week-long continuing medical education conference for up to 40 physicians at a session. This author has been amazed by the impact a week's experience can have. Many of the physicians leave changed. Some leave totally transformed. A major component of the conference is participatory; the attendees themselves experience many of these approaches and modalities. There is also a strong educational component. Although 1 week does not create

expertise, it can provide a sense of appreciation and an understanding for what is possible.

INTEGRATIVE MEDICINE WITHIN THE ORGANIZATION

Administrators will also find that there are simple steps that can be taken within their organization that are realistic and practical. It is important to think about the values of the organizational culture and what will be most acceptable.

Surveying the Staff

One of the best ways to begin is by surveying the staff to determine who has interest and who does not. A survey can provide a baseline and a reflection of where the organizational community stands on these issues, the level of interest and knowledge in the organization, and the organization's degree of openness. The next phase of the program can be shaped by this insight. We performed our survey anonymously; people were not required to sign their names. However, those who were interested in participating included their names so that we could contact them.

Phasing in Integration

If the learning curve becomes too daunting, professionals will walk away from the process. This can create a scenario in which no one is dealing with the real issues. For example, the organization may simply add an acupuncturist to the staff. In other cases, the physicians may learn medical acupuncture and consider that sufficient. In reality, the abstraction of a technique does not encompass an entire system. That does not mean that it is not valuable to learn the technique. However, it is also important to develop an appreciation for the richness and depth of that system, to learn the vocabulary, and to develop an understanding of the core concepts as a basis for communicating with practitioners and referring patients. In other words, all physicians need not be trained in acupuncture. The lines of communication need to be opened, and these different systems need to be integrated in a way that is medically effective.

Evaluating the Range of Options

The integration of CAM occurs across a spectrum. Returning to the example of acupuncture, a practitioner can take a 200-hour acupuncture course and be certified to place acupuncture needles, or he or she can take 4 years of full-time training in Chinese medicine and its practice. There are different ways to approach this training issue, and they are not exclusive of one another; nor is one solution better than another. Similarly, there is more to homeopathy than simply purchasing and ingesting a remedy. It is an entire system, with its own body of theory, logic, and practice wisdom. Like any other skill, its practice can only be developed through training and experience.

Providing the Experience of Integrative Practice

In the Program at the University of Arizona, physicians and alternative care providers work side by side. When the physicians watch the acupuncturist take a case history, they often confide that they are amazed at the difference in approach and perception. What is important in this experience is that the physician have the opportunity to gain a sense of the variations between the two systems, and the substance and depth of traditional Chinese medicine.

On first consideration, it would appear that the case conference is a luxury. However, this model is not intended to be used for all patients—it would be prohibitively expensive. Rather, the team approach is selectively applied to address the most challenging cases. In this context, it offers three important benefits. First, it provides a forum for the discussion of the most difficult cases and access to the resources of the entire integrative team. Second, it is an ongoing opportunity for the team to actually practice integra-

tive medicine. Third, the case conference functions as a cost-effective venue for continuing education in integrative medicine. In the process of developing integrative treatment plans, practitioners are informally educating one another about their disciplines and how they can best be applied in treatment.

Initially, it is possible to integrate using protocols that simply focus on the most benign therapies. In deciding what to integrate and what not to integrate, there are certain therapies that are clearly safe as CAM options in most cases, such as massage and mind-body medicine. If a patient is interested in a particular treatment approach, and the physician feels that it is not going to cause harm, that is fairly easy to support.

Practical Considerations

How are these two approaches to medicine actually integrated? How can the integration process be facilitated?

- *Design a system with a tremendous amount of flexibility.* This is a field that is developing rapidly; both administrators and staff will find that they learn a great deal very quickly. In addition, the more challenging the system, the greater the need for flexibility.
- *Consider hiring a team on a short-term or part-time basis.* I would urge this as a matter of practicality because the right mix of people is crucial. In programs associated with a teaching institution, practitioners and clinicians may be hired for short rotations of a few months at a time; their initial expectations are that they will only be there for a brief period. This has proven to be a practical strategy that provides a structure which enables management to identify and retain practitioners who mesh and work together well as a team.
- *Identify highly capable clinicians:*
  — Work from referrals whenever possible.
  — Perform thorough background checks, comparable to the process any physician would use to identify capable spe-

cialists. The staff member doing the hiring should ask friends and patients and develop a list of capable practitioners, based on those reports. Ideally, the person doing the hiring should talk with the practitioners and patients. In this way, he or she builds up a file of competent practitioners.

— Identify a team leader or staff member responsible for hiring, who is willing to be seen as a patient by these applicant practitioners. Even if the interviewer's knowledge of alternative medicine is limited, the interviewer will gain an intuitive sense of how he or she is being treated and of the practitioners' competence and intelligence. Is the practitioner someone to whom he or she would feel comfortable referring patients? Frequently, those assessments can be made without expertise in a particular discipline.

— Select someone to participate in recruitment who knows the CAM community. This function may be performed by a staff member or an outside consultant. The University of Arizona Program had an advantage in recruiting the multidisciplinary team because Andrew Weil had lived in the community for 25 years and knew many skilled alternative practitioners.

• *Communicate your goals for the program to attract staff with similar values.* Although it sounds idealistic, it is important to articulate the organization's vision. Often people are drawn to this type of program because they want an opportunity to be part of something greater. When they sense that the program is moving in a direction that resonates with their own vision, they are often willing to deal with less-than-ideal circumstances. They are willing to make that commitment if they feel connected to the program at a deeper level. Consequently, those in management pay attention to long-term goals.

• *Encourage dialogue among the team members.* One of the challenges of integrative medicine is that there is not even a common language or a shared vocabulary. This is as true of a conversation between an acupuncturist and a homeopath as it is between physicians and CAM practitioners. Historically, these different disciplines have not had dialogue. In fact, the various CAM disciplines generally know little of one another's knowledge base.

• *Make sure everyone is aligned in terms of their interest in integrative practice.* The organization should identify potential staff who actually want to work on a multidisciplinary team in an integrative environment and who have a high level of commitment to this process. Are all the professionals on the team genuinely interested in integrative medicine?

• *Identify those who can move beyond a focus on their own disciplines.* Some may be tempted to defend their own particular modality. The team will not be successful if practitioners are drawn into turf wars and are not genuinely interested in developing an integrative multidisciplinary approach. As a team, the staff members may have to evaluate how to choose between homeopathy and Chinese medicine and which would be best under what circumstances. A team member who suggests that Chinese medicine is always good for everyone and everything will not be able to participate constructively in this type of dialogue.

• *Make goals clear to members of the team.* Monitor the level of interest to determine what resonates with practitioners. Some will drop out because they are not appropriate for an integrative approach.

• *Communicate the organization's vision and mission to the broader community.* This tends to attract people who are supportive of the program. Staff in our program work in the community to develop the model, provide it exposure, and keep people interested in what we are trying to accomplish.

- *Design in mechanisms for obtaining feedback about the program.* The goal is to institute a process that acknowledges the dynamic nature of program development.
- *Build traditions into the program and the organizational culture.* Once a month the team dines together. We encourage our practitioners to remain conscious of their own health and well-being. We make the effort to infuse what we believe into the day-to-day operations of the program.
- *Reevaluate the relationships in the organization.* It is necessary to evaluate not only the interface between health care providers and patients, but also that between providers and administrators. There cannot be integrative medicine without integrative management.
- *Remember that there are few models in this field, even on a practical level.* For example, there is no widely used standard model for billing. Every aspect of this field is in a state of development, and often requires building from the ground up.

CONCLUSION

Optimally, the integrative approach will be furthered by expanding the continuum of care to include prevention and wellness, engaging mind, spirit, and community as well as the body. This approach is based in a partnership of patient and practitioner within which the best ideas and practices of mainstream and CAM are applied.

However, if the conversation continues to revolve only around complementary therapies rather than the underlying philosophies, an opportunity will have been lost. Specific alternative therapies will gradually be incorporated into the current medical system. There will be more tools in our black bag, but no real change will occur.

The shift in paradigm and practice relies on unprecedented collaboration across health professionals and across disciplines, between medical schools, insurers, hospitals, and most importantly, patients. This new approach to medicine requires a new way of relating, administratively, educationally, medically, and personally. The challenges are many, and the opportunities are great.

REFERENCES

Astin JA. Why patients use alternative medicine: results of a national study. *JAMA.* 1998;279:1548–1553.

Eisenberg D, Davis R, Ettner S, et al. Trends in alternative medicine use in the United States, 1990–1997: results of a follow-up national survey. *JAMA.* 1998;280: 1569–1575.

MANAGEMENT FUNCTIONS

PART II

Practical Strategic Planning

CHAPTER 5

Initial Strategies

5.1   Overview: Evaluating Organizational Readiness

David C. Kailin

DOMAINS OF KNOWLEDGE

Evaluating organizational readiness for integrative medicine involves a synthesis of information from three domains of knowledge: (1) technical, (2) organizational, and (3) personal (Linstone, 1999). Each domain provides knowledge crucial to the initial process of designing the project and developing consensus on its implementation.

David C. Kailin, medical futurist and Chief Executive Officer of Convergent Medical Systems, Inc, Corvallis, Oregon, assists organizations in the development of preferable health care futures. He is currently a PhD candidate in public health at Oregon State University with interests in systems thinking and organizational learning. He is author of *Acupuncture Risk Management* (1997, CMS Press) and is a leading authority on federal regulations of the Occupational Safety and Health Administration and the Food and Drug Administration that impact CAM providers.

Convergent Medical Systems, Inc provides consulting services to health care clients and contributes to strategic planning, mission and values development, and innovative program design. CMS consultants offer expertise in the integration and evaluation of CAM therapies.

Courtesy of David Kailin, Convergent Medical Systems, Corvallis, Oregon.

Technical Domain

The technical domain contains explicit knowledge and quantifiable data about the integrative medicine program under consideration, including organizational resources as well as environmental and informational factors:

- outline of proposed integrative medicine program
- financial plan
- market analysis
- external and internal marketing plans
- service reimbursement plan
- facilities, space, and remodeling plan
- information services integration strategies
- regulatory factors report
- risk management report
- report on qualification and credentialing of providers
- evidence of clinical costs/benefits from integrative medicine
- inventory of expertise and resources.

The technical information will be incomplete, in part because integrative medicine's full clinical potential is not known. An information bias is usually present, in that technologies based in nonconventional theoretic models typically are asked to meet a higher standard of information than many currently accepted technologies. Furthermore, clinical innovations commonly precede reimbursement certainties. Every new step requires a carefully considered act of faith. Complex decisions are usually made with insufficient technical information, a condition accentuated when pioneering a leadership position.

Organizational Domain

The organizational domain refers to the mission and political field of the institution. While primarily an internal matter, the politics of external relationships are also significant. Relevant factors include:

- organizational mission
- strategic plan and environmental forecasts
- comparison with other organizational options
- relationships involving proponents and opponents
- areas of internal conflict and concern
- process for developing organizational informed consensus
- community interests in integrative medicine
- related areas of community conflict and concern
- process for developing community buy-in
- impact on other organizations and external providers

Inquiries may well reveal a tangled web of tacit and explicit power relations, professional biases, and closely guarded turf. Wise observers have noted that there is more competition within organizations than between them. Accordingly, processes to air and resolve conflict are integral to the successful initiation of an integrative medicine program. Even so, some will discover general intractable staff resistance. Moving ahead is not advisable under such conditions, unless the program can be sufficiently isolated or otherwise protected.

Personal Domain

The personal domain refers to the qualities, skills, beliefs, and ideals brought by individual players to the project. The particular perspectives of each of the major participants must be taken into account, including those of the charismatic leader, the vocal patient advocate, the true believers (of any persuasion), and the mediator. Beyond determining political impacts and functional capabilities, the task involves eliciting, acknowledging, comparing, and bridging the conceptual maps of integrative medicine carried by each of the key stakeholders. Cultivating common ground is an uncommonly valuable activity. Creating the conditions for generative dialogue is essential to this process (Isaacs, 1999).

The importance of addressing conceptual maps cannot be overemphasized since they inform, and will ultimately become reflected in the fundamental pattern of the integrative medicine program. Group dialogue and interviews are appropriate methods for revealing the implicit assumptions of the participants. Using a skilled moderator from outside the organization is advantageous since it is often difficult to recognize and evaluate assumptions held in common. Thumbnail descriptions of several typical conceptual maps and their related patterns follow.

Conceptual Map #1: Avoidance Patterns

At one end of the spectrum, certain individuals will conceive of integrative medicine as bereft of clinical merit and/or potential strategic value. When this is the dominant map, projects that reflect an integrative approach are avoided, or sidelined indefinitely, as intrinsically nonviable. Altering this pattern is difficult because it may be rooted in axiomatic disbelief. Transition to a pattern of transformative integration is a long reach.

Conceptual Map #2: Isolated Integration Patterns

When CAM practices are conceived of as marketable, but to be held at arm's length from biomedicine, patterns of isolated integration result. Both biomedical and CAM providers have been known to embrace this map, desiring a marketing association, but not a close working relationship. This diffident arrangement, seen in the development of separate integrative medicine clinics, tends to preserve the status quo of respective providers, thereby making initial mutual approach less threatening. However, professional segregation does not maximize the potential for clinical innovation born of collaboration. Isolated integration is intrinsically conflicted between approach and avoidance.

Conceptual Map #3: Dominating Integration Patterns

When integrative medicine is seen as an errant subset of biomedicine, meant to serve identical clinical functions in the treatment of biomedically defined disease entities, then patterns of dominating integration emerge. CAM providers are situated in highly restrictive roles within extant institutional contexts. While a familiar socioprofessional hierarchy is reinforced in the name of risk reduction, excessive controls can so distort CAM that resultant clinical benefits are markedly diminished. Potential for error resides at both extremes in the delicate balance between the competing goals of preventing harm and providing help (Kailin, 1997).

Conceptual Map #4: Physician Provider Patterns

When integrative medicine is perceived to offer benefit, but nonphysician CAM practitioners are marginalized, then patterns result in which physicians come to serve as the primary CAM providers. Physicians may tend to feel more comfortable referring patients to other physicians than to nonphysician CAM providers, based on the training they have in common. Some patients express greater trust in physicians than in CAM providers (Kailin, 1992). Paradoxically, a major limitation of this pattern revolves around CAM expertise. As specialists, CAM providers often possess more extensive theoretical, perceptual, and technical training

in their alternative discipline, while in some cases, simultaneously exhibiting limitations in biomedical knowledge and practice. Honoring and bridging authentic diversity increase innovative capacity.

Conceptual Map #5: Transformative Integration Patterns

If both biomedicine and integrative medicine are conceived of—not in static terms but in dynamic terms—as engaged in a productive interactive relationship, then transformative integration patterns can occur. Successful collaborative efforts rely on mutual respect, humility, and a spirit of inquiry in the context of close, collegial, working relationships. Participants must be willing to confer, experiment, and adapt their practices based on outcomes. However, the personal qualities necessary to successful collaboration are often in short supply, and must be assiduously cultivated. Transformative integration patterns are the most variable, manifesting the influence of unique local innovations in clinical practices and multidisciplinary arrangements. Moving beyond the divisions of alternative and orthodox, these patterns offer the greatest promise for the reinvention of health services and long-term strategic positioning.

Attention should be directed not so much toward which pattern is right in the general sense, but which pattern is right for a given institution in its particular situation. It is vital at the outset to develop an explicit common understanding of the integrative medicine pattern an organization wishes to attain.

SYNTHESIS

Evaluating organizational readiness requires synthesizing a vast body of incomplete qualitative and quantitative data drawn from the three domains. What tools can assist in the process?

Systems Models

The preliminary work is to develop a rich understanding of the situation within the organization and its environment and its implications for the integrative medicine project and the matrix of relationships that will have an impact on it. Tools for modeling such complex nonlinear situations are drawn from a facet of systems theory known as soft systems thinking, which uses qualitative approaches to description. Patterns of relationship and influence can be depicted with the use of schematics developed through dialogue and analysis.

Qualitative systems diagramming is used to sketch relationships, thereby creating a separate sketch for each of several levels of resolution. This type of diagramming is in the form of a recursive web of feedback loops rather than in a linear chain because it describes a nonlinear

situation. These diagrams are an accessible and frugal method (Checkland and Scholes, 1990).

Fuzzy cognitive maps are similarly useful interpretive devices (Kosko, 1993). These are graphs that depict relational feedback loops and indicate whether the feedback is a positive or negative influence. Both of these approaches graphically depict the dynamic circumstances and cross impacts of the project. Figure 5.1–1 provides an elementary example of a qualitative systems diagram of cross impacts.

Decision-Making Tools

With suitable models in hand, the next task relates to decision making. The core problem

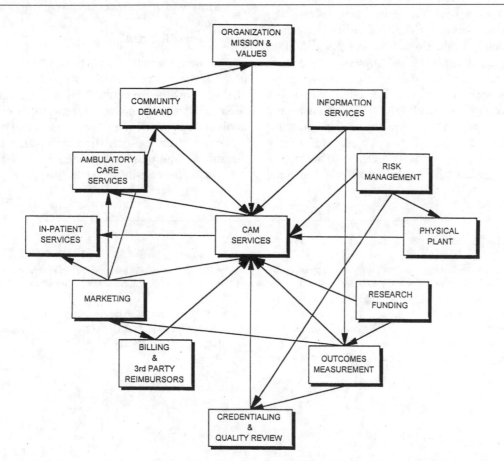

Figure 5.1–1 Systems Diagram of Cross Impacts. Courtesy of David Kailin, Convergent Medical Systems, Corvallis, Oregon.

concerns how to make decisions with incomplete data and conflicting opinions. One of the more promising cutting-edge developments is software that combines relevant quantitative and qualitative data. The software accounts for uncertainty in the data and produces measures of subjective utility. Maximum subjective utility reflects the best choice based on the quantitative data and the included opinions of experts and/or stakeholders; hence subjective factors are also entered in the equation.

Software programs such as ConsensusBuilder (2000), based on the theoretic models of Thomas Bayes (1702–1761), can be used to decrease decision times for complex problems. Expert evaluations of many individuals can be entered into the equations. The conditions can be modified over time in an iterative process. The consensus process is advanced by graphically depicting evaluations from key players, highlighting dimensions and degrees of agreement and disagreement, and charting changes in these parameters as the project develops. While such Bayesian statistical software solutions cannot replace human judgment and accountability for making decisions, they can assist in clarifying the basis and process for decisions. (One can use a program such as ConsensusBuilder to some advantage in decision making even with no understanding of the math, but it should not replace executive judgment.)

EPILOGUE

One can easily lose sight of the focal issues over time, amidst volumes of data and the distractions of other duties. An assessment of organizational readiness methodically elaborates and then evaluates alternative responses to these basic questions:

- Where does the project lead?
- What does the project mean?
- Why it is worth doing?
- Who is ready for the project?
- How will the project be brought to fruition?
- When will it start?

One wants to fathom a complex situation, an array of targets, and pathway options. Facilitated dialogue, qualitative systems models, and decision analysis programs are exceptionally useful tools for comprehension. The development and synthesis of critical data from technical, organizational, and personal domains provide the foundation for well-informed decisions.

REFERENCES

Checkland P, Scholes J. *Soft Systems Methodology in Action.* New York: John Wiley & Sons; 1990.

ConsensusBuilder [computer program]. Corvallis, OR: Camas, Inc; 2000.

Isaacs W. *Dialogue and the Art of Thinking Together.* New York: Currency; 1999.

Kailin D. *Acupuncture Risk Management.* Corvallis, OR: CMS Press; 1997.

Kailin D. *A Survey of Attitudes toward Acupuncture among Seattle Adults* [thesis]. Seattle, WA: University of Washington; 1992.

Kosko B. *Fuzzy Thinking.* New York: Hyperion;1993.

Linstone H. *Decision Making for Technology Executives.* Boston: Artech House; 1999.

5.2   Visioning and Planning

Mary Jo Kreitzer

As consumer demand for complementary and alternative medicine (CAM) has continued to increase, many health systems are faced with fundamental questions. Organizations may wonder whether they should enter the market, and if so, what strategy they should adopt. Given the newness of the complementary medicine market, it is not clear which strategic approaches will succeed over time. What is apparent is that organizations are most successful when they adopt a plan that is consistent with their overall mission and organizational mandates. It is also becoming clear that a standardized one-size-fits-all approach tends to be less successful. Health systems inherently have their own unique strengths and opportunities. Communities and populations served also differ significantly in their needs and expectations.

A strategic planning process designed by Bryson (1995) offers a structure that can be applied in planning for the inclusion of complementary medicine.

DEFINING THE ORGANIZATION

Organizations need to examine critically who they are as service providers with respect to

Mary Jo Kreitzer is Director of the Center for Spirituality and Healing at the University of Minnesota, Minneapolis, Minnesota. Dr. Kreitzer holds a PhD in health services research, policy, and administration as well as BA and MA degrees in nursing. Her research interests include health systems development, quality of life, and outcomes research on complementary therapies and healing practices.

The Center for Spirituality and Healing at the University of Minnesota has quickly emerged as a national leader in complementary, cross-cultural, and spiritual care. The center is involved in a broad spectrum of activities including education of medical and nursing students, an interdisciplinary graduate program, the Mind Body Spirit Clinic, and a variety of research and outreach initiatives.

vision, mission and values, and the environment in which they are operating. A systematic analysis of the internal and external environment allows an organization to identify strengths, weaknesses, opportunities, and threats. An analysis such as this provides a context in which decisions can be made over strategic choices that will guide the organization's planning and implementation of complementary medicine. The following questions may serve as a guide:

- Who are we as an organization?
- What are our mandates?
- What are our values and our mission?
- Which elements in the mandate function as absolutes, defining us as an organization or as a health system?
- What are the key factors in the internal and external environment?
- What are the primary strategic issues and choices?
- How can we develop strategies and actions that will be aligned with our organizational vision?

Figure 5.2–1 illustrates the steps in Bryson's strategic-planning process model.

THE PLANNING PROCESS

1. Initial Agreement on the Planning Effort

The "plan for planning" provides a foundation and legitimacy for the planning effort. At a minimum, it should be clear at the onset whether a planning group is responsible for gathering information, generating recommendations, making decisions regarding organizational strategy, or all of the above. It is important that key stakeholders be involved in the planning effort. Ideally, the design of the integration of

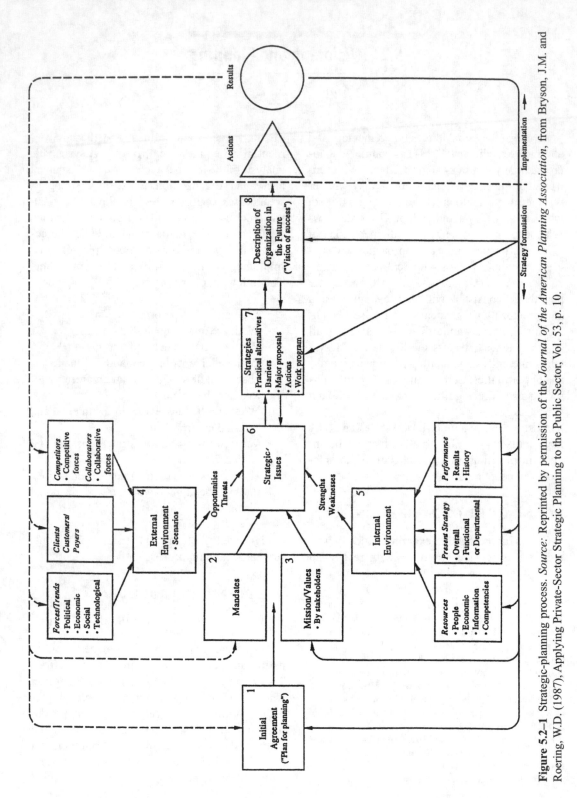

Figure 5.2–1 Strategic-planning process. *Source:* Reprinted by permission of the *Journal of the American Planning Association*, from Bryson, J.M. and Roering, W.D. (1987), Applying Private-Sector Strategic Planning to the Public Sector, Vol. 53, p. 10.

CAM services will involve consumers, board members, physicians, nurses, other biomedical mainstream providers, complementary or alternative practitioners, health care administrators, and third-party payers. Planning efforts often occur within the context of either board or medical staff activities or functions.

2. Identification and Clarification of Mandates

Health systems may have externally imposed mandates—formal as well as informal. These are the requirements with which an organization contends, in order to conform to charters, articles of incorporation, or legislation (in the case of formal legal mandates). Informal mandates may be imposed by tradition or expectations within a community. These mandates may require that a certain patient population be served. In the case of health care systems affiliated with religious organizations, one aspect of the organization's mission may be to ensure that spiritual care needs are addressed. The identification of mandates early in the planning process clarifies any given factors that need to be addressed in making decisions regarding if and how CAM will be introduced within a particular system.

3. Clarification of Mission and Values

A health care system's mission is its justification for existence. The mission and values provide a context for planning that is very useful. For example, the mission of North Hawaii Community Hospital is improving the health status of the people on the northern side of the island of Hawaii. This goal is being put into practice by increasing access to care and providing high-quality services at a reasonable cost. Values or guiding principles shape both the focus and priorities of a health system.

4. Assessment of the External Environment

An external assessment can be useful in clarifying the opportunities and threats that face a health system. The process begins by identifying political, economic, and social trends that impact the organization in general and that would affect the process of integrating complementary medicine. From the perspective of a particular institution, it is important to look at the trends and forces that planners need to track. These trends and forces differ greatly from state to state.

Market Research

Market research will also likely include a detailed analysis of how other health systems and providers in the community are responding to the challenge of offering CAM services. It is important to determine who will be the competitors and who may have the potential of being a collaborator. Based on the external assessment, the health system will evaluate the threats and opportunities posed. Some organizations continue to be concerned about the risk involved in implementing a CAM program. On the other hand, in a community where CAM services are well developed, organizations may be concerned about the loss of market share if CAM services are not offered. A review of the political, social, and economic forces needs to be considered:

- What are the political issues—who are licensed providers and who are unlicensed?
- What are the demographics of the people who will be accessing the services?
- What are the economics? How is health care organized in the environment?
- How much of the system has taken the form of managed care and how much is fee-for-service?
- What are some of the social trends in the community?

Political Climate

The political climate can be evaluated by reviewing the relevant legislative and regulatory patterns within the state. In selecting new therapies, licensure laws will define to some degree which therapies can be integrated, who will be legally allowed to perform them, and what processes are involved in credentialing these personnel. There is an exceptional degree of variability in the licensure laws from state to state. For example, many states license practitioners of acupuncture and massage therapy. In other states, there are no laws or policy guidelines for licensure. Currently, in the state of California, naturopathic physicians are not licensed; they must provide services in another capacity, typically as either nutritional consultants or physician's assistants. Some states, including Minnesota, have statutes that specifically prohibit regulation unless there is risk to the safety and well-being of the citizens.

The extent of existing regulations (or the lack of statutes or policy) has a strong impact on the development of CAM within a state. If licensure is not available, it may be difficult to recruit providers. Clearly, this could decrease the public's access to CAM. On the other hand, it can be argued that regulation in the form of licensure can decrease access because it may limit licensure to practitioners who meet certain standards. It is not uncommon to find a lack of consensus even within a particular discipline as to whether regulation will advance or impede the implementation of its complementary specialty. The political climate is also affected by how professional groups lobby, collaborate, or compete in the public arena.

Economic and Social Trends

Economic and social trends within a community usually have a critical influence on the demand for access to complementary medicine. It is currently estimated that 80% to 85% of the CAM market is financed by out-of-pocket expenditures (Weeks, 1999; Academic Health Center Task Force, 1997). An assessment of the community should include a profile of demographics including age, educational level, income, and employment patterns.

Potential Client Population

The external assessment will also include a detailed evaluation of the potential client base. Many institutions conduct a communitywide market survey to assess the level of interest and the actual readiness of consumers to use complementary therapies. The potential for relationships with third-party payers should also be explored as part of the community assessment.

5. Assessment of the Internal Environment

An assessment of the internal environment begins with a review of the resources, particularly the people within the organization and their interests, readiness, and skills. Such an inventory provides useful information to identify those who presently have training in some area of complementary medicine and those who are interested in obtaining more skills. It may also indicate where pockets of readiness or resistance to complementary medicine exist.

Health systems may seek information regarding perceived patient use of complementary therapies by surveying physicians, nurses, and other health care providers. This type of survey can also provide:

- provider perceptions of referral patterns
- level of interest on the part of professionals in acquiring more information or skills in CAM
- a detailed inventory of the present CAM skills of providers within the system.

It is surprising to learn how frequently staff members are presently providing CAM services either as part of their clinical practice within the system or outside their regular employment. It is also important to evaluate the status of any integrative initiatives occurring within the health system, including any current CAM strategy or planned implementation. In a large health system, certain clinical programs, service lines, or patient care units may have already implemented various CAM approaches. This kind of information is important and helpful to know when a larger organizational effort is being considered.

The assessment of the internal environment will provide an understanding of the strengths and weaknesses of the organization's essential resources—the people and the organization's capacity. This is reflected in the present strategies in progress and in past performance. The history of the organization's response to change is particularly relevant to any integration initiative. This responsiveness will define how much or how little integration occurs, what kind of effort is made, and how it should be implemented.

STRATEGIC ISSUES

The first five steps of the planning process provide the context for moving to the next level: the identification of strategic issues. These are policy questions that affect the health system and include:

- mandates, mission, and values
- level of products or services (both those currently in place and those under consideration)
- mix of clients, payers, cost, financing, and management.

Bryson (1995) points out that strategic issues, by definition, embody conflicts. Conflicts may occur due to:

- the ends (what)
- the means (how)
- philosophy (why)
- location (where)
- timing (when)
- those helped or hurt by various strategic choices (who).

Applied to the implementation of CAM programming, this is the stage in the planning process when the organization decides whether and how to proceed. Several approaches can be used to identify the strategic issues or choices. A health system may identify strategic issues based on a number of criteria. One particular factor may become the predominating value or a number of aspects may simultaneously influence decision making, such as:

- a review of the mandates, mission, strengths, weaknesses, threats, and opportunities
- established goals and objectives of the organization
- description of the health systems' vision of success.

Development of Strategic Planning

The next step of this planning process is the identification of strategies. Bryson (1995) describes a strategy as a pattern of purposes, policies, programs, actions, decisions, and/or resource allocations that define what an organization is, what it does, and why it does it. In implementing CAM in a health system, there are numerous questions to consider including the following:

- Will CAM be implemented in a systemwide effort or incrementally?
- Will services be organized around a core or center within the system or will they be dispersed throughout the system?
- Will CAM be implemented within an inpatient setting, an outpatient setting, or both?
- Will CAM be offered within the system or will the system contract for services from an independent practice association of complementary healers?

An effective strategy must meet several criteria. It must be technically and financially workable, politically acceptable to key stakeholders, and aligned with the organization's philosophy and core values.

A Vision of Success

Based on the strategies identified, all the actions and decisions to implement the strategies must be determined. It is also important to develop an evaluation plan during the initial design of the system for the long-term assessment of results. Bryson (1995) cautions that while the steps are laid out in a linear manner, the process is iterative. At certain stages in the project, planning committees must often repeat steps before further decisions can be made and actions taken.

Not all organizations have a formal statement of their "vision of success." These statements describe what the vision should look like as the health care system successfully implements its strategies and achieves its full potential. The inclusion of this type of affirmative vision can act as an additional organizational rudder, enabling members to retain sight of their ultimate goal.

CASE STUDIES

Woodwinds Health Campus

Woodwinds is a comprehensive health care complex located in Woodbury, Minnesota, that includes a medical office building, a diagnostic and treatment facility, and a 70-bed hospital. It is a collaborative effort between two health systems in the Minneapolis-St. Paul metropolitan area. The vision of Woodwinds is distinct: to be the innovative, unique, and preferred resource for health by fundamentally creating the health care experience in a way that has not been done before. The mission or purpose of Woodwinds is to promote health and healing of body, mind, and spirit for all clients and staff through relationships, choices, and learning. A set of 10 principles is being used to design all processes and systems that support patient care from the ground up. Four of the guiding principles specifically address the importance of embracing change and innovation, as well as care of the whole person:

- Deliver service that is patient- and family-centered while encouraging and supporting active involvement in one's own health care.
- Challenge the status quo and apply innovative thinking by continuously embracing and implementing change.
- Create and sustain a healing environment that promotes health and quality of life, in harmony with nature and spiritual awareness.
- Foster choice by providing a spectrum of care with the integration of selected complementary approaches to health and well-being.

During the strategic planning process, people living in the service area around the Woodwinds Health Campus were surveyed regarding their health and wellness needs. The input of the community was vitally important in making decisions about the care and services to be offered.

The intent is to fully integrate complementary approaches into care throughout the Campus. Each of the facility's health care teams designs the manner in which care will be delivered within their given area, such as preoperative services, labor and delivery, nutrition services, and intensive care. The institution's guiding principles are used to shape the health care experience. The teams evaluate which complementary approaches are most appropriate to integrate.

North Hawaii Community Hospital

Located on the Big Island of Hawaii, North Hawaii Community Hospital (NHCH) in Waimea, Hawaii, is positioning itself as a site that integrates high-tech Western medicine along with complementary approaches to healing. The mission of the hospital is to improve the health status of the people of the community by increasing access to care and providing high-quality services at a reasonable cost. The intent is to provide care that is genuinely patient-centered within a total healing environment and empower patients and families to become actively involved in their own health care choices.

NHCH offers a full spectrum of acute care hospital services with a commitment to care that is attentive to the whole person—the mind, body, and spirit. Complementary services provided include naturopathic medicine, chiropractic, acupuncture, massage therapy, healing touch, clinical psychology, and native Hawaiian healing. The pharmacy includes a variety of herbal remedies.

Significant attention was focused on the design and construction of the physical environment and the building, so that they too become instruments of healing. Patient rooms have natural lighting and garden views as well as doors that open onto gardens. Every aspect of the site has been considered in order to gain full advantage of the natural setting and mountain vistas that surround the hospital. The interior design incorporates warm colors, textures, and native art. NHCH is widely recognized as a prototype of an institutionwide integration effort.

Virginia Piper Cancer Institute

The Life Choices in Healing Program is located in Abbott Northwestern Hospital in Minneapolis. The program is available to patients faced with a diagnosis of cancer and to their families. The institute provides access to a variety of custom-designed programs in the arts, humanities, and complementary therapies. These approaches are designed to empower patients by giving them the tools to perform their own research on choices in healing and to experience their own discovery process. They are supported in making the choices that seem most appropriate for themselves and their families.

Resources available include a healing coach who serves as a facilitator and guide, as well as support groups. A variety of complementary therapies oriented to physical healing are provided, including nutritional counseling, acupuncture, acupressure, massage, and relaxation techniques. Healing the mind is encouraged through the use of music, poetry and art therapy, as well as educational programs. Modalities focused on the healing of the spirit include meditation, prayer, and the sacraments.

The program has two other unique elements: the Garden of Hope and a resource center known as the Living Room. The garden provides a year-round sanctuary of life and beauty that facilitates conversation, reflection, and a sense of peace. The Living Room offers a vast array of information through books, journals, videos, audiocassettes, CDs, brochures, and the Internet.

CONCLUSION

These case studies illustrate the variety and creativity of programs that are emerging within health systems. Each of the three organizations faced the same key strategic issues: what, how, why, where, and when to implement. Each responded in a unique and different manner:

- The Virginia Piper Cancer Institute resides within a large, complex tertiary care system that has not embraced or integrated complementary therapies systemwide. Yet, within the product line of oncology services, it serves as one of the most exceptionally imaginative and comprehensive programs developed to date.
- North Hawaii Community Hospital provides care to a rural population that is ethnically diverse. The nature and scope of services delivered reflect the unique community and environment of the Big Island of Hawaii.
- Woodwinds has capitalized on a rare opportunity to create a new health system, designed to be as responsive as possible to the community it serves. Systems and processes have been developed to maximize the patient-centered focus, and staff recruitment has focused on attracting health professionals and caregivers whose values are congruent with the organization's philosophy.

REFERENCES

Academic Health Center Task Force on Complementary Care. *Transforming Health Care: Integrating Complementary, Spiritual, and Cross-Cultural Care*. Minneapolis: University of Minnesota. Feb. 1997.

Bryson JM. *Strategic Planning for Public and Nonprofit Organizations: A Guide to Strengthening and Sustaining Organizational Achievement*, 2nd edition. San Francisco: Jossey-Bass; 1995.

Weeks J. CAM and the public health: Opportunity for alliance? *The Integrator*. 1999;3(10):1–2.

5.3   Checklist: Critical Success Factors

Robert E. Christenson

What are the critical success factors in the market of CAM? There are certain resources that must be available if an organization is to achieve its business objective. A self-evaluation will indicate whether these capabilities and resources are in place or whether they must be developed. The organization needs to determine the ideal realization and fulfillment of each success factor as well as define what is minimally acceptable. If the organization meets all the minimal standards, it will have a measure of stability. If the ideal realization is met, there is the potential to become highly profitable and it will likely achieve a leadership position.

Other stakeholders in the field should be interviewed to determine their perceptions of the essential elements of success. These factors will be different for each organization. They must be in congruence with the organization's mission, vision, and long-term strategies. If they are not, it will either be necessary to find another way to access that particular resource or else to redefine the organization's strategy.

It is most ideal if the CAM program is integrated well within the organization. Many health systems bring in CAM, but set it aside as a separate enterprise. If there are economic shortfalls or problems, the CAM unit is one of the first programs to experience cuts in budget or staffing. This is most likely to occur when the CAM program is outside the primary mission and strategic plan of the organization.

Robert E. Christenson is the cofounder and Senior Principal of CAM Consults, a consulting firm in Minneapolis, Minnesota, that advises clients on approaches to the integration of conventional and alternative health care. He is also cofounder and moderator of the Minnesota Health Care Roundtable and cofounder of ThoughtCast.com.

THE SUCCESS FACTORS

- *Establish access to clients.* It is essential to create an efficient pipeline to patients with an interest in alternative medicine, who will do business with the organization and purchase services and products. This upstream connection to clients could be a clinic, hospital, or large employer.
- *Identify sources of reimbursement.* This is essential. By definition, alternative medicine is an entire industry that has very minimal reimbursement. To date, no one has quite figured out how to obtain insurance coverage commensurate with conventional medicine, so fee-for-service business is an integral aspect of providing CAM services. Since both clinics and network development represent a major investment, it is important to develop a creative, yet realistic, payment mechanism utilizing both task and reimbursement methodologies.
- *Devise a flexible and portable payment system that does not compromise the length of visit or the quality of care.* For example, success does not necessarily mean opting for network participation if deeply discounted reimbursement rates force clinicians to cut the length of office visits. CAM is a consumer-driven paradigm. Patients want time with practitioners. Shortened treatment time will compromise the aspect of the service that is attracting clientele.
- *Obtain sufficient capital.* Start-up funds must be available on a long-term basis. It is essential to have a source of capital that will wait 3 to 5 years before requiring any return on investment.
- *Develop an effective infrastructure to manage risk.* This field entails a different

kind of risk, but it is risk just the same. Good management involves credentialing to high standards, ongoing monitoring, and quality assurance initiatives. It is prudent to have patients sign releases and agreements for binding arbitration or mediation to minimize the risk of litigation. Some aspects of risk management are unfamiliar to practitioners in CAM, but are well known in the mainstream.

- *Form friendly alliances with conventional medicine facilities and practitioners.* It is important to establish formal linkages with clinics, hospitals, managed care, and other health systems, as a basis for sharing information and working jointly on projects that gather data.
- *Recruit a stable of loyal practitioners, willing to cross-refer to one another in-house.* Team loyalty among practitioners should be developed through mechanisms such as equity ownership, compensation based on production, participation in management decisions, and individual marketing. The integrative center should be marketed, but also advertise each individual practitioner.
- *Position the organization advantageously in its particular market.* The name of the organization must call up a highly favorable image. Consider participation in projects for public benefit as a way to obtain good coverage from the press.
- *Develop a relationship with a research facility.* Strategic liaisons should be formed, and the organization should be identified as a potential site for clinical or outcomes research. Association with a respected mainstream organization can potentiate cobranding.
- *Provide the therapies most desired in the organization's market, offering a carefully chosen selection.* For each market, the choice and combination of disciplines will be different. Those known to receive the highest utilization in the context of the locale should be evaluated. The most popular therapies typically include chiropractic,

acupuncture, massage, herbal therapy, and nutritional medicine. It is not economically practical to offer "one of everything." A lesser known modality can be added, but the primary therapies should be included first in order to attract sufficient business.

- *Empower patients.* Patients should be provided with knowledge, options, control, and health improvement tools, so that they can take personal responsibility for their own health. This style of practice is what differentiates a complementary approach from a conventional one. Clients value opportunities for self-education and empowerment. Since they are paying cash, it is especially important to please them and offer what they want to build their loyalty.
- *Consider health care a business, and guide operations with that in mind.* Practice management for CAM providers is not vastly different from that of physicians. It is vital to track overhead, market well, and be very good at collecting and analyzing data. Stay at the leading edge of information technology by using the Internet and computer technology.
- *Identify one or more champions in the organization who are highly regarded by all constituents—someone who is looked up to by physicians with respect.* A champion can be key to the success of the integrative process and the organization.
- *Obtain a strong endorsement from the board and top management.* When problems arise, someone with power and authority must be able to step in and arbitrate the issues. It is essential to have the confirmation that the organization has made an investment in this project and is going to stand by its investment. If opponents know that strong support from leadership is lacking, they have the leverage to sabotage the integrative program.
- *Develop an extensive education program that serves all stakeholders.* Most people learn about CAM through anecdotal evidence and the media. Clients should be in-

formed about the organization's services, how they work, why they are important, how alternative therapies can interface with conventional services, and how integrative medicine can enhance their care and their health.

- ***Emphasize effective communication.*** This is important for any organization, whether a hospital, network, or freestanding medical center. Within the health system, clear channels of communication should be built and maintained to keep constituents apprised of new developments and long-term strategic goals, their rationale, and their benefits. The step-by-step integration of initiatives should be communicated clearly.
- ***Use media to link staff and stakeholders.*** Communications can be maintained through newsletters, a Web site, regular meetings, e-mail, fax, and phone trees. Everyone should be included in the communications; those who feel left out will not be supportive and may work against the goal. In particular, board and administrative leadership, every doctor and nurse, and the entire medical staff should be kept informed.

CHAPTER 6

Phasing in Integrative Medicine

Roger Jahnke

Health care is in the midst of a profound transformation. All organizations are confronted with constant change. Complementary and alternative medicine (CAM), while perceived by many as a history-making innovation, has also been seen as a fad and a distraction from the core business of delivering good medicine.

Like many health maintenance organizations (HMOs), medical centers, and clinical practice groups across the country, your organization is probably receiving requests from members, patients, and consumers to offer a wider range of services, particularly complementary medicine. In response, your health system may be considering the inclusion of CAM services and therapies.

Numerous major health plans now offer access to complementary medicine through discount products and networks of CAM providers. In health systems, medical schools, and teaching hospitals, there is a readiness to move forward with CAM initiatives. These efforts include research units, the addition of complementary therapies in certain departments, and in a few cases, new "bricks-and-mortar" facilities. However, in other organizations, there are varying degrees of resistance to the integration of complementary medicine.

If the integration of complementary therapies has created a challenge for your organization, there may be value in considering a model for phased integration. A phased, modular approach can be accomplished over time, and paced to the specific needs of your health system. In this model, the organization evolves through the integrative process in at least three stages. This can eliminate some of the pitfalls known to occur in implementing complementary medicine. The phases can be introduced in any order or paralleled, in response to the level of interest in the organization.

- *Phase 1*—Maximize health promotion
- *Phase 2*—Expand the infrastructure
- *Phase 3*—Integrate complementary therapies

Many major providers have successfully accomplished the task of bringing CAM into the discussion and even into the delivery mix. However, in most organizations, the integrative process is taking place gradually. It is clear that full integration—the creation of a comprehensive and integrated health care delivery system—is a developmental process that will occur over time.

An initial emphasis on prevention, health improvement, and disease management can provide a window of opportunity for the later inclusion of CAM. Much of the infrastructure

Roger Jahnke, CEO of Health Action, Santa Barbara, a consultant, and futurist, has assisted numerous health systems in the design of comprehensive health care delivery strategies. He has facilitated initiatives in the phased implementation of health promotion programming in numerous health systems and the inclusion of evidence-based complementary therapies. As a lecturer and author, he has presented to the American College of Healthcare Executives, the American Hospital Association, and Catholic Health Association, and is the author of *The Healer Within* (HarperCollins, 2000). The Health Action Group is a consulting and training organization in Santa Barbara that collaborates with large health care organizations to build market share, improve health outcomes, and create new or expanded revenue streams. See http://HealthAction.net.

Courtesy of Roger Jahnke, PhD, OMD, Director, Health Action, Santa Barbara, California.

necessary to integrate these types of programs will be relevant in implementing complementary medicine as well. Since health improvement is a perspective inherent to most fields of CAM, such as Chinese medicine, naturopathy, nutrition therapy, and herbal medicine, this is a logical programmatic association.

AN OVERVIEW OF PHASED INTEGRATION

To develop a comprehensive and fully integrated delivery system, first evaluate the programs and services you currently have in place that reflect a focus on wellness and health enhancement. Many hospitals and health plans offer programming in exercise, nutrition, stress management, and risk reduction. Inventory the services you offer that are considered complementary, such as support groups, biofeedback, or health education. Also identify services and environments in your organization that are congruent with CAM therapies, such as the physical therapy department, comprehensive cancer programs, cardiac prevention initiatives, or a fitness center. Survey your staff to determine who already has expertise and training in wellness strategies or complementary therapies. Assess the needs and desires of the community. Then apply the principles of good strategic planning.

Phase 1—Maximize Health Promotion

First upgrade health promotion programming to the state of the art. In organizations where there is resistance to complementary medicine or a misunderstanding of its benefits, initial services can be focused on wellness, prevention, and disease management. Introducing CAM therapies at a later stage will allow time for the benefits of a more comprehensive approach to become apparent. This staged integration can increase receptivity and help create the infrastructure for the further development of the model. The full implementation of alternative therapies can be reserved for Phase 3 and paced according to the requirements of the organization.

Phase 2—Expand Infrastructure

The refinement of the infrastructure of delivery has value in its own right and also prepares the organization for the future integration of CAM. As a deeper understanding of complementary medicine evolves, substantive discussion about integrative programming becomes less focused on adding new therapies into the clinical mix, and more centered on the comprehensive integration of health care delivery at large. When complementary therapies are viewed just as add-on features in addition to conventional medicine, the integration is less complete and more fraught with pitfalls. Ideally, *complementary* means "the integration of safe and effective services across the full continuum of delivery." It is through the process of carefully evolving the infrastructure that true integration of services occurs.

Phase 3—Integrate Complementary Therapies

As more research data accrue, it has become increasingly clear that many complementary therapies meet the criteria of safety, clinical effectiveness, and cost-effectiveness. Interventions such as acupuncture offer the potential for improving clinical outcomes, increasing fee-for-service income, and creating cost savings. The integration of alternative therapies is best seen in the context of the entire organization and its development. Then planning, design, and implementation can be integrated into a larger, more logical framework. In this way, CAM becomes less a peripheral issue and more a relevant piece in a comprehensive approach to the process of carefully designing, or redesigning, health care delivery.

INVENTORY EXISTING PROGRAMS AND SERVICES

One of the surprises in this process is the discovery of assets that already exist within your organization. As you carefully assess the programs and services available throughout your system, you will find that some of the components of health improvement and CAM programming are already present. In the area of health promotion, your organization probably provides exercise and nutrition classes either for the general community or in conjunction with specific programs such as diabetes education or cardiac rehabilitation. The CAM activities most often available in health systems are mind-body services, such as support groups, counseling, stress reduction classes, or biofeedback. Some hospitals already provide massage (for example, in pain reduction programs); there may also be the opportunity to offer Therapeutic Touch since many nurses have this training. Support groups that make use of a health coach, facilitator, or guide can be advertised in tandem with other health promotion activities (available either on an outpatient or inpatient basis) to meet consumer-driven demand for new options and alternatives in the delivery mix.

At each phase of the integrative model, careful planning and design will optimize the benefits to the organization and eliminate errors in the process. This conceptual phase should include input from important stakeholders such as the health system's board of directors, administrators, physicians, CAM providers, and consumers. Throughout this process, it is vital to remain responsive to new information. The most significant tool in the design of delivery for the emerging new era of health care is not the addition of alternative therapies, but the application of "alternative thinking" to create a comprehensive delivery system.

PHASE 1—PROMOTE HEALTH IMPROVEMENT PROGRAMS

If the integration of complementary medicine is viewed as an aspect of the multifaceted shift in the delivery of health care, one primary strategy logically involves expanding the continuum of care to include a focus on health. This suggests wellness programming, health promotion, and population-based health enhancement initia-

tives. These programs typically take the form of nutrition, exercise, stress reduction, and risk reduction (for example, smoking cessation). This emphasis on health improvement is actually more important to clients than the inclusion of any single therapy or technique.

Consumers want a focus on health even more than they want alternative medicine. In 1993, the seminal Eisenberg survey (Eisenberg et al, 1993) was published in the *New England Journal of Medicine* on the use of nonconventional medicine. The data suggest that more than two-thirds of the respondents who indicated the use of alternative approaches were actually using self-care activities such as relaxation techniques or products such as vitamins. Less utilization focused on specific CAM therapies such as acupuncture, chiropractic, and massage than on self-care. In 1998, similar findings were reported twice in the *Journal of the American Medical Association* (Eisenberg et al, 1998; Astin, 1998).

In Phase 1, health promotion programming is enhanced on several levels:

1. Maximize and promote existing programs.
2. Develop new programs and market them dynamically.
3. Integrate these programs throughout the system.

Phase 1-1: Maximize Existing Health Promotion Programming

Across the health care industry, organizations are reengineering to integrate health education, expand prevention services, and implement disease management. Today, many hospitals and health plans are also applying these concepts in community outreach, in their delivery networks, and within their own systems.

The implementation of a dynamic health promotion program, targeted at well populations as well as those at risk or acutely ill, is becoming a key component of comprehensive delivery. This critical component of health care can be funded through a range of sources, including fee-for-service, the marketing budget, and in some cases

Case Study: Innovative Group Services

St. Charles Hospital in Bend, Oregon, offers symptom reduction support groups for people with chronic illness, focused on reducing medical symptoms through basic health enhancement activities such as healing exercise, good nutrition, breath practice, meditation, and massage. The program serves people with a range of diagnosed conditions, all working together in a single group, each focusing on their own individual health improvement. The program functions as a form of social support for participants, to reinforce the behavioral goals they set for themselves. Outcomes data indicate that these clients experience measurable improvements in their health.

community health improvement grants or third-party reimbursement. Health enhancement programs provide a means of increasing satisfaction for current customers and also a venue for attracting new customers. The research suggests that health improvement programs are viable complements to conventional clinical services.

Organizations can utilize and train expertise within the system including:

- health educators and medical social workers, with expertise in mind-body paradigms
- occupational and physical therapists, frequently knowledgeable regarding movement therapies or medical massage
- nurses, who often have training in Touch Therapy, visualization, and relaxation.

Other staff, including physicians, may have educational backgrounds that make them appropriate candidates for additional training. This will allow the system to upgrade expertise without necessarily bringing in new staff. In other cases, it will be more practical to draw on local experts from the community as outside contractors to provide specific health improvement services.

Phase 1-2: Develop New Health Promotion Programs

In the emerging paradigm with its emphasis on health, the patient consumer population has shifted and expanded to encompass larger numbers, in a much broader client base. When programming focuses on health improvement, "the client" is redefined to include asymptomatic members or clients. The new goal includes promoting and maintaining the health of those who are at risk but not currently in need of medical intervention. This approach to health care fulfills the promise in the term *health maintenance organization*.

The programmatic goal in Phase 1 is to create new initiatives that promote health improvement and behavioral change. This could include health education, such as adjunctive programs for patients with cardiac conditions, diabetes, or cancer; community outreach; or new offerings in mind-body medicine.

Examples of options for health promotion programming include:

- exercise classes, yoga, T'ai Chi, Qigong, movement therapy, and therapeutic exercise
- nutritional counseling, cooking classes, and diets for special conditions

Case Studies: Multifaceted Programs

Kaiser Permanente Medical Center of San Francisco has developed a large health education center that offers a rich array of courses, support groups, and workshops that include all these examples and more. The Riverside System in Virginia, with several hospitals and ambulatory care centers, includes six fitness centers that are available to both clients and the community (see Chapter 48). The Mercy System in Cincinnati has also opened several impressive "healthplex" facilities that offer a comprehensive and diverse menu of health improvement programming.

- health education courses, such as childbirth coaching or diabetes management
- healing techniques, such as massage
- relaxation and stress reduction classes, including meditation
- risk reduction (for example, smoking cessation, blood pressure reduction, and osteoporosis management)
- support groups for patients with conditions such as breast or prostate cancer, for at-risk populations, and for health improvement in its own right.

A health resource center is another means of promoting health in the community. This could be as simple as providing a bookcase of health resource information in the corner of a hospital clinic or practitioner's office or as elaborate as a freestanding library. Some centers have annual budgets in excess of a million dollars a year, while others operate without a budget, using donated materials.

User-friendly resource centers empower clients with information on self-care, preventive services, and treatment options. By cultivating interest in health promotion and complementary

---

The Health Information Resource Center

California Pacific Medical Center in San Francisco has a library and resource center that provides books, medical journals, and other sources of information on self-care, health promotion, and complementary medicine. Their services include an extensive library and several computers, Internet and database access, as well as videos, audios, and resource information. Volunteers and trained staff are available for assistance. The resource center also offers literature searches at an affordable cost on specific medical conditions. Classes and monthly lectures are sponsored by the associated Institute for Health and Healing that feature local and national experts in complementary medicine.

---

medicine, they position the organization for the integration of complementary therapies. In the case of California Pacific, years after the creation of the resource center, a CAM component was developed within the hospital campus. The Health and Healing Clinic offers integrative medicine, acupuncture, homeopathy, and massage (see Chapter 39). The new clinical health center has become a logical extension of the health resource center and its growing community of support.

Another developmental model is used at Union Hospital near Boston, part of the Atlanti-Care system. The medical library, historically used by physicians, now has an area set aside as a health resource center that can be accessed by both physicians and the public. An on-site staff member is available to guide inquiring patients and perform literature searches. This project is a cost-effective initiative that is part of programming that includes a highly refined cardiac prevention and rehabilitation program, a women's clinic, and a classroom setting with a spacious atrium.

Phase 1-3: Integrate Health Programming throughout the System

Health promotion programming should be implemented systemwide to serve patients at all levels of need—from those who are well to those who are acutely ill. This means making health promotion and existing complementary services available to serve patients throughout the system by integrating them with both the clinical and business model.

Cost-Effective Strategies

Participation by skilled physician extenders can make health promotion programming more cost-effective and accessible. This may involve professional staff, as well as adjunct providers and consulting professionals with particular expertise. Currently, health promotion services are typically ordered and reimbursed only on the basis of medical necessity (for example, exercise programs for cardiac patients or physical ther-

---

Case Study: The Ornish Program for Reversing Heart Disease

The Ornish Program for Reversing Heart Disease is an example of health promotion principles applied to the needs of acutely ill and high-risk patients. This lifestyle program has been documented for its dramatic reduction of heart disease symptoms. Yet it costs less than 40% of the typical expenditures for coronary artery disease, with accompanying decrease in human cost. The program involves careful screening, health education, coaching, and monitoring. Participants learn new ways of eating, exercising, and reducing stress. They also participate in support groups with others, which reinforces their efforts. Many patients in the program have experienced not only improved health and quality of life, but also the actual regeneration of heart tissue, which has been documented in PET scans. The Ornish Program is an important innovation that meets consumer demand for options and a powerful focus for a unique marketing program (see Chapters 9 and 40).

Systemwide Integration and Dynamic Marketing Power

It is important to inform consumers of the services you currently provide that are patient-centered and holistic. Advertise any new health promotion services and, in tandem, promote existing complementary services such as mind-body therapies and massage. In this way, your organization can expand its emphasis on health and on familiar complementary therapies, in a context that is compatible with the culture of the organization. Conscious use of this type of programming can promote a natural progression to the inclusion of complementary medicine in Phase 3 and is a powerful marketing strategy.

Internet Innovations for Health Promotion and Marketing

An interactive Web site can be both dynamic and cost-effective. Health promotion on-line, when carefully designed and managed, can address consumer desire for information and at-

apy activities for stroke patients). In the future, health enhancement activities will be provided through preventive programming that reduces potential medical costs and is funded by employer groups and third-party payers.

Community-Based Programming

Health promotion strategies can also be provided outside the health care environment in collaboration with employers, public health centers, and community-based organizations. This type of activity has been the foundation of the Healthy Communities movement, in which health care institutions and local organizations collaborate to reduce risk and improve health by collaborating with agencies, schools, and churches in the community.

Case Study: Seton Good Health School

At the Seton Healthcare System of Hospitals in Austin, Texas, clinical programming and community outreach have focused on the provision of services to schools, nonprofit agencies, and corporations. A major health education program with a diverse focus, the Seton Good Health School offers everything from classes in nutrition and diabetes management to yoga and energy healing. One of the most impressive aspects of this initiative has been its response to the challenge of funding. Seton elected to offer these programs as a form of marketing to increase community awareness of the health system. A major portion of the marketing budget was dedicated to the implementation of a multifaceted campaign. In a single strategy, Seton met consumer demand, integrated health promotion, and funded the initiative.

tract new clients. Sponsorship of the Web site also allows the institution to retain control of the integrity of on-line information.

A variety of dynamic Web site strategies are available. An on-line newsletter provides a relevant forum that can focus on general health improvement or cardiac, cancer, or diabetes care. Interactive on-line conferences or chat rooms create opportunities for the public to query experts in real time or by e-mail. These venues can be hosted by members of the health system's medical staff and health educators. On-line support groups can also be provided, thereby allowing small groups of participants to exchange resources and discuss their personal health issues with the guidance of a staff member. Web-based care coordination (case management) can be combined with on-line appointment setting and referral to providers throughout the system.

Implementing Phase 1 can be as simple as reaching out to the community through courses or programs that enhance health. It is a way to make friends, obtain new customers, and demonstrate a robust understanding and commitment to the new paradigms of health care. This creates the foundation for an organization's abil-ity to integrate complementary therapies, either as a parallel phase, or at a later time. Clinical outcomes, customer satisfaction, and medical cost reduction can be accelerated significantly with a coordinated approach to health promotion programming.

PHASE 2—ENHANCE INFRASTRUCTURE

Most health care organizations are in the process of creating a more cohesive infrastructure across the delivery system. Examples include the application of proactive triage and the redefinition of care management, as well as the use of comprehensive clinical pathways and multidisciplinary teams.

These infrastructure upgrades will facilitate the integration of prevention and health promotion services and the eventual integration of CAM. Program enhancements can be implemented in any order. The inclusion of health promotion programs from Phase 1 typically requires the infrastructure improvements of Phase 2 in order to achieve authentic program integration. In tandem, these enhancements expand the power of an organization to provide comprehensive health care delivery.

It is useful to inventory and assess the current status of your system's development in terms of infrastructure innovations. Your organization may already be upgrading some of these approaches to service delivery. This expansion of capacity makes possible more comprehensive delivery and fosters the organizational and clinical infrastructure necessary to accommodate integrative medicine.

Phase 2 involves the expansion of infrastructure to provide more comprehensive service in areas such as:

- proactive triage
- case management and care coordination
- care pathways
- expanded multidisciplinary teams
- networked digital patient records
- outcomes tracking and research.

Case Studies: The Internet

Two examples of the many innovative health care Web sites that make intelligent use of the Internet include LifePath <www.mylifepath.com>, which is a program of Blue Shield of California, and HealthWorld <www.healthworld.com>. Both sites offer information and referral to CAM providers. The sites also serve as a form of advertising for the site sponsor. Numerous other Web sites that are associated with hospitals, HMOs, and wellness organizations provide an immense amount of information that can help to prevent disease, reduce medical visits, link consumers to CAM services, and help to decrease medical costs.

Phase 2-1: Proactive Triage

In an emergency department (or on the battlefield where triage originated), triage is the decision-making process used to evaluate what to do and when to do it. It asks questions such as, "Does this person need to be treated immediately?" and "What is the most appropriate form of treatment?" Historically, the benefits of triage are impressive.

In the emerging new paradigm, the focus is at the other end of the delivery spectrum. Rather than limiting triage to acute cases, the new emphasis is on implementing triage with broader populations to prevent disease before it occurs and to reduce preventable medical demand. Optimally, this means that the system includes mechanisms for addressing people's need for health care when they are well or first identified at risk.

Assess your organization's current level of triage. Then design pathways and methods that are more proactive. This upgrade implies the need for new professionals in health care who have the cross-disciplinary training to evaluate a wide range of cases and suggest strategies in prevention and health improvement, as well as in the clinical context.

Proactive triage should now be applied to patients with nonacute needs. This involves the use of decision making to carefully target services for at-risk clients who are not in acute clinical situations and who will benefit from health improvement services. Proactive triage evaluation is based on all the indicators available from the client record including health and family history, laboratory testing, economic or social limitations, the client's readiness to learn, areas of interest, and former program participation. When members enter the system through health enhancement programming, proactive triage provides a means to address their needs before they present for a medical visit; they are triaged into appropriate categories and into programming that is suited to their level of risk.

Whenever there is risk, there is the potential for consequences to both the patient and the provider, in terms of human cost and medical expenditures. The goal, in the context of comprehensive delivery, is to continually encourage clients toward health through prevention and risk management, rather than waiting to react later to catastrophic illness. When proactive triage and innovative care management are prevalent within the system, an entire new superstructure for the delivery of services becomes available. This superstructure can foster the authentic integration of health promotion, and clinical services with complementary therapies.

Phase 2-2: Case and Care Management

Assess the current extent to which your organization has developed the case management model and then add the role of care coordinator to encompass a more comprehensive domain of options. This will include proactive triage with a broader range of choices, including health promotion, self-care activities, and CAM therapies, in addition to medical specialties. As health promotion activities develop and become better integrated within the fabric of the organization, care coordination becomes less focused on conventional clinical and social services, and more associated with the comprehensive inclusion of preventive and health-improving activities.

The mechanisms for case management are familiar: evaluate, refer, monitor, and follow up. This approach also includes active periodic review of individual cases. Upgraded case management, sometimes called care coordination, simply expands the domain of management. Rather than managing only the patient's medical case, care coordination also has the capacity to link the client with a coordinated interaction of primary care, prevention services, health promotion, and potentially CAM. These added services are relevant to customers who are relatively well and want to maximize their health, those who are at risk, and those who want assistance in coordinating their medical treatment with health promotion activities.

In care coordination, the focus is to provide clients access to cost-effective preventive resources that involve them in health promotion, educational programming, the use of support groups, various forms of mind-body interventions, and alternative treatment. The inclusion of case management or care coordination in the infrastructure allows for a more focused comprehensive, health-based system of delivery. Upgraded case management is a key to integrating health improvement strategies within the system. It may also take the form of support groups that make use of a health coach. Another example is parish nursing, which provides care coordination outside the health care institution. As complementary therapies are included in the

---

Case Studies: The Health Guide

At the Mercy System in Cincinnati, the Mercy Caring Program features health guides who bring health promotion into all levels of the continuum, from health maintenance and prevention to acute and chronic disease management. Since the focus is on health in expanded populations, as well as acute and chronic care, this is a multidisciplinary role rather than a medical one. Care coordinators function as part of the multidisciplinary team. When the team addresses cases that are medically complex, they are led by specially trained care coordinators.

In the leading-edge programs of the Riverside Health System in Virginia, care coordinators provide proactive triage to clients who wish to participate in health improvement programming. The coordinators also assist in managing clinical demand by triaging minor clinical cases. For the health care system of the future, it is too early to tell who will be the proactive triage manager. Currently, in some settings, nurses and medical social workers have this role. In the context of integrative medicine, this role might be fulfilled by a new form of specialist, with in-depth dual training in both conventional and complementary medicine.

---

system, they can be accessed through referrals from the care coordinator.

Innovative Telephone and Internet Centers

Certain aspects of care coordination and proactive triage can be implemented by phone; doing so can provide clients with an array of beneficial services. The concept is to initiate, manage, and maintain a relationship between the organization and the client/customer/patient on a proactive basis, in order to minimize his or her medical needs. Many hospitals are building these relationships by reaching out to the community, using an 800 number, call center counselors, and an Internet site that people can contact when they have questions or concerns. These inquiries are often practical requests for information; in other cases, they are initiated by patients asking, "At what point should I come in to see the doctor?" For parents with young children and older people with complex health and medication issues, this kind of accessibility can provide greater peace of mind. Increased accessibility is patient-friendly medicine that builds good will. In some "nurse on the phone" centers, anyone can call in, whether they are a client or not. This type of phone or Internet resource service functions as a marketing tool, an entry site for new customers, a proactive triage tool, a strategy for case management, a means of enrolling participants in classes, a strategy for building and managing relationships with clients, and even a mechanism for performing market research.

Phase 2-3: Care Pathways

The concept of critical pathways indicates a set of prescribed steps that a team of medical experts has agreed upon as the best clinical protocol for a particular condition. The pathways serve as a type of expert system that suggests a variety of treatment options for all the associated symptom patterns at each stage in a given condition.

Most health care organizations develop critical pathways (care pathways) to maximize the continuous improvement of clinical outcomes. Typically, a task force or committee oversees this process. Assess the current status of the care pathways in your organization and consider a redesign of your process to include a stronger focus on:

- earlier contact with the customer
- health and risk assessment
- health improvement strategies.

This focus provides the foundation for the inclusion of CAM therapies in a context in which systemwide consensus has been reached on how the therapies will be integrated into the care pathways.

In the future health care system, clinical pathways for health promotion and risk reduction will also maximize the integration of complementary and mind-body therapies. For example, a client recently experiencing depression may be referred to pharmacological therapy, but also be offered the option of learning meditation, going to yoga or stress reduction class, becoming involved in a fitness and weight training program, seeing a nutrition counselor, or exploring low-dose herbal therapy. The options would depend on the pattern of the presenting symptoms and the patient's own preferences. Care pathways that are agreed on by the Critical Paths Committee can leverage the inclusion of adjunctive programming. They are one of the most important tools for the authentic integration of both health promotion programs and CAM therapies.

Phase 2-4: Multidisciplinary Teams

The integration of multidisciplinary teams is standard in health care delivery. On the most basic level, a physician, a nurse, and a physical therapist working together are a functional example of a multidisciplinary team. To prepare for integration, assess the makeup of the delivery teams in your organization and redesign them to expand their capacity. In more comprehensive delivery, a wider spectrum of services becomes available throughout the system. Conceptualize the multidisciplinary team in the broadest sense. The health improvement focus will bring health educators, care coordinators, and specialists in nutrition, exercise, and mind-body methods onto the team. It is important to carefully craft mechanisms for team communication as well as service coordination. This upgraded approach to health care delivery teams creates the foundation for the integration of CAM services. The focus here is not just medical. Spiritual, emotional, and psychosocial aspects of the case are explored, as well as the physiological.

On a fee-for-service basis, this type of care would be prohibitively expensive. However, cost-effective models are available. In health systems in which the providers are salaried, disease management can be implemented by the multidisciplinary team without incurring high cost. Another model, the Health Medicine Forum in Oakland, CA, uses volunteer providers who participate in multidisciplinary case conferences one afternoon a month, in return for the opportunity to have their patients seen by the team and to participate for professional enhancement.

Phase 2-5: Implementation of the Networked Digital Patient Record

Much discussion in health care has focused on the networked patient chart. It has been the information technology "pie in the sky." The goal has been to make the same information available to all practitioners—the physician, physical therapist, case manager/health counselor, and others. The digital record is one of the tools that will facilitate true clinical integration. In current practice, one of the major pitfalls of CAM is the lack of communication between mainstream and alternative providers (for example, between the doctor and the acupuncturist). When the networked patient record is in place, some aspects of this problem will resolve quite easily.

If the physician and the CAM provider are making entries into the same chart, they are actually involved in a form of communication that enables more integrative treatment of the patient. There is an opportunity for the exchange of information that can lead to open discussion. One of the problems with alternative medicine in the past has been that it occurred completely outside the system, so that the records were not available to the primary care physician, nor could the alternative practitioner obtain precise information on medications and allopathic treatment prescribed. The digital medical record can be used to coordinate the use of prescription medications and herbs or nutritional supplements, as occurs when Chinese medicine is used in conjunction with conventional treatment.

The issue of confidentiality has been the most challenging barrier to the implementation of the digital record. Advances in encrypted files, electronic record security, and client PINs (personal identification numbers) now afford a more secure context and will allow for the expanded use of the digital record.

Issues of confidentiality are in the forefront of most successful AIDS programs. In the San Francisco area, centers such as the Quan Yin Healing Arts Center provide protocols that include mainstream multidrug treatment, Chinese herbal therapy, nutritional supplements, acupuncture, support groups, and other mainstream and alternative therapeutics. Good communication is vital to the success of this treatment, and is not problematic to achieve in the intimate environment of a small clinic. However, as complementary therapies are included in larger health systems on a broad scale, the digital record will become an invaluable tool. Despite the convenience of the digital record, this is an innovation that must be implemented with judicious planning in order to ensure the privacy of patients. If these issues are addressed, the digital chart can become a powerful strategy to support proactive triage, multidisciplinary treatment, and outcomes tracking.

Phase 2-6: Outcomes Tracking and Research

There are no more prominent concepts in health care than evidenced-based medicine and outcomes research. Outcomes-based planning has become the gold standard in much of the industry. On the administrative side of health care, the outcomes revolution looks largely at the data on volume such as dollars, members, and demographics. In clinical medicine, outcomes has been translated into the use of data to refine the provision of care through evidence-based medicine. This approach to planning provides a means of obtaining further information on therapeutic approaches that have a history of safety and effectiveness. Outcomes-driven planning creates a solid foundation for the inclusion of preventive services and CAM. As well-designed studies demonstrate safety and effectiveness of new approaches, they become integrated into conventional delivery.

Assess your organization's current model and methodologies for tracking outcomes. Explore their redesign to gather evidence of program efficacy in every arena: health promotion, complementary therapies, and clinical biomedicine. In cardiac disease, evidence-based outcomes identified preventive behavioral interventions as superior and more cost-effective than acute medi-

---

Case Study: Tracking Data on Cost Savings

A study of work site health promotion programming for a Procter and Gamble facility in Cincinnati reviewed the health care expenditures for approximately 8,000 employees. One half elected to participate in health improvement programs for a 3-year period. The other half of the employees in the study elected not to participate.

By the third year of the study, the employees participating in health promotion averaged almost $400 less per person, due to fewer hospital admissions and fewer days of hospital care compared with nonparticipants. In one year of the program, Procter and Gamble saved approximately $1.6 million on just those 4,000 employees (Goetzel et al, 1998). (For more detailed information, see Chapter 49.)

cal interventions (Ornish, 1998) (see Chapter 40). Clinical evidence provided the basis for the 1997 National Institutes of Health (NIH) Consensus Statement on the safety and efficacy of acupuncture (NIH, 1997).

This is an example of the meaningful data that can be useful in tracking health promotion and CAM programming. A major argument against CAM has been the lack of evidence for efficacy. With carefully designed outcomes research methods, the evidence that health systems and health plans require will become available. In the presence of robust data, one of the major barriers to the integration of complementary medicine can be removed.

PHASE 3—INTEGRATE COMPLEMENTARY THERAPIES

With the implementation of health promotion and the infrastructure for integrative delivery in place, the structure for the authentic integration of complementary therapies is secure. For organizations in which complementary therapies are already operational, the purposeful implementation of the earlier phases—wellness programming and infrastructure upgrades—will ensure that these complementary services are integrated throughout the system.

In Phase 3, the administrative goals include a series of action steps:

1. Plan the integration process for complementary and alternative therapies.
2. Develop strategies for credentialing and implementation.
3. Select key therapies and apply credentialing protocol.
4. Initiate complementary programs.
5. Integrate programs and providers into the system.

In organizations in which CAM implementation is already in progress, Phase 3 can be initiated parallel to Phase 1 that promotes health improvement and Phase 2 that expands the infrastructure. In environments where there is not yet a consensus on the benefits of complementary thrapies, Phase 3 can be deterred until a later time. The inclusion of CAM could also begin simply, for example, through the addition of programs on which there is consensus and positive evidence-based research, such as therapeutic massage or biofeedback. In either case, the first steps to fully integrated CAM activity are vision, planning, and careful design.

Phase 3-1: Plan the Integration of Complementary Therapies

The first priority in planning is the identification and involvement of key players and stakeholders. Probably the worst error that can be made in CAM initiatives is to proceed without a broad base of support. Initiate a task force of stakeholders who can create a working plan for the integration of new therapies. The blueprint for integrative medicine should be circulated for input to key decision makers and participants within the system to develop consensus. A broadly inclusive process will encourage buy-in. If the organization is not at a complete state of readiness, failures in implementation can occur. Problems may also result if this buy-in step is not exercised. Historically, in such cases, integrative medicine programming has become isolated or fragmented because it has not been fully integrated into the system.

Broad representation on the integrative task force is essential if the task force is to reflect the desires of the entire community. The task force must act as a bridge and accept input from mainstream providers, administrators, trustees, CAM practitioners, and the public. This process will require political savvy, particularly in the initial stages. Later, the task force can guide and monitor the implementation process. This entails troubleshooting to ensure that full integration within the infrastructure has actually occurred and is as comprehensive as possible. Once the planning task force has been created, a logical step is to produce an inventory of existing CAM-related services and expertise within the system.

Case Study: Phased Integration

St. Charles Medical Center in Bend, Oregon, has done an excellent job of phasing in an integrated delivery model. Early on, staff adopted a mission of patient-centered care. Programs in health improvement were developed and implemented. The Symptom Reduction Program, including self-healing methods and support groups, reflects a complementary medicine philosophy, but did not initially include alternative therapies. An inclusive, team-based approach to decision making was initiated, and several task forces were created, including one to foster CAM. Following on the NIH consensus that acupuncture is safe and effective, they identified acupuncture for inclusion by developing a protocol that defines its use in care pathways for specific diagnoses (NIH, 1997).

An inventory of existing expertise and services within the organization often reveals that successful steps toward complementary delivery have already been taken. Many organizations currently offer therapies from mind-body medicine, such as support groups and lifestyle counseling. Frequently, massage is available as well. Offering these therapies is a natural step in the development of a comprehensive CAM program. In certain cases, staff providers within the organization may be selectively trained with the goal of upgrading staff credentials. Practitioners outside the system can also be credentialed as appropriate.

Phase 3-2: Develop Strategies for Credentialing and Implementation

The next step is to target the key modalities not formally credentialed. Include any CAM therapies that have generated significant levels of interest. By performing a survey throughout the organization and community, the planning group can prioritize the list for the therapies most requested by the public and providers. In order to retain forward momentum in the process, it is helpful if modalities are agreed upon by primary stakeholders both within the organization and in the community.

The task force can then design the credentialing process once consensus development and political buy-in are in place. A consultant may be utilized to clarify organizational values and mission. The group can also elect to bring in an outside credentialing consultant; in that case, the task force has the charge of identifying the funding stream and defining the scope of work. The use of an outside credentialing team is not an unrealistic possibility. In a 1999 survey, Landmark Healthcare found that 50% of all health plans providing CAM used adjunctive organizations to provide credentialing services (National Market Measures, 1999).

Case Study: Complementary Therapies in a Hospital

North Hawaii Community Hospital is a state-of-the-art hospital. Although CAM practitioners do not participate directly as hospital staff, they are granted privileges to see patients who have been hospitalized; these practitioners are credentialed to the hospital's standards under the same type of process as other adjunctive medical professionals and specialists. Consequently, patients can receive services such as acupuncture while in the hospital. Although the introduction of these adjunct professionals has been gradual, it has been made possible by a thorough credentialing process that provides greater assurance of quality services. Presently, 5% to 10% of the patients admitted to the hospital receive consultations from licensed CAM practitioners and over 60% of the patients admitted receive some form of mind-body-spirit therapy such as healing touch, guided imagery, or prayer.

Phase 3-3: Select Key Therapies and Apply the Credentialing Process

Carefully prioritize the preferred therapies. Focus on the modalities on which there is agreement by all stakeholder groups at this time and select the credentialing parameter. The variety of disciplines typically evaluated for integration encompass a wide range of philosophies, each with its own knowledge base, protocols, and practice wisdom. Acupuncturists, osteopaths, chiropractors, massage therapists, herbalists, naturopathic physicians, and homeopaths are each involved in practices that are very different. Consequently, since there is an immense variety of factors in the design of credentialing, the developmental criterion for CAM new providers will require attention and patience. A credentialing process already exists in most all hospitals and provider organizations today. (For additional information, refer to Chapter 17, *Credentialing Demystified*.)

Surveys of hospitals and medical centers have found that in most new on-site programs, one of the first therapies to be added is acupuncture. The 1999 Landmark survey found that 31% of HMOs offered acupuncture (National Market Measures, 1999). Numerous surveys of hospitals and HMOs name acupuncture as the number one priority for CAM inclusion in the near future. The official Consensus Statement of the NIH in 1997, indicating the safety and effectiveness of acupuncture, has done much to bolster confidence in the use of this therapy (NIH, 1997). The acupuncture profession is licensed in more than 40 states (AOMA, 2000), and there are accredited schools of acupuncture nationwide, including several training courses within medical schools such as UCLA (ACAOM, 2000). Within managed care networks and workers' compensation programs, chiropractic is the most widely integrated discipline; in 1999, 65% offered chiropractic benefits (National Market Measures, 1999).

Frequently, it is easier to initiate a program in stages, particularly if outcomes or evidence-based progress is desired. While there is no reason to limit implementation to one or two key therapies, typically acupuncture and massage are logical choices for the first stage of integration. Within hospital health systems, therapeutic massage is highly favored because of links to physical medicine and physical therapy, its applications in the treatment of pain, and reimbursable status already defined through the CPT (Current Procedural Terminology) codes. It is best to choose therapies that both the public and the providers agree are desirable. Invite practitioners to apply for participation and credential them to fill the positions that have been targeted throughout the system.

There are a number of questions that will need to be answered carefully in order to successfully implement CAM therapies:

- Is there existing insurance coverage for any, some, or all of these services?
- Will they be available as core benefits, through a rider, a discounted program, or a fee-for-service basis?
- Which environment, department, or program within the system will be the most conducive to host this therapy?
- How can CAM services be positioned so that they will be fully integral and not simply add-ons?

In hospitals, a logical environment for a complementary medicine program may be the physical medicine department, with its attention to pain management and palliative care. In a health plan, it will be important to consider how CAM benefits can be included with seamless interface. How can CAM services be made available to consumers in a way that fosters prevention and early intervention, thereby protecting the health of the customer and saving money for the funder?

Phase 3-4: Initiate Programs in Complementary Therapies

This is the stage at which the therapies are actually made operational. For example, in a

**Case Study:
Mind-Body Techniques in a Surgical Unit**

Located in New York City and associated with Columbia University, Columbia-New York Presbyterian Hospital provides mind-body therapies that are integrated into the services of the coronary care unit. In preparation for surgery, patients are taught meditation, breathing exercises, and a variety of relaxation and imagery techniques. Massage, healing touch, and soothing music are available to minimize anxiety before surgery and to promote healing following the procedure.

hospital environment, the integration of complementary therapies requires that there is an infrastructure in place to accommodate new providers and new therapies.

Phase 3-5: Integrate New Providers into the System

This stage engages the infrastructure put in place in Phase 2, maximizing the role of new providers through triage and referrals, clinical care coordination, and care pathways.

Case Study: Care Guidelines

In Washington state, where insurance coverage has by law been expanded to include CAM services, health systems have developed care pathways that include the use of complementary medicine. Group Health Cooperative of Puget Sound, a large, managed care organization, implemented its guidelines through a consensus process that involved CAM practitioners and its own clinical management staff. The team has defined a series of algorithms that identify conditions for which CAM referrals can be made; the guidelines also stipulate the level of care to be provided (see Chapter 33).

In hospitals and health systems that provide CAM, complementary therapies are offered in a variety of environments, including:

- self-contained integrative centers within major hospitals, such as Hennepin County Clinic in Minneapolis and Memorial Sloan Kettering Cancer Center in New York
- wellness and fitness facilities, such as the Mercy System of Cincinnati, Ohio, and Riverside of Hampton Roads, Virginia
- rehabilitation units, where integrative services are being planned in hospital health systems in Boston and the San Francisco Bay area.

As discussed earlier, complementary providers can be integrated into the system through multidisciplinary teams. Clinical teams are currently being redefined in many hospital systems. At the appropriate point in the integrative process, the role of the team can be expanded to include the participation of alternative/adjunctive providers. In the future, this will make possible the utilization of alternative therapies on hospital health care teams in a fully integrated delivery context. In acute care settings, it is probable that direct service delivery to patients will continue to be provided by physicians and other professionals with dual credentialing. For example, in the health care system of the future, physicians trained in acupuncture may serve as adjunctive anesthesiologists on the surgical team. Nurses trained in hypnosis may also participate on these teams. In staff model, managed care environments, multidisciplinary teams will have the capacity to provide state-of-the-art disease management (see Chapter 38 for an example of an integrative spine center that utilizes a multidisciplinary approach).

In managed care environments, CAM services are frequently accessed through specialized provider networks, which have been seen by some as evidence that the integration of CAM has been accomplished. However, these projects may not be fully integrated into service delivery throughout the system and may be isolated from

---

**Case Study: Complementary Therapies
in the Rehabilitation Unit**

In health systems such as Kaiser of Northern California, Vallejo, CAM services have been successfully integrated in an orthopedic rehabilitation unit. Services include the use of acupuncture, massage, and hypnosis for the reduction of chronic pain. Rehabilitation medicine programs are an example of existing environments that can be expanded to accommodate the integration of complementary services.

---

the organization, plan, or facility that created them. Clearly, full integration is an ongoing process that is likely to occur over time.

Similarly, when CAM therapies are provided in health systems, they can become isolated within the CAM unit. They may not be integrated across the continuum of care or with the health system infrastructure. The level of communication between providers throughout the system may be low, even if communication within the CAM unit is high. The creation of a comprehensive health care delivery system demands that complementary services be authentically integrated into both the business and clinical structure.

In order to successfully implement a staged approach, the rollout of Phase 3 should reflect a balance between the organization's impetus to be responsive to consumer demand, the health system's internal need for integrated infrastruc-

ture, and the level of acceptance within the physician and provider communities.

In summary, to achieve the most effective outcomes, Phase 3 must reflect the values of the major stakeholders:

- the institution and its mission
- the consumer
- the provider community

A NEW ERA OF HEALTH CARE DELIVERY

Ultimately, most organizations will consider the inclusion of complementary medicine and an integrative model of delivery. If your organization elects to pursue this phased approach, it is important and practical to build on your organization's assets. Progress according to your organization's mission through a judicious process that involves planning, scientific review, and market research. Too much innovation and too little planning can be disastrous. Too much planning with too little creativity may stifle the process. The careful design of infrastructure will foster the emergence of the most effective and comprehensive system of delivery.

Throughout the health care industry, there is broad recognition that the focus must be on core business. In the emerging marketplace, this business mission must satisfy customer interest, improve clinical outcomes, and build market share. A sound strategy to meet these needs can be achieved by linking health promotion, complementary therapies, and conventional medicine across the continuum of services through a practical, phased approach.

REFERENCES

AOMA (Acupuncture and Oriental Medicine Alliance). Legislative Update. Olalla, WA: AOMA; 2000, May.

ACAOM (Accreditation Commission for Acupuncture and Oriental Medicine). Accredited and Candidate Programs. Silver Spring, MD: ACAOM; 2000, May.

Astin J. Why patients use alternative medicine: results of a national study. *JAMA*. 1998;279(19):1548–1553.

Eisenberg D, Davis R, Ettner S, et al. Trends in alternative medicine use in the United States, 1990–1997: results of a follow-up national survey. *JAMA*. 1998;280(18):1569–1575.

Eisenberg DM, Kessler RC, Foster C, et al. Unconventional medicine in the United States. *N Engl J Med*. 1993;328(4):246–252.

Goetzel RZ, Jacobson BH, Aldana SG, Vardell K, Yee L. Health care costs of worksite health promotion participants and non-participants. *J Occup Environ Med*. 1998;40(4):341–346.

National Institutes of Health (NIH). *Consensus Statement* [on Acupuncture]. 1997 Nov 3–5;15(5):1–34.

National Market Measures. *The Landmark Report II*. Sacramento, CA: Landmark Healthcare; 1999.

Ornish DM. Avoiding revascularization with lifestyle changes: The Multicenter Lifestyle Demonstration Project. *Am J Cardiol*. 1998;82(10B):72T–76T.

CHAPTER 7

Strategic Planning in the Integration of Complementary Medicine

Lisa K. Rolfe and Karen A. Hohenstein

The development of a successful integrative medicine strategy must be grounded in a detailed market and competitor analysis and include a thorough understanding of how this approach fits within the context of the organization. At Tiber Group, we believe that an integrative medicine initiative must be relevant to overall organizational strategy, contribute to the primary mission, and leverage the organization's strengths. Developing a complementary medicine program as an isolated initiative could compromise its ability to contribute to the organization. Hospitals and health systems that will be most successful in this emerging field will be those that:

- View integrative medicine as a strategic investment.

Lisa K. Rolfe is a founding member and Partner at Tiber Group. With over 15 years of health care consulting experience, she is a leader in designing state-of-the-art health strategies to address the challenges of the evolving health care marketplace. Her expertise includes organizational strategy, physician integration, medical group formation, physician compensation design, and service line and ambulatory care planning. She is a graduate of the University of Chicago's Graduate School of Business and Stanford University.

Karen A. Hohenstein has over 10 years of experience in health care consulting and leads Tiber Group's integrative medicine product line. Her client work includes organizational strategy, service line planning, physician integration, and ambulatory care development. She holds a master's of management from the J.L. Kellogg Graduate School of Management at Northwestern University and an undergraduate degree from Ohio State University.

- Have a plan of action that reflects the role of integrative medicine in the context of their greater vision.
- Have an understanding of the type of infrastructure necessary to support this form of integration and growth.

EVALUATING THE OPTIONS

Although an integrative medicine center is frequently the first option that health systems consider when entering this market, the development of a freestanding center is not the only approach to complementary medicine. There are a number of other options that are less capital-intensive than a freestanding center, yet still enable the health system to differentiate itself, meet market-driven needs, and remain consistent with it mission, vision, and organizational strategy. A broad range of initiatives can be successfully implemented. (See Figure 7–1.)

Integrative medicine services can complement a health system's strategy in a number of ways that are not necessarily dependent on a "bricks-and-mortar" approach. Integrative services can become a strategic platform or can be developed to augment existing programmatic offerings in ambulatory care, customer service, or specific service lines, such as obstetrics-gynecology, cardiology, oncology, orthopedics, or geriatrics. Integrative medicine can also offer the health system a new way to collaborate with physicians in the community.

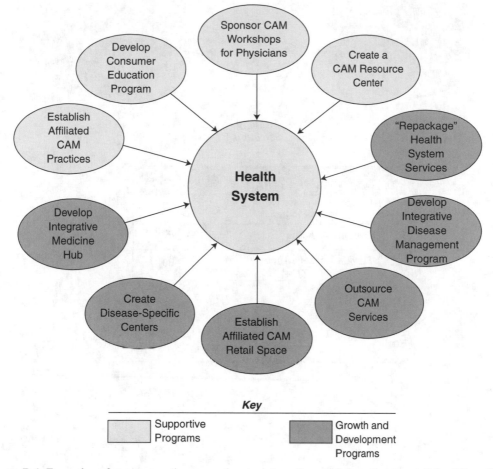

Figure 7–1 Examples of programmatic approaches to integrative medicine. Courtesy of the Tiber Group, Chicago, Illinois.

While any one of these initiatives or a combination of them can be used, selecting the most effective approach for an organization can be challenging. We recommend an evaluation process that assesses both the market and the organization to determine the optimal course of action (see Figure 7–2).

Before initiating this process, an organization should identify a sponsor group composed of 8 to 10 individuals that will oversee strategy development. The sponsor group should include physicians; other clinical disciplines, such as pharmacy and nutritional services; and representatives from management. The group will be responsible for guiding the planning efforts, reviewing analysis, weighing options, and ultimately making recommendations on how the organization should proceed with regard to complementary medicine. It is important that the committee reflect a range of opinions within the organization. Participants who are open but skeptical of the delivery of complementary medicine should be included. Involving physicians who have reservations about the initiative can

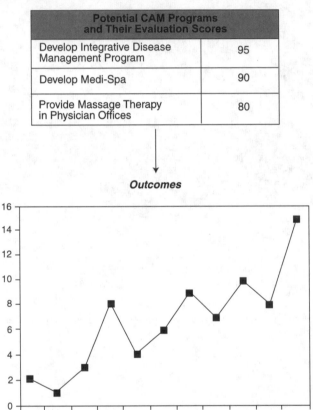

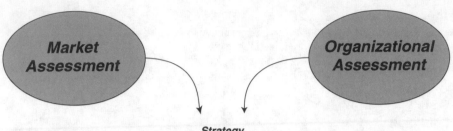

Strategy
Selection

Potential CAM Programs and Their Evaluation Scores	
Develop Integrative Disease Management Program	95
Develop Medi-Spa	90
Provide Massage Therapy in Physician Offices	80

Outcomes

Figure 7–2 CAM planning process. Evaluation score determined using the scorecard (Exhibit 7–1). Courtesy of the Tiber Group, Chicago, Illinois.

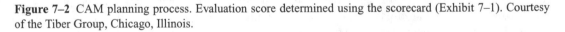

have a significant influence on the organization and the rest of the medical staff. If these skeptics become part of the process, their peers and colleagues may be less inclined to view the comple-

mentary medicine initiative as the work of a fringe element.

The key steps in the development of an integrative medicine program include market analysis, organizational assessment, strategic selection, and performance measures.

Market Analysis

A comprehensive market analysis will assist the organization in identifying the population's receptivity to complementary medicine and provide insights into specific programmatic initiatives of potential interest to the community. The results may indicate an environment that is not conducive to complementary medicine or, conversely, may suggest more opportunity than originally anticipated. When we work with health systems, we typically build in a "go/no-go" decision point after the market analysis has been completed. Either way, this evaluation provides a health system with a strong foundation upon which it can base decisions. The following elements should be part of a thorough market analysis.

Demographic Analysis

Demographic characteristics that are important to assess include the age, gender, income, and education levels of the population, as well as ethnic diversity within the market. Figure 7–3 summarizes the demographic profile of complementary medicine users indicated by the research of Eisenberg and colleagues (1998).

In addition to basic demographic information, it is helpful to use tools that combine traditional demographic measures with psychosocial and socioeconomic characteristics such as Prizm Clusters or HCIA/Sachs Group population categories. The use of these population groupings enables more accurate prediction of health care utilization patterns and the potential use of complementary medicine. This information provides a basis for identifying the kinds of complementary medical services that would best correlate with any particular demographic profile.

For example, services provided to empty nesters (midlife couples whose children no longer live at home) are likely to be very different from those selected by a population composed primarily of young families. The empty nesters may be receptive to massage therapy, stress reduction, and anti-aging medicine, while the families may be more inclined to use chiropractic, alternative allergy treatments, and wellness programming. Regardless of the target population, the strategy must incorporate the priorities of that specific group and provide services in a

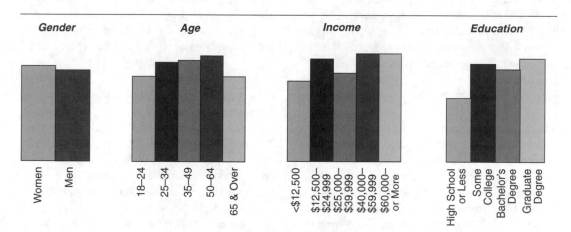

Figure 7–3 Percent of U.S. population using CAM services in 1997. *Source:* Data from D. Eisenberg et al., Trends in Alternative Medicine Use in the United States, 1990–1997: Results of a Follow-Up National Survey, *Journal of the American Medical Association*, Vol. 280, No. 18, p. 1574, © 1998, American Medical Association.

manner that is sensitive to the group's needs, desires, and cultural values.

Epidemiological Data

Epidemiological data will provide insight into the prevalence of specific disease conditions within the community. In determining which services or programs to offer, it is important to be objective in understanding what the population may require. Tiber Group has had clients who have built integrative medicine centers to provide disease management for populations within the community with specific health care needs. For example, one health system developed an AIDS alternative medicine center to respond to a very high-density population of HIV-positive patients. This facility serves its clients by providing alternative treatments such as massage therapy, nutritional counseling, stress reduction, and spiritual programs. They have had enormous success in reaching out to their target client group. The analysis of epidemiological data provides another way to define *who* is being served and *what* is trying to be achieved.

Competitor Assessment

No strategic planning exercise would be complete without an understanding of competitor positioning, strengths, and weaknesses. The challenge of assessing alternative medicine competitors lies in the fact that the competition can be very diverse and difficult to identify. Unlike the hospital industry, there is no database of complementary medicine facilities. There are no readily available resources to identify providers and their services, volume, or market share. The strategic planner must consider as competition not only hospital and health system programs and freestanding integrative medicine centers, but also fitness facilities, solo practitioners, weight loss centers, spas, pharmacies, health food stores, book shops, and recreation centers. In addition, physicians (both primary care doctors and specialists) may be providing some of these services within their office setting. Since many complementary medicine providers do little advertising or marketing, tapping into a word-of-mouth network may be the most suc-

cessful method of identifying and assessing the competition. Although the intent of this analysis is to understand how competitors are positioned and what markets they are reaching, the analysis may also serve a dual purpose as a useful study of potential joint venture partners.

Payer/Employer Analysis

Before embarking on a strategy for an integrative medicine initiative, the planner should evaluate current insurer coverage, as well as the potential for local and regional employers to offer alternative services.

Payer coverage of complementary medicine has major implications for the development of integrative medicine programs. Some payers are now including alternative services such as acupuncture, chiropractic, and massage therapy in their realm of services. However, these services are not typically covered benefits and are more commonly offered as discounted affinity products that are available through complementary medicine networks. Markets in which there is a high level of payer competition and fragmentation are ripe for complementary medicine inclusion because payers will attempt to attract new members with this perk. While increased insurance coverage may boost utilization of complementary medicine, a lack of coverage should not derail new programmatic efforts. On the contrary, a lack of payer coverage in a market with strong demographic characteristics could indicate a sizable cash-based opportunity.

A survey of employers in the market can also provide insight into the potential acceptance and future coverage of complementary medicine services. The presence of large, employee-friendly companies may provide the impetus for payers to offer coverage for certain services. In a tight labor market, complementary medical benefits can be a successful enticement for employees. Even if they do not offer these services through their benefit plans, many of the more progressive employers are supporting the use of on-site services such as massage therapy, nutritional programs, and stress reduction classes. For example, in Chicago, the Quaker Oaks Company offers a stress reduction program that includes yoga and meditation. Understanding the employment and payer profile of the market will also provide insight into the appropriate integrative medicine strategy.

Consumer Research

Focus groups and surveys often provide an effective means of tapping into the consumer mindset. These resources are usually used in two ways: (1) during preplanning and (2) as a concept-testing tool. In a preplanning mode, consumer feedback can be used to augment market demographic analysis and provide unique and valuable insights into market demands. However, at Tiber Group, we prefer to use focus groups and consumer surveys at a later stage in the market research when participants can respond to a preliminary vision or concept developed by the sponsor group. Using consumer feedback mechanisms in this manner allows us to refine the concept and generate more specific feedback, which can then can be applied to fine-tune the preliminary strategy.

The market analysis is a primary element in the foundation upon which an organization builds its integrative medicine program. Consequently, the analysis should be a thorough, well-planned effort conducted at the outset of the process, particularly since the steps that follow will be built largely on the data gathered during this phase.

Organizational Assessment

The goals of the organizational assessment are to determine how integrative medicine fits within the health system's strategy and if the organization is ready to tackle a potentially controversial program. The organizational evaluation can ultimately determine a strategy's success to an even greater degree than the market analysis. While the *market* might be ripe for development, if the organization and particularly the physicians are unable to support the concept of health system–delivered alternative care, the program will probably be unsuccessful. A number of considerations are important in an assessment of the organization.

Mission Consistency

To ensure the success of an integrative program, an organization should carefully define how such an initiative would relate to the organization's mission and vision, taking into account the health system's sponsorship, core beliefs, and values. We have found that the delivery of alternative medicine can fit well in faith-based organizations since these systems are likely to address the spiritual needs of their patients and many alternative medicine therapies include a significant spiritual element. On the contrary, academic medical centers tend to have a more difficult time with these programs since they are devoted to the science of medicine and can be somewhat reluctant to embrace therapies viewed as unsubstantiated due to the lack of scientific research. However, some community hospitals and health systems are well positioned for the delivery of specific aspects of complementary medicine, particularly wellness programming.

Strategic Fit

Assuming compatibility with market and mission, an integrative medicine strategy must fit into the long-term vision and goals of the organization. We firmly believe that complementary medicine can be integrated into a range of health system initiatives. For example, some of our clients have designed their alternative medicine strategy as a means of augmenting an ambulatory care program, by developing outpatient centers that combine traditional and complementary medicine therapies. Others have used integrative medicine as a complement to an organizational focus on key service lines, such as women's health, cardiac care, oncology, geriatrics, or orthopedics. In these programs, complementary medical services are designed and focused within the context of the medical specialty.

Some health systems have viewed complementary medicine as a way to enhance the performance of their employed medical group by adding complementary therapies to physician offices, or through partnerships in the co-development of an outpatient center. Complementary medicine can even be used to penetrate a new market. Other organizational strategies may focus on health and wellness initiatives with Healthy Communities 2000/2010 targets.

Many times complementary medicine can provide the glue that holds together a number of different strategic initiatives. For example, one health system we worked with defined the following strategic objectives:

- To penetrate a new market through a distinctive service offering.
- To provide oncology programs regionwide.
- To develop closer alignment with independent physicians.

To address all these objectives, the system developed an ambulatory care cancer center in a previously untapped, adjacent geographic area. The center integrated traditional oncology services such as physician care and chemotherapy with complementary therapies such as acupuncture, massage therapy, stress reduction, guided imagery, and an education component. These complementary services are provided in partnership with physicians. The health system owns the center, but physicians were hired to provide management and supervise complementary medicine providers.

Ultimately, it is important to think about complementary medicine not as an isolated initiative, but, rather, as one that is integral to the overall strategic plan for meeting defined organizational objectives.

Organizational Culture

Despite a fit with market, mission, and strategy, the effort to provide complementary therapies can be compromised if there is not sufficient support within the organization. Programs that will succeed in one health system may be denounced in another. Resistance can be found at the conceptual level or in relation to specific disciplines or types of treatment. It is important to understand not only management's position with regards to these services, but also the perspective of physicians and other clinical staff. For example, one organization we worked with had overwhelming support for a complementary medicine initiative from management and nonphysician clinical staff, but physicians were strongly resistant to the concept.

To determine the organizational culture and prevailing attitudes toward complementary medicine, we typically begin the assessment process with a number of interviews, which should include a cross section of senior management, service line administrators, physicians (such as primary care providers, specialists, staff physicians, and independent providers), as well as other clinicians (for example, pharmacists, nutritionists, and physical and occupational therapists). Medical staff surveys are another useful tool to gauge physicians' perceptions of complementary services. However, we have found that these surveys are most beneficial if they are developed around a preliminary concept to which the physicians can respond.

The information gathered from the market and organizational assessments should provide enough background to develop a complementary medicine strategy that is sensitive to the community and the internal dynamics of the organization.

Strategic Selection

Once these evaluations have been completed, the organization should be able to create a preliminary list of initiatives that could be pursued. Ideas for the list should flow from the work created to date. In our experience, we have seen preliminary lists range from 15 to more than 60 potential initiatives. The next step is to prioritize the initiatives. One tool we have successfully applied is the scorecard. This format can be used to evaluate each potential program across 8 to 12 measures. Examples of criteria to be measured include consistency with the organization's mission, improved access to care in the community, the level of capital required, operational complexity, and potential physician support. The *criteria* are weighted based on their importance to the organization (high numbers equal high value). A numerical weighting scale from 1 to 5 is typically used.

Each potential *program* on the list is then scored, based on how it meets the evaluation criteria, typically on a scale of 1 to 3; again, higher numbers indicate higher value. Points are calculated by multiplying the criteria's weight (importance) by the assigned score (the value of a particular program to the organization, in the context of that measure—for example, the level of capital investment required). Tallying the scores allows rank ordering of the initiatives.

Clearly this tool should not prescribe the strategy and initiatives, but it can provide critical insight as to the direction the organization should pursue. The sample scorecard (see Exhibit 7–1) provides an example of the types of potential evaluation criteria and how they are applied.

Performance Measures

Regardless of the approach adopted, it is imperative that the organization clearly articulate its expectations. The development of an integrative medicine strategy is likely to involve significant capital investment, require the use of political clout, and affect the organization's public image. Consequently, it is important to consider how the success of such a program will be measured.

Given the thin margins experienced by health systems in the current market, financial performance cannot be overlooked. However, it is wise to also consider measuring the success of the new complementary medicine program from a broader perspective. For instance, consumer awareness of the organization, patient satisfaction, and community health measures could contribute as much, if not more, to the organization as having these services perform initially in the black. Clearly, these nonfinancial objectives cannot supplant profitability, but they should also be considered when evaluating the success of the new initiative.

No matter which performance expectations are deemed appropriate, evaluating program success over time requires that management clearly define the indicators to be tracked. For example,

when the primary goal is profitability, management must determine the necessary targets for return on investment, specifically identifying the volumes and cost ratios that are required to achieve the defined targets. If, on the other hand, the goal is to improve community health status and the management of particular diseases, management will need to define the specific indicators that will be used as benchmarks of success, such as increased use of preventive services and decreased incidence of morbidity.

In complementary medicine, as in most health-related services, the development process includes a certain amount of unpredictability, and the implementation of these programs does not always follow the path initially outlined financially, operationally, or in terms of consumer reaction and physician participation. The uncertainty of the future success of these outcomes does not necessarily result in negative outcomes; in some cases, the project exceeds expectations. It is essential to remember that this is a relatively new product/service with a fluid nature for which data are limited. Consequently, we suggest regularly scheduled reviews including checkpoints at the 6- and 12-month marks. These checkpoints will not only allow a review of progress, but also afford the health system an opportunity to scan the environment for changes that may have occurred since the program's development. Trends and assumptions that supported the strategy should be reassessed and verified on an ongoing basis. Changing environmental factors should be carefully evaluated, such as new players in the field or regulatory issues, and incorporated into the implementation phase.

PLANNING THE INTEGRATIVE MEDICINE CENTER

The following is a compilation of Tiber Group's experience in planning and operationalizing these types of facilities. Given that these centers are on the cutting edge of health care services, there are currently few examples of health system–sponsored centers that have been

Exhibit 7–1 The Scorecard: A Sample Evaluation Tool.
Formula: weight × score = Points.
Score: 1 = low, 3 = moderate, 5 = high.

Domain / Evaluation Criteria	Mission Measures — Contributes to Organization Mission (Weight 5)		Access Measures — Expands Continuum of Care (Weight 2)		Access Measures — Increases Clinical Efficiency/Quality (Weight 5)		Receptivity Measures — Community Receptivity/Demographic Fit (Weight 3)		Receptivity Measures — Ease of Integration with Physician Profile (Weight 4)		Competitive Position Measures — Enables Market Differentiation (Weight 3)		Competitive Position Measures — Leverages Hospital's Programmatic Strengths (Weight 4)		Financial Measures — Impact on Financial Performance (Weight 5)		Financial Measures — Level of Investment Required* (Weight 2)		Implementation Measures — Ease of Implementation (Weight 1)		Total Points
	Score	Points	Score	Points	Score	Points	Score	Points	Score	Points	Score	Points	Score	Points	Score	Points	Score	Points	Score	Points	
Potential Initiatives																					
Activities that Support CAM Integration																					
Provide physicians and community on-line access to CAM information (such as WebMD)	3	15	5	10	3	15	3	9	3	12	5	15	5	20	3	15	3	6	3	3	120
Credential CAM practitioners in community as a referral point for physicians	1	5	3	6	3	15	3	9	1	4	3	9	1	4	3	15	3	6	1	1	74
Develop physician in-office questionnaire/health assessment product	3	15	3	6	3	15	3	9	3	12	3	9	3	12	3	15	5	10	5	5	108
Integrative Clinical Programs																					
Develop integrative CAM Rehabilitation Program	3	15	5	10	5	25	3	9	3	12	5	15	5	20	3	15	3	6	3	3	130
Develop integrative CAM Pain Management/Anesthesiology	3	15	5	10	5	25	5	15	3	12	5	15	3	12	3	15	1	2	3	3	124
Develop integrative CAM Cardiac Program	3	15	5	10	5	25	5	15	5	20	5	15	5	20	5	25	1	2	3	3	150
Facility-Based Initiatives																					
Develop a CAM program for women such as a medi-spa	3	15	3	6	5	25	3	9	5	20	5	15	5	20	3	15	1	2	3	3	130
Develop a primary care-based integrative medicine center	3	15	3	6	3	15	3	9	1	4	3	9	1	4	3	15	3	6	3	3	86
Develop a retail outlet in the fitness center	3	15	2	4	1	5	3	9	3	12	3	9	3	12	5	25	3	6	3	3	100

Courtesy of the Tiber Group, Chicago, Illinois.

operational long enough to be performing profitably. Consequently, careful planning and implementation are even more critical elements for the ultimate success of such a center.

Scope

Organizations should consider starting with a small scope of operations. Granted, there are certain situations that warrant the development of a large freestanding building in which the entire staff can work together. However, starting small allows the organization to test the concept, the reaction of the physician community, the desirability of the services selected, and the volume of business actually experienced. Starting small also enables the health system to limit the initial capital investment and to fine-tune the delivery model and operations before committing substantial capital. For example, one center we assisted initiated its project with approximately 900 square feet located in an existing medical office building. The center offered a limited number of services on a part-time basis. The new program did exceptionally well despite limited marketing, reluctant physician support, and limited organizational backing. This testing period allowed the health system to evaluate community and physician response with limited risk. As the center became more established, the positive response of the community became apparent. The system expanded the facility and offered a broader range of services. Currently, the center occupies more than 6,000 square feet and offers a wide variety of therapies, products, and classes.

Starting small can provide another benefit in the development of an integrative practice. Patients who use alternative medicine are generally attracted to low-tech, personalized environments. They tend to seek out complementary care because it involves a different approach and offers a different kind of relationship with providers. As a result, it can be counterproductive to place too much emphasis on the facility. The development of a big new building with all the bells and whistles may not create the more personal environment desired by patients.

The primary focus should be on developing the right style of practice and creating a comfortable atmosphere for patients. Starting small can ensure that the focus stays on the care model and not the facility.

Design Considerations

Several architecture and interior design firms specialize in the design of integrative medicine centers. These firms provide choices in aesthetics and planning in terms of color, layout, and use of space. Some of the architects' designs reflect sensitivity to the use of sounds, smells, and light, and "fung shui" or energy flow throughout the center. Regardless of the size or location of the facility, efforts to avoid the institutional or strictly medical environment and to emphasize the qualities that promote a sense of healing are well founded. All these considerations are important in the final design of a center and its ultimate success (see Chapter 43 on designing the integrative medicine center).

Products and Services

The decision regarding the inclusion of a product line, be it a therapy, service, or retail products, should be based on many dimensions, including the primary goals of the center and how it relates to the overall organizational strategy, physician input, community interest, and supporting research. Since service selection can sometimes be a contentious process, it may be helpful to let a subset of the sponsor group oversee this process. This subcommittee can guide the selection and ensure that the process is responsive to the issues raised by various constituents and stakeholders.

A major decision for the organization is whether to include retail products, such as herbal remedies, vitamins, and other nutritional supplements. Strong arguments can be made for both perspectives—the inclusion or exclusion of these types of products in a center sponsored by a health system. On the positive side, the organization can play a role in validating the quality and reliability of the products. Given the unregulated status of these products, this can be of benefit to the consumer. Conversely, some believe very strongly that physicians and health systems should not be distributing these types of products because it raises the issue of conflict of interest. Compounding the issue is the fact that retail products have been found to be one of the more profitable segments of alternative medicine, and are, in some cases, one of the drivers that keep independent integrative medicine centers afloat. Ultimately, this decision-making process must be worked through by the organization with input from physicians and complementary practitioners.

Many of the centers that we have seen developed are focused around primary care services, treating a broad array of patients and conditions, but there are other models of care that are also worth exploring. For example, if a strategy called for women's health program development, the integrative medicine center could be built around a medi-spa concept. A medi-spa incorporates traditional medicine (obstetrics-gynecology, primary care providers, dermatology, aesthetic services, diagnostics, and testing), complementary therapies (massage, acupuncture, and stress reduction), as well as spa-like services (facials, manicures, and body scrubs). Medi-spas are becoming increasingly popular in urban markets because they create an environment that is uniquely attuned to women and their wants and needs. These programs are just one example of how the design of a center can be fine-tuned based on objectives.

Care Delivery Model

The very term "integrative medicine center" implies that traditional and complementary therapies will be delivered in concert. However, this integration can be a complex process because it involves human emotions and belief systems. To some degree physicians and complementary medicine practitioners are skeptical and apprehensive of one another. Currently, we estimate that there are as many complementary practitio-

ners who are opposed to integrative medicine as there are physicians who oppose this initiative. Establishing common ground can be difficult from both perspectives. The task of the organization is to identify providers who see advantages to using the best of both forms of medicine and are open to participation in mainstream environments. They tend to see integration as an opportunity, driven by consumer interest, to expand the practice of their disciplines and provide value to a larger population of patients.

The care delivery model defines the structure under which traditional and complementary services will be brought together. Models can vary widely. In arrangements with less integration, practitioners are in business for themselves, and merely lease space in an integrative medical center. Under this model, physicians and practitioners could have little if any interaction. We are aware of one center in which physicians' offices are on one side of the building and complementary medicine providers on the other, with virtually no interaction. In a more fully integrated approach, complementary medicine practitioners participate on multidisciplinary teams with physicians, meeting regularly to review charts and discuss treatment options for patients. It is important to define the desired degree of integration and how the primary care physicians and specialists involved with the center will interact with alternative practitioners.

Health systems and physicians may be inclined to develop a physician-managed approach, in which physicians have oversight of the complementary medicine practitioners. While this model can work, our experience indicates that this approach can frustrate and stifle complementary providers. A more effective approach is the establishment of a physician medical director who is thoroughly knowledgeable in complementary medicine and can set the direction and monitor quality for the center. Typically, this kind of oversight is coupled with a team approach to care delivery. Under this model, physicians and practitioners communicate regularly about patients and work collaboratively to achieve desired outcomes. This model, although difficult to implement, can satisfy the organization's desire for physician oversight, while simultaneously addressing provider need for a balance between participation and autonomy.

Defining the care delivery model is a very important component of the center design and planning. Too much oversight can inhibit productivity, but a lack of integration can add little value for the patient seeking a total solution.

Physician and Practitioner Staffing

Once services have been selected and the care delivery model defined, the next step is to identify physicians and practitioners to participate in the center. Incorporating highly qualified, respected complementary medicine practitioners will facilitate greater support from both the medical community and skeptical administrators.

Credentialing is the first step in the selection process and ensures the selection of qualified practitioners. The credentialing process involves verifying the education, training, and experience of the complementary medicine providers. In addition to checking references and validating certifications and experience, the credentialing process should include site visits to the practitioner's current operation. The site visit will allow the organization to see how the practitioner functions in the practice environment and interacts with patients and staff.

Training is not the only important consideration. In addition to having appropriate educational certification, and experience, it is important to find providers who are comfortable working within the defined care delivery model. Interviews can be used to advantage in the hiring process by probing potential candidates to determine their "fit" with the center's operational model. We have found that it is wise to perform extensive interviews with practitioners as part of the evaluation and hiring process. A practitioner who has good credentials on paper may not always be the right choice since he or she may not mesh well with the medical staff, or may

not be comfortable with a biomedical approach to care. Not everyone can bridge both worlds and function well in an environment in which mainstream medicine is delivered hand-in-hand with complementary therapies.

To learn more about the practice style of the applicant, we suggest the use of a case study, which can involve a fictitious patient with a predefined medical condition and a complex history. Asking the practitioner how he or she would address this case can yield firsthand knowledge of both philosophy and approach. It often reflects the practitioner's level of comfort with integration, physician-colleagues, and the mainstream delivery system. The interview and case evaluation can be useful tools to quickly identify those candidates who will best fit in the center. It is essential to go beyond the basics of credentials and capabilities. Finding the right mix of providers may be time-consuming, but the payoff of a well-functioning center is worth the investment.

Employment Arrangements

Complementary medicine practitioners can be offered a variety of employment arrangements including:

- contracting
- direct employment
- transitional approach

The method chosen will depend on the scale of operations and the organization's risk tolerance. Practitioners who are idle while receiving a salary can cripple the performance of a center. Consequently, under an employment model, the center is at risk for low patient volumes. On the contrary, contracting with complementary practitioners limits the downside risk of low volumes, but may also limit the upside potential. Contracting can raise issues of loyalty with practitioners. If the providers have practices at other locations, they may be inclined to funnel patients to these other sites. Depending on the market, the organization should consider a transitional model in which practitioners start as contractors with the expectation of becoming direct employees over time. This is a workable strategy that has been successfully used by several of our clients. The transitional approach is consistent with the "start small" mind-set and limits the organization's risk exposure in the start-up phase. This type of arrangement provides an assessment stage in which the organization can become familiar with the practitioners and physicians, and verify that practitioners mesh well with the rest of the multidisciplinary team before incorporating them into the center on a full-time basis.

Salaries and Compensation

Compensation programs must be based on a number of factors including productivity, quality service provision, and patient satisfaction. In addition, some centerwide incentives should be included to decrease competition between providers and encourage appropriate cross-practitioner referrals. Just as physician compensation has many nuances in terms of incentive programs, the compensation of complementary and alternative medicine practitioners requires careful thought and planning.

Monitoring Clinical Outcomes

The need to track and monitor outcomes is fundamental to an integrative medical practice. When an integrative center is developed in conjunction with a major health system, the program is usually under tremendous scrutiny. Patients may be highly enthusiastic about their care and believe wholeheartedly that they are benefiting from treatment, but physicians, administrators, and other key stakeholders will want to see measurable results. There will be numerous requests for data to evaluate efficacy and cost-effectiveness, and to compare with other programs and treatment approaches.

The outcomes monitored can be based on several indicators. For some organizations, monitoring can occur through patient self-reporting, using instruments such as the SF-36, the Beck Depression scale, and others. Minor modifications (made with necessary approvals) to some standard measurement tools can make them more applicable to the integrative medicine environment. The center can also track the effectiveness of certain therapies for identified conditions (for example, the use of acupuncture to treat chronic sinusitis). Private and government sources for funding research in the efficacy of complementary medicine are worth investigation.

The collection of data and research studies can have a major impact on the center's credibility with the community, medical staffs, and patients. Therefore, it is important that a strategy and process for monitoring outcomes should be developed early on in the planning and implementation phase.

MANAGING THE INTEGRATIVE MEDICINE CENTER

From an operational perspective, there are aspects of managing this type of business that are radically different from the operation of a hospital and even from the management of traditional physician offices. Some issues tend to be much more challenging; others are simply dissimilar. Areas that need to be handled differently from traditional practice include billing, hours of operation, scheduling, and marketing.

Billing

In an integrative center, billing and collections can be either very complicated or very easy. Requiring payment at the time of service is a widely accepted practice in complementary medicine because patients are accustomed to paying out of pocket for these services. Although insurance coverage is becoming more available for alternative therapies, the process of obtaining payment from a third-party payer can be time-consuming and lengthy. If the center chooses to bill the insurer, the center assumes the risk of collecting from the patient at a later time. The iterations and delays inherent in insurance billing can significantly tie up a center's cash flow.

If insurance billing is preferred, it can be helpful to outsource billing functions to a practice management service with specific experience in alternative medicine billing. Because these services are relatively new on the market, they still require careful monitoring. There are also very well designed software packages such as Alternative Link that can support record keeping and billing functions. The key issue is to provide a seamless interface with insurance companies and managed care organizations, which could alleviate unnecessary delays in payment.

Hours of Operation/Scheduling

Clearly, the goal of these types of centers is to provide a high level of patient service and to minimize stress. Emphasize convenience by making services accessible to your clients. Another related issue is that many of these therapies require multiple or extended appointments. Patients cannot simply drop in and leave. As a result, extended hours are often more important for an integrative medicine center than for a physician's office.

Maximizing the use of the treatment rooms and offices is integral to achieving cost-efficient operations. A multipurpose treatment room can be used by a number of practitioners, for example, a massage therapist, a chiropractor, or an acupuncturist. The room can be converted quickly and easily, at substantial savings to the organization. This type of arrangement requires creativity and cooperation on the part of the staff.

In an integrative medicine center, scheduling tends to be more complicated because of the varied amount of time required for different procedures. For example, a recheck or a chiropractic treatment may only require 15 minutes, whereas a new patient visit or an acupuncture treatment requires up to an hour. As a result, the scheduling process can be much more complicated than that in a physician's office, or in a single specialty practice in complementary medicine. To ensure a smooth flow of patient services, the scheduling process must be handled by highly capable staff.

Marketing and Community Outreach

There are several differences between developing a physician practice and an integrative medicine center. One of them is marketing. The use of traditional forms of advertising may be effective (for example, the use of direct mail or an advertisement in the yellow pages). However, the center can reach a more receptive population by advertising through different media, publications, businesses, and events. This requires an awareness of the resources available within the community and the identification of those used by target clientele. For example, advertisements in city-based magazines or journals that focus on alternative medicine provide an excellent opportunity to tap into a market predisposed to integrative therapies.

By addressing these issues from the onset instead of through trial and error, the organization can facilitate the success of the integrative medicine center.

CONCLUSION

Regardless of the program design selected, we encourage all organizations to consider this powerful consumer-driven trend that has the potential to change the way health care is delivered. The integration of complementary medicine into health systems can be challenging, but can provide a sustainable competitive advantage if executed carefully.

REFERENCE

Eisenberg D, Davis R, Ettner S, et al. Trends in alternative medicine use in the United States, 1990–1997: results of a follow-up national survey. *JAMA*. 1998;280(18): 1569–1575.

CHAPTER 8

Integrative Medicine Programs in Hospital Environments

8.1 New Hospital Programs in Integrative Medicine
  Neil Sol with Nancy Faass
8.2 Briefing: A Consultant's Strategies for Hospitals and Integrative Medicine Centers
  H. Phil Herre with Nancy Faass

8.1   New Hospital Programs in Integrative Medicine

Neil Sol with Nancy Faass

THE ECONOMIC ENVIRONMENT

Hospitals are redefining their roles in health care. In order to continue to be the health resource center of the community, many hospitals are participating in new approaches to service delivery. For example, health systems in all regions of the country are becoming involved in the development of exercise and medical fitness centers and in wellness programming. These programs tend to attract consumer support, and some have proven to be substantially profitable. As a result, forward-thinking hospitals are increasingly becoming involved in these trends.

Under the current system of reimbursement, medical care provided in hospitals is paid for primarily by insurance companies and the federal government. Payment may originate from a number of sources, including capitated managed care, Medicare, Medicaid, indemnity insurers, and other payers.

Payment is frequently set at negotiated rates that are deeply discounted. To remain economically viable in this environment, hospitals must find new markets. Currently, insurance companies and government continue to lower payment schedules through a variety of policies that limit reimbursement, such as diagnosis-related groups (DRGs) and prospective payment. Future Medicare payments will also be affected by the Balanced Budget Act of 1997, which will have an impact on outpatient reimbursement as well. In an effort to accommodate the discounts of payers, hospitals may inflate their retail prices to obtain sufficient reimbursement. In addition, hospitals are challenged by the need for big capital in order to replace technology and to respond to fluctuations in the market. Consequently, there has been a movement within the hospital industry to diversify product lines.

Neil Sol, PhD, has been a leader in the fields of health enhancement and fitness for the past two decades. He has extensive experience in creating, managing, and marketing health-related products and services in academic environments, the commercial fitness industry, and hospital health systems. He has diversified traditional health care institutions to include and realize the promise of health promotion services as a profitable venture. Currently, he is Vice President of Outpatient Services at Valley Care Health System in Pleasanton, California.

Major Trends in the Hospital Industry

The Expanded Continuum of Care

Hospital systems now provide products and care in the context of a continuum, which has expanded to include preventive services, as well as acute care and rehabilitation. The goal is to stay within the realm of the continuum, adding products the public will pay for at a fair out-of-pocket price, including services such as exercise and fitness and alternative therapies. In the past, hospitals have not been oriented toward these types of services. Rather, their models and mindset have traditionally focused on reimbursement through insurance and Medicare.

Enhanced Customer Service

Hospitals are developing an expanded customer-service orientation to the patient:

- Hospitals are becoming increasingly responsive to market demand.
- They are operating from the premise that patients must become return customers. Because many physicians practice at more than one hospital and insurance plans are linked to more than one hospital provider, patients can now choose where they receive care.
- Hospitals are marketing from the perspective that a great deal of promotion actually occurs informally through word-of-mouth.

Business Orientation

In many ways, hospitals are also coming to be seen as businesses. On an economic level, they really are businesses. In the current economic environment, they must function successfully to survive. Hospitals become more viable when they diversify their products to meet market demand.

New Sources of Income

At present, there is a movement among progressive hospitals to consider products that will generate dollar-for-dollar increases in income. Wellness, fitness, and preventive services are growing aspects of the industry. Community and group education is an additional area of consumer interest that can also provide sources of revenue to the hospital. Alternative medicine is also becoming an attractive market because it entails services and products that are typically provided on a cash basis. This appears to be a sizable market. Although estimates vary widely, several studies suggested that as much as 40% of the American population has participated in alternative treatment of some kind (Eisenberg et al, 1993; Astin, 1998). Acupuncture, chiropractic, and massage are the therapies that seem most congruent with traditional Western health care in its current form. These are the modalities that appear to be the most easily fused into the medical model of traditional health care as practiced in hospitals. Most of these therapies are paid for directly by consumers out of pocket at the time service is rendered.

Alternative Therapies on the Hospital Campus

Hospitals are realizing that alternative therapies can be integrated in their service offerings in a number of ways. Practitioners can be brought into the hospital environment. Alternative practitioners would locate their private practices within the hospital campus, with roles comparable to those of adjunctive medical staff. The credentialing process would enable alternative providers to open offices and in some cases apply for hospital privileges. They would pay a rental fee as other providers do once they are credentialed by the hospital. In this type of arrangement, the hospital can offset square footage expense and make a profit.

The mission of the hospital can be expanded to include integrative medicine healers in the continuum. This type of arrangement would tend to work reciprocally, just as it does for providers in more traditional disciplines. Although there may be few opportunities for referrals to inpatient care, some of the alternative providers would refer patients for diagnostic services such as radiology, blood work, or MRIs (magnetic resonance imagings). These reciprocal relationships, which tend to evolve over time, have the potential to be economically beneficial to the hospital. While some referrals to complementary therapies would not be reimbursable, an increasing number of services will become eligible for coverage as insurance for integrative medicine continues to expand.

Complementary Practitioners as Hospital Staff

Another strategy is to hire complementary practitioners as part-time or full-time employees. The hospital can retain alternative practitioners as staff to provide services such as chiropractic (for example, in a spine clinic or physical therapy program) or acupuncture (in orthopedic pain management). The practitioners would provide services for which the hospital collects dollar-for-dollar revenue based on the procedures delivered. The hospital may establish productivity expectations of complementary practitioners just as they do of any other providers. The level of integration of these services would depend on the state of acceptance of integrative medicine at a given hospital.

Greater Provision of Specific Products and Services

Hospitals are becoming involved with other aspects of alternative care that are based on cash reimbursement. These include a variety of services and products ranging from vitamin and herbal therapies to expanded massage services such as reflexology and Reiki.

Author's comment: I personally conduct two chat rooms on the Internet in the area of health and fitness. I have found that many people search alternative medicine Web sites to find information they cannot obtain from their physicians, because their doctors no longer have the time to provide teaching and explanations. There is clearly a need for public education on complementary medicine. This industry is being driven by consumer interest and an explosion of information available to the public through the Internet, the media, and the publishing industry.

Public Education and Information

There is a significant public demand for courses and other forms of information. These topics range from therapeutic exercise such as yoga, T'ai Chi, and Qigong to the management of serious conditions such as diabetes and heart disease.

Increased Insurance Coverage

Another trend that is developing in the insurance industry is the expansion of coverage for the delivery of chiropractic, acupuncture, massage, and other alternative services. Health systems see an opportunity to participate in a business that generates as much as $50 billion per year. They have incorporated this perspective into their thinking as an extension of the health care continuum. As insurance coverage increases, this market is predicted to continue to expand rapidly.

Physician Perception of Alternative Medicine

Recent proprietary information from focus research reflects physician willingness to refer patients to alternative practitioners. A very large percentage of doctors indicated that they already make these referrals because they know their patients are currently using therapies such as massage and acupuncture.

We found that patients want their doctors to help them integrate different forms of treatment. Some patients want more information from their doctors about commercial herbal products such as St. John's Wort, Ginkgo Biloba, or Echinacea, and many are now buying these products at the corner drug store. It is important that doctors become familiar with the implications of this emerging field. An expanding segment of the medical profession is beginning to view alternative practitioners as colleagues with whom they can interact. This is a result of the demand by the consumer, who is the impetus for this trend.

A Major Period of Growth for Chiropractic

Increasingly, there is perceived value in these services, not only by the community at large, but also by some traditional physicians. Five years ago, physical therapy departments in hospitals received few referrals from chiropractors. Now, there is an increase in the referral base to physical therapists from chiropractors and also in referrals back to chiropractors and acupuncturists by physicians and orthopedic surgeons. These are practitioners who would never have considered making such referrals in the past—an indicator that a change is taking place.

The level of acceptance of complementary medicine will evolve over time. Some disciplines such as homeopathy and naturopathy are still not well understood. Other therapies are rapidly gaining acceptance, such as chiropractic, acupuncture, and massage. The fact that these disciplines have national standards for certification or licensure probably adds to their credibility. In many environments, nutritional and herbal therapies are also becoming more widely utilized. In the near future, every hospital is likely to consider including these services if they are not already doing so.

INCORPORATING WELLNESS AND FITNESS INTO THE MODEL

Wellness programs and medical fitness centers represent potential cash business for the hospital. If operated correctly, they can generate 10% to 25% at the bottom line. Membership can be structured as a contractual membership business, comparable to private fitness centers. The client or patient would elect membership on a yearly basis.

Hospitals have a unique advantage as providers of fitness services. Interesting data have been gathered on the fitness industry, comparing a hospital-based wellness center to a commercial athletic or health club. Researchers found that hospitals actually appeal to a much wider audience, with potentially greater market universe. Typically, a commercial facility serves approximately 6% of the adult population within a 12-minute drive of any given facility. When a medical fitness center, wellness center, or athletic club has hospital sponsorship, that number will increase to 12% or 15%. The data suggest that there is a market of people who would like to join commercial health clubs knowing they would benefit, but who ultimately do not join. Many of these people choose to join when they are offered the same services under the auspices of a hospital.

In 1989, a major study called the One Percent Solution was conducted through the fitness industry (McCarthy, 1989). The International Health, Racquet, and Sports Association (IHRSA), a national trade association for commercial health clubs, interviewed 1,500 people over the age of 35 who were not currently members of any fitness center. They asked respondents why they had not joined a health club. In 99% of the responses, people said they were concerned that the employees of commercial fitness facilities lacked the expertise to deal with their special health needs, which revolved around asymptomatic problems such as hypertension, diabetes, arthritis, and obesity.

People felt that if they were going to exercise, they wanted to go to a facility where they could receive guidance regarding their special health needs and where medical care could be provided if something happened to them—in essence, a hospital. The association asked these respondents what it would take to get them to join a fitness program. In response, 75% said it would require an affiliation with a health care system. When the results of this survey are applied to the service offerings of a hospital in the area of health and fitness, that translates into an increase in market universe from 6% to 15%. Based on the experience of the new hospital-affiliated fitness centers that are developing across the country, it is becoming apparent that there are many consumers who will become proactive and join a health club once a hospital lends its expertise and credibility to such a facility.

This is a logical and legitimate business for a health system because it is ultimately an extension of the continuum of care. In capitated health care, the goal is to keep people healthy and out of the hospital. Capitation pays the provider one price for each person per month per year, regardless of health care costs. The key is to minimize utilization, not by restricting services, but by promoting health and wellness.

Another advantage of participation by the hospital in the fitness industry is the opportunity to generate income that is not encumbered reimbursement. A gross income of $5 million in a dollar-for-dollar facility is the equivalent of $15 million in a reimbursement-covered facility. As a result, hospital participation in the fitness industry is increasing rapidly.

Superb integrative models have been developed. An integrative program typically includes medical therapies such as cardiac, pulmonary, and rehabilitation services, physical therapy, nutritional counseling, and weight control. This also provides an optimal environment in which to integrate complementary medicine (see Chapter 46).

A medical fitness center can provide exercise in both a preventive and a rehabilitative model. In integrative facilities, economies of scale are achieved through the dual use of personnel, equipment, and space. This type of center typically offers preventive exercise with a simple health focus, but also the entire range of therapeutic exercise. In the context of the continuum of care, this type of facility provides a very positive environment in which to offer rehabilitation services.

CONCLUSION

In the 1980s, hospitals explored fitness and health promotion programming. They began providing these services to build good will in the community and enhance their image as health-oriented institutions. However, most of those

---

Providing the Continuum of Services for Cardiac Patients

A patient in Phase 2 of cardiac rehabilitation typically receives rehabilitation services with telemetry monitoring. Patients remain in that program for 12 weeks, and services are reimbursed at a moderate level. At that point, many patients are ready to progress to Phase 3, which consists of rehabilitation services without telemetry monitoring. These services are paid for out of pocket by the client, who is usually willing to invest in this phase of service because he or she is highly motivated to become healthy again and participate in a more normal life. Typically, they remain in the program for another 12 weeks. In the past, clinicians have attempted to motivate the patient to make the transition from this Phase 3 rehab to secondary prevention through fitness center membership. After someone has had an occurrence, he or she definitely wants to prevent a second episode.

Typically 60% to 75% of patients continue in some form of fitness program. For people who have had a cardiac event, hospital-based fitness is ideal because medical monitoring and support can easily be incorporated. Patients begin under the supervision of the physiologists, who help them get started in Phase 2. Once they make the transition into the traditional fitness component of the facility 24 or 27 weeks later, they can still come to the same facility and continue to receive support and feedback from the same physiologists on an as-needed basis. In addition, there is a bond and a friendship that remains even though the physiologist is no longer working directly with that patient. As a result, patients with a history of an acute life-threatening condition logically have a greater sense of security because the physiologists who already know their history are available for questions or monitoring.

programs failed because they were operated by staff unfamiliar with the fitness industry and lacking a consumer-service orientation. At this point in time, these services are being seriously reconsidered. Major commercial fitness chains are exploring partnerships with hospitals nationwide because they understand that these joint ventures will increase their market universe beyond the 6% of the population typically attracted by commercial fitness facilities. More and more hospitals have become attuned to this trend and are adding some form of fitness facility, as well as other nontraditional services. All the data, research, and feasibility studies indicate that some excellent models have been developed. This diversification beyond inpatient care is essential for the economic health of hospitals.

REFERENCES

Astin J. Why patients use alternative medicine: results of a national study. *JAMA*. 1998;279(19):1548–1553.

Eisenberg DM, Kessler RC, Foster C, et al. Unconventional medicine in the United States. *N Engl J Med*. 1993;328(4):246–252.

McCarthy J. *The one percent solution*. Club Business International. International Health, Racquet, and Sports Association (IHRSA). 1989, Feb.

8.2   Briefing: A Consultant's Strategies for Hospitals and Integrative Medicine Centers

H. Phil Herre with Nancy Faass

PROGRAM DEVELOPMENT

A number of hospital systems have asked East-West Health Centers to perform the feasibility study for a potential integrative medicine center. The development of a strategic business plan typically involves an assessment of the community, interviews with physicians and practitioners, and an analysis of potential locations and space requirements. Recommendations include capital and operating budgets and operating statements that project the first 5 years of operations. Other assignments have focused on making existing integrative medicine centers profitable and financially viable.

Outsourcing

There are certain aspects of program design that are of special importance to hospital systems. Hospital administrators and hospital systems are accustomed to providing all aspects of service. In developing a complementary medicine program, there are some functions that are better left to others.

Billing is one of the functions probably best provided through outsourcing. Billing and collections can be contracted with an outside

H. Phil Herre is the Chief Executive Officer of East-West Health Centers in Denver and one of the organization's owners and founders. He has extensive experience in hospital management, having served as the chief operating officer of HealthOne, a three-hospital health system that is the largest in Denver. For more than 15 years, he was chief executive officer of Aurora Presbyterian Hospital in Aurora, Colorado.

East-West Health Centers is a large multispecialty group practice combining Eastern and Western medicine under one roof, thereby providing the best of both medicines for the benefit of the patient.

agency, particularly an agency that provides that service for physicians and alternative providers. It is important to use a billing agency that knows how to bill workers' compensation and auto injury cases. This is the type of coverage patients will be using most frequently when they see chiropractors and massage therapists. Many hospital administrations are not structured to do this type of billing, particularly auto injury coverage.

Credentialing is another function that is usually provided by the hospital administration. Hospitals should consider outsourcing the credentialing of staff to organizations with expertise in alternative medicine. Since alternative practitioners are not seeking hospital privileges, the credentialing that is performed for the center should be different from that normally applied to physicians and specialists providing inpatient services. Credentialing guidelines must be developed, and qualified providers must be evaluated and hired in each of the disciplines. The credentialing process can be developed in-house or relegated to an outside vendor. (See Chapter 17, *Credentialing Demystified*.)

Organizational Structure

The center can succeed only when there is an entrepreneurial spirit associated with its development and the flexibility to act quickly and to respond to the market and to specific opportunities. The organizational structure and the relationship of the center's management to the system are also vitally important. In a large health system, organizational demands may inhibit the ability of the center to move as quickly as it should. Consequently, although a complementary and alternative medicine center can be managed under the auspices of the hospital, if the hospital has 100% control, it may be problematic.

Whether a hospital is nonprofit or for profit, most have a for-profit arm. The integrative medicine center is best placed in that for-profit unit, probably in a partnership arrangement in which the hospital owns a part of the center, but not all

of it. There must be partners who may be other alternative providers who work in the center in a profit-sharing or other partnership arrangement. It may be difficult for some hospitals to entertain the notion of not owning the entire operation, but that is an approach that should be explored.

One option is to develop a partnership with an outside organization that manages the hospital-based center. In such an arrangement, the outside vendor takes on many of the tasks that are difficult for the hospital. For example, a consultant can run interference with medical staff. In almost any hospital system, there will be staff members who will criticize the health system for bringing in alternative medicine. However, hospitals will find that they must consider including complementary approaches because of the high level of consumer demand. The majority of the 5,000 to 6,000 hospitals in the United States will need to develop strategies for dealing with integrative programming. It can be highly advantageous to involve an outside vendor with the expertise to create a successful program.

Initial Assessment

As consultants to hospitals wishing to establish or revitalize their integrative centers, we use a variety of strategies. These typically include:

- Interviewing members of the medical staff and the management to gain a sense of their openness toward alternative medicine.
- Looking at the resources of the area to determine a good location/site, and evaluating the area in terms of demographics including income levels, college education, and the potential client base (typically identified as women between 25 and 49).
- In the case of an existing center, reviewing the hospital's financial statements and assessing how it has positioned and marketed the center.
- Evaluating the range of services provided in the center.
- Developing a list of the alternative providers located in the area; information can be

gained through membership associations and other resources.

Selecting Therapies for Inclusion

In designing the center's programs, one important consideration is the choice of therapies to be included. It is a fact that the most widely used modality in complementary medicine is chiropractic (Eisenberg et al, 1993, 1998). Although 65% of managed care organizations are reported to offer chiropractic (National Market Measures, 1999), traditionally, most hospitals have not credentialed chiropractors or included them as part of the medical staff. A hospital must overcome this mind-set if it is going to develop a successful integrative center.

Chiropractors provide 94% of the spinal manipulation procedures in the United States (Shekelle, 1994), which are intended to address back pain. Back pain is one of the two most frequent medical complaints in our society, second only to the common cold (Hurwitz et al, 1998). Osteopathy could be substituted for chiropractic, but osteopaths have a different practice style. Although chiropractors and osteopaths both perform manipulation, chiropractors receive much more in-depth training in spinal manipulation. State-of-the-art spine care provides an important resource for employers and workers' compensation clients, addresses the public health need for options in the treatment of back pain and injury, and is also financially viable. (See Chapter 56 on the cost-effectiveness of chiropractice and Chapter 57 on safety research.)

ADDITIONAL ASPECTS OF PROGRAM DESIGN

Hospitals will want to initiate continuing medical education programs in complementary medicine for their staff. Ultimately, it is as important to market this program to the medical staff as it is to market to the community. This is best done through education. In addition, it is important to provide physicians with information on how the credentialing process is being performed, so that they are aware of the high standards to which alternative practitioners are being held. Having a staff of practitioners sanctioned by the hospital will ultimately benefit the physicians, by creating a pool of credentialed providers to whom they can refer their patients with assurance. Patients will appreciate expanded access to practitioners; they will know the providers have been evaluated for their level of excellence by the hospital.

It is also important that physicians and other stakeholders in the system gain an experiential understanding of the major therapies. This is best accomplished by providing them with hands-on experience of the therapies. When I first learned of acupuncture, I thought of the needles as comparable to those used to draw blood. It was not until I received an acupuncture treatment that I learned that the needles are generally painless and very fine—as thin as hair. Most people who actually experience acupuncture find that the treatment is exceptionally relaxing, comparable to the sense of well-being produced by a good massage. That is the kind of education that must occur in hospital systems with the medical staff and with the patients. Hospitals will want to begin by making these services available to their own employees. Patients could have access to education on complementary medicine through a number of venues, including the closed-circuit television channels.

Benefit Design

Many hospitals are self-insured and are able to design their own benefit plans. These institutions have the option of initiating the integrative process by including alternative medicine in the treatment regimen for certain diagnoses and conditions. For example, surgery for carpal tunnel syndrome is an expensive procedure that may cost as much as $15,000 to $20,000. In some cases, the technique of neuromuscular release can successfully address this condition and should be tried before electing expensive surgery (NIH, 1997; Branco and Naeser, 1999). Treatment using neuromuscular release may require ten $50 treatments; when appropriate, that is a good first option. Over time, health care and the hospital field will expand the various care pathways for treatment to include these types of effective, cost-saving options. Ultimately, outcomes research will make it apparent that some conditions are better treated with alternative therapies first and others are better treated using Western modalities first. As more research data are gathered, these results will be documented and provide the basis for standard protocol.

It can be useful to open this dialogue with the insurance companies with whom the hospital has good business relationships. The basic issues include how to improve acceptance levels and how to expand coverage for complementary services. An example of a viable integrative approach is the provision of integrated pain management. Physicians currently provide the majority of pain management. Most often they are anesthesiologists who use drugs and administer pain blocks for patients in severe pain. How useful it would be if there were a multidisciplinary pain management program that included options ranging from acupuncture to anesthesiology. Such a program could provide a tremendous marketing advantage to a hospital, thereby attracting patients who prefer not to use medication, those who are unable to tolerate medica-

tion, and those who are in chronic pain. There are many elderly people who suffer chronic pain, yet would never go to an acupuncturist. However, if acupuncture were provided in a center under the auspices of a hospital and recommended by their physician, they would be more likely to consider this as a viable medical option.

CONCLUSION

Progressive hospitals are beginning to view integrative medicine as a viable product in their continuum of services. New programs are likely to take many forms. They may involve credentialing or hiring practitioners to provide treatment on site or the development of referral relationships with the most highly qualified practitioners in the community. It is possible that many hospitals will eventually seek an ownership role in the integrative medicine center model, just as many health systems currently have a partnership role in diagnostic facilities. As outcomes research and cost-effectiveness studies provide an expanded foundation for evidence-based medicine, more hospitals will want to become involved. In the future, the majority of the 5,000 to 6,000 hospitals in the United States will consider the inclusion of adjunctive and complementary therapies in some form.

REFERENCES

Branco K, Naeser MA. Carpal tunnel syndrome: clinical outcome after low-level laser acupuncture, microamps transcutaneous electrical nerve stimulation, and other alternative therapies—an open protocol study. *J Altern Complement Med*. 1999;5(1):5–26.

Eisenberg D, Davis R, Ettner S, et al. Trends in alternative medicine use in the United States, 1990–1997: results of a follow-up national survey. *JAMA*. 1998;280(18): 1569–1575.

Eisenberg DM, Kessler RC, Foster C, Norlock FE, Calkins DR, Delbanco TL, et al. Unconventional medicine in the United States. *N Engl J Med*. 1993;328(4):246–252.

Hurwitz EL, Coulter I, Adams A, Genovese B, Shekelle P. Utilization of chiropractic services in the United States and Canada: 1985–1991. *Am J Public Health*. 1998;88(5):771–776.

National Institutes of Health (NIH). *Consensus Statement* [on Acupuncture]. 1997 Nov 3–5;15(5):1–34.

National Market Measures. The Landmark Report II. Sacramento, CA: Landmark Healthcare; 1999.

Shekelle PG. *The Use and Costs of Chiropractic Care in the Health Insurance Experiment*. Santa Monica: RAND Corporation; 1994.

CHAPTER 9

Case Study: Needs Assessment and Strategic Planning—The Ornish Program

Glenn Perelson

Intensive lifestyle modification often can improve the clinical status of patients with moderate to severe coronary heart disease. Clinical trials by Dean Ornish, MD, and colleagues at the nonprofit Preventive Medicine Research Institute (PMRI) have shown that utilizing a lifestyle program can in some cases slow, stop, or reverse the progression of heart disease. Once the research data made it clear that this was a viable approach, it became necessary to develop a strategic process in order to replicate the program at other sites.

DEVELOPING INSURANCE COVERAGE

When PMRI first took its research findings to the health plan community, insurers quickly perceived the value of the approach. However, at that time, insurance companies were not interested in paying for what they perceived to be only a preventive program. Given the high turnover in their memberships, they did not want to pay for a service to members who might not be with them in a year. At that point, PMRI

reframed the discussion to focus on the program as a treatment option. The program has always been utilized as a legitimate form of treatment for people awaiting a more intensive procedure. For health plan members anticipating surgery who choose this program, there are substantial cost savings, particularly if they find they no longer require the surgery.

The PMRI team worked closely with insurers to create inclusion criteria that made the program economically beneficial for both insurers and for host sites providing the intervention. In order to design a successful protocol, the team had to determine the kind of program delivery system that would best fit the core criteria of the insurer. Highmark Blue Cross Blue Shield of Pittsburgh, one of the nation's largest health insurers, became the first plan to offer it directly to its subscribers at on-site facilities. They have been an active partner in helping PMRI shape the program so that it appeals to the broader health plan community.

Highmark is also noteworthy for the excellence of its clinical implementation of the Ornish model. Of more than 350 Highmark members who have participated in the Ornish program since its inception, only one has required a surgical procedure. None have suffered heart attack or stroke. No participants have required bypass surgery, and only one has had an angioplasty. In addition, one of the participants has been able to avoid an anticipated heart transplant.

Highmark and the PMRI, in April 2000, created a new company, Lifestyle Advantage, to provide a platform for the expansion of nationwide access to the Ornish program and other

Glenn Perelson is Director of Network Development at the Preventive Medicine Research Institute founded by Dean Ornish, MD, and has been active in the marketing efforts and program development of more than 16 Preventive Medicine Research Institute program sites over the past 6 years. A graduate of the University of California, Berkeley, he has more than a decade of substantial experience in marketing and organizational development for two major retail and service-oriented businesses. He also has several years of experience in financial planning.

Courtesy of Glenn Perelson, Ornish Preventive Medicine Research Institute, Sausalito, California.

lifestyle-related interventions. These programs will continue to partner with leading health care delivery systems to deploy strategically intensive risk-factor modification services as alternative or complementary therapies for coronary artery disease. This approach will also be applied to the treatment of other chronic conditions, such as diabetes and arthritis, for which research has documented effectiveness.

ASSESSING POTENTIAL SITES

The Importance of Strategic Planning

In the creation of the Multicenter Lifestyle Heart Trial, sites were selected so that they would represent geographical and socioeconomic diversity. Some were private hospitals; others were public hospitals and teaching university hospitals. In looking back at the demonstration network, all the sites performed effectively from a clinical perspective, but some sites were not as financially viable as others. From these experiences, PMRI staff learned that a response to any invitation to join the program network must involve in-depth strategic planning (that is, the development of a market analysis, community needs assessment, and prospective program). PMRI staff have found that it is important to make no prior assumptions.

Evaluating Key Elements for Prospective Sites

All prospective sites need to be evaluated for the key elements of success before they can participate in the program effort. Potential sites are assessed by a team of three primary staff members:

1. *A business analyst* who looks at the area health plans from the perspective of potential reimbursement and the willingness of area health plans and employers to fund sufficient numbers of qualified patients. The analyst also evaluates the level of effort and expenditure that would

be required to market the program in a particular community.

2. *A medical director*, whose goal is to assess the level of physician support, understanding, and enthusiasm for an intensive lifestyle modification program and the potential for physician referrals.

3. *A clinical evaluator* who inventories community resources.

Through these analyses, PMRI is better able to determine whether a community has the readiness and resources for this type of program. Only through time and testing has the Institute been able to identify the benchmarks that typically predict whether a particular program will succeed.

Based on the experience gained from the multicenter demonstration project, there are a number of major areas that are evaluated in any community in order to determine its potential viability as a program site. One important aspect of the interface with the potential host site is the identification of resources essential to the success of the program.

- *Potential patient population*:
  — Do standard demographic measures reflect a population in need of this type of treatment program, based on hospital discharges and epidemiological analysis?
  — Among those patients with coronary artery disease, is the self-pay patient community large enough to suggest a sizable program population? Interviews are conducted with physicians to estimate the percentage of patients who would potentially be motivated to work with the Ornish program. Interviews with complementary programs focus on whether cardiac patients in that community might be interested in the program.
- *Administrative support:*
  — Is the administration bringing the program on board because it fits the mission

to promote wellness within the community and to expand the continuum of care?

— What is the administration's commitment to support the program during the initial 3 years and for the long term?

— Is the administration willing to introduce the program to the physician community?

- *Physician referrals to the program*:
  — What is the level of interest and potential for referrals to the program within the physician community?

- *The potential for reimbursement*:
  — Will health plan coverage be available to some of the participants? The financial success of the program is dependent in part on long-term relationships with health plans and self-insured employer groups.
  — Are the resources in place to provide reimbursement for patient participation? Typically, half the participants in Ornish programs pay out of pocket. Thirty to 40% receive some form of health plan reimbursement for their participation. The balance is made up by foundation support.

- *The availability of foundation support:*
  — Is foundation funding available to provide scholarships for underserved individuals in the community who do not have health plan coverage and cannot pay out of pocket for services?
  — Is foundation funding available to assist the host institution in underwriting program start-up costs?

- *The presence of complementary programming within the system:*
  — Will the Ornish program interface well with existing programs or compete with them?

- *Community resources:*
  — Is fresh, healthful food accessible at a reasonable price?
  — Are there a sufficient number of health-

ful restaurant choices available, given that many people eat out?

The first on-site meeting is a presentation to the key stakeholders of the host institution, outlining the Ornish program, its potential benefits to their community, and the scope of the assessment process. At a second visit, additional on-site meetings and interviews are scheduled to evaluate each of the key elements of success described above. During the course of these meetings, PMRI staff assess the level of interest and the potential support for the program. This is a multifaceted process. The meetings also provide a venue for educating the community about the nature of the treatment program and serve as opportunities to plant seeds for future success.

Key Qualities of Prospective Clients: The Model of Readiness to Change

When evaluating the population of a typical community, research suggests that approximately 5% to 10% will be ready for change. For this receptive segment of the population, simply being provided with good information enables them to begin a process of change. Whether they buy a book or obtain information on the Internet, they will initiate the changes by themselves.

Another 5% to 10% of the people on the other end of the spectrum are unlikely to make any change. Then there are the 80% in the middle; 40% are typically moving away from change, and 40% are moving toward change. Unless something dramatic happens, those moving away from change will probably not reverse their behavior. However, they may become motivated to change through a catastrophic life event, for example, learning that a family member has heart disease or discovering that they have it themselves.

The Ornish program focuses on the 40% of any population who are moving toward change. These are well-intentioned people who have tried various exercise programs and different diets without success because, like most of us, they really need a support structure to make major changes in their lives. Otherwise, they usually do not succeed on their own.

People who are highly motivated tend to do very well in this program. Those who are participating simply to please their family have a much harder time than those who are self-motivated.

Assessing the Readiness of the Community

An important aspect of the community evaluation is this readiness-to-change model. When PMRI develops a program, staff consider the general level of receptivity. This is a significant factor that must be in evidence not only in patients, but also in the community culture.

- Is a significant proportion of the community ready for change?
- What are the unique circumstances presented here?
- How should the program be introduced at this particular site?
- What are the keys to success in this particular environment?

PMRI has been fortunate to be invited into communities by people who fundamentally understand population-based wellness programming. They realize that the goal is to provide resources so that people can take their health into their own hands, working with the support of the program.

IMPLEMENTING THE PROGRAM

Adapting the Program to the Community

PMRI recognizes that each community has a distinctive dynamic. Therefore, although the core program does not change from site to site, the specifics are adapted to fit the culture of the community. For example, in the nutritional component, foods served in the program are selected from those typically eaten by people in that community or region. The transition to a healthier diet begins with these choices. When there is a predominant ethnic component to the community, our nutritionists and executive chef work with the on-site nutritionist and food service provider to determine how to modify recipes to make them healthier, yet still taste familiar.

The culture of the community dictates how the program will be taught although the components remain fundamentally the same. They remain the same because the research has shown that if patients participate in these core components, they are much more likely to positively affect their disease. For example, if there is a predominant religious orientation in the community, the stress management component provides the option of incorporating familiar prayers from that religious culture into the meditation exercises.

Training the Staff

The quality of the staff who implement the intervention will make or break a program of this kind. The program's design requires a multidisciplinary team that is cross-trained with a flat, decentralized structure in which team members collaborate and make decisions with an attitude of shared responsibility and leadership.

In a typical medical environment, these staff members are frequently separated by geography, proximity, and organizational structure. After the patient sees the physician, he or she may be referred to a nutritionist, an exercise physiologist, or a cardiac rehabilitation program. However, often there is less opportunity to integrate care. The value of having a team that works together includes the opportunity to provide case conferences in which staff can focus as a team on the progress of the patients. This integrated, multidisciplinary team approach can provide practitioners with additional insight into the medical needs of the patient, thereby allowing providers to further tailor interventions for each individual.

Training is provided for the new site by staff members from PMRI. Practitioners at the host facility are trained in order to be licensed to offer the program. They receive classroom education and participate in a week-long residential retreat. Through these experiences, they become immersed in the culture of the program very quickly and become attuned to the transformative qualities of this approach.

The program is implemented by practitioners at the host site trained by the Institute. They typically include an exercise physiologist, a nutritionist, a support group leader, and a stress management instructor. In addition, there is a case manager, a program director, a medical director, and at some sites, one person who coordinates marketing activities and oversees data collection. Some practitioners are cross-trained and function in two different roles.

This type of support is exceptionally important for clients who are making lifestyle changes. A 1999 study on heart disease and lifestyle factors among nurses found that those who had a healthy lifestyle had an 82% better chance of avoiding heart disease than their contemporaries. However, the research confirmed the tremendous difficulty in actually implementing this kind of lifestyle. Only 1% of the nurses in the study fully maintained all health behaviors such as eating a healthy diet, exercising regularly, not smoking, and managing stress.

These same needs have been identified in the clients who have participated in PMRI studies. It is clear that for most people, basic lifestyle changes will probably not occur unless there is a rich support structure in place. Clearly, it serves agencies and providers who are developing programming to include support structures that enable people to make and maintain healthy lifestyle choices.

Adapting the Protocol to Client Needs

The first demonstration project was basically a one-size-fits-all program. The initial protocol required 1 full year of program participation. Clients came for a weekend retreat, then attended three times a week for 12 weeks. After the initial immersion in the program, clients participated once a week for the remainder of the year.

Based on the key learnings from the demonstration project, PMRI created a second-generation model. The goal of that model has been to maintain the clinical integrity of the program, while customizing the protocol to fit the needs of the clients, in response to the severity of their condition and the needs of their lifestyle. This more flexible approach has increased the financial viability for host institutions. PMRI created a risk-stratified model in which clients participate for 3 months, 6 months, 9 months, or 1 year. The duration of participation depends on the severity of the participant's condition or risk, his or her adherence to the program, and fundamental understanding and compliance—whether the participant "gets" the program. People may be in the program for as little as 3 months or as long as a year. Even if an individual is only in the program for 3 months, he or she is still monitored and receives case management services for a full year. The case management component is essential.

Providing Client Support

Support is one of the key ingredients provided in the program. As mentioned, an exceptional professional team is available to support change. An even more important factor is the support of the group. This is the community of people who go through the program together as a cohort. The support of the group helps each individual remain involved and committed to the program. They find that they develop deeply meaningful connections with others who are also facing the same challenges. This sense of connectedness often occurs on a level they have never before experienced.

In addition, participants begin observing tangible improvements in their own health early in the program, such as diminished angina pain, the increased ability to exercise, and clarity of thinking. These changes can provide surprisingly rapid benefit. If patients did not experience the tangible benefits they gain from the program early on, they would not be motivated to stay with the program. In fact, one spectacular statistic is that the attrition rate is only 10% per year. *The low attrition rate is the result of several factors:*

- Program sites screen potential patients carefully to determine their level of motivation.
- A substantial professional support environment is maintained.
- As patients go through the program together in a group, the group dynamic provides an impressive level of support and reinforcement.
- Patients experience significant and dramatic tangible changes that make it clear that if they continue to maintain this new lifestyle, they will have less pain and more energy.

Participants are also kept motivated by the data that serve as concrete indications of progress. PMRI obtains in-depth data at every stage of the program. Consequently, staff can objectively demonstrate the health status of participants at baseline and at any stage throughout the program. PMRI obviously cannot promise that all adherents will reverse their heart disease, but the outcomes data are very encouraging.

When PMRI staff meet former patients face-to-face who are healthy and vibrant, with no sign that they have ever had heart disease, it is very gratifying. Efforts in the program tend to be fairly abstract rather than clinical, focused on research, the development of treatment protocols, and planning strategies. Meeting participants reconnects staff with the program in a more direct way and reminds them of the ultimate motivation in this work.

CONCLUSION

Within the challenging world of health care delivery, it is incumbent on programs with a lifestyle-treatment orientation to use professional business methodology, to ensure the success of their delivery system and the continued expansion of programs. For this reason, PMRI and now Lifestyle Advantage have chosen to use this type of systematic approach with any new community or organization that wants to make lifestyle programs available to its members. This orientation includes all the traditional forms of demographic research, economic analysis, and resource assessment that would be included in any planned business development. These efforts are intended to provide a foundation for the clinical component, which can then be implemented and individualized to meet the needs of the community and its clients.

BIBLIOGRAPHY

Dienstfrey H. What makes the heart healthy? A talk with Dean Ornish. *Advances.* 1992;8:25–45.

Gould KL, Ornish DM, Kirkeeide R, et al. Improved stenosis geometry by quantitative coronary arteriography after vigorous risk factor modification. *Am J Cardiol.* 1992;69(9):845–853.

Gould KL, Ornish DM, Scherwitz L, et al. Changes in myocardial perfusion abnormalities by positron emission tomography after long-term, intense risk factor modification. *JAMA.* 1995;274(11):894–901.

Ornish DM. Avoiding revascularization with lifestyle changes: The Multicenter Lifestyle Demonstration Project. *Am J Cardiol.* 1998;82(10B):72T–76T.

Ornish DM. Can life-style changes reverse coronary atherosclerosis? *Hosp Pract.* 1991;26(5):123–126, 129–132.

Ornish DM. Lessons from the Lifestyle Heart Trial. *Choices in Cardiology.* 1991;5:24–27.

Ornish DM. Lifestyle Heart Trial. *Cardiovascular Risk Factors.* 1992;2(4):277–281.

Ornish DM. Reversing heart disease through diet, exercise, and stress management: an interview with Dean Ornish. *J Am Diet Assoc.* 1991;91(2):162–165.

Ornish D, Brown SE, Scherwitz LW, et al. Can lifestyle changes reverse coronary heart disease? The Lifestyle Heart Trial. *Lancet.* 1990;336(8708):129–133.

Ornish D, Scherwitz LW, Billings JH, et al. Intensive lifestyle changes for reversal of coronary heart disease. *JAMA.* 1998;280(23):2001–2007.

CHAPTER 10

Pursuing Integration: A Model of Integrated Delivery of Complementary and Alternative Medicine

Charles A. Simpson

integration *n.* **1.** the act or instance of combining into an integral whole. **2.** behavior in harmony with the environment. (Stein, 1975)

A MODEL OF HEALTH CARE INTEGRATION

Stephen Shortell and colleagues (1996) have studied the development of integrated delivery systems through the lens of community health care management. Shortell's model defines and describes the dimensions of system integration in integrated health delivery systems. His analysis is fully relevant to the processes of integration that are occurring within complementary and alternative medicine (CAM) as it becomes a part of mainstream health care. By necessity, these processes must continue if CAM is to become an integral part of the health care system.

Shortell's model considers integration from three perspectives:

1. administrative integration
2. practitioner-system integration
3. clinical integration

Charles A. Simpson, DC, has been a practicing chiropractor for over 20 years. He is a founder and currently the Chief Medical Officer of Complementary Healthcare Plans (CHP) of Portland, Ore. CHP provides integrated acupuncture, chiropractic, naturopathic medicine, and massage therapy services for health plans, health maintenance organizations, and preferred provider organizations in Oregon and Washington state.

Administrative Integration

Administrative or functional integration is the administrative platform on which clinical integration and the integration of practitioners in the system can occur. Shortell defines administrative integration as "the extent to which key support activities are coordinated so as to add the greatest overall value to the system." This concept identifies the primary functional components most reflective of the level of integration within the organization such as financial management, human resources, information systems, strategic planning, and continuous quality improvement (total quality management). High levels of "systemness," in his words, define the higher degrees of integration. Shortell and colleagues believe "that a system's vision, culture, strategic orientation, and leadership will be positively associated with its degree of functional [administrative and organization] integration." It is the administrative platform on which practitioner-system and clinical integration can occur. In order for CAM to become an effective part of the health care delivery system, CAM and its practitioners must be integrated at these three fundamental levels.

Practitioner-System Integration

Practitioner-system integration reflects "the extent to which physicians and other practitioners are economically linked to a system, use its facilities and services, [and] participate in its planning, management and governance." The nature of the linkage between each practitioner and the health care system will set the stage for how the practitioner sees and executes his or her role in the system. Whether the system is viewed as a partner or an adversary can have a significant impact on general health care outcomes, as well as specific clinical outcomes. The impact of cohesion or friction in the system may well determine the effectiveness of complementary medicine provision within the health care system and ultimately be reflected in both cost and patient outcomes.

Clinical Integration

Clinical integration is defined by Shortell as "the extent to which patient care services are coordinated across people, functions, activities, and sites so as to maximize the value of services delivered to patients." Administrative and practitioner-system integration underpin clinical integration. The foundation of clinical integration is the integration of administrative/organizational functions and the integration of the provider into the system. In order for patients to maximize the benefits of integrated CAM services, care providers, both mainstream and alternative, must function as a team. Shortell's idea of clinical integration brings into focus the elements that must be coordinated to create a functional health care team.

The Value of Integration

Shortell and colleagues (1996) cite the Institute for the Future for its view of an ideal health system. In "the perfect world of a fully integrated medical system, each clinical decision—whether it be a decision regarding drug therapy versus surgery, ambulatory care versus hospital admission, or nutritional counseling versus psychological counseling—would be determined by answering the question: 'How can we, the providers and the system, restore the patient's health using the smallest amount of total resources?'"

CAM interventions offer meaningful options in the effort to restore health effectively while using the fewest resources. Complementary therapies typically provide minimalist, noninvasive approaches to early-stage and chronic health conditions. These therapeutics can be one of the rational first steps in many protocols that address nonacute conditions. CAM treatments with a demonstrated history of effectiveness are coming to be seen as viable options in medical treatment and clinical care pathways. Used appropriately and knowledgeably, successful CAM therapeutics meet the criteria for safety, efficacy, and cost-effectiveness.

Evidence on the use of CAM services suggests that in the current system, it is patients who integrate CAM through their own personal strategies for obtaining medical care. Eisenberg et al (1993), for example, reported that 83% of patients who sought CAM treatments for serious medical conditions saw mainstream practitioners as well. However, more than 70% of patients did not inform their mainstream practitioners regarding their use of CAM services (Eisenberg et al, 1993)

The lack of integration between CAM and mainstream practitioners has effectively forced patients to integrate their own care. Patients currently determine when to use CAM and when to choose mainstream care. The question for practitioners and health care organizations becomes: Can CAM and mainstream practitioners, working together in integrated systems, provide meaningful assistance to patients for the integration of their health care? In this context, pursuing the integration of CAM and mainstream therapies has the potential to improve outcomes for patients, enhance treatment protocols for practitioners, and provide strategic market advantages for health plans.

To fulfill this potential, it will become important that complementary therapies become better integrated into the clinical offerings of the health care system in a manner that is meaningful and effective. This will require sound information and training, well-linked communication, and the alignment of incentives throughout the system.

In the real world, however, imperfect information, incomplete communication, conflicting incentives, and organizational/professional biases tend to hinder the process of seamless integration—particularly the integration of disciplines that have historically been polarized. The purpose of integration is to improve communication, resolve conflict, prioritize incentives, and eliminate biases. An integrated system's goal is to provide technical support and offer positive and negative sanctions that can counteract negative influences. This is a valuable model that can be used to evaluate the effective incorporation of complementary and alternative approaches into systems of health care delivery.

Trends in Integration

Enthusiasm for integration among industrial and business organizations has ebbed and flowed over the past several decades. Feverish periods of corporate mergers and acquisitions are often followed by divestiture and return to core competencies. The creation of virtual organizations is another strategic approach that attempts to achieve the benefits of consolidation but avoid the creation of ponderous and inefficient organizational structures. Ongoing trends toward outsourcing and downsizing are evident, with the goal of achieving greater efficiency and productivity.

However, the trend in health care may well be in the other direction, toward higher levels of integration. Within CAM, significant trends toward integration are also evident. In just a decade, CAM has rapidly evolved from an enterprise practiced by sole practitioners or in small group practices to disciplines included in organized networks, expanding medical centers, and certain institutional environments.

Examples of both virtual and bricks-and-mortar strategies abound. Health plans typically have had to decide whether to buy or build networks of CAM practitioners. The virtual organization of network model health maintenance organizations (HMOs) can be readily adapted to incorporate CAM practitioners. Other success-ful models also exist. Many plans, hospitals, and medical groups are now seriously considering bringing CAM and mainstream practitioners into bricks-and-mortar arrangements in full-scale, interdisciplinary facilities.

Financial and Organizational Incentives for Integration

From a broad perspective, Shortell and others (1996) identify two key elements that seem to be driving a "rush to integration" in health care: complexity and financial incentives. Shortell's work is focused primarily on large integrated delivery systems, usually hospital-based. The features of complexity and the nature of new financial arrangements combine to drive health care into increasingly "organized" systems.

In order for most patients to have access to CAM services, it is important that CAM practitioners and CAM organizations develop the strategies and technologies that can effectively navigate this rush to integration. Moving from isolated sole-practitioner, cash-based models of practice to network and group models with insurance-based reimbursement presents significant challenges to both the consumer and the organization. It also presents dynamic opportunities to make the benefits of CAM available to the majority of the population.

The health care enterprise is exceedingly complex and interdependent. The restoration of a patient's health often requires the combined expertise of many different practitioners, particularly in the context of integrative medicine. When patients have chronic or acute conditions, care may be provided in a variety of environments or facilities, by different practitioners, using numerous technologies. The outcome of the process can be significantly affected by factors outside the direct control of any particular caregiver. The ultimate outcomes (the products of health care) can be extremely difficult to measure. Shortell observes that this complex and interdependent nature of health care demands a "high degree of integration" to be as successful as possible. In this context, the coordination between mainstream and complementary disciplines is as relevant and important as that which occurs elsewhere in health care.

Integrating the delivery of health care and its financial aspects brings into focus the need to achieve efficiencies by the elimination of duplicative or unnecessary services, clinically inappropriate or conflicting interventions, and the use of the least intensive setting and least invasive procedure appropriate for effective care. Again, this perspective is pertinent to the integration of CAM. One of the primary concerns of insurers is whether and when CAM therapies will be provided *in addition to* conventional care, rather than *in lieu of* mainstream medicine. Greater understanding and coordination of CAM technologies could enhance protocols and therapeutics without wasteful duplication. Economic constraints make these considerations more important than ever. Capitation adds further fuel to the fires of integration in health care.

Systems Integration As the Impetus for Innovation

As Hertzlinger (1997) suggests, the most successful organizational responses to the need for system integration incorporate systems perspectives, integration through strategic partnership, and technological innovations such as reorganized work teams, employee empowerment, and information sharing. Successful organizations move away from "big is beautiful" and "top down" strategies. She is convinced that this same approach can be utilized to create "integrated, efficient, and focused systems of health care." Complementary and alternative medicine can be seen as another form of innovation that applies primarily low-tech medical technologies and styles of practice.

While Hertzlinger and Shortell tend to have quite different pictures of effective health care delivery organizations (virtually integrated health care versus integrated delivery systems), both theorists indicate the need for successful strategic integration. In the delivery of CAM, each of these models of delivery has become relevant—in the networks and panels that are essentially types of virtual systems, as well as in the more highly integrated freestanding medical centers. Shortell's work also provides an appropriate framework for evaluation when considering the integration of CAM into organized systems of health care.

ADMINISTRATIVE INTEGRATION

Administrative or functional integration is the extent to which key support functions work together within the system; these include financial management, the business side of the infrastructure, information systems, the technologies of contracting, organizational leadership, strategic planning, and the organization's commitment to total quality management. Administrative integration really means the way that all these different elements fit together across the organization to drive the quest for value, effectiveness, and efficiency.

Strategic Vision

The strategic vision of the organization is a fundamental component that contributes to administrative integration. The goals that the system is trying to achieve set the tone and direction for administrative functions and activities. In health care, strategic vision rightfully includes perspectives on the health needs of the populations served and the difficult chore of meeting those needs with the resources that are available. For an organization contemplating the integration of CAM, how CAM is incorporated into the strategic vision of the organization will be reflected in the ultimate success of the endeavors in complementary medicine. The extent of integration may predict whether the CAM initiative will be able to realize its full potential within the organization. This will involve factoring in the unique perspectives that CAM and CAM practitioners bring to health care.

The Influence of Leadership and Organizational Culture

Effective leadership by both administrative and clinical leaders is crucial to the successful integration of CAM within an organization. In fact, until there is clear buy-in from the leadership, it is possible that the best course of action is to wait to initiate CAM programming. The most effective leadership in the integration process will come from those who have had clinical or personal experience with CAM therapies and consequently perceive their value in improving patient health. Leaders who view CAM as strictly a market-driven add-on to a health plan are likely to perceive CAM much differently than leaders who understand the clinical value of CAM services. The extent to which an organization's leaders buy in to CAM integration will determine how well (or how poorly) CAM interventions will be implemented. This will ultimately be reflected in program success and patient outcomes.

The character of the organization's culture will also have an impact on the degree of integration of CAM. Cultures that encourage inquiry, objective evaluation, and evidence-based activity are more likely to incorporate the innovations of CAM health care delivery. Systems that are driven by performance measurement will be able to recognize and leverage the effectiveness of appropriate CAM treatment strategies and further the incorporation of them into health care practices.

PROVIDER-SYSTEM INTEGRATION

Linking CAM Providers with the System

Highly integrated organizational and administrative systems tend to support the interface of practitioners with the system. Corporate cultures that value collaboration and partnership are much more able to see all practitioners as partners. This collaboration will have an impact on performance, outcomes, and economics. The alignment of incentives among all stakeholders in the health care enterprise (payers, practitioners, and patients) holds the best possibility of maximizing the value of the health care dollar.

The effective delivery of health care is an interdependent endeavor. This is no less true of integrative medicine. When patients present with complex or chronic conditions, the restoration of health often requires the combined expertise of many different practitioners and facilities across the continuum of services. In order to realize the potential benefits of CAM in arenas such as disease management, these services and the practitioners that render them must become an integral part of the health care team.

Practitioner integration typically is considered in terms of the economic linkages between health care providers and the system; access to and use of facilities; and participation in planning, management, and governance (Shortell et al, 1996). The discussion here focuses on each of these components as they relate to CAM providers and to the unique challenges and barriers to effective integration of nontraditional health care providers into managed care and health systems.

Aligning the Incentives

Long-term success in the managed care arena requires rationalizing and balancing the often competing goals and objectives of the parties at the managed care table. Practitioners, patients, and payers each have unique and sometimes conflicting needs. Providers seek professional compensation and maximum autonomy. Patients look for empathy and results. Payers are interested in the highest quality for the lowest cost (the search for maximum value). To be successful, managed care organizations must achieve an appropriate balance among these sometimes opposing desires.

The extent to which practitioners are committed to and supportive of the goals of a managed care enterprise can have a significant impact on the success of that enterprise as it seeks to satisfy the needs of all stakeholders. Practitioner loyalty frequently hinges on the extent to which managed care organizations achieve effective integration of those practitioners. Shortell and others (1996) propose a model of physician integration that presents a continuum of integration ranging from independent practice associations to more fully organized group practices, physician hospital organizations, staff model HMOs, and equity model managed care organizations. This continuum is also relevant to CAM services, with more complete integration occurring in risk-bearing networks and staff model integrative medicine clinics. The array of organizational models and integration strategies that currently exists provides the means for health plans to begin the process of bringing the benefits of CAM services to plan members. How a plan chooses to engage with CAM practitioners can determine in part the potential for effective integration.

The underlying strategy in provider integration is realignment of incentives. For example, in managed care organizations, sharing financial risk with CAM providers emphasizes the need for practitioners to make treatment decisions carefully. Rather than "doing everything possible," the clinical focus becomes "doing what is effective and efficient."

CAM Provider Access to Managed Care Services

Another dimension of CAM provider-health care system integration is the ease of using, and extent to which CAM providers use, the other health care services of the health plan in caring for that health plan's members. The degree of integration is reflected in access to conventional medical providers for diagnostic and specialized therapeutic services in managing their patients' conditions. Diagnostic imaging, for example, is often ordered by chiropractors, naturopathic physicians, and other CAM providers. Clinical laboratory testing is also a routine part of many CAM treatment programs.

Fully integrated primary care and specialist providers in managed care are usually constrained by contract to refer to hospital, diagnostic and ancillary treatment facilities, and services in their own networks or systems. Similar relationships between CAM providers and managed care services have yet to develop fully. This aspect of integration is inhibited by lack of more coherent financial integration. In the absence of incentives like those which drive clinical decisions by integrated providers, there is little that can convince managers of a health plan that diagnostic and ancillary services use by CAM providers will be appropriate and cost-effective.

The typical carve-out arrangements in CAM often provide for certain diagnostic services within the structure of the CAM benefit. Radiography services, for example, are usually covered by chiropractic benefit packages. Members attending a contracted chiropractor can receive radiographs either taken in the chiropractor's office or at a contracted facility. These diagnostic tests are available without the need for the CAM provider to send the patient back into the system for a primary care referral for that test.

In this type of arrangement, utilization can be controlled through a risk-sharing arrangement between the health plan and its network of providers. Consider the example of a chiropractic network in an HMO that offers a capitated carve-out chiropractic rider with coverage for radiographs. Practitioners within the network are at risk for diagnostic services including radiographs and other relevant laboratory tests. Practitioners who have radiographic facilities in their own offices are reimbursed out of the capitation pool according to a schedule. Practitioners who must refer out for laboratory or radiographic examinations remain at risk for the cost, either paying for the testing themselves or striking an arrangement with the facility to accept the network's fee schedule.

In the network described, overutilization of certain services is also controlled through a gatekeeper mechanism. The network has not contracted for risk with regard to more advanced imaging services such as computed tomography (CT) scans or magnetic resonance imaging (MRI). Chiropractic practice often makes use of these imaging modalities, although much less frequently than radiographs. Patients who require advanced imaging must be referred back into the system to the member's primary care provider, who in turn must decide whether to make the referral for the diagnostic test. Great care is required on the part of the chiropractor's office not to create unwarranted patient expectations.

Practitioner Participation in Planning, Management, and Governance

Medical practice has historically been characterized by individual practitioners plying their trade in relative isolation. Within orthodox medicine, growing professionalism initiated a trend toward group-based peer relationships that has tended to create a more homogeneous profession. Starr (1984) documents the rise of medicine from its historical beginnings to its position of sovereignty and cultural authority in the twentieth century. He points out that the tension between medicine's professional dominance and the economic imperatives of the business of health care came to be accommodated largely through the reorganization of medical practice. Starr notes, ". . . underlying tension continues today—between a medical care system geared toward expansion and a society and state requiring some means of control over medical expenditures . . . controlling expansion means redrawing the contract between the medical profession and society, subjecting medical care to the discipline of politics or markets or reorganizing its basic institutional structure."

The reorganization growing out of the conflict between professional autonomy and socioeconomic imperatives has resulted in the "corporatization" of health care. The willingness and abilities of physicians to participate in corporate medical life may spell the difference between professional survival in reorganized health care and relegation to a more marginalized role as simply a provider of health care services. While many physicians decry corporate medicine, others see participation in the planning, leadership, and management of health care as the only available avenue to advocate for maintaining quality health care and, not incidentally, respectable measures of continued professional autonomy.

Inglehart projected in his 1992 essay that ". . . the basic challenge of managed care plans is to create systems in which physicians are delegated the responsibility for managing care and then held accountable for their performance . . . well-run managed care schemes have considerable potential for allowing physicians to use their clinical skills as full partners in the quest to allocate scarce health care resources effectively." Full partnership extends to direct participation in management and governance of managed care organizations.

Many managed care organizations recognize the strategic advantage that can be realized by effective integration of physician-providers into management roles. A commitment to effective integration of CAM providers into managed care systems would do well to follow this same model. CAM providers who share the same commitment will develop a deeper understanding of the challenges and opportunities presented with the potential of becoming more competent managed care leaders. An indicator of CAM-system integration would be the extent to which CAM professionals confront the challenges and seize these opportunities.

CLINICAL INTEGRATION

Patient-Centered Health Care

Shortell and colleagues (1996) define clinical integration as "the extent to which patient care services are coordinated across people, functions, activities, and sites so as to maximize the value of services delivered to patients."

Shortell's study focuses on integrated delivery systems and identifies several indicators that are relevant to clinical integration of CAM into health care systems. These include clinical protocol development, medical records uniformity and accessibility, outcomes data collection, shared clinical support services, and perceived clinical integration. To this list can be added the opportunities for research in the areas of health services and cost-effectiveness.

Clinical Integration and Competitiveness

Successful clinical integration, from Shortell's perspective, is a patient-centered approach that is consistent with the strategy of "mass customization" as advocated by Peters (1994) and others. The idea of mass customization recommends that business focus intensively on the needs and desires of its customers. Rather than producing goods and services designed to meet the needs of the average customer, business can realize a significant competitive advantage by having the capability to produce on demand goods or services that meet each customer's needs more exactly.

The extent to which the plan recognizes the unique needs and preferences of each member and then positions itself to meet them can have a large impact on that plan's ability to attract and retain customers. Plans traditionally have sought to offer attractive arrays of orthodox medical and allied services in an attempt to meet the health care needs of their prospective members and to differentiate themselves in the marketplace. The public's intense interest in CAM services has penetrated thinking in health plans to make these formerly invisible and unorthodox methods of healing seem attractive. At the present time, the attraction of CAM therapies may be primarily on the basis of their popularity among patients and members. As the integration of CAM proceeds, the focus will shift to the use of the most effective of these technologies through the identification of the most highly efficacious therapies. This focus is likely to occur in the context of disease management for specific diagnoses

and disorders, ideally individualized to meet the unique needs of patients, given their orientation to health and their preference for health care interventions.

Successful clinical integration from the patient's perspective—from the knowledgeable CAM users' point of view—will be a clinical encounter that is marked by medically appropriate and effective combinations of CAM and orthodox procedures. Patients value care that reflects smooth coordination among orthodox and CAM providers, efficient transfer of information among providers and facilities, and clinical outcomes that are better both in terms of satisfaction and health status. Health systems that can achieve effective integration of CAM into the mix of services for patient care will realize a significant advantage in meeting the needs of patients who do use CAM. As Eisenberg (1998) and Astin (1998) both have noted, this is a significant percentage of the population.

The Potential Benefits of CAM Research

Clinical integration holds the prospect of producing health care services that are even more effective, strategically applied, and thoroughly integrated, as data are accrued through expanded research efforts. The integration of CAM in health systems creates significant opportunities for research. Traditionally, in settings outside of insurance-based reimbursement, CAM data collection was almost impossible; even the aggregation of the most basic data on CAM, its users, utility, and outcomes was very difficult. Data have simply been inaccessible. The integration of providers into the system enhances the development of data streams that can be analyzed for information that will contribute to outcomes assessment, health services research, and cost-effectiveness studies. These investigations will help clarify for health plan managers and clinicians the clinical conditions that benefit most from CAM interventions, where CAM services may lower cost through effective forms of care, and where the most value is to be derived in the allocation of health care resources.

Once this type of data and information are available to financial and medical managers, the basis for CAM inclusion is likely to change. Business decisions to provide CAM services in a health plan's offerings will be based on CAM's demonstrated cost-effectiveness and not simply on its market appeal. Clinical decisions to render CAM treatment will be on the basis of sound, evidence-based clinical practice. CAM will be a part of health systems not only because of its popularity among certain client populations, but also because of its cost-effectiveness and clinical efficacy.

Clinical Cost-Effectiveness

In a sense, managed care has become the surrogate for the public's desire to restrain health care costs. The advent of managed care in all its various forms can be seen as a response to the pressure inflated health care costs have brought to bear on public and private resources. As a result, managed care organizations have had to wrestle with each of the forces that tend to drive up health care costs: the oversupply of physicians and providers, expanding technological innovations, increasing patient and public expectations, and demographic factors.

From an individual provider's perspective, most of the cost inflation pressures appear to be beyond the reach of effective control. An individual practitioner has little ability to moderate the public's demand to do "everything possible" in the pursuit of restoring health or extending life. These are generic problems across all types of health care that affect most all practitioners. Every practitioner is confronted periodically with patients and families who want the maximum level of care.

Another example of trends that practitioners find difficult to manage is the proliferation of direct-to-consumer advertising of prescription drugs, hormones, herbs, and nutritional supplements. Yet this type of marketing thrust has a great deal of effect on consumer demand and also ultimately on cost. The most potent leverage that individual practitioners have to restrain cost

is the reduction of medically unnecessary care. Some element of control can be exercised by providers to create efficiencies, without sacrificing quality, in the elimination of care that is duplicative, inappropriate for the patient's condition, or delivered in a setting or form that is more cost-intensive than necessary.

The primary threat to clinical efficiency may be unexplainable variation in the way in which health care is delivered. Wennberg's seminal work (O'Connor et al, 1999) on regional variation in surgical rates in hospitals unleashed a veritable flood of studies fully documenting wide variation in health care practices. CAM practice has largely escaped inspection for variation because of lack of data about CAM service delivery. Most CAM services have been paid for out of pocket outside of health care systems. Consequently, these services have not been evident in data sets that are typically included in the economic analysis of health care services research. Developing and using these data in health systems is necessary to reduce variation in CAM practice and improve its cost effectiveness.

MODELS FOR MANAGERS

As physicians have become more fully integrated into health care systems, they have encountered the mixed blessing of greater requirements for leadership and management capabilities. CAM providers who anticipate similar degrees of provider-system integration must prepare to meet similarly high expectations for performance in managed care and health systems.

Within the fields of health care, foremost among the several competencies necessary for an effective CAM manager is a clear vision of managed care philosophy. CAM managers are challenged to articulate this vision and communicate it to practitioners on the one hand and to managers on the other. Yet this skill is the necessary complement to a coherent managed care philosophy. Communication skills also necessarily include the ability to listen effectively. Clinician-managers are frequently in the role of the go-between, listening to the concerns of providers and translating them into terms understood by managers and, conversely, explaining the concerns of management to practitioners.

There is an ongoing balance of opposing perspectives that must be reconciled within health systems: the autonomy of providers in making health care decisions and the system's drive to maximize value for purchasers. It can be suggested that practitioners themselves have the ideal vantage point from which to resolve the seeming clash of cultures between the business of health care and the traditional orientation of providers as advocates for their patients' needs. The goal is commitment to a vision of health care that can achieve objectives of both high-quality health care delivery and rational allocation of health care resources. This is the well from which effective clinical leaders can draw credibility and authority.

REFERENCES

Astin JA. Why patients use alternative medicine: results of a national study. *JAMA*. 1998;279(19):1548–1553.

Eisenberg D, Davis R, Ettner S, et al. Trends in alternative medicine use in the United States, 1990–1997: results of a follow-up national survey. *JAMA*. 1998;280(18): 1569–1575.

Eisenberg DM, Kessler RC, Foster C, et al. Unconventional medicine in the United States. *N Engl J Med*. 1993; 328(4):246–252.

Hertzlinger R. *Market Driven Health Care*. Reading, MA: Perseus Books; 1997.

Inglehart J. Health policy report: managed care. *N Engl J Med*. 1992;327:742–747.

O'Connor GT, Quinton HB, Traven ND, et al. Geographic variation in the treatment of acute myocardial infarction: the Cooperative Cardiovascular Project. *JAMA*. 1999;281(7):627–633.

Peters T. *The Pursuit of Wow!* New York: Vintage Books; 1994.

Shortell SR, Anderson D, Erickson K, Mitchell J. *Remaking Health Care in America*. San Francisco: Jossey-Bass; 1996.

Starr P. *Social Transformation of American Medicine*. New York: Basic Books; 1984.

Stein J, ed. *The Random House College Dictionary*. New York: Random House; 1975.

PART III

Reimbursement, Marketing, and Policy

CHAPTER 11

Reimbursement and Funding

11.1 Strategic Planning for Reimbursement

Linda L. Bedell-Logan with Nancy Faass

Complementary and alternative medicine (CAM) has created a shift in patient utilization of medical services. In the past decade, this expanded patient demand has been validated through new research indicating that CAM therapies are being utilized more often and that more money is paid out of pocket for these therapies than in the primary care arena (Eisenberg et al, 1993; 1998). Since 1991, there has also been an increase in the allocation of federal research dollars for CAM therapies with the establishment of the Office of Alternative Medicine and its

expansion as the National Center for Complementary and Alternative Medicine (NCCAM, 2000). Preliminary outcome studies focusing on chronic pain and disease and the use of CAM therapies are very promising. In this environment, managed care organizations and health systems are endeavoring to respond to patient interest in alternatives. The resultant expansion of integrative solutions within health care has been the impetus for a range of programmatic efforts.

AN EPIDEMIOLOGICAL APPROACH TO DISEASE MANAGEMENT

One of the most effective strategies in developing CAM programs is the use of epidemiology in program design. From region to region and state to state, the incidence of disease differs, and as a result, the primary medical needs of the population are different. The profile of any given community depends in part on the environment, lifestyle, genetics, ethnic belief systems, and other factors. In order to design a viable program, the prevailing medical needs of the community should be evaluated in an effort

Linda L. Bedell-Logan, President and CEO of Solutions in Integrative Medicine, attended the University of Southern Maine and has worked in health care administration for Medicare and the private sector. She initiated her consulting and billing practice 10 years ago, after the death of her 25-year-old sister from cancer and her 33-year-old brother from AIDS, viewing her own losses as a catalyst to work for change. Her firm has consulted on the development of more than 65 integrative medicine centers to date, including those of major universities and hospitals such as Harvard, Stanford, and Yale. A nationally recognized speaker, she has also participated in research studies and continuing medical education with the team of David Eisenberg, MD, at Harvard/Beth Israel Deaconess Medical Center in Boston.

to design regionally unique disease management programs.

Obtaining Baseline Data on the Community

The U.S. Public Health Service indicates that 70% of health care dollars go to 30% of patients. To develop a program, epidemiological data should be used to identify which diseases are affecting the 30%. In Pennsylvania, it could be diabetes and diverticulitis. In Southern California, it might be cancer and asthma. Across the country, the medical needs of the population vary widely. In designing a complementary medicine center, the programmatic response to these needs not only focuses on disease management, but also on prevention and wellness programs that provide continuity in the area of longevity and quality of life beyond symptomatology.

Identifying Relevant CAM Therapeutics

Once the medical needs of the community have been identified, emerging CAM technologies can be applied to address these needs. Assume, for example, that asthma, migraines, and cancer are the conditions resulting in the highest utilization of medical care in a particular region. Having identified the diseases causing overutilization, one can use the research to determine which types of therapies are relevant to the needs of the community, based on the evidence for effectiveness in the peer-reviewed medical literature (evidence-based medicine). The specific treatments and services to be offered can then be selected. For example, the plan may be to manage asthma through an integrative approach that includes acupuncture, alternative allergy testing, environmental evaluation, biofeedback, and nutrition. The types of therapies and practitioners that will need to be available within the integrative team have been identified based on the evidence. As the center develops, further analysis of outcomes will allow the team to refine evidence-based treatment protocols. The goal is to achieve the maximum medical outcomes in the most cost-efficient manner.

Specifying Risk

Insurance companies set rates based on health risk in the cities and regions they cover. If insurers are suffering the economic burden of having to meet the needs of overutilization, this approach will be relevant to them as well. An epidemiological approach to disease management provides a rational way to open the dialogue with insurers. It makes more sense to target services, for example, than to ask the insurer to cover innovative cancer treatments in a region with low cancer rates. Basing decisions on in-depth data increases the potential for positive insurance partnership.

TRACKING OUTCOMES

The term *evidence-based medicine* implies the inclusion of a research component. This industry's development is at the point at which everyone wants outcomes: NCCAM at the National Institutes of Health (NIH), insurers, managed care organizations, physicians, and consumers. In conventional medicine, there are electronic medical record systems in place to assist in tracking clinical and financial outcomes. In complementary and integrative medicine, electronic medical records that track CAM therapies such as traditional Chinese medicine do not yet exist or are in the process of development. Retrospective data are available, but they are difficult to interpret at this preliminary stage.

A major component of practice management involves putting systems into place to track the center's clinical outcomes. Such data are vital for internal decision making, insurance negotiations, and marketing. In the future, statistical delivery-based feedback will shape the industry in a way that clinical research alone has not been able to accomplish. This approach builds the business model with the clinical model, instead of one driving the other.

Documenting Treatment

There is value in being able to demonstrate treatment successes: the number of chronic conditions resolved, the therapies applied, and the duration of treatment. For example, if in 6 months or a year X number of cases have been resolved using acupuncture and X number of cases using craniosacral therapy, the next step is to evaluate the treatment more specifically. The most well-developed outcomes tools available should be employed. The SF-36 is good, but there are many others as well.

It is also important to include objective findings whenever possible, typically in the form of subjective objective assessment and plan (SOAP) notes. Ideally, objective findings are measured with various types of functional testing. Without the inclusion of an objective measure, the notes are essentially anecdotal reporting. The assessment and plan define the symptoms and assess what should be done, based on the practitioner's expertise. Many complementary practitioners are not trained to measure objective findings, but in an integrative setting, the skills of the more conventionally trained providers can be enlisted to help collect these data.

Applying Outcomes Data

Identifying the Most Effective Therapy

In the future development of integrative medicine, quality data will be invaluable in shaping clinical care, protocols, and disease management. A practical example is a clinically based study of patients with low-back pain receiving workers' compensation benefits who saw either a chiropractor, a massage therapist, or an acupuncturist. The expenditure required to reach maximum medical improvement through chiropractic treatment was $1,200. The maximum required for acupuncture and massage was $2,200. However, when another group of patients went to all three providers in a coordinated team program, the maximum medical improvement dollars totaled just $800. This study demonstrated that in some cases, CAM therapies are most effective when provided in a coordinated protocol.

Identifying the Most Effective Treatment

Comparative data can also be used to identify the most effective approach within a particular discipline. For example, in tracking various types of acupuncture to resolve carpal tunnel syndrome, outcomes of treatment by acupuncturists trained in Five Elements style, Japanese style, and a medical training program may be monitored. If each practitioner saw 100 patients with carpal tunnel, these cases can be followed, and the treatment resolving the most conditions can be identified. Treatment protocol can then be refined.

Compromised Clinical Data

There are a number of factors that have the potential to encumber research. Consequently, it is vital to be careful about how data are gathered.

In many programs and practices, data are lacking on CAM therapies because the majority of CAM transactions occur on an out-of-pocket basis, without an electronic billing system. If bills are not generated electronically, there is no easy way to aggregate the data. Without an electronic tracking system, outcomes are buried, and there is no practical way to monitor them.

Capturing Data in a Clinical Setting

Mechanisms for tracking clinical and financial outcomes are already in place for those centers that process accounts receivables through a billing agency or an internal electronic billing system. There are also existing standard software packages that can be used or adapted to track data on services and expenditures. It is important to look at not only clinical outcomes, but also cost-effectiveness, known as cost-offset.

THE CURRENT STATUS OF INSURANCE COVERAGE

Many of the patients who use CAM are managing a chronic condition. For these people, the situation with insurance coverage is often complex.

Case Study: Migraine Headaches

If a patient with migraine headaches tries to resolve his or her headache using alternative therapies (such as acupuncture, stress reduction, or chiropractic), the patient is likely to find that none of these services are covered. However, if the patient remains on medication and periodically visits the emergency department, insurance will continue to cover the medical charges. Coverage for the treatment of migraine headaches by insurers can average as high as a $6,500 a year. Migraine patients tend to be in and out of the emergency department, take a variety of medications and narcotics, see physicians frequently, see specialists, and may require computed tomography (CT) scans. Unfortunately, the outcomes data suggest that none of the $6,500 expenditure per patient resolves the headaches. The money is primarily spent on rule-out diagnostics and pain and symptom management. On the other side of the equation, $6,500 will purchase a great deal of integrative medicine. This is a classic example of why more data are needed in order to develop sound, evidence-based protocols for debilitating (and expensive) conditions.

The Insurer's Perspective

Insurers are still determining how to handle CAM coverage because they believe these services represent additional and increased costs, rather than replacement for other services with a resulting decrease in utilization and cost.

The experience of staff at Solutions in Integrative Medicine is based on the data of its billing company, which show that in many cases costs go down. For example, acupuncture is a highly effective ancillary treatment for patients with cancer receiving chemotherapy. It helps patients maintain adherence to the chemotherapy regimen; allows them to complete it with fewer interruptions; and allows them to use fewer additional pharmaceuticals to overcome nausea, dizziness, or side effects. In many cases, these medical issues can all be handled using one intervention, acupuncture. This decreases pharmaceutical expenditures and, in some cases, costly inpatient stays. Acupuncture is an additional service, but one that appears to be more effective and less expensive than traditional adjunctive treatments dealing with the effects of chemotherapy. This type of data can be tracked through the billing and electronic medical record process.

Overutilization can be a concern with CAM, as in other areas of medicine. In the evolution of integrative services and expanded coverage, it is the practitioner's responsibility to set reasonable limits on utilization. Solutions in Integrative Medicine has received billing from practitioners who treated patients under workers' compensation coverage for thousands of dollars worth of care before deciding that the therapy was no longer helping. It is important for the practitioner to set reasonable treatment parameters and define the range of individual variation typically seen for any given patient, disease, or treatment. Sound disease management, provided in any setting, should take into consideration cost-effectiveness, efficacy, and patient satisfaction. In the experience of Solutions in Integrative Medicine, the majority of CAM practitioners offer good value and reasonable treatment. In a market as competitive as today's, most would never have survived if they did not provide competent service with discernible health outcomes.

Compromised Insurance Data

Numerous issues are involved in designing coverage. One important factor in developing guidelines is the very individual nature of disease and recovery. Although a standard protocol may provide 12 treatments for a particular diagnosis, one patient may require 18 treatments in order to fully recover, and another, only 5. There is a need for guidelines that are realistic and flexible.

Incomplete Data

Data on treatment outcomes are skewed when patients are lost to follow-up. In some cases, this can result from a flaw in the program design. For example, an insurer may cover only 8 of the 12 acupuncture visits considered necessary to resolve a painful fibromyalgia condition. Since those last four visits are not reimbursable, the data are never submitted to the insurer. In other cases, the patient may end the treatment prematurely for financial reasons once reimbursement is discontinued. The patient and the data will be lost to follow-up. The progress notes in the insurer's files on both cases will indicate that at the end of eight visits, the condition was not yet resolved. If the insurer's record is incomplete, there will be no way to determine whether the condition ever fully resolved. When protocols are based on a preconceived guideline or on the incomplete medical record, rather than the actual outcome achieved in treatment, the data can be skewed. In addition, without data on treatment in conventional medicine for comparable conditions, it will be difficult to compare the financial outcome.

Expanding Coverage

Insurance coverage is one of the keys to the future survival of the integrative medicine center. When organizations read the Eisenberg studies (1993; 1998) and the Landmark data (Interactive Solutions, 1998; National Market Measures, 1999), some become interested in CAM for reasons of financial motivation. What they may not realize is that the billions of dollars of out-of-pocket expenditures paid for a wide variety of services and products including numerous self-help activities and over-the-counter vitamins. The total expenditure documented in the research was not only for CAM providers. A number of clinics have had to close their doors over the past 5 years because they were unable secure the patient volume they needed, in part due to lack of insurance coverage.

At Solutions in Integrative Medicine, we are advocates for increasing the involvement of insurance companies, because doing so will create access to CAM services across all economic levels. At that point, CAM will not just be the

medicine of those with disposable income. We serve as advocates on behalf of organizations or individuals with insurers to obtain coverage for CAM services. Administratively, the first step in developing an advocacy position is an assessment and a review of all the literature and specific treatment options for a particular diagnosis. Peer-reviewed research literature provides background and baseline information that is not generally available or has not previously been applied in protocol development. For example, the insurance company may or may not pay for acupuncture, and it may not cover acupuncture for a particular diagnosis. Solutions in Integrative Medicine initially bills for the services and then takes the request through a hearing process. The approach is to document outcomes through the creation of efficacy manuals that contain the research. In some cases, the manuals range from 350 to 500 pages and contain peer-reviewed literature, as well as information on coding and reimbursement.

Solutions in Integrative Medicine also assists insurance companies in implementing new policy to expand coverage, through a similar approach. Currently, many insurers do not have the specialized expertise in CAM or the human resources available to perform this type of research. In some states, insurance companies are receptive to CAM and are prepared and able to participate in pilot projects. In other areas, standards may be relatively conventional and somewhat less flexible, and there is less receptivity to new insurance products. Reimbursement is also affected by whether the focus is on more familiar, accessible types of complementary medicine such as massage therapy, acupuncture, and chiropractic.

Providing Data to Referring Physicians and Insurers

Practitioners have found that it can be constructive to work collaboratively with a physical therapy center in the evaluation of complex chronic conditions. Before treatment begins, patients can be scheduled for a functional assessment with an evaluator or physical therapist to establish baseline performance and the degree of disability. At the midpoint evaluation, the evaluator provides objective findings and specific indications of progress (or lack of progress). At that time, a reevaluation is also performed by the medical staff at the integrative center, including both objective and subjective findings. The data are then shared with the patient's referring primary care physician. These evaluations are also performed at discharge.

This approach, where appropriate, tends to be more integrative. It involves an outside observer as well as objective findings. Providing periodic evaluation can enhance communication with the mainstream medical community and establish the basis for mutual referrals. It can also avoid accusations of overtreatment and provide legitimate feedback for insurance purposes.

Keeping physicians apprised of progress through periodic evaluation reports can be important in obtaining coverage. The insurance company may contact the primary care physician to ask, "We have a referral here for acupuncture; why did you send this patient to acupuncture?" By the time the insurance company calls the provider, he or she may no longer recall the details of the encounter. The provider will pull the chart and read in the fine print that the patient has coercively obtained an acupuncture prescription (which may be what actually happened). In this context, the provider is not likely to advocate for coverage for the acupuncture services. At this point, the patient may already have had four or five visits with the acupuncturist and is now responsible for out-of-pocket payment.

However, if the physician finds that the chart contains good documentation from the acupuncturist—an initial evaluation, a midpoint reevaluation, and a discharge summary—the recommendation can be justified to the insurer. The physician will be able to advocate for treatment based on the documentation that the clinic reported back. With the report in hand, there is the ability to advocate for the decision and for the patient and the integrative medicine center, all in one telephone call. Whereas, if the insurer decides that the primary care provider was misinformed in referring the patient to acupuncture, the service will not be covered. The most important education in CAM is taking place right now in the community through a process of feedback and information exchange. This approach involves complementary and conventional providers, focused on evidence-based medicine and includes insurers in the dialogue.

CONCLUSION

The integration that is taking place within medicine will continue to bring a greater number of players to the table to create an infrastructure that will introduce CAM to mainstream medicine. In the future it is foreseeable that in an effort to reduce the cost of health care, more managed care organizations and insurers will allow reimbursement for modalities that address chronic pain and illness. This in turn has the potential to reduce the overutilization of services through increased access to preventive programs, early intervention, and integrative disease management services.

REFERENCES

Eisenberg D, Davis RB, Ettner SL, et al. Trends in alternative medicine use in the United States, 1990–1997: results of a follow-up national survey. *JAMA.* 1998;280:1569–1575.

Eisenberg DM, Kessler RC, Foster C, et al. Unconventional medicine in the United States—prevalence, costs, and patterns of use. *N Engl J Med.* 1993;328:246–252.

Interactive Solutions. *Landmark Report I on Public Perceptions of Alternative Care.* Sacramento, CA: Landmark Healthcare; 1998.

National Market Measures. *The Landmark Report II.* Sacramento, CA: Landmark Healthcare; 1999.

National Center for Complementary and Alternative Medicine (NCCAM); Web site <http://nccam.nih.gov>.

11.2   Perspective: Funding Sources for an Alternative Medicine Clinic

Debra Canfield with Nancy Faass

The Hennepin County Medical Center is a 600-bed inner-city hospital in Minneapolis, one of the teaching hospitals of the University of Minnesota School of Medicine. The Alternative Medicine Division is a unit of the Department of Medicine and has three components: clinical services, research, and education. The clinical component includes the Alternative Medicine Clinic, an ambulatory care facility located in a professional building near the hospital where approximately 1,000 patients are seen per month. In addition, approximately 2,000 clients are served monthly off-site in a variety of addictions treatment programs. The following are key aspects of the Clinic:

- The Clinic is accredited by the Joint Commission on the Accreditation of Healthcare Organizations (Joint Commission), which indicates that very strict standards have been met.
- The program is hospital-based, so the clinic has also met exceptionally high internal standards.
- The alternative medicine program has been in place for more than 13 years and has a reputation for stability.
- The clinic is under the supervision of a medical director who is a physician.
- As part of a major hospital, the Alternative Medicine Division participates in institutionally supervised research.

Debra Canfield has been operations coordinator since 1996 for the Alternative Medicine Division at Hennepin County Medical Center in Minneapolis. She has also served as public information specialist for the NIH-funded Center for Addictions and Alternative Medicine Research and as a supervisor in the home care division of Caremark of Minnesota. She has presented in national forums on the topics of operations and quality improvement in integrative medicine.

ASSESSING POTENTIAL INSURANCE REIMBURSEMENT

It is easier to obtain reimbursement once an organization is fully accredited and rigorous credentialing is in place. It is important to have someone on staff who will review insurance policies from major insurers to determine how to obtain reimbursement in as many cases as possible. This typically means "thinking outside the box." We found that we could learn to evaluate coverage in new ways. The process may involve accumulating various policies from a number of insurers to assess potential coverage. In some cases, it may require calling the insurance companies to ask specific questions about coverage. For example, some policies will cover acupuncture if it is provided in a hospital-based program. Others are written to cover acupuncture if it is supervised by a physician, which is also true of our program.

In addition, we have been able to identify the medical billing codes that are relevant to the conditions we treat and the practitioners we have on staff. It has been productive to have the acupuncturist and massage therapist review the CPT codes with the administrator to define specific services the practitioners provide and identify the conditions for which their treatments are effective. Through this evaluation process, they found that they were certified in a number of areas that were reimbursed by insurers. For example, therapeutic massage services are typically not covered by insurance; however, our massage therapists are trained in the specific massage technique of neuromuscular reeducation and services that involve that particular method are billable. The service is identified by a CPT code that is most often used in conjunction with physical therapy billing; it is also legitimately used in conjunction with services by massage therapists who are specifically trained in that method. In addition, we have practitioners who are trained in myofascial release and in acupuncture. All three of these therapies have CPT codes and can be reimbursed if they are billed within the appropriate guidelines.

The following are additional considerations to keep in mind when working with the insurance companies:

- Insurers should be provided with all the relevant information regarding the program, its accreditation, credentialing, and the level of supervision.
- All providers in the program should be credentialed and privileged, if possible.
- Training, licenses, and certification held by providers should be documented, as well as their scope of practice as defined by state law and their level of competence.
- Clinical codes (ICD-9 and CPT) should be reviewed to identify the diagnoses most frequently treated and the services most frequently provided. For example, some insurers cover a broad range of complaints related to pain conditions. It is important to identify as many of these qualifying factors as possible before initiating the billing process.
- All providers should be trained in documentation. Insurers are most responsive to documentation they can understand, which is one of the essential keys to reimbursement. Good documentation is also important when insurance companies perform periodic audits.
- Ideally, one employee on staff should be identified to serve as liaison with the insurance companies to maximize good communication. Knowledge of standards and regulations will be as important as clinical knowledge.
- If an insurance company does not cover a particular therapy, the program may request that it make an exception. The documentation and research evidence are then provided to the insurer to demonstrate the efficacy of the therapy for a specific complaint.

Insurance companies do make exceptions in some cases if the provider can show that the treatment is safe, efficacious, and cost-effective. Acupuncture, for example, can be more cost-effective than pharmaceuticals or surgery for the treatment of certain conditions.

- There can be value in requesting a formal meeting with the insurer. This may provide the groundwork for coverage in the future. In some cases, the insurer may be willing to work with an integrated clinic to perform pilot studies on cost benefits.

OTHER SOURCES OF REIMBURSEMENT AND FUNDING

Workers' Compensation and Accident Insurance. These are very specific types of coverage that tend to reimburse complementary medicine services. To a certain extent, these types of coverage tend to be very broad. At the point at which the insurer deems treatment should be completed, the company will refuse further payment, but while it is providing coverage, almost all complementary services may be reimbursed. In many cases, the insurer pays close to full reimbursement, approximately 90% to 100% of the amount billed.

Medicare. Medicare covers chiropractic under certain conditions and that coverage was expanded in 2000, but at the time of this writing, it does not yet cover most other CAM therapies either explicitly or indirectly.

Medicaid. Every state has its own laws and policies regarding Medicaid. The center has developed a very reasonable working relationship with Minnesota Medicaid. The approach has been to contact the Minnesota Medicaid agency, provide information on the patient's diagnosis and the relevant services the center offers, and request information on available coverage. For example, under Medicaid rules, the center is allowed to treat acupuncture patients for up to 10 office visits without prior authorization. After that, prior authorization and additional documentation are required. Medicaid pays only a percentage of the cost of services, so the Clinic must absorb some of the cost of treatment. The availability of this service has been very beneficial for our Medicaid patients because they were not able to access these services as private pay patients.

Charity Care. The mission of the institution enables the Clinic to accept clients whom other facilities may not be able to serve. The Medical Center is an inner-city public health hospital and, as part of its mission, provides charity care. The Clinic treats people who will benefit from its services and then writes off or absorbs the expense.

Fee-for-Service Clients. Fee-for-service clients are an important part of the center's patient population. The primary demographic population is clients identified by research as the highest users of CAM services: Caucasian women who earn $50,000 or more and who can pay for their own services if and when necessary.

Off-Site Treatment for Clients with Addictions. The Hennepin County Alternative Medicine Division includes leadership and staff with specialized expertise in the treatment of addictions. The Clinic contracts with mental health and addictions programs to provide acupuncture in treatment facilities. Auricular (ear) acupuncture service is provided in group settings, and the contracts are written for reimbursement at an hourly rate.

A number of alternative and integrative medicine centers across the country have developed particular aspects of their program by providing specific expertise in a particular field such as adjunctive services for patients with AIDS, cancer, or other types of chronic or degenerative disease. In some situations, these programs qualify the center for special funding streams, such as foundation money, or attract specific types of donors.

Research Funding

The research component of the Alternative Medicine Division has focused primarily on research in the field of addictions. A number of innovative research programs for addictions treatment have been developed here in the Minneapolis-St. Paul area, and the Alternative Medicine Division has participated in the majority of these studies. The research arm of the Alternative Medicine Division also serves as a national center for addictions research, under the auspices of the NIH Center for Complementary and Alternative Medicine, which has recently refunded the addictions research project here. Patricia Culliton, the program director and co-founder, was co-investigator on the original project, which was one of the two first NIH CAM research centers in the country. In the clinical trials performed by the research center, patients are recruited and participate under specific protocols of the studies. These individuals are not seen in the Clinic or at the off-site addictions treatment programs.

In addition, the center participates in a number of studies on other topics, such as the multisite cocaine Alternative Therapies Study, through Yale University, which has received government funding. The Alternative Medicine Division is also affiliated with research performed here by UCLA and other studies as well (see Chapter 28.2 on research).

ADMINISTRATION

Data Management

The Clinic uses CPT codes as well as ICD-9 codes in insurance billing, and information is tracked in the Clinic's database by these codes for future access and outcomes data aggregation. The Clinic also provides outcomes data to insurance companies that request further justification for a particular approach to treatment. Patient outcomes have been tracked on an ongoing basis since the program's inception, and periodically insurance companies request information regarding the potential benefit of complementary therapies for specific chronic conditions. For example, an insurer might ask about a particular patient with fibromyalgia who experiences chronic pain and for whom no therapy has been successful. In order to respond to such a request for treatment information, staff draw from the Clinic's databases that track treatment outcomes by diagnostic ICD-9 codes. The database enables the center to provide written documentation on aggregated outcomes data and examples of various treatment approaches.

Some types of insurance require long-term tracking. For instance, some coverage may stipulate an annual total or a lifetime limit. Consequently, the Clinic monitors those cumulative totals and alerts patients as appropriate. The goal is to avoid a situation in which patients suddenly receive a bill for services because they have unknowingly exceeded their limit.

Supervision

All of these insurance and research programs require oversight, including workers' compensation, Medicare, Medicaid, and other types of insurance and research protocols. In addition, it is important to monitor utilization, scheduling, and other aspects of the program. It is also essential to have at least one person who provides administrative oversight, with experience in planning, risk management, quality improvement, secondary research, and report writing. Many of these functions are integral to the maintenance of any integrated medicine clinic and similar to those faced by Western clinics as well. Although the content differs, the basic functions and services are comparable. The Clinic must meet the standards of regulatory agencies such as the Joint Commission and government funders such as Medicare, and be responsive to the policies of insurers. We also see our patients getting better and responding with appreciation to the services offered them. In the final analysis, that is what is important.

CHAPTER 12

Marketing Integrative Medicine

12.1 Marketing and Incorporating Integrative Medicine Programs

Marla Jane Orth

MARKETING COMPLEMENTARY AND ALTERNATIVE MEDICINE

The complementary and alternative medicine (CAM) industry in the new millennium finds itself in a most enviable position. Consumer demand and utilization of CAM services continue to grow at a remarkable rate. Consumers are availing themselves of CAM services and products and continue to be willing to pay substantial sums for them out of pocket. More employers are choosing to offer CAM services and products on an insured basis, thereby forcing insurers to innovate and provide CAM product offerings despite their reluctance in some cases to do so.

The future demand for CAM has been clearly documented to be strong in both the purchaser and consumer sectors. In fact, the CAM industry is the single, fastest growing sector in the health care industry today. What was not long ago a fringe movement has emerged in less than a decade as a well-respected and profitable industry in its own right.

To understand this emerging and ever-evolving industry, one needs to look at the drivers motivating various constituents and to carefully examine what the data indicate about the developing trends. For organizations that desire to successfully market CAM products, it is important to have in-depth information on what customers want in terms of type of service, cost, and access. The popular perception of the CAM market is that "if you build it, they will come." This is not necessarily a realistic perspective. To establish the feasibility of launching a product or service of this type, demand must be documented, and the availability of credentialed providers must be ascertained.

Marla Jane Orth, MS, MPH, a 25-year health industry veteran, has provided health management, organizational development, and capital investment expertise to a broad array of constituents including legislators, regulators, venture investors, health systems providers, payers, purchasers, and consumers. Ms. Orth also served as a consultant, board member, and the president/CEO of Landmark Healthcare, Inc., a Sacramento-based provider of complementary and alternative health care products and services. During her more than 5-year tenure, the company's service provision expanded from one product in a single-state service area to nine products offered in 20 states, serving more than 10 million members. Ms. Orth recently returned to her 15-year-old San Francisco Bay Area consulting practice, Dimensional Health Systems, Inc., to provide strategic planning and capital formation via angel, traditional venture capital, and initial public offering (IPO) strategies for emerging growth companies.

Establishing a Profile of the Market

As the former chief executive officer of Landmark, I was a strong proponent of the use of research to guide product and program development. Landmark utilized third-party researchers to survey its customers, members, practitioners, and the public at large. It surveyed purchasers including insurers, self-insured employer groups, and unions. Landmark thoroughly evaluated the demographics of the practitioner community to ensure that there were adequate numbers of well-trained and credentialed practitioners to serve members. Based on all of the collective data, the products were designed from the ground up and specifically to the stated needs of customers. From the research, Landmark learned a great deal about its market. For example, the 1998 surveys published in the *Landmark Report on Public Perceptions of Alternative Care* indicated that:

- 42% of consumers had used some type of alternative care in the preceding year. In addition, Landmark delineated the field much more narrowly than previous and subsequent studies to define CAM more clearly from a centrist perspective and to avoid fringe elements.
- Almost 50% of consumers indicated they were willing to pay additional monthly premiums to have access to insured CAM therapies.
- 67% believed that the availability of alternative care was an important factor when choosing a health plan.

These findings came as a considerable surprise to the insurance community, which had heretofore believed that CAM was only a passing fad. Not only did the data suggest that CAM was not simply a phase, it also provided strong indications of trends toward increased acceptance and utilization in the future. Soon after the release of these findings, many insurers voluntarily added CAM products and services to their portfolios of insured product options,

as evidenced by Landmark's subsequent rapid growth.

Changes in the Market

Why are these changes and shifts occurring in consumers' purchasing patterns and what are driving these trends? The incentives vary for each constituency.

Consumers

The public is looking for options in health care. As customers, they are better educated and more empowered to make their own decisions than past cohorts. There has been a significant and very fundamental change in the way people look at their health care. Generally, most people no longer simply go to their doctors and follow their advice. Patients now ask, challenge, and question. They also research and educate themselves as evidenced by the burgeoning use of health care Web sites and the proliferation of alternative medicine publications.

The subtle but significant trend of increased consumer demand has sent an influential message to purchasers (predominantly the employer community), which in turn has demanded that the insurance community provide access to CAM products and services. Virtually every study that has been conducted in the past 10 years has substantiated this significant upward trend in utilization and the likelihood of increased usage (see Chapter 2).

What is interesting to note is the identity of the representative consumer of CAM. Landmark found that, typically, it was a female in her early 40s, well educated, working at a managerial or professional level, and not coincidentally the household decision maker for health care options for herself and her family. These consumers are not the fringe element that many critics would have people believe.

However, as more of these products and services are made widely available, particularly as insured products, there is likely to be a significant trend toward expanded diversity in the demographics of the user community. A shift will occur from those who can afford to pay for these products out of pocket to include those who have access to them at an affordable price through their jobs, and with greater ease of availability. Hispanic cultures, for example, are very supportive of chiropractic; and as they participate in the American workforce in growing numbers, they will be a major constituent in the next wave of consumerism.

Consider that many consumers have had some limited exposure to chiropractic and acupuncture under workers' compensation legislation and third-party liability (auto and accident insurance coverage). If these services are appropriate for work and accident-related injuries, why not include them as regular medical benefits?

It is also interesting to note that nearly three-fourths of the adults who reported that they used CAM used it conjunction with traditional care. Of these, 30% reported a decrease in visits to their traditional doctor, suggesting major cost benefit (InterActive Solutions, 1998).

Employers

Why would an employer add CAM to its medical coverage? Why would an employer be interested, given that the conjecture has been that it will cost more? The primary motivations for an employer are straightforward. The increasing number of employers who are adding these services indicates burgeoning interest in CAM. A self-reported survey of employers and their representative/consultants is summarized below.

Attracting Good Employees. Offering alternative medicine products and services tends to attract and retain high-caliber employees. This is particularly significant in tight job markets in which employers are in intense competition with one another. Increasingly, employees want access to CAM, and employers are offering these services in response. The inclusion of CAM in the benefits package gives an employer a distinct advantage in recruiting and retaining valued employees.

Satisfying Employees. The data suggest a very high degree of employee (patient) demand and apparent satisfaction associated with complementary and alternative medical services. Landmark has conducted two significant CAM studies (InterActive Solutions, 1998; National Market Measures, 1999). Findings show that nearly one-half of adults in the U.S. say they would be willing to pay more each month to have access to complementary alternative care, and more than two-thirds believe the availability of complementary alternative care is an important factor when choosing a health plan.

Employees also seem to be unequivocal in their desire to avail themselves of therapies that are closer to their values, beliefs, and lifestyle views (Astin, 1998). Astin used a number of demographic and psychographic variables to help predict acceptance and use of alternative therapies to examine this premise.

It has also been documented that employees have increasing levels of satisfaction with the use of complementary and alternative care therapies. Data from the *Landmark Report on Public Perceptions of Alternative Care* found that four out of ten adults say that their attitudes toward complementary care have become more positive in the past 5 years, primarily because they have learned more about it or had a favorable experience with it. In the case of chiropractic care, the vast majority of patients who receive chiropractic treatment are satisfied with their care: 73% are "very satisfied," and 23% are "somewhat satisfied."

Why do consumers report high satisfaction? These therapies can be very effective in the treatment of certain difficult-to-manage conditions, particularly chronic illness and pain. For example, chiropractic has a track record of effectiveness for low-back conditions (see Chapter 57) and acupuncture has been found beneficial in pain management (see Chapter 52). The use of CAM expands the options available to patients.

Alternative medicine tends to be very nurturing, hands-on, and personalized. Practitioners typically spend more time with the patients; spending more time enhances the patient-practitioner relationship. Practitioners not only empower their patients but also educate them in the improvement and maintenance of their health and well-being.

Controlling Costs. Employers want to control costs. They are finding that CAM is cost-effective, for example, in the treatment of chronic neuromusculoskeletal conditions. In the majority of states, chiropractic, for instance, is less expensive than the services of a physical therapist and can certainly be less expensive than the care of a traditional physician (see Chapter 56).

Offering Options. Employers have traditionally wanted to avail their employees of options that would promote good health and well-being. In order to remain competitive, employers want improved and consistent productivity from their workforce since the cost of labor is generally the single most expensive factor in running a company. Frequently, staffing is 50% or more of overhead costs when salary, benefits, and taxes are included. Research suggests significant cost savings and higher productivity by healthy, empowered, and positive employees. The tremendous cost of ongoing health care expenditures is also an ever-present issue. These expenses are clearly compounded in employee populations with chronic illness (see Chapter 3 on demand).

Mandates. With growing frequency, states are mandating the inclusion of alternative medicine into benefit coverage requirements. For example, New York, Arizona, and Georgia recently mandated the inclusion of chiropractic as a basic health care benefit to join the ranks of other states.

Insurers

Many of these same factors are also motivating insurers to include alternative medicine in their benefit designs. However, their drivers differ somewhat. They are summarized below.

Staying Competitive. If other health plans are providing greater offerings in CAM, they gain competitive advantage at open enrollment. This is particularly the case since many plans are very similar in terms of the design of the medical benefits and the practitioners who are providing services.

Satisfying Client Needs. If health plans do not offer CAM services, clients may go elsewhere. There is nothing worse than having a stated demand and not addressing that demand. By offering new and exciting products, health plans wish to be perceived as being on the cutting edge and responsive to client and member needs. Early adopters have earned the opportunity to publicly document their responsiveness. The inclusion of CAM therapies and products into benefit designs has yielded tremendous positive publicity and considerable goodwill in the purchaser, practitioner, and client communities. Being the first in the marketplace creates a very real competitive advantage.

Collecting and Analyzing Member Data. Many plans are interested in offering exploratory CAM products and services because they are curious about member demand, want to document member utilization and cost of services, and want to evaluate member satisfaction with product offerings. At the end of the day, health plans want to be able to document the cost and clinical effectiveness of CAM therapies in the context of their own membership. They need to have sufficient data to be able to conduct their own analyses, which will guide their clinical and benefit design decisions in the future.

There is a strong likelihood that an increasing number of health plans will offer CAM. The 1997 *Landmark Report II on HMOs and Alternative Care* (InterActive Solutions, 1998) substantiated that many plans are offering CAM in response to consumer demand. Among health plans, 38% of the respondents indicated they believed offering CAM would increase their plan enrollment; 58% of the plans confirmed their interest in offering a CAM benefit within the next 2 years, in response to the consumer demand and the need to stay competitive.

Brokers

Why would brokers, consultants, and general agents want to offer these products? It is a variation on the above. As consumer demand and clinical research on CAM gain the attention of insurers and employers, professionals in the field such as brokers, general agents, and consultants have increased their support and promotion of these therapies to their clients. The ability to offer access to CAM services gives the broker community a distinct marketing advantage. In addition, offering CAM products and services provides another source of commission revenue that is very attractive in an era of declining commissions and increased competition from Internet-based brokerages.

BASIC BENEFIT DESIGNS

Some states mandate exactly what and how much of a benefit or service can be offered and to whom it will be offered. Typically, however, the offerings fall into several broad categories.

Discounts

Discounts range from 5% to 25% (or 15% on average) off usual, customary, and reasonable charges. Practitioners are willing to provide discounts in order to avail themselves of a larger patient base. Not all practitioners have been known to abide by their discount arrangements, however. Plans are finally getting smart about documenting the real value of the discount. Consumers are not realizing a value at all in some cases. Many insurers want to offer discounted services because they require a minimum of administrative involvement. There is less risk to the insurer, and it is the easiest and least expensive way to get a CAM product into the market quickly.

Supplemental Coverage

A typical supplementary benefit package might include 20 to 30 visits per benefit year and a $5 or $10 copayment per visit. Benefits can be offered as a stand-alone (such as chiropractic services only) or in combination (such as both chiropractic and acupuncture in one benefit package). For example, in 1999, Landmark Healthcare pioneered a new combination product that included chiropractic, acupuncture, and medical massage that was very well received.

The insurer (or self-insured employer group) has the option of developing and managing the network of providers or subcontracting them to a specialty health plan. The contracted networks are typically reimbursed on a per-member-per-month capitated basis, although some insurers reimburse the networks on a standard fee-for-service basis (with or without risk-sharing features between the insurer and the network).

Core Coverage

In the provision of core coverage, the benefit design is similar to that of supplemental coverage. The only significant difference is that core benefits are offered to all members of a health plan, not just those who choose to purchase additional coverage. The CAM services are offered as a basic medical benefit much like physical therapy or other specialty services. As a result, core coverage is typically less expensive coverage because the risk (the utilization and cost of services) is shared across the entire membership and not just within select employer groups. Therefore, the likelihood of higher than normal utilization is greater, due to self-selection factors in noncare benefit designs.

Many health plans already offer alternative medicine riders that supplement their regular medical benefits. In fact, all California plans offer chiropractic to their members, and many offer acupuncture and herbal remedies as well. CAM is not only a California phenomenon, however. While regional pockets nationwide appear to embrace more CAM than others, the acceptance and usage of these services are widespread. The Landmark surveys did not indicate any statistical variances between different states or regions of the country.

INCREASING REGULATION ON THE HORIZON

Many states, like California, already heavily regulate the health insurance industry, and others are likely to follow in their stead. Few networks and plans can meet the stringent requirements established in the statutes and the regulations. Many provider panels and some plans are ill-equipped to handle the assumption of financial risk. They may not have the infrastructure necessary to manage a mini-insurance company with all of its requisite requirements.

For example, the state of California requires that a qualified management team be in place to discharge all the legal, financial, medical, marketing, servicing, and contractual responsibilities of the licensee. A financial structure must be in place that includes checks and balances over financial accounting methods, fidelity bonding, reserves, and evidence of financial viability. This also means a licensee must have a reliable and timely management information system and processes to manage administrative, medical, and financial information.

Practitioners must be credentialed and formally contracted directly with the licensee and be of sufficient number as to adequately serve the enrolled membership. For example, the standard of accessibility for acupuncturists and chiropractors must be one practitioner per 5,000 enrollees. Other standards of accessibility also apply, involving travel time and distance. In addition, there are a number of complex requirements for the accumulation of tangible net equity. Licensees must demonstrate that they have adequate deposits on reserve to cover projected medical and administrative expenses. Fidelity bonding and insurance coverage must be in place for protection against an event of insolvency, as well as insurance coverage for errors or omissions on the part of officers and directors. The licensee must substantiate sufficient capitalization to achieve and maintain financial breakeven and fiscal solvency on a continuous basis.

Networks and plans that fail to develop or maintain the sophisticated infrastructure necessary to support these complex requirements and continuous demands are ill-equipped to manage risked-based business. Risk sharing via capitated or risk-sharing arrangements between a health plan and network has become the standard contracting approach in the industry. Health plans are eager to cap their financial risk exposure and to minimize their administrative burden, and are increasingly subcontracting network and benefit management to existing specialty networks with proven track records.

EXPANDING INSURANCE COVERAGE FOR CAM

The integration of CAM is most likely to occur once it has become a core benefit that is offered side by side with all other creditable clinical interventions. As long as CAM is seen as a supplement to health care (or in some cases regarded as fringe medicine), rather than as a core benefit in the design of medical coverage, genuine integration will not likely take place.

Cost-Effectiveness

Change will occur once there is broad recognition that CAM therapies are not only clinically efficacious, but also provide cost benefit. CAM services will necessarily have to be cost neutral or cost saving to receive widespread acceptance in the traditional insurance model. The research literature currently includes data on the cost-effectiveness of complementary medicine. For example, Branson's review of studies from a 15-year period comparing chiropractic and biomedicine found chiropractic to be cost effective (see Chapter 56).

A dramatic example is the treatment of the arthritic knee. Osteoarthritis is typically a very difficult disease state to manage. The conventional wisdom has been to treat the condition first with drugs and physical therapy. When those interventions fail, the treatment of choice is a surgical arthroscopic procedure. In very severe cases, knee replacement may be necessary, which is expensive and requires extensive rehabilitation.

The least invasive arthroscopic procedure usually costs thousands of dollars per patient, which does not take into account lost productivity. The more invasive knee replacement costs tens of thousands of dollars, not including the protracted rehabilitation period. This is a significant burden for both the insurer and beneficiary to bear.

However, many people with osteoarthritis respond well to the intervention of acupuncture and can be managed very satisfactorily (Berman et al, 1999; Berman et al, 2000; Osiri et al, 2000). In fact, my husband is one of those people who had an exacerbated osteoarthritic knee and was told nothing more could be done. He was considered an inappropriate candidate for a knee replacement because he was too young, despite the fact that he was in constant severe pain. At one point it became difficult for him to sit, stand, or lie down. Having tried multiple standard approaches with no relief, he tried acupuncture with excellent results. We paid out of pocket because it was not a covered benefit under his health plan. All told, he managed to obtain relief and return to functionality for approximately $400 over a treatment course of 8 months. He has had no surgery or medication nor has he required prescribed anti-inflammatory drugs since the acupuncture treatment nearly 3 years ago. This is a fairly profound example of cost benefit, yet it is far from being an isolated story.

Access to CAM Data

Positive results from CAM therapies will always be considered anecdotal evidence for treatment that has not been subjected to large double-blind studies.

Data in many well-respected publications suggest that CAM is efficacious, produces good clinical outcomes, can be cost-effective, and engenders a high degree of patient satisfaction. This is ironic given that 85% of Western medical interventions have not been subjected to similar levels of scrutiny. With CAM, there is not yet a basis for performing valid statistical analyses on large populations from which objective outcomes could be derived. Until there is access to extensive cost-effectiveness research on CAM interventions, it will be impossible to convincingly prove that there is economic benefit. More time and resources need to be committed to collaborative research and objective evaluation.

Clinically Based Research

To obtain good data, it is vital to have effective tracking mechanisms in place. Objective, quantifiable, bottom-line results in terms of costs, the number of interventions, and patient outcomes (both self-reported and clinical findings) are needed. Researchers need to employ standardized collection materials with tools that make it possible to evaluate CAM in comparison with conventional interventions for comparable diagnoses on an objective and consistent basis. Ideally, research is best performed by an impartial third party. This will, however, require the complete cooperation of health plans, practitioners, and patients in order to collect the data necessary to evaluate various interventions impartially, reliably, and objectively. As the health care industry accrues and analyzes more data, more insurers are likely to voluntarily offer CAM products and services. Bias-free analysis could provide the basis for the adoption of the most highly effective treatment protocols.

Best Practices

A commitment must be made to best practices. The entire medical profession has an ethical and fiduciary responsibility to understand what patients are doing to their bodies and to evaluate and make available options most suitable to patient needs. Health plans also have a stake in this dialogue. To remain competitive, they must stay abreast of best practices and offer appropriate options to their members.

Currently the field of complementary medicine is largely consumer-driven. The majority of health plans remain skeptical about CAM and its integration into mainstream Western medicine. Insurers and providers offer these products and services primarily because their members want access to them and/or because they are looking for a way to differentiate themselves from other insurance industry offerings.

Protocol development and insurance coverage can most effectively be guided by best practices. Clearly, if a traditional intervention can produce better results for a certain disease for a particular patient, then that person should be referred to that practitioner to obtain the most effective results. However, if a CAM intervention or non-traditional approach is the most appropriate, the treatment protocols and referral processes must be redefined and expanded. Over time, a sorting-out process will occur in which the most effective and cost-effective interventions, applications, and protocols are identified. As a result of this evaluation process, not every alternative intervention will become part of conventional medicine, but those that are most beneficial are likely to be adopted. The same should also be true of more traditional medical interventions.

To establish best practices in CAM, it is necessary to examine the clinical literature on a worldwide basis with exacting thoroughness. Consensus should be developed through unbiased expert panels of practitioners from a wide range of disciplines. Expert evaluation necessarily includes physicians, nurses, and pharmacists, as well as naturopaths, acupuncturists, chiropractors, and herbologists. Clinicians are needed who can evaluate the data from a perspective of expertise with a degree of healthy skepticism. If the data are valid, they should be applied in a context that will achieve maximum outcomes for the patient regardless of which discipline provides the care. If this can be accomplished on a cost-neutral basis, then these approaches will become more widely accepted and integrated into the continuum of care.

Integration and the Global Medical Record

Another issue that impedes integration is the question of how one integrates the medical records. Complementary and mainstream medicine operate from different philosophies and in essence speak different languages. To open and maintain the dialogue and truly effect integration, education needs to occur among all practitioners to create a common nomenclature so that everyone will be using the same terminology and have similar understandings about the same patient. Until the professions can adopt a common language, it will be difficult, if not impossible, to effectively case manage patient care and achieve a best practices approach.

Currently, there is little integration of the medical record due to that lack of common nomenclature and the fact that there has been little opportunity until very recently to offer the services of complementary and traditional practitioners under one roof. In fact, some of the more integrated clinics do not yet share a common medical record, nor are practitioners given copies of consults and treatment plans. In centers in which practitioners work independently, individual cases are not evaluated through team case conferences because it is often too expensive and impractical. Another problem is that allopathic providers frequently reject the inclusion of CAM consults and treatment plans due to fears of increased malpractice exposure.

In order to provide quality medical care, practitioners need to be informed about any and all health care services the patient is receiving, including all medications, vitamins, herbs, and supplements. That is essential in order to monitor the appropriateness of care and the ultimate impact on the patient. Without the integration of the medical record, open lines of communication among practitioners and honest dialogue with patients about treatment and outcomes cannot be effectively or responsibly coordinated. Without such collaboration and cooperation, the already-fragmented health care delivery system will be exacerbated and perpetuated.

The development of the integrated medical record will occur over time. Insurance companies can promote the sharing of medical records in peer review processes and procedures by standardizing consult and treatment formats, nomenclature, and coding of services. Once there is true economic integration and practitioners are rewarded on the basis of optimal patient outcomes, change will occur quickly. Only then will the lines be erased that now divide traditional interventions from CAM.

Comparative Outcomes

Currently, the widespread perception is that CAM is cost inflationary. This is an area that bears further scrutiny because there are sufficient studies that indicate cost savings through CAM. Additional quantitative and qualitative data analysis is required. A very simple but precise study would be the evaluation of a common diagnosis such as osteoarthritis. Using standard intake data, patients could be assessed for their severity of disease and other contributing factors so that all patients in the study have similar medical profiles. Then patient care, its frequency, and cost would be objectively monitored. Consults, medications, and treatments would be tracked over the course of a year or more. At the end of the study period, all the costs of the care provided would be calculated. In addition, lost productivity would be calculated using a standardized questionnaire, and patients would be asked to evaluate their perception of the clinical outcome and their satisfaction with the intervention. Practitioners would complete a standardized exam form that compares the pre- and postintervention clinical findings. This would provide the objective and subjective data to compare costs and outcome in a standardized, unbiased approach. These data could then be used to develop best practice approaches and treatment protocols.

If the data suggest that patients have good clinical outcomes from CAM therapies that are equal in cost or less expensive than biomedical interventions, then everyone wins. When such comparative data are gathered, there will be a stronger basis for referral to CAM services. Information that offers concrete evidence of cost savings and cost-effectiveness would provide the incentives for the rapid expansion of CAM coverage. Then CAM will have earned its place at the table, and the debate about it will be transformed into dialogue on how better to improve patient care and outcomes.

REFERENCES

Astin JA. Why patients use alternative medicine: results of a national survey. *JAMA*. 1998;279(19).

Berman BM, Singh BB, Lao L, et al. A randomized trial of acupuncture as an adjunctive therapy in osteoarthritis of the knee. *Rheumatology*. 1999;38(4):346–354.

Berman BM, Swyers JP, Ezzo J. The evidence for acupuncture as a treatment for rheumatologic conditions. *Rheum Dis Clin North Am*. 2000;26(1):103–115.

InterActive Solutions. *Landmark Report I on Public Perceptions of Alternative Care*. Sacramento, CA: Landmark Healthcare; 1998.

National Market Measures. *The Landmark Report II*. Sacramento, CA: Landmark Healthcare; 1999.

Osiri M, Welch V, Brosseau L, et al. Transcutaneous electrical nerve stimulation for knee osteoarthritis (Cochrane Review). *Cochrane Database Syst Rev*. 2000;4:CD002823.

12.2   Effective Marketing of CAM Services

Cheryl E. Stone

Traditionally, the marketing discipline addresses issues related to product design, placement (distribution), pricing, and promotion. Those who are introducing complementary, alternative, or integrative medicine in a hospital or health system setting will need to address these four aspects of the marketing mix. In addition, while many of the usual considerations apply in developing the marketing plan, the very nature of CAM suggests the consideration of unique approaches to marketing.

MARKET RESEARCH

Marketing complementary medicine successfully requires careful attention to the selection of the target market. Potential clients can be identified through market research that focuses on delineating the optimal market segments, which are homogeneous groups of individuals who share common characteristics regarding their likelihood of utilizing CAM services and the way in which they make purchasing decisions. Identifying those segments also may require some nontraditional thinking. For exam-

ple, it often is assumed that the typical early adopters of CAM services in the community are the first and easiest segment to target. In fact, this population, which is accustomed to using CAM services in community-based, alternative settings, may feel co-opted by the concept of CAM within a traditional health care setting. In contrast, the "worried well," who have been following the story of CAM in women's magazines and the consumer health press, may be a more likely target for CAM services under the roof of the traditional health care establishment. Effective segmentation—identification of the market cohort—is highly market-specific. The types of segments will vary depending on the sociodemographic composition of the market, the current market environment, and other factors. CAM providers need to ask these questions of their local markets through methodical market research.

Measurable Objectives

The best marketing plans are designed to achieve measurable objectives. Incremental growth in volume, income, market share, and reputation are key among these types of objectives. The planning process involves setting measurable objectives for the marketing of CAM services, and then monitoring their achievement. This is not necessarily a straightforward process because the types of data typically used as a baseline for a marketing plan or campaign are not readily available for CAM services or providers.

For example, when developing a marketing plan for a heart center, one usually obtains data on market size and market share. The size of the market for heart care services can be estimated by combining age- and gender-specific population data with future use rates that project for-

Cheryl E. Stone, MSPH, is Senior Vice President at Rynne Marketing Group. Ms. Stone consults with health care provider organizations nationwide on the development and marketing of health services, focusing on women's health and heart care programs. She holds a master's degree in health policy and management from Harvard School of Public Health, and is on the board of the National Association for Women's Health Foundation.

Rynne Marketing Group is a health care consulting firm located in Evanston, Ill. Since 1983, the company has provided market research, marketing and business development planning, and marketing communications services for hospitals, health systems, and other health care organizations throughout the United States.

ward the recent trends in utilization. This type of demographic information generally is available through the Bureau of the Census or private data houses. Hospital and health care service use rates are available through government sources such as state health data consortia, the National Center for Health Statistics, and the National Institutes of Health. Use rate projections can be obtained from private vendors who may offer sophisticated models of the market. Information on market share—for hospitals as well as for individual physicians or medical groups—often is available through state health data consortia or state hospital associations. Data are even available that project the potential to shift the market for a particular type of service, through primary market research studies such as statistically projectable consumer surveys. This type of customized research may address an institution's reputation for a specific type of service as well as the market's willingness to shift providers under a variety of conditions.

While the general rate of CAM use by the American consumer has been documented, providers do not have access to the level of detail on the market that is available for more established treatment modalities, such as market share or use rates by condition, age, gender, and type of service. Primary research to assess the potential utilization of CAM modalities by consumers requires a high degree of sophistication. The research needs to be formulated to facilitate a sensitivity analysis, by exploring consumers' responses to a range of realistic scenarios with respect to the cost, accessibility, degree of insurance plan coverage, and out-of-pocket payment. Establishing a baseline on market share or market penetration and then monitoring progress requires more time, resources, and creativity for the CAM provider than for the provider of traditional health care services.

Volume and income are more readily measured by the provider. Volume is initially defined in terms of number of visits or patients served. Once programs are well established, the percentage of new patients coming into the program every month or quarter also is an important mea-

sure of marketing success and a testament to the program's sustained viability.

However, it may be difficult to assess the impact of CAM services beyond simple measures of volume. Some CAM programs may generate a revenue stream through direct billing; these typically include services such as acupuncture, chiropractic, massage therapy, nutritional counseling, or a homeopathic pharmacy. However, even when it is possible to track the immediate revenue stream for these CAM services, there are concerns about the cost-benefit ratio of these programs and the extent of coverage by third-party payers. Simply put, the costs of operating these programs in a traditional health care setting may not be offset by the direct revenue after subtracting the contractual allowances of third-party payers or bad debt. The gap between costs and income may be exacerbated in the first years of the program, when the market is being developed.

PROGRAM DESIGN

In some settings, selected CAM services may be offered as loss leaders, that is, programs that are designed to attract a particular segment of the market to the provider, under the assumption that this segment will also use other revenue-generating services. This is particularly true for services such as educational programs on CAM therapies that add value to traditional services, but cannot be coded and billed. Providers also may offer selected CAM services, such as massage therapy or nutrition counseling, at a reduced loss leader rate to introduce the services to the market and build the customer base.

Eventually, however, health care organizations tend to require that even loss leader programs demonstrate value added. It is important that the managers of CAM programs be able to track the referrals they generate to other providers and services in the organization, as well as the revenue impact of the services for which they have referred patients. Tracking the referral path and its associated revenue is technically straightforward but politically difficult.

The cooperation of information systems staff is required to develop and maintain an updated record of referrals generated by the CAM program. The vigilance of schedulers and receptionists is needed to consistently ascertain the referral source for patients who utilize the CAM program. Effective tracking suffers, however, because there often is little incentive for the practitioners and services that receive the referrals to provide confirmation of the business they have received from the CAM program.

Health care marketers need to grapple with the extent to which selected CAM services can function as "investments in customer development," and need to ensure that the tracking systems are in place to determine whether the utilization of CAM services actually leads to referrals to other services within the system, or to enhanced patient satisfaction and retention.

Developing Integrative Programs

In the silo approach, each service is provided independently of others, and is solely responsible for generating its own patient base and revenue. This approach has been typical of much of the product design in health care settings. In some health systems, there has been a tendency toward the isolation of CAM services, rather than multidisciplinary efforts. In the recent past, for example, cancer care had its own programs, staff, and facility, and behavioral medicine had a separate locus within the hospital or health system; it required a tour de force to meet the needs of cancer patients who required counseling and other forms of psychosocial support.

Increasingly, organizations are moving beyond this isolated programming. Women's health, oncology, cardiovascular care, behavioral medicine, and many other service lines increasingly function in matrixed systems that involve a multidisciplinary approach. Despite these gains, however, health care organizations continue to introduce CAM as a stand-alone service. The CAM program may not belong to any of the established service lines, and as a result does not benefit from cross-referrals and integration

with traditional health services. Consequently, the marketing of CAM services on a stand-alone basis may be less effective. Comarketing of synergistic traditional and CAM services is a much more powerful statement than the promotion of each service individually.

Some successful approaches that overcome insular tendencies include:

- Incorporating CAM into an existing department or practice. For example, more hospital-sponsored women's health programs now offer comprehensive primary and preventive care to women, including massage therapy, mind-body medicine, and other CAM services in tandem with internal medicine, family practice, and obstetrics and gynecology. The CAM services benefit from the additional exposure when marketed in association with traditional health services, and both types of providers benefit from cross-referrals. Examples include the Center for Women's Health at Evergreen Hospital Medical Center, Evergreen, Washington; Wellspring Women's Center of Community-General Hospital in Syracuse, New York; and the Women's Health Center of Christ Hospital and Medical Center, in Tinley Park, Illinois.
- Supporting cross-training of providers in traditional and complementary skills. Some hospitals, including Watertown Area Health Services in Watertown, Wisconsin, offer the services of anesthesiologists who also are certified in acupuncture or other alternative pain management techniques. The provision of these services by mainstream professionals in the community can help to generate awareness and acceptance of complementary modalities.
- Offering value-added services that increase consumers' loyalty to the sponsor. Academic medical centers are uniquely poised to provide information and resources for consumers and providers. Johns Hopkins Medicine, for example, offers a pharmacological hotline that consumers and provid-

ers can call to address their concerns over the potential interactions of medications and supplements or herbs.

These approaches have been found particularly successful in generating acceptance from other providers (and potential referrers) within and outside the sponsoring organization. From the administrator's perspective, however, programs that do not directly generate revenue may appear to have less accountability because it is difficult to trace the volume and revenue they generate.

PLACEMENT/DISTRIBUTION

Placement refers to the distribution of a product or service and the way it gets from the provider to the consumer. For CAM services, the placement element of the marketing plan may refer to the types of sites in which CAM services are provided, the distribution of CAM services in the community, and the way in which they are packaged with other types of health care services.

Rynne Marketing Group's extensive focus group research conducted throughout the United States with consumers substantiates the national statistics on the use of CAM services. Much of this utilization is at the consumer's own discretion, and much is currently paid for out of pocket.

However, focus group participants consistently articulate their preference for "one-stop shopping"—an integrated approach that would include both traditional and complementary medicine services. Many would like to see CAM services go beyond a side-by-side approach with traditional medical care. Ideally, they prefer that their mainstream providers become knowledgeable about CAM practices and incorporate them directly into their own treatment protocols. Failing that, they would like their providers to be aware of CAM's capabilities, and be able to make informed referrals to such services. Many consumers remain hesitant to inform their physi-

cians about the types of CAM services they are using.

From a marketing perspective, the services with strongest appeal are those offered by physicians who are well trained in CAM modalities. Second in appeal is offering conventional medicine and CAM services side by side, in a setting where the two types of providers cross-refer and consult cooperatively or co-manage patients. Third in appeal is offering a stand-alone CAM program in a traditional medical setting (such as a hospital's office building). Other methods, such as the placement of stand-alone CAM programs in the community, are likely to attract a following among the early adopters, but less likely to attract the larger mainstream market.

PRICING

Concerns about the pricing of CAM services offered within a traditional health care setting include:

- the determination of appropriate pricing for what has essentially been a retail service, when offered in a setting that includes the high overhead of a mainstream health care provider
- consumers' willingness to pay for CAM services out of pocket, which appears to diminish in proportion to the degree to which the setting is a mainstream health care setting, thereby reflecting the assumption that such services should be covered
- payers' lack of willingness to cover many CAM treatments, as well as the deep discounts required of practitioners for those services they do cover.

There is another aspect of price, however, that has not been addressed. In today's hectic work world, consumers continually make tradeoffs of time and money. In the health care setting, there is a segment of consumers who are willing to pay more for accessibility and convenience—typically in the form of extended hours in the early mornings, evenings, and weekends, nearby parking, on-time appointments, and one-stop shopping for multiple services. Health care providers that meet consumers' heightened expectations for accessibility through their CAM programs or the integration of CAM and other services may attract an audience that is prepared to invest in prevention and personal well-being.

PROMOTION

There are two major audience segments for CAM services:

1. those who have sought out such services on their own in the past (early adopters)
2. those who have not yet done so.

In developing the promotional plan for CAM services, it is important to consider the paths that each of these consumer segments take when choosing health care services and providers. How do established CAM patients choose when and from whom to obtain such care? How do consumers of mainstream health services decide when and where to seek care? Promotional efforts need to be grounded in an understanding of these patterns of patient decision making and appropriate ways of marketing at the decision points along the path.

The first consideration should be given to the role of internal marketing. Positive word of mouth and testimonials from satisfied patients are important and can be harnessed in the promotional plan and reflected in paid advertising as well as press releases. Another important source of referrals is the organization's own staff, including frontline staff and the office staff of physicians and other providers. Physicians often rely on their office staff to channel the patient to specific providers, once the referral for a particular treatment has been made.

Educational information can be provided informally through lunchtime presentations by the CAM practitioners. Paycheck stuffers, Intranet announcements, and discounted visits to CAM services provide employees the opportunity to become more familiar with the CAM services and spread the word in their communities. Variations of this type of promotion also can be provided to the community. For example, one women's health center builds the base for its CAM services by offering coupons for its massage therapy program to patients whose physicians are delayed in seeing them for their scheduled appointments. The free service functions as a token of apology and generates return patients for the massage program.

The second stage is to expand the size of the market by creating new audiences for CAM services. Based on Rynne Marketing Group's experience introducing new health services to the market, the greatest impact has resulted from a multistage promotional plan that includes:

- broadcast media (radio, TV, and cable) to generate initial awareness of and interest in the program
- print and direct mail to generate inquiries and utilization of services.

The third consideration is the development of relationships among high-potential prospects, to keep them apprised of new developments and offer them successive opportunities to utilize the program, through:

- direct mail
- Web sites
- broadcast e-mail
- newsletters, including direct mail and e-mail versions.

The Ornish program for lifestyle modification is an example of a program that can readily be incorporated into the scope of services offered by a mainstream health care provider. Rather than market this program as a stand-alone, one hospital (St. Francis Hospital and Health Center in Blue Island, Illinois) decided to market the program as an integral component of its cardiac services. The program was offered directly to consumers and also to physicians who might generate referrals. The centerpiece of the marketing campaign was a newspaper advertisement that featured a testimonial by the president of the hospital, who had benefited from the Ornish program personally. This paid advertising was complemented by public relations that included a radio interview with the medical director of the program and several feature stories in the lifestyle and food sections of area newspapers. To further develop the referral pool, letters describing the program were sent to primary care physicians in the area.

CONCLUSION

CAM services are entering a market of untold potential, as consumers become increasingly focused on prevention, wellness, and enhancement of their quality of life.

The checklist for CAM marketers is brief:

- Research the local market: evaluate market potential and predisposition among consumers, referral sources, and payers.
- Identify the demographic and psychographic segments of the market with the greatest potential.
- Develop measurable marketing objectives. Ensure that the systems are in place to monitor progress.
- Look for synergies and cross-marketing opportunities. Provide introduction to CAM services through women's health, the cancer center, the fitness center, or senior services, and share the marketing budget with them.
- Identify value-added and customer service opportunities that will help position the organization as a resource for credentialed CAM services, such as the pharmacy hotline program.
- Build the referral network for CAM services with likely and unlikely allies. Consider not only primary care physicians and specialists, but also the local health food stores, natural foods grocery stores, fitness facilities, bookstores, and community service organizations.
- Maximize the power of internal marketing.
- Support paid advertising with equal attention to its public relations potential.

Marketing CAM services is not business as usual; yet there is much to learn and apply from the traditional marketing discipline. The most effective approaches to the provision of CAM services are those that integrate multiple disciplines. Similarly, the most effective means of promoting CAM services are those that build synergies with a health care provider's traditional marketing vehicles and go one step beyond.

CHAPTER 13

Perspectives on Insurance Coverage

13.1 Considerations in the Design and Pricing of a Complementary and Alternative Medicine Benefit
    Thomas Snook
13.2 Field Report: Indemnity and Rider Products in Complementary Medicine
    James E. Connolly with Nancy Faass

13.1   Considerations in the Design and Pricing of a Complementary and Alternative Medicine Benefit

Thomas Snook

INTRODUCTION

Traditionally, health insurers in the United States have not provided coverage for most alternative medicine services. Now, however, as a response to public demand, health plans are increasingly beginning to offer coverage for these services.

CAM, also sometimes called alternative medicine, complementary medicine, or unconventional medicine, is defined as modalities of care neither taught widely in medical schools nor generally available in U.S. hospitals. Examples of CAM include chiropractic, acupuncture, herbal medicines, and naturopathy.

CAM was very popular with Americans in the 1990s, and the trend shows no sign of abating. One study estimates that the total number of visits to alternative providers exceeded the total number of visits to primary care physicians during 1997 (Eisenberg et al, 1998).

This is new territory for health plans, in the sense that most do not understand the CAM marketplace and the different types of services available. In addition, health plans do not have enough experience with these services to know what constitutes a well-designed benefit, or to accurately estimate the cost associated with such a benefit. Thus, while health plans may be starting to include coverage for these services, they are largely proceeding slowly and cautiously.

The purpose of this report is to outline issues plans face in designing a CAM benefit, and to present some of the key assumptions actuaries must make when pricing such a benefit.

BENEFIT DESIGN ISSUES

Scope of Coverage

The key issue a health plan faces when considering a CAM benefit is the scope of services to be included in the coverage. There is a very

---

Thomas Snook is a Principal and Consulting Actuary in the Phoenix office of Milliman & Robertson, Inc. His area of expertise is managed care and health insurance; clients include HMOs, insurance companies, hospitals, physician groups, and others. He is a 1983 graduate of Rice University.

Source: Copyright © 2000, Milliman & Robertson, Inc.

broad range of services that fall under CAM, some of which are thought to be more mainstream and accepted by the general public than others are. Examples of CAM services that have been covered by health plans include:

- chiropractic
- acupuncture/acupressure
- naturopathy
- massage therapy
- Chinese medicine
- hypnosis/hypnotherapy
- homeopathy
- biofeedback
- Ayurveda
- natural medicinals/herbal therapy

There are a number of factors a health plan must consider when choosing which services to include under a CAM benefit.

Market Demand

Because they are largely responding to perceived public interest in CAM, presumably in hopes to gain market share, health plans should carefully consider which benefits are likely to be most popular. The more mainstream CAM modalities such as chiropractic are likely to generate more market interest than the more exotic services such as Ayurveda. In addition, the demographics and geography of the target market will play a role. Men may have different interests than women, the elderly have different needs than a younger population, and what sells in California may not be of interest in Rhode Island.

Legal Requirements

State-mandated benefit requirements need to be considered in determining the scope of services to be included in the CAM benefit. Many states have mandated coverage for chiropractic services. The state of Washington garnered headlines a few years ago when that mandate was expanded to include other forms of CAM, including naturopathy. Health plans also need to consider legal restrictions on certain CAM services. Not all CAM modalities are legal in all states.

Network Building and Credentialing

Managed care plans looking to contract with a network of alternative providers may choose between contracting with an existing network of providers, or building their own. Because building a network from scratch can be a time-consuming and expensive process, contracting with an existing network may have some appeal. However, many of the alternative provider networks available today often have a bias toward one or a few alternative care modalities (for example, a network may have a preponderance of acupuncturists and little or no representation of other alternative disciplines). The health plan considering contracting with such an alternative provider network will need to consider whether the scope of services provided by the network is consistent with the perceived market demands and other considerations.

A health plan may encounter some difficult issues in the provider credentialing process. A full discussion of the credentialing of alternative providers is beyond the scope of this chapter. However, it should be noted that licensure and continuing education issues, to name two examples, are often not nearly as clear-cut for alternative modalities as for mainstream allopathic or osteopathic medicine. Thus, the amount of effort and risk involved in credentialing CAM providers may play a role in determining the scope of services covered under the benefit.

Self-Referral versus Primary Care Physician Referral

Managed care plans will also need to decide if they will permit members to refer themselves to an alternative care provider, or if the member is required to get a primary care physician (PCP) referral first. Requiring PCP approval has the potential to significantly damage the market appeal of the CAM benefit, but will likely result in substantially less benefit cost than a self-referral plan.

Risk Issues

The ability and desire of a health plan to assume risk on largely unknown and potentially costly benefits will impact the scope of alternative services it covers. A more risk-averse plan will likely place greater limits on the services covered than will a plan more inclined to assume additional risk.

Moreover, a health plan will want to carefully consider any potential increased legal liability associated with covering CAM. A number of states have passed medical malpractice liability laws for health maintenance organizations, thereby allowing them to be sued for the practices of their physicians. Providers of CAM are not immune from malpractice lawsuits, and in fact some may face greater exposure due to the lack of widespread acceptance of some alternative care modalities.

Copayments and Limitations

Another issue in designing the CAM benefit is the member cost-sharing and internal benefit limits. CAM services can be considered to be largely elective in nature, in the sense that an individual can go through an entire lifetime without accessing care from a CAM provider. Consequently, copayments and annual maximum benefits are common in CAM benefits since they can discourage frivolous utilization and put some limit on the health plan's exposure to risk.

Many CAM benefits include member cost-sharing (copayments or coinsurance) that is greater than that which the health plan requires for visits to a traditional physician. Annual benefit maximums vary, but typically range between $500 and $2,500 per year.

In designing a CAM benefit, a health plan will need to strike a balance between the market appeal of a rich benefit with low member cost-sharing and high benefit maximums, and the reduced exposure to risk of a less rich plan with higher cost-sharing and lower maximums.

PRICING OVERVIEW

Actuaries develop estimates of the per member per month (PMPM) cost of any set of health care service (alternative or traditional) by building

actuarial cost models, which include assumptions as to the utilization rate and average cost per service. Utilization assumptions are typically expressed as "per 1,000 per year," meaning the number of services expected to be provided to 1,000 members in 1 year. The impact of copayments, coinsurance, deductibles, and annual benefit maximums must also be taken into account in the cost model.

Actuarial cost models are built up from relatively homogeneous types of service, with separate utilization and cost assumptions for each. The total PMPM cost for a given scope of services is then equal to the sum of the PMPM costs developed from these component pieces. The narrower the definition of the line item types of service in the cost model, the more line items are needed to cover the entire scope of services. For example, an actuarial cost model for traditional medical benefits could have one line item for all inpatient admissions, or several line items for groupings of diagnoses, or a very detailed set of line items by diagnosis-related groups (DRGs). Thus actuarial cost models can vary in their level of detail depending on the degree to which the entire scope of services to be priced is subdivided into smaller types of service line items.

To price a CAM benefit, therefore, the actuary must make assumptions as to the rate at which the covered scope of services will be utilized and the average provider charge for these services. The determination of the line item types of service will be a function of the desired level of detail in the model and the degree to which detailed data are available.

The average charge per service is the easier of the two sets of assumptions. Managed care plans contracting with a network of providers will have a set fee schedule that defines the fee (or sets a maximum fee) for each service for the providers in the network; this fee schedule will then form the basis of the average charge assumption. The actuary will, however, need to make some assumptions as to the relative frequency of use of each service for which there is a separate fee.

For indemnity plans, the average charge assumption is not so straightforward. The company will need to research published information on provider fees or conduct a survey of provider fees (in a geographic area) to make this assumption. Unlike traditional medical services, however, a standard of usual, customary, and reasonable charge levels does not exist for most alternative care modalities. Therefore, the indemnity carrier may find it beneficial to establish a set fee schedule for the scope of services it is providing in its CAM benefit.

Utilization Assumptions for CAM

The most difficult aspect in the pricing of the CAM benefit is the determination of reasonable utilization assumptions for an insured population. Useful, credible data regarding the utilization of CAM services are sparse at best. The actuary usually must exercise a great deal of judgment in setting the utilization assumptions.

There are generally three different sources of data available to use in the determination of utilization assumptions for CAM:

- insurance company experience
- uninsured data
- provider network data

Each of these data sources has its strengths and shortcomings, which are discussed below.

Insurance Company Experience

The ideal data source for pricing a CAM benefit is utilization experience under similar insurance programs. However, there is currently very little good insurance data available to make use of in setting CAM utilization assumptions. These data will likely emerge in time as CAM benefits become more popular and have been around long enough to generate several years of statistically credible experience data. As the data do emerge, however, it may be difficult for plans that have not already begun to offer a CAM benefit to access the information since such data will be proprietary in nature. It remains to be seen the extent to which good, insurance-based

utilization data will be made publicly available. (Milliman & Robertson is in the process of gathering insurance-based utilization data for CAM services. The advantage of using a consultant for this information is that it avoids the proprietary issue altogether.)

An important exception to the statement above relates to chiropractic care. Chiropractic coverage is mandated in many states and has been available as an insured benefit for a number of years. In 1997, about 18% of individuals seeking chiropractic care reported having complete insurance coverage for such treatment, and another 38% reported having partial coverage.

The 1999 *Milliman & Robertson Health Cost Guidelines* contains the utilization information listed in Table 13.1–1 for chiropractic care for insured populations that do not require primary care physician referral.

The *Health Cost Guidelines* information also shows a wide variation in utilization rates based on the age and sex of the member. The highest utilization rates are for older female adults and are nearly three times the utilization rates for young adult males. In addition, significant variations in chiropractic utilization rates exist by geographic area as well.

If a managed care plan requires PCP referral for chiropractic visits, the Milliman & Robertson data show a substantial reduction in utiliza-

---

Table 13.1–1 Chiropractic Care Utilization*

Demographic Category	Number of Visits per 1,000 Insured Members
All employees	1,119
Male employees	972
Female employees	1,306
All spouses	1,254
All children	162
Composite, all members	815

*Indemnity plan with self-referral—loosely managed health care delivery system.
Source: Copyright © 2000, Milliman & Robertson, Inc.

tion. The data indicate that PCP referral requirements can result in utilization rates that are 75% less than in plans that allow members to self-refer to chiropractors.

Uninsured Data

Uninsured data are utilization data available on the general population, which, by and large, does not have insurance coverage for CAM services. There are a number of different sources of uninsured utilization data available. Probably the best sources are the two papers by Eisenberg et al (1993, 1998).

The 1998 paper includes a great deal of detailed information, including estimated adult visit rates for each of 16 different alternative therapies. The paper also includes estimates of the proportion of the population that has visited an alternative practitioner, and the average number of visits per user per year. Table 13.1–2 summarizes some of the utilization data in the paper.

Other interesting highlights of the study include the following:

- Use of at least 1 of 16 alternative therapies during the previous year increased from 34% in 1990 to 42% in 1997.
- Forty-six percent of users of alternative therapies visited an alternative practitioner in 1997.
- The therapies increasing the most in that period were herbal medicine, massage, megavitamins, self-help groups, and energy healing.
- A little under 40% of individuals who seek alternative therapies disclose the fact to their physicians.
- The proportion of users paying entirely out of pocket for services provided by CAM providers declined from 64% in 1990 to 58% in 1997 although the sample size for this information meant that this comparison was not statistically significant.
- Extrapolations to the U.S. population suggest a 47% increase in the total number of visits to CAM practitioners.

Table 13.1–2 Eisenberg et al (1998) Data

Type of Therapy	Number of Visits per 1,000 per Year, 1990	Number of Visits per 1,000 per Year, 1997
Relaxation techniques	219.3	521.2
Herbal medicine	20.7	53.0
Massage	422.8	574.4
Chiropractic	904.8	969.1
Spiritual healing	54.9	n.a.
Megavitamins	35.7	112.1
Self-help group	180.0	402.8
Imagery	90.1	114.3
Commercial diet	193.8	138.8
Folk remedies	n.a.	2.6
Lifestyle diet	36.5	9.0
Energy healing	34.7	201.9
Homeopathy	13.5	9.0
Hypnosis	12.1	21.1
Biofeedback	13.3	19.5
Acupuncture	140.2	27.2

Source: Adapted with permission from D. Eisenberg et al., Trends in Alternative Medicine Use in the United States, 1990–1997: Results of a Follow-Up National Survey, *Journal of the American Medical Association*, Vol. 280, No. 18, P. 1574, © 1998, American Medical Association.

- The total number of visits to CAM practitioners in the U.S. in 1997 was 629 million, exceeding the total number of visits to all U.S. primary care physicians in the same period.

The data in the 1998 Eisenberg report are probably the most complete, credible, and up-to-date information available regarding utilization rates for CAM services. However, even this quality data set poses a number of problems for use in pricing a CAM insurance benefit.

First and most significantly is the question of the applicability of uninsured data to an insured population. Put simply, the question is this: How will utilization rates for CAM change when the person seeking the service has little or no out-of-pocket expense associated with using the benefits? As noted above, CAM treatment is largely elective in nature. Absent insurance, an individual considering an alternative therapy may be dissuaded by the out-of-pocket expense. When insurance is present, that dissuasive factor disappears, and utilization rates will likely increase. The size of the increase cannot be accurately estimated until credible insured data emerge, which will likely be several years after CAM coverage becomes more common.

A related issue is the degree to which utilization patterns will change in the presence of insurance. In other words, will alternative practitioners be more likely to prescribe more expensive courses of treatments to their patients whom they know have insurance coverage for CAM therapies? Again, in the absence of a financial dissuasive factor, one can expect some shift in utilization to more expensive or elaborate courses of treatment. However, the magnitude and impact of that shift will not be known until good insured data on alternative therapies emerge.

In addition, it should be noted that the data in the Eisenberg studies reflect utilization rates for the adult population at large, including (presumably) people of all income levels, age (excluding children), and geographic location. Nearly all of the CAM insurance benefits offered today relate to commercially insured populations, that is, the working population and its dependents. The population underlying the Eisenberg data includes the commercially insured population, plus the elderly, the uninsured, and the poor or unemployed. The Eisenberg data also exclude children, which would be included in the commercially insured population. Therefore, it is evident that a significant demographic mismatch exists between a commercial group population and the population that underlies the Eisenberg study.

The significance of geographic area needs also to be considered. Material variations in utilization patterns exist from one region of the country to another. In fact, because many alternative modalities have little or no degree of standardization of practice, the geographic variation in alternative therapies may be greater than it is for traditional medicine. The Eisenberg study is national in scope and does not consider these regional variations.

In summary, then, the actuary should use a great deal of caution when using data from population-based studies of CAM utilization. Significant modification to the data in these studies is probably warranted in most cases when pricing a CAM insurance benefit.

Provider Network Data

An often-overlooked source of utilization data is the information in the alternative providers' office files. While this information is not perfect, or adequate to completely derive utilization assumptions, it can provide some good insight into the specific practice patterns of the providers in the network. A typical study of alternative provider office data might proceed as follows:

1. Determine the experience period to be studied.
2. Pull data on all patient visits during the experience period. Preferably, this would be computerized data although data can be compiled from paper files.
3. Map visit data to unique patient identifiers over the course of the experience period. For each patient, then, the data will show the number of visits and different types of treatments rendered.
4. Compile these data to determine average number of visits per patient, average number of different treatment types per patient, etc.

This procedure will allow the actuary to determine historical utilization patterns for a given alternative provider network. The advantage of this approach is that it is specific to the practice patterns of the providers who will be providing the care in the insured benefit plan. As mentioned previously, there is a lack of standardization of practice in many alternative modalities, and so this information can be very important.

To make use of these data, however, the actuary will still need to make an assumption about the rate at which people will present for care to an alternative provider. In addition, note that the data gathered in this sort of study are still, by and large, uninsured data; no information is provided as to how the providers' practice patterns may change in the presence of an insurance benefit. And, of course, this type of study is possible only with the cooperation of the providers in the network.

Setting the Price for a CAM Benefit

Although the actuary may have completed an actuarial cost model for the scope of alternative benefits in question, the pricing work is not done. There are a number of other factors that must be considered in determining the final price (premium rate) for the CAM benefit.

Impact on Traditional Medical Costs

The actuarial analyses described in the preceding sections do not include consideration of the impact of a CAM benefit on the utilization of traditional providers. The question is, to what extent are visits to alternative providers in lieu of, rather than in addition to, visits to a traditional provider? Is the presence of a CAM benefit likely to reduce utilization of traditional services? The complete answer to this question will not be known until insurance coverage of CAM becomes more widespread.

CAM proponents also argue that since many CAM therapies are preventive in nature, covering CAM will encourage its use and result in a healthier population less likely to consume medical resources. However, even if one accepts this hypothesis without skepticism, the timeframe over which this healthier population will emerge is much longer than the typical 1-year group health insurance contract period.

Administrative and Other Costs

As for any other medical benefit, the actuary must load the anticipated claim cost estimate to reflect administrative and other costs. Administrative costs for CAM benefits could conceivably be greater in proportion to claim costs than

they are for traditional medical benefits for the following reasons:

- cost of building and/or credentialing a network of alternative providers
- training of sales, claims paying, and other administrative staff
- marketing cost of getting the word out about the CAM benefit
- claims paying cost is likely to be higher due to the relatively high-volume, low-cost nature of the CAM benefit.

In addition, the actuary will need to consider what reinsurance cover is available (particularly for stand-alone CAM plans) and the cost of that reinsurance.

Risk Loading and the Degree of Conservatism Desired

It may be appropriate for a health plan to add a substantial risk loading to the CAM benefit premium rate. The scant nature of the data available and the high degree of actuarial judgment required in setting pricing assumptions mean there is a higher probability that the actuarial claim cost estimate may be materially understated. A larger risk loading will reduce the chance of underpricing the benefit. The decision as to the level of risk loading to add to the premium will ultimately depend on management's desired degree of conservatism in the rates. Note that the risk of a material underpricing is much greater for a stand-alone CAM benefit than it is for an integrated CAM benefit. Consider the following example:

Total cost of traditional medical benefits:
$100.00 PMPM
Actuarial estimate of CAM benefits:
$1.00 PMPM
Actual experience cost of alternative benefits: $1.50 PMPM

In this example, the CAM benefit has been underpriced by $0.50 per member per month. Taken as part of the total cost of both the traditional and alternative benefit cost combined, the error is relatively small, roughly on the order of

0.5%. However, looking at the estimate of the cost of the CAM benefit only, the error is 50%.

Thus, the risk associated with adding a CAM benefit to an existing plan of traditional medical benefits is substantially less than the risk associated with offering CAM benefits by themselves. A corollary to this statement is that the risk to a health plan of providing a CAM benefit integrated with its traditional benefit plan is substantially less than the risk the same benefits pose to capitated alternative providers. A 50% error in the capitation rate calculation can mean the difference between solvency and insolvency for an alternative provider network.

Of course, the opposite relationship exists for the health plan itself. A 50% error in the estimate of the cost of alternative benefits (in this example) represents an underpricing of less than 0.5% in total. In other words, the magnitude of the risk of alternative benefits to a health plan is relatively small. This relatively small magnitude of risk, coupled with market demand for the product, are the factors which have encouraged health plans to consider adding CAM benefits.

Final Considerations in Pricing

Ultimately, the market demand for CAM services will determine the price a health plan can charge for these benefits. The results of all actuarial analyses and risk issues must be tempered with an understanding of how much the market is willing to pay for CAM benefits. In this sense,

then, the analyses and considerations described in this report really constitute an outline of a feasibility study for a profitable CAM benefit, rather than an absolute pricing methodology.

CONCLUSION

There is little debate as to the popularity of CAM in the United States, and that the trend is toward more, not less, alternative care. A recent study concluded that "the majority of CAM users appear to be doing so not so much as a result of being dissatisfied with conventional medicine but largely because they find these health care alternatives to be more congruent with their own values, beliefs, and philosophical orientations toward health and life" (Astin, 1998)."

Health plans considering offering a CAM benefit are in a bit of a Catch-22 situation. Reliable data to use in pricing such benefits will not be available until the benefits are insured, but the lack of useful data discourages health plans from offering such coverage.

A debate as to the relative clinical merits of the various alternative therapies is outside the scope of this paper. From a strictly financial standpoint, a health plan's decision to offer CAM benefits means that it has determined that the financial gain to be had (via increased revenues attributable to greater market share) outweighs the additional risk of losses (due to inadequate data with which to price the benefit).

REFERENCES

Astin JA. Why patients use alternative medicine: results of a national survey. *JAMA.* 1998;279(19):1548–1553.

Eisenberg DM, Davis RB, Ettner SL, et al. Trends in alternative medicine in the United States, 1990–1997: results of a follow-up national survey. *JAMA.* 1998; 280(18):1569–1576.

Eisenberg DM, Kessler RC, Foster C, et al. Unconventional medicine in the United States—prevalence, costs, and patterns of use. *N Engl J Med.* 1993;328:246–252.

Milliman & Robertson Health Cost Guidelines. 1999 ed. Seattle, WA: Milliman & Robertson; 1999.

13.2   Field Report: Indemnity and Rider Products in Complementary Medicine

James E. Connolly with Nancy Faass

Over the past decade, significant change has occurred in the coverage of complementary and alternative medicine (CAM). In the early 1990s, endorsements to cover chiropractic care were available, and in some areas of the country, acupuncture was covered as a core medical benefit. However, little mention was made of massage therapy or naturopathic medicine. Today, through both legislative initiatives and to some extent public demand, CAM coverage is becoming more commonplace.

COVERAGE FOR CAM

The most common rider design for alternative medicine is typically a coinsurance product in which a predefined percentage of charges is covered. However, in managed care, the most common benefit design for alternative medicine is one that has a copayment or visit charge. Charges would typically be either $10 or $15 for most services such as acupuncture, chiropractic, and naturopathic medicine, with a greater charge for massage therapy. When considering

coverage for massage, it is important to differentiate between medically therapeutic massage prescribed to treat a particular symptom for a patient with a specific diagnosis versus massage simply provided for relaxation. Due to the potential for high utilization of massage therapy, riders for massage are typically limited to a certain predefined number of benefits. Medically therapeutic massage is also frequently categorized as a subset of physical therapy, which may allow 20, 40, or 60 visits a year, or some other type of visit limitation.

There is also the integrated benefit (of the type available in Washington state). Occasionally, true indemnity plans are available that pay an amount such as $20 per visit, up to a maximum of 20 visits for CAM. A few programs of that nature have been developed by Regence BlueCross BlueShield of Oregon when requested by client groups. However, in general there are only a few types of CAM insurance products currently available. A large percentage of CAM is still paid for out of pocket and is not covered by health insurance.

The primary geographic area in which CAM is available as a core benefit is Washington state, due to the legislation that requires insurers to provide this coverage. Chiropractic services are covered, as well as naturopathic medicine, acupuncture, massage therapy, nutrition, and other therapies which are included in core benefits. One might anticipate greater utilization because there is less financial barrier.

Generally speaking, there are a very limited number of riders for CAM at the time of this writing. Those that are available are primarily chiropractic riders or a comprehensive benefit generally called an alternative medicine or complementary medicine rider. Comprehensive

---

James E. Connolly, MBA, Assistant Vice President for Allied Products at Regence BlueCross BlueShield of Oregon, holds a bachelor's degree in business administration from Seattle University and a master's in business administration from the University of Portland. He has held a variety of positions with Regence over the past 27 years, and his experience encompasses more than 10 years of working with ancillary products that include dental, vision, and complementary medicine. He is a member of the Healthcare Financial Management Association and is a certified managed care executive.

The views expressed in this chapter are those of the authors and may or may not reflect the position of Regence BlueCross BlueShield of Oregon.

Courtesy of Regence Blue Cross Blue Shield of Oregon, Portland, Oregon.

riders can be available on an indemnity basis or sold through some type of managed system on a capitated basis. Groups that acquire managed riders provide their enrollees with services limited to practitioners from a panel available through the insurer for a capitated premium.

BASIC DEFINITIONS

A *rider* is additional elected coverage, reimbursed through an added premium charged for a very specific benefit. Typically, the most common riders are vision or dental care riders. Since a rider is generally sold to a group, the individual does not have the option to opt in or out for a rider, such as chiropractic. Riders are also termed an endorsement to the contract.

Indemnity coverage historically has been used to describe products that pay benefits as a flat dollar amount. Usually, both the employer and the employee contribute to that payment. As time goes on, the price per visit increases, and the patient pays a greater portion. However, more recently, the term *indemnity coverage* has come to mean any traditional plan that provides benefits for usual, customary, and reasonable charges covered under the plan. This is in contrast to health care organizations and preferred provider organizations.

Managed Care CAM Benefits

Of all CAM insurance products, managed CAM has grown the most rapidly throughout the country. This coverage is provided by firms that have assembled panels of practitioners that they manage. These organizations have developed expertise in selecting practitioners through careful credentialing. The organizations have also become skilled in utilization management and quality assurance, to ensure that the CAM services delivered are cost-effective and of high quality. Such organizations are attractive to third-party payers because they provide an all-

in-one package and because they have the expertise to manage that package.

In many of these arrangements, CAM health care services are provided to the insurer or self-funded group on a capitated basis (a specific amount per member per month), rather than a fee-for-service basis. As the demand for CAM has increased and as the expertise in these managed CAM firms has increased, they have become quite successful. This is a field that will continue to grow over the coming years. It expanded significantly in the 1990s and this is anticipated to continue to grow in the next decade.

Although many managed care health plans are not fully capitated, they often include some form of risk-sharing model in which providers of care are at risk. In other words, they may be paid a certain agreed-upon fee, but 15% of the fee will be held in a risk pool to ensure that utilization stays within the target. If utilization does remain within the target, then at year-end that risk pool is returned. If it does not, the risk pool is used to offset the added cost of additional utilization. Consequently, utilization is still definitely an issue, even in managed care organizations that are not fully capitated.

Coverage for Programs in Wellness and Prevention

One focus of third-party payers in recent years has been on preventive medicine. Historically, insurance was designed as catastrophic coverage for people who were facing disease. Self-help programs have not been included in third-party coverage for a number of years. There is a fine line between what is considered a self-help program and what is defined as prevention. In either case, these types of services are not universally included as core benefits, but are most often paid for out of pocket.

From the third-party payers' perspective, the market is going to drive the demand to some degree. In the 1980s, a considerable amount of good information became available on wellness. Some of that information was incorporated into everyone's everyday thinking although people may not actually be aware of the changes. Tremendous changes have taken place in lifestyles over the past 15 or 20 years. Twenty years ago, for example, more people smoked and ate in a less healthful manner.

Presently, there is not a broad demand for wellness coverage, except for product development for employers who request custom-designed programs. Usually those who elect these programs are entrepreneurs who have worked to develop a substantial business. Regence BlueCross BlueShield of Oregon has worked with employers on some innovative wellness programs, but to date, they have all been primarily prototypes (one-of-a-kind efforts).

There are a number of ways in which a wellness program can be structured. Flexible spending accounts allow employers to offer pretax dollars to people who want to use some types of wellness services.

Flexible Spending Programs

This type of program is based on a flexible design in which funds can be applied to payment for a variety of services, including CAM. This is not a "medical savings account" because such a program may take many forms. In the flexible spending account, the member can set aside a specific amount per month to pay for medical services. That money is not taxed. However, there are several limitations. If the plan member does not use the money on medical expenses by the end of the year, he or she loses it. When an employer offers these accounts, employees can elect the amount of money they want to put in. For example, a plan member may decide to put aside $50 a month. He or she can use that money to pay the deductible or copayment charges, or for eye glasses, CAM, or other noncovered medical or dental services. In the current design, at the end of the year, the member loses any unspent money. This arrangement forces employees to be reasonable and conservative in their contributions. The amount should be low enough that the member will use it entirely on a variety of essential health care needs. Flexible

spending accounts have the potential to be a more widely used product to pay for CAM services. Currently, many people do not have any kind of benefit or even a rider to provide CAM coverage. With this type of product, they can put their own money aside before taxes to pay for CAM.

CAM Products of Regence BlueCross BlueShield of Oregon

Regence BlueCross BlueShield of Oregon offered its first CAM product approximately three decades ago with a rider for chiropractic services. The demand in Oregon in the chiropractic market has resulted in approximately 380,000 enrollees (of 1.1 million medical enrollees) with a Regence BlueCross BlueShield chiropractic rider. The products have often been limited by either the yearly allowance (which is 20 visits) or $20 per visit (the insurer covering $20 of the cost of each visit).

In the early 1990s, another type of product was developed that differed from a classic indemnified chiropractic rider. This capitated chiropractic benefit is available through ChiroNet, an Oregon-based preferred provider network. The indemnity product, however, also continues to survive and thrive with more than 340,000 enrollees. At this time, chiropractic is the primary complementary rider offered by Regence's plan. There have been other value-added CAM services offered by Regence BlueCross BlueShield of Oregon and by others in Oregon (much like discount affinity programs), but not as indemnity business.

EXPANDING CAM COVERAGE

What types of information and data do insurers want as a basis for expanding CAM coverage? It is important to realize that insurers are a reflection of the market in which they operate. Whether an insurer decides to offer new coverage depends on the demand on the part of employers, who are the primary purchasers of health insurance. If the market demand is there for CAM, a much stronger CAM benefit will be offered in the future.

Certain parallels can be drawn to the provision of routine vision coverage. Vision coverage riders or endorsements to medical coverage contracts have been common for some time. Today, with an emphasis on preventive care, health maintenance organizations often cover routine vision exams as part of their core medical benefit and sell only eyewear as a rider. Other health plans offer value-added or discount arrangements to access routine vision care services and suppliers. In some areas of the country, these programs include services that direct-mail contact lenses to the client's home or arrange for substantially discounted laser surgery to correct refractive error. This expansion is a reflection of a market, which for health plans is primarily the employers, looking for greater value for their health care dollars.

It is still very difficult to convince an underwriter that including CAM will not result in additional costs as opposed to resulting in reduced costs saved in another arena. An underwriter might suggest that if the number of providers of care to which an individual has access is increased, utilization will go up. If people use CAM and that does not resolve their conditions, they will seek traditional treatment. If they seek traditional treatment and that is not successful, they may seek additional complementary care. If they have access to a greater number of providers of care, the cost will go up.

Another factor that insurers believe has caused CAM to grow in the last decade has been the very strong economy in the United States.

People have disposable income, and with that income they have chosen CAM in many circumstances. If the country goes into a recession, CAM could experience a downturn as disposable income evaporates. It is likely, however, that the more people who become involved with CAM services, the more people will probably continue to use them.

Similarly, for employers to seriously consider integrating CAM benefits, good data are needed that demonstrate the effectiveness of CAM, and employees will need to request and expect CAM coverage. The industry is interested in reliable CAM outcomes data. Additionally, insurers and their clients want to know more about the practice profiles of the practitioners. Data are essential for the substantial expansion of CAM coverage.

CONCLUSION

The financial barriers to CAM continue to be overcome through a variety of methods. Today CAM insurance products are becoming more common, as are value-added products, which make costs predictable. Additionally, flexible spending programs permit employees to set aside pretax dollars to pay for many CAM benefits. State legislation has required CAM coverage in a few states, and the strong U.S. economy has increased incomes, thereby resulting in discretionary dollars available for spending on CAM services. Combined, these factors could be expected to lead to the expansion of the CAM industry.

CHAPTER 14

Coding and Software in Support of CAM Claims Processing: Alternative Link

Melinna Giannini

CODING AND SOFTWARE FOR CAM DATA CAPTURE

Alternative Link has captured over 13 million units of information in a database tied to coding to facilitate the reimbursement of complementary and alternative medicine (CAM) practitioners by third-party payers. The system describes procedures performed, services ordered, and supplements prescribed, in a way that is clear and logical to both providers and payers. Three products were developed to meet these needs:

Melinna Giannini is a co-founder, President, and CEO of Alternative Link, Inc., system developers for industry-compatible insurance claims coding and e-commerce processes for CAM and nursing services. She was instrumental in the concept development and formulation of a CAM coding product and in obtaining its patent. As director of product development, she is involved with the customization of insurance products, is editor of a series of coding manuals for CAM and nursing forthcoming from Delmar Publishing, and oversees the development of research projects. Ms. Giannini is a faculty member of the Kaiser Institute; she has testified before the National Committee for Vital and Health Statistics (U.S. Dept. of Health and Human Services), presented at national health care conferences, and is a board member of the Computer-based Patient Record Institute.

Alternative Link is a privately funded company that has spent the last 5 years in research and development to build the business tools necessary for alternative providers and nurses to interface with insurance companies. This work has resulted in the development of CAM codes for electronic billing for capturing data on pricing and treatment patterns. The company has developed a database of information on relative pricing and state scope-of-practice laws that contains more than 6 million units of information.

1. supplemental software to verify the legality of each service provided
2. a database of state scope-of-practice laws and regulations
3. a database of relative values for pricing, linked to each code.

CAM Codes

The coding system was developed to meet the need for electronically compatible codes to describe and support coverage for chiropractors, acupuncturists, massage therapists, midwives, homeopathic physicians, holistic physicians, advanced practice nurses, and naturopaths. Until CAM codes were developed, there had not been a way to capture unique data about the services of alternative practitioners, to track whether their treatments are affordable, or to determine how many visits are required to resolve particular conditions. Insurance companies require this type of information before they can underwrite CAM benefits.

The development of this type of electronic system has been necessary because currently there are no actuarial data on CAM to support broad-based coverage and reimbursement. In conventional medicine, there are now more than 30 years of data available. The data provide the parameters for clinical protocols and the basis for insurance reimbursement and define the normal ranges of cost and treatment patterns for any given diagnosis. With CAM, we do not yet have sufficient historical data to provide the basis for analyzing and underwriting claims.

It is necessary to wait until the data have accumulated and treatment patterns emerge. In the meantime, if an alternative treatment protocol is contested, the payer must spend an average of $150/hour to have the claim evaluated through a medical review process by a highly paid expert. If many of the claims for CAM required medical review, CAM services would not be affordable and could not be covered. For this reason, payers currently carve out services by counting claims or counting dollars, but they are not likely to fully underwrite services to CAM providers without cost and outcome data.

A uniform national standard code set, coupled with precise definitions of treatments, has been needed to communicate services and electronically capture data from large patient populations across multiple legal boundaries. Conventional coded information is used by Medicare and Medicaid, Veterans Affairs, CHAMPUS, and national carriers such as Aetna and United HealthCare to calculate exposure and underwrite health plan benefits. Relative values for coded services allow these agencies to compare cost outcomes for each disease no matter what the prevailing rates are for a given area. Coverage issues and payment for conventional physician services are not thwarted by different scope-of-practice laws from state to state. In contrast, major insurers are not yet able to provide full-scale benefits for CAM services due in part to differences in state laws, lack of information on the patient encounter, and the absence of relative values to calculate the costs of services. Insurance companies also require verification that CAM practitioners are allowed to provide specific services in their particular jurisdiction.

This entire range of information will make it more practical to gather CAM data and eventually to underwrite plan benefits. The following are various applications of the CAM codes:

- Facilitation of claims processing
- Allowing automated data capture using existing industry claims processing software
- Enabling sorting and aggregation of outcomes data that are provider-specific

- Facilitation of comparative analysis contrasting alternative treatment with conventional treatment patterns, by provider type and by diagnosis

For example, an acupuncture practitioner, providing dental anesthesia with acupuncture needles, has no CPT (Current Procedural Terminology) coding or description to define what that service is, how long it should take, what type of training the practitioner has, and whether it is legal within the scope of practice of the licensing regulations in that state. In order to obtain reimbursement, practitioners need the tools to communicate this type of information effectively with insurance companies. Both parties need a systematic way to verify scope of practice by state. There is also a need for a means of automatically attaching further documentation to any claim being filed to verify the legality and training requirements for each procedure used. Exhibit 14–1 indicates the categories for practitioners currently tracked by the system.

Exhibit 14–1 ABC Codes for Practitioner Types in Alternative Link

AN = Advanced nurse practitioner
CN = Clinical nurse specialist
DC = Doctor of chiropractic
DO = Doctor of osteopathy
MD = Holistic medical doctor
MT = Licensed massage therapist
ND = Naturopathic doctor or physician
NM = Certified nurse midwife
OM = Doctor of Oriental medicine
PA = Physician assistant
PN = Licensed practical nurse
RM = Registered midwife
RN = Registered nurse

Courtesy of Alternative Link, Las Cruces, New Mexico.

Claims Processing Software

The Alternative Link software application is designed to be electronically interfaced with existing claims processing software and runs simultaneously with any of the major claims processing systems. The Alternative Link database (rules engine) includes the legal citations that describe CAM scope of practice and therefore legitimize and justify medical claims for various CAM services on a state-specific basis. The database can be accessed by conventional software and currently includes over 13 million up-to-date units of information. The legal provision of health care services in the 50 states for each category of CAM practitioner can be sorted by practitioner, code, and/or by state. The system provides a wealth of information that facilitates the processing of a claim for CAM services, by describing scope of practice for licensed providers, as well as clinical procedures, laboratory tests, nutraceuticals, and care pathways. The rationale for appropriate treatment and payment is accessed by attaching information from the database/rules engine to claims. Documentation is further enhanced by supplying explanations of services and descriptions of the training required for each licensed provider according to each state's law.

The software and database(s) provide a variety of important functions in claims processing:

- facilitation and expedition of claims processing and payment
- delineation of the scope-of-practice reports by providing documentation that verifies the range of services allowed by state laws for each provider type
- facilitation of decision support by documenting each service, thus eliminating the need to create or interpret written reports
- delineation of training standards that describe the education required for any given patient service in any state
- attachment of credentialing standards based on state regulation.

Pricing Attached to Codes—Relative Value Units

Relative values are numerical values attached to each code to establish fees for professional medical services, including CAM and nursing. This mechanism allows the practitioner to use a single dollar multiplier to define or price any coded service. The relative value for any given service is based on measurable criteria such as training required, the degree of difficulty of the service provided, malpractice insurance rates, and the expense of specialized equipment that may be used for each procedure. Relative values are adjustable. The dollar multiplier can be adjusted up or down to reflect different insurance contracts, to allow for cost of living increases, or to reflect regional variation. The relative value scale in the system is verified by Relative Value Studies, Inc. Over 80% of insurance companies set fees for services using relative values.

Relative values support the integration of CAM practitioners and:

- facilitate fee negotiations with insurance companies
- allow cost comparisons with conventional medical services
- predict the cost of underwriting CAM services
- provide a necessary tool for utilization management of premium dollars.

INFORMATION CONVEYED BY THE CODES

The Use of Codes To Describe CAM Service Provision

The continued shift to electronic commerce is altering the way in which insurance claims are filed. The Health Insurance Portability and Accountability Act (HIPAA passed in 1996) demands more accurate assessments of the patient encounter. Providers are required to report in precise terms the treatments they provide patients. HIPAA also requires this information to be delivered in standard electronic formats to reduce paperwork. The Alternative Link system was built to meet both of these requirements. It further enhances this communication by supplying state-by-state legal edits. (See Exhibit 14–2.)

The codes provide the following information:

- *UI*—Unique identifier that allows historical tracking of procedures
- *The ABC© Code*—A 5-character alphabetical code attached to each procedure that includes both the practitioner code and modifier
- *Practitioner Modifier*—A 2-character alphabetic code indicating the type of practitioner providing the service (see Exhibit 14-1)
- *RVUs*—The relative value unit that provides pricing information relevant to the pricing of the service.

Information Fields

Service Provider. The modifier field of this code set defines the practitioner with a two-letter alphabetical modifier, such as "MT" for massage therapist and "ND" for naturopathic doctor. The current version of the Alternative Link system supports state-by-state coded reports (defining which practitioners are allowed to do what procedures) for 13 different types of licensed practitioners in all 50 states and the District of Columbia as described in Exhibit 14–2.

The developers of Alternative Link mapped the various terms used in state law to indicate each type of practitioner. For example, "nurse practitioner" has eight different variations in state law, although these descriptors all define the same training. In the Alternative Link software, nurse practitioner is indicated by the modifier "NP." Massage therapists have nine different names in state law, such as massage therapists, certified massage therapists, licensed massage

Exhibit 14–2 Services That Only Acupuncturists or Certified Oriental Medicine Practitioners Are Trained To Provide

CAM-NET™ MIS Code Sample

Examples of codes without a good CPT™ Crosswalk.

Colorado Scope of Practice
Subcategory: Oriental Medicine

UI	ABC© Code	Description	CPT Code	RVUs	DC	MT	MD	OM	ND	DO	NM	RM
261	CAAAA	Dental, Anesthesia, Oriental Medicine, Practice Specialties	01999	5.98				✓				
262	CAAAB	Surgical, Anesthesia, Oriental Medicine, Practice Specialties	01999	20.8				✓				
263	CAAAC	Induction of Labor up to one hour, Delivery, Anesthesia, Oriental Medicine, Practice Specialties	59899	7.63				✓				

Courtesy of Alternative Link, Las Cruces, New Mexico.

practitioner, and licensed massage therapist/technician. Massage therapists are categorized under the modifier "MT" for massage therapy.

The practitioner codes provide access to information that can be attached to claims, such as the state law on training. That allows everyone with the same training to be identified by scope of practice laws. (See Exhibit 14–3 for an example of the training standards provided by the software.) This two-letter modifier is placed at the end of the code to indicate the practitioner. This allows the claims adjuster to call out all the information about the provider as captured in the patient encounter. It also allows comparison of the service provision of two providers (for example, comparing treatment of low-back pain by a massage therapist with that of a chiropractor).

Additional Training

The data also list additional training that may be required of a particular practitioner in order for his or her services to be reimbursable when providing a particular treatment. For example, in Hawaii, physicians are required to have the full 3 years of training certification as an acupuncturist in order to provide moxibustion treatment to patients. The software's code set correlates additional information from the HCFA 1500, as an electronic claims attachment, thereby expanding the information available to the claims adjuster. In summary, information is provided on the alternative treatment (Exhibit14–4), the practitioner, his or her training, and the licensing requirements.

Scope of Practice. The legal scope of practice has been linked to the code as an indication of whether a particular alternative treatment is legal for that practitioner in the state in which the service was provided, thus allowing the provider's claims to be electronically verified or adjudicated. As long as the service is within legal guidelines, the electronic edit will facilitate payment.

SOFTWARE TO SUPPORT ELECTRONIC CAM BILLING

Use of the Alternative Link coding and systems provides a national language for communicating claims while ensuring that the claims are legal and

Exhibit 14–3 Training Standards

ABC© Code	Required Naturopathic Doctor Training
CEAAD Pelvic Exam with PAP Smear, Midwifery	If practicing in a regulated state, territory or possession of the United States, licensure, certification or registration as required by law and licensed as a midwife in that state or hold current active Midwifery certification by the American College of Naturopathic Obstetricians. If practicing in an unregulated jurisdiction, current active certification by and passing scores received on Naturopathic Physicians Licensing Exam, NPLEX, in Naturopathic Medicine; or current licensure, registration or certification as a Naturopathic Physician in another state, territory or possession of the United States; and licensed as a midwife in another state, territory or possession of the United States; or hold current active Midwifery certification by the American College of Naturopathic Obstetricians.

Training standards for different practitioner types are also contained in machine-readable format by code.

Courtesy of Alternative Link, Las Cruces, New Mexico.

Exhibit 14–4 Expanded Definitions

ABC© Code	Description	Expanded Definition
CAAAB	Surgical Anesthesia, Anesthesia/Stimulation, Oriental Medicine, Practice Specialties	Administration of any acupuncture or oriental medicine modality or modalities or of any herbal medicines, when any of the same are for purposes of providing anesthesia and/or analgesia for one or more surgical procedures performed on a single occasion. No other oriental-medical procedures or modalities are billable for any services provided in relation to such surgical procedures if such services could reasonably have been provided within one hour of conclusion of such surgical procedures. For up to two hours in attendance by provider, regardless of complexity. Usually not billable when performed by the same provider who is qualified and is also performing the surgery. For additional time requirements, see code CAAAE.

The expanded definitions also keep providers from bundling or unbundling services.

Courtesy of Alternative Link, Las Cruces, New Mexico.

are within state legal scope-of-practice definitions The coding and data create the capacity for capturing outcomes. When an insurance company receives the data, it can query by diagnosis and compare cost for alternative treatments with those of conventional treatments for the same health problem (using ICD-9 codes, procedure codes, and relative pricing information).

Software Functions

State-by-State Documentation To Justify Claims

State laws vary tremendously regarding every aspect of licensure and scope of practice for alternative practitioners. In order to meet this need for state-specific regulatory information, the data warehouse of the software includes the legal descriptions of scope of practice for every state for 13 different types of practitioners. The information is referenced on a code-by-code level, based on the discipline of the provider, the state in which he or she practices, and the service provided. In addition to the legal definitions and citations, training standards for each discipline are also available in the database.

Interface with HCFA Forms

Currently, conventional claims are filed on a HCFA 1500 form (generated by the Health Care Financing Administration and the only form accepted by all payers). That form contains the diagnostic rationale for treatment, using the ICD-9 (International Classification of Diseases, Ninth Edition) codes and the HCPCS (Health Care Procedure Coding Systems) codes (Level I to III) to describe the procedures that were performed on the patient for the treatment of a specified diagnosed disease or problem. (Hospitals use a similar standard form called the UB-92.)

Alternative Link coding is designed to be compatible with the HCFA 1500 form and the UB-92, and data from these forms are captured in conjunction with the existing ICD-9 descriptors and diagnoses. The coding was created to fit into the procedure coding fields of these forms and current coding software systems. The CAM codes of Alternative Links are distinct, in that they are all alphabetic. These alpha codes provide information on procedures that are unique to CAM using the procedures-reporting features of the HCFA 1500 form and the UB-92 (based on the Uniform Bill, 1992) and are thus compatible with industry standards.

Applying CAM Codes to the Super Bill

Most conventional practitioners use a super bill to invoice their patients. The super bill is a patient encounter form on which practitioners can simply check off the services they normally provide. They also have the option of writing in any unusual service on that form. Physicians have super bills that automatically translate into coded HCFA 1500 forms. Although CAM providers sometimes use super bills, they are also required to attach doecumentation to explain services because CPT codes are not precise descriptors of CAM services.* Alternative Link facilitates electronic billing and the development of super bills so that CAM providers have the same efficiency as conventional physicians.

EXPEDITING PAYMENT

When forms can be electronically transmitted, payment is reimbursed in 14 days, rather than the average of 51 days for paper claims. This is now possible for alternative medicine using the CAM codes. Most all claims processing software reviews provider documentation on the HCFA 1500 to verify that the form is filled out correctly. For each field, the system edits the form for logic, completeness, and accuracy. Consequently, attaching the CAM coding system to a claims processing system reduces the time required to process CAM claims and thus makes them affordable. The CAM software provides the same type of completeness and accuracy for processing CAM claims that are available to physician services.

Facilitating Documentation

The documentation provided by the software adds weight to claims from providers by supplying precise definitions and boundaries of service

---

*CPT™ is a registered trademark of the American Medical Association.

not previously included in CAM claims. Consequently, even a claims adjuster who knows nothing about CAM services will now have complete access to the legal and regulatory documentation needed to process claims. Alternative Link coding is compatible with standard message formats in HCFA 1500 and UB-92 claim forms, and all of these attachments can be interfaced with the claims processing software of the payer or claims adjuster.

Case Study: Processing a Claim

Consider a case in which a chiropractor in New Mexico provides a patient with advice on nutrition and recommends a botanical regimen to follow for an arthritic condition. The HCFA 1500 form would specifically indicate:

- The state in which the claim was filed: NM = New Mexico.
- The procedure used by the chiropractic practitioner: nutritional education (AE-BAC—individual holistic nutritional education 15 minutes).
- Allowed or disallowed practice: The legal citation is attached. The reader is referred to the New Mexico statute under the New Mexico Chiropractic Act, 6.4-4.2A, Regulatory Board, New Mexico Board of Chiropractic Examiners Rules and Regulations, 16NMAC4.1.7.1. A summary of that legal citation indicates "Chiropractors may counsel and recommend nutraceuticals." The statute allows this clinical practice. Therefore, it would be approved by a claims adjudicator because the adjudicator is provided with the legal citation that allows a chiropractor to provide counseling on nutritional supplements and advice regarding diet.

Facilitating Interface with the Router and the Payer

Once the HCFA 1500 form has been completed, it is forwarded electronically to the router, a company that forwards claims to the payer and translates the electronic claim so the payer's system can read it. The data are automatically formatted to fit the payer's system. The router is able to forward the information to any payer. Once it is received by the payer, the claim will be evaluated electronically. The payer will be able to use the codes to determine whether that coded service is allowed in the plan's benefit.

Interfacing with Multiple Payers

In some cases, there is more than one payer. If Medicare is paying a portion of the bill, and the Medicare supplemental policy is paying another portion, there must be some coordination between the payments. At each point in the process the information is checked. Then the claim goes on to the next level of the edit. An automated system asks if the provider is contracted with a preferred provider organization, a health maintenance organization (HMO), or an independent practice association (IPA). If the provider is not contracted with an HMO, the claim is rejected. The Alternative Link data warehouse provides the state-specific information that verifies the provider's credentials. If the practitioner's services are covered, the next question is whether this provider has supplied a service that is appropriate to his or her credentials and scope of practice, as defined by state law. A copy of the statute is attached electronically to the claim, verifying the legal appropriateness of the service. If the service is not legally appropriate, the claim is rejected.

Additional Reporting

The Automatic Provision of Additional Documentation. If a CPT code ends in the numbers "99," a written report is required from the practitioner. Normally, this can be problematic. If the attachment is logical and the claims adjuster finds it acceptable, the claim will be approved. However, if the claims adjuster does not find the attachment acceptable, the claim will be returned, requiring additional information. The

software can avoid this potential problem by supplying electronic attachments that include treatment protocol. This can potentially save significant amounts of time for both providers and payers.

AGGREGATING COSTS AND OUTCOMES DATA

The coding creates new opportunities for outcomes research. The Alternative Link software facilitates the capture of cost and outcomes data. Historically, insurance providers have relied on double-blind studies and reports of patient satisfaction. The coding provides data to the payer's underwriting department and indicates how many visits were needed to alleviate the condition and stop the claim; it also specifies the total cost of treatment. The coding provides a basis for sorting and aggregating empirical data on CAM. This expands the basis for underwriting claims. Consequently, it gives the payer the ability to compare cost data on alternative therapies with the cost of conventional interventions for the same diagnosis, using the payer's current software system.

FUTURE TECHNOLOGY

The average processing time for paper claims from CAM providers can require as long as 51 days to determine whether a claim will be paid. The clearinghouse router technology requires 14 days. Currently, Internet technology is still in development, but once it becomes more advanced, processing could require as little as 2 or 3 days before reimbursement is transferred into the practitioner's bank account electronically.

Standards development in the insurance industry has been ongoing. Common electronic language has now been developed for the health insurance industry as it was several years ago for the banking industry. The organization that coordinates these efforts is the American National Standards Institute X-12 Committee (American National Standards Institute, 1999). By a vote of consensus, Alternative Link has been included in the implementation guide as an optional field. CPT codes are also included in the guide, as well as code sets developed by the American Dental Association, HCPCS Level II codes developed by HCFA, pharmaceutical coding, and other codes used to process health care claims.

Alternative Link has sought through government involvement to make the CAM codes an electronic standard for processing claims for CAM. The original vision remains: to include access to CAM services for everyone because we believe that CAM is one of the key solutions in the reduction of rising health care costs.

REFERENCES

American Hospital Association. *International Classification of Diseases: Ninth Edition.* Chicago, IL: AHA; 1998.

American Medical Association. *Current Procedural Terminology CPT™ 2000.* Chicago: American Medical Association; 2000:8.

American National Standards Institute. American Standards Committee. X12N, *Implementation Guide Version 004*, Release 2, Subrelease 2 (004022). New York, 1999.

CHAPTER 15

Federal Initiatives and Resources in Complementary Medicine

15.1 Programs of the National Center for Complementary and Alternative Medicine and the National Cancer Institute, National Institutes of Health (NIH)

Congressional Testimony by Stephen E. Straus and Edward L. Trimble

OVERVIEW

The need for scientifically valid information about CAM (complementary and alternative

---

Source: Excerpts from a statement by Stephen E. Straus, MD, Director, National Center for Complementary and Alternative Medicine before the Senate Appropriations Subcommittee on Labor—HHS—Education and Related Agencies on the Fiscal Year 2001, President's Budget Request for the NCCAM, Thursday, March 30, 2000. <http://nccam.nih.gov/nccam/ne/appropriations-s.html> Accessed 4/00.

*Excerpts from a statement by Edward L. Trimble, MD, Head, Surgery Section, Division of Cancer Treatment and Diagnosis, National Cancer Institute, National Institutes of Health. Hearing before the House Committee on Government Reform. June 10, 1999. <http://nccam.nih.gov/nccam/ne/appropriations-s.html> Accessed 4/00.

medicine) therapies is heightened by the potential for benefit as well as for risk. These benefits and risks can result from use of the preparations and procedures alone or as a complement to conventional therapies. However, evidence for the balance of benefit and risk is not available for most CAM approaches. The ongoing development of the National Center for Complementary and Alternative Medicine (NCCAM) will provide an expansion of research and information dissemination.

NCCAM's work reflects the growing public interest in CAM and the belief that various CAM therapies may play a role in improved public health. Approximately 42% of U.S. health care consumers spent $27 billion on CAM therapies in 1997. CAM enjoys particular popularity among baby boomers. A number of practices, once considered unorthodox, have proven safe and effective and assimilated seamlessly into current medical practice. Diet and exercise are today commonly used to prevent and control disease. Acupuncture is routinely applied to manage chronic pain and nausea associated with chemotherapy. Some of our most important drugs—digitalis, vincristine, and taxol—are of botanical origin. Additional CAM practices have the potential to prevent and treat chronic disease, to improve understanding of how healing works, and to be integrated into the routine practice of medicine. Absent definitive evidence of effectiveness, however, alternative practices may impart untoward consequences for large numbers of people.

As CAM use by the American people has steadily increased, many have asked whether reports of success with these treatments are valid. It is critical that untested but widely used CAM treatments be rigorously evaluated for safety and efficacy. It is similarly important to identify promising new approaches worthy of more intensive study. The promising areas for future investments are numerous.

In order to best seize these opportunities, our strategy must differ from that used by other NIH institutes and centers. Other projects are usually driven by basic science discoveries. In contrast, the NCCAM must focus first on definitive clinical trials of widely utilized modalities that, from evidence-based reviews, appear to be the most promising. Credible, not anecdotal, data must be provided to the public, and we must educate conventional medical practitioners about the panoply of effective CAM practices so that they can be integrated into patient care. In recognition of these needs, Congress responded in 1998 by elevating the NIH Office of Alternative Medicine (OAM), expanding its mandate, creating NCCAM, and affording it administrative authority to design and manage its own research portfolio. Five strategic areas have been identified: investing in research, training CAM investigators, expanding outreach, facilitating integration, and practicing responsible stewardship.

CURRENT NCCAM RESEARCH

In its first year, NCCAM has developed a diverse research portfolio in partnership with other NIH institutes and centers, in support of some of the largest and most definitive Phase III clinical trials ever undertaken for a range of CAM therapies. These include therapies for a number of conditions.

Herbal Therapy for Dementia

For centuries, extracts from the leaves of the *Ginkgo biloba* tree have been used as Chinese herbal medicine to treat a variety of medical conditions, including age-related decline in memory. A new NCCAM study, in collaboration with the National Institutes on Aging (NIA), may help resolve these questions. This study includes four clinical centers and will enroll almost 3,000 participants who will receive either *Ginkgo biloba* or a placebo.

The Treatment of Arthritis

In collaboration with National Institute of Arthritis and Musculoskeletal Diseases (NIAMS), NCCAM has mounted two critical clinical trials for the treatment of osteoarthritis. One is the first U.S. multicenter study to investigate the dietary supplements glucosamine and chondroitin sulfate, two natural substances found in and around joint cartilage. The other study is an evaluation of acupuncture for the treatment of pain associated with osteoarthritis.

Herbal Therapy for Depression

A study sponsored by the NCCAM, National Institute of Mental Health (NIMH), and the NIH Office of Dietary Supplements (ODS) represents the largest and most rigorous assessments of the effectiveness and safety of St. John's wort to date. A recent study reported in *The British Medical Journal* showed that St. John's wort is more effective than placebo in treatment of depression, and perhaps as effective as an older generation antidepressant drug, imipramine. NC-CAM's study, which is considerably larger than the European trial, compares St. John's wort with placebo and with Zoloft, currently one of the most commonly used antidepressants.

Treatment of Benign Prostatitis Hyperplasia (BPH)

Anecdotal reports suggest that the botanical product saw palmetto decreases prostate swelling. To determine the validity of these observations, NCCAM, in collaboration with National Institute on Diabetes and Digestive and Kidney Diseases (NIDDK), is supporting the first rigorously designed, placebo-controlled study to evaluate the effect of saw palmetto extract on symptoms and quality of life in men.

Cancer Therapies

Both shark cartilage and a diet/dietary supplement approach have found considerable support and use in the nonmedical and medical communities, but the scientific evidence is sparse. Two large trials are being supported by NCCAM and are being conducted by the National Cancer Institute (NCI).

Intervention for Liver Disease

NCCAM has planned a collaboration on the treatment of liver disease with the NIDDK and the National Institute of Allergy and Infectious Diseases (NIAID). The project will examine the efficacy of milk thistle extract, *Silybum marianum*, when used to treat hepatitis C and other hepatic diseases.

COLLABORATIVE RESEARCH

NCCAM has already begun a number of activities that will serve to facilitate the integration of validated CAM therapies into conventional medical practice. The NCCAM plans to make awards to foster incorporation of CAM infor-

mation into the curricula of medical and allied health schools and continuing medical education programs. Also, the NCCAM must educate eager medical students about CAM so that they may knowledgeably guide an avid patient base toward safe and effective CAM applications. We must also work to overcome the reluctance of conventional physicians to consider validated CAM therapies and to assimilate proven ones into their practices. The center has established a Clinical Research Curriculum Award (CRCA) to attract talented individuals to CAM research and to provide them with the critical skills that are needed.

Intramural Research Program

The NCCAM will establish an Intramural Research Program that will develop a critical mass of CAM research to stimulate collaboration in the NIH Clinical Center with other institutes and centers, our federal research partners, and others. The intramural program will serve as a focus for training future CAM researchers.

Collaboration with the NCI

The collaboration with the NCI affords an efficient means of utilizing the resources and expertise of the Cancer Therapy and Evaluation Program. Importantly, this collaboration between NCI and NCCAM is being expanded with the development of a Cancer Advisory Panel for Complementary and Alternative Medicine. This panel will evaluate and recommend future studies and diminish the misunderstanding and controversy surrounding CAM therapy in cancer. The trials should indicate which therapies have value, which do not, and what are the safety and adherence issues.

CAM Research Centers

A center program was initiated by the Office of Alternative Medicine 5 years ago with the goal of developing a core of resources, researchers, and collaborators that would investigate promising clinical observations and develop pilot studies aimed at building a base for larger and more definitive clinical trials. The centers' program is being expanded under NCCAM to include new areas of interest and to increase support for individual research projects that will move the research toward evidence-based statements of CAM practice. The centers have brought together researchers from the CAM community and experienced scientists with strong methodological skills. The CAM research centers focus on cancer, cardiovascular disease, HIV/AIDS, pediatrics, musculoskeletal disorders (with emphasis on rheumatoid diseases and osteoarthritis), neurological disorders and stroke, substance abuse, and problems associated with aging.

Interagency Endeavors

The important scientific assistance provided by them will continue by having a designated liaison scientist for each institute and center. These liaisons attend scheduled meetings that also include liaisons from other health agencies. These interagency scheduled meetings began in 1997 and have fostered interagency agreements with Agency for Health Care Policy and Research (AHCPR) and the Centers for Disease Control and Prevention (CDC). The evidence-based practice centers program of AHCPR will be tasked to develop evidence-based reviews of selected CAM practices as designated by NCCAM. CDC has an agreement to conduct field investigations of practice experiences with CAM and to report their findings. In both instances, the unique resources of these agencies are being used to complement studies supported by NIH, and this information provides direction for future studies.

Multicultural Research Collaborations

The development of culturally sensitive studies will enable NCCAM to establish method-ological feasibility and strengthen the scientific rationale for proceeding to full-scale, randomized, clinical trials on the application of traditional indigenous systems. The ability to validate some of these therapies will also expand health care options for those who are primarily consumers of conventional medicine. The international character of CAM necessitates that the NCCAM develop a broad-based international research program. That process will ensue with the appointment of a director for International and Traditional Medicine Studies who will develop a long-range plan for the pursuit of studies on a global scale. NCCAM support has already been authorized, in collaboration with the National Institute of Child Health and Human Development (NICHD), for international studies of traditional medical approaches to the health of women and children.

Grant-Supported Research

NCCAM reviews and funds investigator-initiated research grants using the usual NIH peer-review system. These investigator-initiated studies include basic investigations of mechanisms, field investigations, or reported therapeutic successes, and exploratory studies and small trials. The NCCAM will also continue to benefit from the interest and active participation of staff from other institutes and centers at NIH and from collaboration with other agencies.

Research Training

Research training has a critical role in advancing research in CAM. Both the conventional and CAM communities have expressed an interest in conducting CAM research. Both groups need training in design and conduct of clinical research and in addressing the unique issues presented in studying CAM modalities. The centers' program has facilitated training by bringing together a critical mass of CAM investigators and projects. Training and fellowship awards have been made to trainees working in the CAM research centers and as supplements to other grants. The intramural research training program began in 1998.

NCI PROGRAMS*

The NCI is steadily building an environment that fosters the convergence of ideas from traditional and alternative approaches to the goal of eradicating cancer.

Human Papilloma Virus

Studies have revealed that approximately 90% of cervical malignancies are linked to infection with human papilloma virus (HPV). NCI is sponsoring a Phase II trial to determine whether a carotenoid-rich diet can be effective in reversing mild cervical lesions. Changes in HPV status will be concurrently monitored.

Complementary Cancer Therapies

The NCI is moving ahead with a number of research efforts that involve the evaluation of CAM approaches to cancer-related problems. NCI, along with NCCAM, is supporting an evaluation of Dr. Nicholas Gonzales's nutritional therapy at Columbia Presbyterian Medical Center, one of the NCI-designated comprehensive cancer centers. Another interesting area of potential research activity is the evaluation of green tea as a cancer prevention strategy. Among the many other research efforts are projects examining the therapeutic value of vitamins and minerals in cancer treatment and prevention, studies in stress and pain management to enhance the quality of life for cancer patients, and studies examining the effect of natural inhibitors of carcinogenesis.

Angiogenesis

A number of angiogenesis inhibitors that arrest tumor expansion by curtailing the formation of new blood vessels and subsequently the delivery of oxygen and nutrients to the tumor site are undergoing testing in clinical trials. One of the agents set to be evaluated this year in a Phase III trial cosponsored by NCI and NCCAM is Neovastat, a preparation of shark cartilage.

Collaborative Activities with NCCAM

We have collaborated with NCCAM on the establishment of a Cancer Advisory Panel (CAP-CAM). The CAP-CAM meets two to three times a year and draws its 15 members from a broad range of experts from the conventional and CAM cancer research community. This group will review and evaluate summaries of evidence for CAM cancer claims submitted by practitioners, make recommendations on whether and how these evaluations should be followed up, and communicate the results of any ensuing studies.

Natural Products Research

Since 1955, the NCI has screened samples of plant, marine, and microbial origin for activity against cancer, and several clinically effective anticancer drugs, including vincristine, vinblastine, etoposide, topotecan, adriamycin, actinomycin, bleuomycin, and taxol, have emerged from this program. Since 1986, the NCI's Developmental Therapeutics Branch has performed collections of over 50,000 plants and 10,000 marine organism samples in over 30 countries located in tropical and subtropical countries worldwide through contracts with botanical and marine biological organizations.

15.2 The White House Commission on Complementary and Alternative Medicine Policy*

Press Release by the President of the United States

Today, I am pleased to announce the appointment of the Chair and the first members of the White House Commission on Alternative Medicine. This commission, created by an executive order on March 8, 2000, is charged with developing a set of legislative and administrative recommendations to maximize the benefits of complementary and alternative medicine for the general public.

Each year, tens of millions of Americans receive alternative therapies. The great potential and possible perils associated with the use of complementary and alternative medicine have been well documented. There is no doubt that these therapies should be held to the same standard of scientific rigor as more traditional health care interventions. If we are going to hold complementary and alternative therapies to an appropriate standard of accountability, we need to invest in research so health care professionals and consumers can make informed judgments about the appropriate use of these services. In that vein, we have worked with Senator Harkin and a bipartisan coalition of members of Congress to establish the NIH Center for Complementary and Alternative Medicine to invest resources in scientific analysis to make such information available.

But we need to do more. We need to be able to use information about alternative therapies to set the national agenda for the education and training of health care practitioners in this field and provide recommendations for advisable coverage policies for alternative therapies. I particularly want to applaud the leadership of Senator Tom Harkin, Senator Barbara Mikulski, Senator Arlen Spector, Senator Harry Reid, and Congressman Peter DeFazio in advocating for and finding funding for this commission. There is no question in my mind that we would not be making this announcement without their tireless efforts. I also want to thank Secretary Shalala for her commitment to explore all avenues of scientific discovery to help ensure that Americans have access to the most accountable and responsive health care system possible.

As we enter into the 21st century, we need to get better information to ensure American families have access to the best and most cost-effective health care. I know I join the Congress, the policy makers, and the American public in saying how much we look forward to the results of the commission's work.

MEMBERS OF THE WHITE HOUSE COMMISSION

The following members have been appointed to the White House Commission on Complementary and Alternative Medicine Policy: chair: James S. Gordon, MD; George M. Bernier, Jr, MD; David Bresler, PhD, LAc, OME, Dipl Ac; Thomas Chappell; Effie Poy Yew Chow, PhD, RN, Dipl Ac; George T. DeVries, III; William R. Fair, MD; Joseph J. Fins, MD, FACP; Veronica Gutierrez, DC; Wayne B. Jonas, MD; Linnea Signe Larson, LCSW, LMFT; Tieraona Low Dog, MD, AHG; Charlotte R. Kerr, RSM; Dean Ornish, MD; Conchita M. Paz, MD; Buford L. Rolin; Julia R. Scott; Xiaoming Tian, MD, LAc; Donald W. Warren, DDS.

Source: Reprinted from The Federal Register, July 14, 2000.

15.3   Federal Initiatives in Chiropractic

Jay Witter

CHIROPRACTIC LEGISLATION

Recent Initiatives

Recent and forthcoming legislation that will expand the scope of chiropractic in federal programs include several initiatives.

Medicare Initiative. On January 1, 2000, the mandatory radiographic requirement for chiropractic services in the Medicare program was removed. Under the revised legislation, Medicare beneficiaries who seek chiropractic services will not be required to obtain a radiograph from a physician or medical center before obtaining chiropractic treatment. This provision eliminated an artificial barrier to chiropractic services and allows doctors of chiropractic to determine whether or not an x-ray is appropriate. Prior to this legislative change, Medicare covered chiropractic services involving manual manipulation of the spine to correct a subluxation only when demonstrated by a diagnostic x-ray. Medicare regulations prohibited payment for the x-ray either if performed by a chiropractor or ordered by a chiropractor. This mandatory requirement was included in the Medicare program in 1972 as an intentional barrier to chiropractic services.

U.S. Department of Defense (DoD) Chiropractic Initiatives. In 1995, the U.S. Congress approved a Chiropractic Health Care Demonstration Project authorizing the DoD to conduct a pilot program to demonstrate the feasibility of integrating chiropractic services into the U.S.

Jay Witter is Vice President of Government Relations for the American Chiropractic Association, a professional organization representing doctors of chiropractic, whose mission is to preserve, improve, and promote the chiropractic profession.

military health system. The legislation was further modified in 1998 to include the provision of chiropractic care on a test basis at a total of 13 military treatment facilities within the United States.

In 2000, the DoD released a final report on the results of the pilot program. Data in the DoD report clearly demonstrated:

1. higher levels of patient satisfaction with chiropractic care
2. superior outcomes for patients receiving chiropractic care for neuromusculoskeletal conditions
3. fewer hospital stays for cases treated by chiropractic care
4. significant improvements in military readiness due to the inclusion of chiropractic care due to a large reduction in lost duty time.

H.R. 4205 (Public Law No. 106-398)— Chiropractic Benefit for Active Duty Military Personnel. As passed by Congress in 2000, H.R. 4205 requires access for active duty military personnel to "a permanent chiropractic benefit . . . which includes, at a minimum, care for neuromusculoskeletal conditions typical among military personnel on active duty." This legislation requires that full implementation of the benefit be phased in over a five-year period, throughout all three service branches of the military. When the phase-in has been completed, all active duty personnel stationed in the United States and overseas are to have access to the chiropractic benefit. A full "implementation plan" will be developed in 2001. The legislation also includes a provision that required the DoD to consult with the Chiropractic Health Care Demonstration Project's (CHCDP) Oversight Advisory Committee, which includes doctors of chiropractic, regarding the development and implementation of the phase-in plan.

U.S. Department of Veterans Affairs Conference Report Chiropractic Provision. The Veterans Millennium Health Care Act, P.L. 106-117, signed by President Clinton on November 30, 1999, contains a provision requiring the Department of Veterans Affairs (VA) to develop a policy regarding the utilization of chiropractic care in the VA health care system.

15.4　Ornish Program: Medicare Lifestyle Modification Program Demonstration

HEALTH CARE FINANCING ADMINISTRATION

In September 1999, the Health Care Financing Administration announced plans to implement a demonstration project to determine whether a comprehensive lifestyle program may be a safe and cost-effective alternative to conventional medical treatments for selected Medicare patients.

The demonstration project is designed to study up to 1,800 selected Medicare patients with severe coronary artery disease who have elected to follow Dr. Dean Ornish's Program for Reversing Heart Disease as an alternative to bypass surgery and angioplasty. This demonstration will be implemented at medical facilities around the United States that have been trained and licensed by Dr. Ornish and his colleagues at the nonprofit Preventive Medicine Research Institute in Sausalito, California.

DEPARTMENT OF DEFENSE REPLICATION STUDY

Congress has appropriated $2.5 million through the U.S. Department of Defense for the Preventive Medicine Research Institute to train health professionals at the Walter Reed Army Medical Center. This program is funded to implement a replication study of the Ornish Program, which will be offered to active and retired military personnel.

15.5　Federal Resources in CAM

INFORMATION DISSEMINATION AT NCCAM AND NCI

NCCAM has several publicly available information sources.

- ***The NCCAM Information Clearinghouse*** develops and disseminates fact sheets, information packages, and publications to enhance public understanding about CAM research supported by the NIH. The NCCAM Information Clearinghouse provides information for those who call the toll-free number (888-644-6226); operators can respond to inquiries in English or Spanish.

About 1,500 inquiries are handled each month, and the number continues to grow.

- **The NCCAM's Web site** (<http://nccam.nih.gov>), established in 1998, reflects the NCCAM's growth in size and stature. Averaging more than 460,000 visits per month, the site includes links to NCCAM program areas, news and events, research grants, funding opportunities, and resources.
- **The CAM Citation Index (CCI)**, assembled by NCCAM from the National Library of Medicine's MEDLINE database, affords the public access to approximately 175,000 bibliographic citations searchable by CAM system, disease, or method. The CAM Citation Index can be accessed on the NCCAM Web site through the consumers' homepage, which lists complementary and alternative medicine databases, or directly on the Internet at <http://156.40.172.112>.
- **The Combined Health Information Database (CHID)** is another federally supported service in which NCCAM participates, which includes a variety of materials not available in other government databases. CHID aggregates health information for the public on numerous topical areas related to health and disease. The CHID database can be accessed through NCCAM on the page of databases or directly on the Internet at: <http://chid.nih.gov>.

Information materials on CAM cancer therapies are being revised cooperatively with the NCI, available at the Web sites of both NCI and NCCAM.

A series of town meetings to facilitate outreach to the general public has also been initiated; the first was held in March 2000 in Boston, in conjunction with the Center for Alternative Medicine and Education of Beth Israel Deaconess Medical Center.

NCI PUBLIC INFORMATION ABOUT CAM

Detailed CAM summaries are being prepared on cancer therapies identified by the Cancer Information Service (CIS) and the NCCAM Information Clearinghouse as being of public interest. The development of these summaries will follow the same model as those for conventional therapies and include specific trial results and references to the published literature. These summaries will also be sent to experts in the CAM community for review and comment before they are made available on the NCI Web site.

The primary avenues NCI uses to communicate with the public and the health care community are on its Web site (www.nci.nih.gov). An addition to NCI's Web site is the CancerTrials site (www.cancertrials.nci.nih.gov). Through this site, patients, health care professionals, and the public can learn about ongoing NCI-sponsored trials, the most recent advances in cancer therapy, and resources related to cancer treatment.

CIS provides up-to-date cancer information to patients and their families, the public, and health care professionals in every state through 19 offices located in NCI-funded cancer centers and by dialing 1-800-4-CANCER.

There is now an Office of Cancer Complementary and Alternative Medicine (OCCAM) within the National Cancer Institute. The website of OCCAM can be accessed at: <http://occam.nci.nih.gov>.

Federal resources in general can be accessed through the federal Web directory on First Gov on the Internet at: <http://firstgov.gov>.

CHAPTER 16

State Initiatives in Complementary Medicine

16.1   Field Report: The Coverage of Complementary and Alternative Medicine in Washington State

Lori L. Bielinski

The Washington state legislation on complementary and alternative medicine (CAM) was enacted as part of a comprehensive health care reform effort. The reform was inspired by the Health Care Commission, which held statewide meetings on health care reform in 1992. Consumers and providers of health care of all types testified to the Commission regarding what they wanted in terms of health care reform and in a health care package. Grassroots advocacy was also instrumental in this process because the meetings of the Commission were open and held throughout the state, even in isolated, rural areas.

The Commission made recommendations to the legislature, and when the legislature passed the health care reform laws in 1993 their recommendations were included in the reforms. In 1994, a new legislature was elected, and the new body repealed many of the reforms, although leaving the most popular changes in effect. One component of the reforms that remained intact was the "Every Category of Provider" law. It prohibits insurers from excluding, by category, providers who are licensed and treating conditions covered in the basic health plan, in accordance with their scope of practice. However, insurers may limit provider pools and establish condition-based protocols/guidelines on utilization, cost control, documentation, gatekeep-

---

Lori L. Bielinski, LMP, has served as Senior Policy Analyst to the Washington State Office of the Insurance Commissioner (OIC), Health Policy Division since 1996, working with a broad range of issues including complementary and alternative health care integration. She managed the Clinician Workgroup on the Integration of CAM (CWIC) of more than 50 professionals from the health care, insurance, and academic sectors, whose directive was to evaluate insurance coverage issues facing providers and payers.

Courtesy of Office of the Insurance Commissioner, State of Washington.

ers, administrative issues, scope of practice, and other issues.

In 1995, the State Insurance Commissioner, Deborah Senn, held meetings for providers and insurers on the implementation of CAM coverage, so that all stakeholders would know what the commissioner expected regarding compliance with the law. These were also open meetings, intended to promote discussion of issues affecting both providers and consumers. The goal of the rule process has been to define the specific parameters of the law.

The law requires that:

- Providers must work within their scope of practice.
- Providers must be credentialed with the health insurance carrier or its designated network.
- There must be a medical necessity for the coverage to be authorized through a referral from a primary care provider, with an attached diagnosis or condition.
- Coverage is only required for conditions covered in the basic health plan (a state model set of health care benefits identified by law). The benefits list does not indicate conditions covered, but it does state service exclusions.
- Providers must be licensed or certified by the Department of Health. If there are several providers who can appropriately treat a particular condition (for example, back pain), then patients should be allowed to select the kind of care they want for treatment and the type of provider.

The pros of implementing this law are increased access to CAM providers and complementary approaches that expand the continuum of care. This provides consumers with increased choice and treatment options. It also has the potential to enlarge the regular client base for CAM providers. Insurance consumers (employers or individuals) also have the option of purchasing a rider for additional benefits that cover a specific type of provider, or condition, or visits with a self-referral benefit.

In terms of the negatives, the law makes it more difficult for insurers to set premiums, to predict utilization, and to define the rules of care in order to set limitations on the number of patient visits.

Despite the challenges, other states are currently working on ways to offer this coverage to their consumers. One of the limitations, however, is that there is not currently licensing for all of the alternative disciplines in all 50 states. That makes it more difficult to credential providers to ensure public safety and to meet National Committee on Quality Assurance (NCQA) standards that insurers must follow. Many insurers are developing a set of coverage options outside the context of a legislative expansion of coverage.

To some degree, the public perception of CAM tends to differ from geographic area to area. The level of familiarity is partly dependent on the number of training programs and CAM providers available in the area. This increases consumers' comfort level, since they have the opportunity to experience the therapies more frequently. Some cities have launched their own diverse integrative medicine programs, such as the King County Natural Medicine Clinic in the Seattle area.

How does this law actually affect consumer choice? If an individual has low-back pain, and his or her primary care provider diagnoses the condition, the provider should treat the condition or refer the patient to another practitioner. The provider should offer a method of treatment, or discuss with the patient additional options, such as chiropractic, massage, osteopathy, or orthopedic care. Back pain is a good example because it can be treated by many CAM providers. The choice of practitioners would depend on the type of injury or the condition and its severity. The law on expanded coverage ensures that a range of choices is available to the patient.

The costs of CAM coverage continue to be an unknown at this time since there has been no research on the current experience of coverage in Washington state since the law was passed. There has been coverage at different levels for the past 3 years, but the experiential data are proprietary and have not yet been released by the carriers. However, the carriers have indicated that they are willing to release the data to a reputable research project with collaborative princi-

pal investigators who will conduct the research. There is also a collaborative team of providers who are willing to serve as an advisory panel to the research project to assist in the process (see Chapter 16.2).

16.2 Field Report: The Clinician Workgroup on the Integration of Complementary and Alternative Medicine

Office of the Insurance Commissioner, State of Washington.
Report edited by Lori L. Bielinski and Robert D. Mootz

EXECUTIVE SUMMARY

This report documents the establishment and work of the Clinician Workgroup on the Integration of Complementary and Alternative Medicine (CWIC). This 3-year process initiated by the Office of the Insurance Commissioner (OIC) represents a constructive partnership between the public and private sector as well as health insurance carriers and providers. Participants included complementary and alternative medical health care providers, conventional medical providers employed in health insurance companies, primary care providers (PCPs) working in primary care organizations, educators of complementary and alternative medical students, and representatives of state regulatory agencies. One of CWIC's charges was to identify the many issues related to insurance coverage for services that may be considered complementary and al-

ternative to conventional medical services. One of the most powerful outcomes from CWIC was the positive working relationships that developed between the various participant communities.

FORMATION OF THE WORKGROUP

Background

In 1993, health care reform legislation was enacted by the Washington State Legislature that included provisions ensuring consumers in Washington could buy health insurance even if they were sick or had changed jobs. Several provider groups pursued inclusion of all licensed providers in the state for insurance reimbursement of services within their respective practice scopes. To preserve the insurers' ability to select competent and efficient providers, the final legislation settled on the term for every category, or type, of licensed provider being reimbursable, without mandating inclusion for every individual practitioner. Subsequent revision to the law preserved these aspects of reform and the OIC promulgated administrative rules to implement the legislative intent. Concurrent with and following court challenges, efforts were made by the OIC to pursue nonadversarial processes to identify issues, barriers, and solutions for implementing legislatively mandated changes.

The Office of the Insurance Commissioner (OIC) regulates insurance companies that do business in Washington state. When the Washington State Legislature creates laws that affect insurance, the OIC must enforce those laws and write relevant policy, rules, and regulations for those laws. The OIC is also oriented toward the needs of consumers, providing them assistance in receiving proper coverage.

Courtesy of the Office of the Insurance Commissioner, State of Washington.

The first attempts at initiating these processes included discussions about coverage options for complementary and alternative medicine (CAM) services as well as how carriers would credential providers for their networks. These meetings were initially legally focused and were shifted to a more clinical direction after the agreement to include outside facilitation was made.

Format of Workgroup—CWIC

The OIC's health policy staff and outside facilitators met with provider groups to identify those categories that would be most affected by this law. A series of informal discussions with health care practitioners helped identify those categories considered CAM, licensed by the Department of Health, and caring for patients with health conditions covered by the Washington State Basic Health Plan. Simultaneously, facilitators conducted face-to-face and telephone interviews with potential participants to further refine issues of interest and concern.

A representative group of payer medical directors and CAM providers was established using criteria that ensured balance and emphasized provider experience. Exhibit 16.2–1 summarizes primary participants. External independent facilitation was arranged and funded privately by the group participants themselves. In-kind OIC staff resources were provided, but the majority of direct costs for this effort were borne by the carriers and providers themselves.

ACTIVITIES OF THE WORKGROUP

1998 CWIC Activities

An aggressive agenda was proposed to address coverage decisions, technology assess-

---

Exhibit 16.2–1 The Clinician Workgroup on the Integration of CAM

Health Insurance Carriers
- Aetna U.S. Health Care
- Community Health Plan
- Group Health Coop of Puget Sound
- Pacificare of Washington
- Premera Blue Cross
- Qual Med Washington Health Plans
- Regence BlueShield
- United Health Care

Physician Organizations
- Hall Health Primary Care Center
- Multicare
- Providence Health System
- Providence Seattle Medical Center
- University of Washington Physicians
- Valley Medical Center
- Virginia Mason Health Plans

Network Providers
- Alternate Health Services
- American Complementary Care Network
- American WholeHealth Network

CAM Provider Associations
- Acupuncture Association of Washington
- American Massage Therapy Association, Washington Chapter
- Midwives Association of Washington State
- Washington Association of Naturopathic Physicians
- Washington State Chiropractic Association
- Washington State Dietetic Association

Educational Institutions
- Ashmead College
- Bastyr University
- Brenneke School of Massage
- Brian Utting School of Massage
- Northwest Institute of Acupuncture and Oriental Medicine
- Renton Technical College
- Seattle Midwifery School

Courtesy of the Office of the Insurance Commissioner, State of Washington.

ment, medical necessity, data collection, and the gathering of literature on costs and practices, exploration of holistic health care versus condition care, and integration of CAM services. (Holistic health care was defined as "of or relating to wholism, emphasizing the importance of the whole and the interdependence of its parts." For the purposes of this chapter, the use of the word "holistic" should be considered to include health promotion, disease treatment and prevention, and wellness. The term does not fully reflect the range of differences in paradigms between CAM disciplines.) A variety of approaches were used, including didactic presentations by outside experts or group participants, workshops and training, literature and survey research, group discussion, and/or facilitated decision making. For obvious logistical and efficiency reasons, experts within Washington state were used.

1998 CWIC meeting topics included inventory of existing standards for CAM practices, status of coverage, and use of CAM services by carriers and physician groups; carrier procedures for technology assessment; medical necessity determinations and coverage decisions; survey of CAM patients' views of perceived benefits; clinical guideline training; CAM as add-on versus replacement to conventional care in high-cost conditions; and CAM integration into conventional delivery settings.

1999 CWIC Activities

The next full year of CWIC was directed at exploration of existing successful integrated CAM and conventional medical (CM) practices and development of draft clinical care pathways, algorithms, and protocols by participant CAM organizations; training of participant representatives in written clinical care pathway development; development of draft examples of clinical care pathways for conditions that the respective CAM providers might commonly address; identification of possible next steps for the group or future spin-offs; and research opportunities. Dedicated training was aimed at using evidence

review as well as expert and community-based consensus development to draft written protocols in a way that non-CAM providers could apply within their respective professional communities.

1999 CWIC meeting topics included multidisciplinary clinic presentations; discussion on insurable practices; clinical care pathway and algorithm training; CAM practices survey project presentation; discussion on high-cost conditions; research planning with University of Washington and Bastyr University; researchers' interest in CAM; presentations from Bastyr University, University of Washington, and CWIC participants; presentation of draft algorithms by participants; and summarizing of CWIC experience and review of material and information for the final report.

INSURANCE COVERAGE

Variations in Coverage Strategies for CAM

There are currently several different coverage models for CAM services used in Washington state. No preferred or "right" ways of including these benefits are being recommended by CWIC or OIC. *Each approach has advantages and limitations for various constituencies:*

- *Dollar Cap.* This coverage applies maximum dollar expenditure per coverage year for a set range of CAM services.
- *Condition-Based.* This CAM coverage model bases benefits on allowances related to specific clinical diagnoses or conditions. The covered benefit may require specific clinical regimens to have been followed prior to referral for CAM services.
- *Gatekeeper Method.* Characteristic of managed care coverage. Use of CAM requires direct referral from PCP gatekeeper, and benefits follow a medical necessity model. Some carriers include naturopathic physicians as PCPs.
- *Open Access Model.* Built on integration and coordination without a gatekeeper. This

design allows a member to access network providers of all categories without the requirement of a PCP referral.

- *Self-Referral and Preventive Care.* This model is usually structured as a rider to a core benefits package and usually follows a medical necessity model for coverage decisions. This could include patient access to a set number, or amount, of services without PCP referral, but require referral for additional coverage.
- *Discount Networks.* Some carriers have negotiated with CAM providers to provide discounts to their members, but do not provide reimbursement for the members' expenses for the services. This approach attempts to enhance access to CAM providers, but does not reimburse for any of the services.

CONCLUSIONS OF THE GROUP

Lessons Learned

- Better understanding of each other's language and philosophies is needed.
- A forum of insurers and providers is a valuable environment for discussing coverage, payment, and cost concerns.
- Creation of resources is needed for use in other like forums.
- Building trust and relationships breaks down barriers.
- The CWIC process increased awareness of the multifaceted nature of the current health care delivery system.
- Payers began to see the value in CAM delivery experience; providers gained understanding of managed care systems and payer issues.
- CAM providers could benefit from broader application of quality improvement protocols to reduce variation and document improvement in patient progress and overall outcomes.
- Many of the changes in health care have resulted from marketplace factors that are

frequently beyond the direct influence of providers, payers, and regulators.

Next Steps

- Research should be a top priority. Specifically, cost data, claims experience, utilization appropriateness, and other health services research issues will need to be better understood to assist in making coverage decisions.
- Care management considerations need to be explicitly addressed. Clinical guidelines and condition-specific care pathways will assist CAM providers in conveying clinical rationale and the need for coverage determinations. Attention to these issues can also help CAM providers better understand their approaches and address practice variation.
- Education was an important byproduct of the CWIC experience, and a forum to allow that to continue should be considered. CAM providers who can communicate well and can be made available should be identified.
- A collaborative forum for communication between payers, CM providers, CAM providers, and regulators should be established, perhaps at the national level.
- Integration of CAM and CM services was an ongoing theme throughout the CWIC process. Additionally, members felt that options and approaches for integration should be explored and inventoried.
- Delineation of care thresholds, financing mechanisms, and the qualification of cost-benefits for CAM and other preventive services will need to be prioritized.
- In general, sources of funding and resource support need to be identified for all of these activities.

Key Issues Regarding Integration

- *Relationship Development.* Mutual respect and recognition of perspectives are essential.
- *Speaking Different Languages.* Patience and openness are required regarding dif-

ferences in training and experience, hence the syntax used for communicating each other's views and needs.

- ***Learning Each Other's Paradigms.*** Attitudes toward healing, intervention, and care coordination may vary between CAM approaches and compared to CM approaches. Appreciation for how this impacts approaches to care is essential for coordination and integration.
- ***Algorithms and Guidelines.*** Recognition of these tools for both improving quality and outcome of care, along with communicating CAM care decisions and thresholds, is important. Documentation of recognized limitations and strategies for preventing inappropriate use are essential.
- ***Research Support.*** The absence of research in support of a particular intervention's effectiveness should not by default be treated as though there was scientific evidence demonstrating ineffectiveness.
- ***Members' Different Needs.*** Each constituent, payer, CAM provider, CM provider, and regulator has different perspectives, needs, and accountable bodies that must be recognized. A forum for constructive engagement and problem solving is essential.

Recommendations of CWIC for the Integration of CAM

- Individual CAM professions should work closely with carriers to assist them in knowing when to cover their services for a specific condition, and so provide clinical algorithms to assist in supporting the claim.
- Insurers should involve the respective CAM professionals when establishing CAM benefits packages.
- Participants in CWIC and their organizations should explore ways to maintain an informal network and consider seeking broader, perhaps national, support for establishing an ongoing forum for dialogue and problem solving.
- Educational strategies should be adopted for enhancing cross-fertilization and understanding of the issues of payers, CAM providers, and CM providers. Recognition of areas of mutual interest should be made explicit, and areas of divergent needs and priorities should be acknowledged and engaged constructively.
- Explore opportunities to use technology and communication to keep members aware of various methods to integrate CAM and CM.

16.3   Case Studies in Complementary and Alternative Medicine for the Underserved

Sita Ananth

INTRODUCTION

The landmark Harvard study (Eisenberg et al, 1993) on alternative medicine usage patterns created a flurry of interest in hospitals and health maintenance organizations (HMOs) to explore ways to capitalize on the burgeoning consumer demand and market for complementary and alternative medicine (CAM) services. While the primary motivations to offer these services are intended as revenue generators and are most often delivered fee-for-service or as a health plan rider, there are several institutions and organizations that are dedicated to making these services and therapies available to everyone regardless of ability to pay. While the literature addresses the practical and business aspects of integration of these services into the traditional medical setting, very little has been written about the availability of CAM to clients of low income.

The question of access is one that is rarely addressed when the subject of CAM integration is discussed. CAM, which is, in general, lower in cost to deliver, less invasive, with minimal or no side effects or risks, has become the medicine for the affluent and middle class only. One has to either have a generous health plan benefit that includes a rider for chiropractic or acupuncture or massage therapy or have the disposable income to be able to afford visits to private practitioners.

Sita Ananth, MHA, is Associate Director of Education for Health Forum/AHA, a subsidiary of the American Hospital Association. She is responsible for the design, content development, and implementation of the Health Forum's Leadership Summit, an annual meeting attracting more than 1,000 senior-level health care leaders. In addition, she is responsible for developing the complementary and alternative medicine strategy for Health Forum/AHA.

The purpose of this chapter is to showcase several unique organizations: a public inner-city hospital, a volunteer-run clinic, and a nonprofit community clinic. Each serves the needs of its distinct patient population by offering the best fit of CAM therapies and modalities.

A HOSPITAL-BASED ACUPUNCTURE PROGRAM FOR ADDICTION TREATMENT

Lincoln Hospital
349 E 140th Street
Bronx, NY 10454
Michael Smith, MD, DAc
Director
Phone: (718) 993-3100

Lincoln Hospital, a city-funded hospital in the impoverished South Bronx, introduced acupuncture in 1974 as an alternative to the methadone program for treating heroin addiction. Over the last 25 years, it has grown to become the largest medically supervised, drug-free outpatient treatment center for drug and alcohol addiction in the country. Dr. Michael Smith, program director, has been with the center since its inception and describes the program's four pillars as:

- acupuncture
- individual counseling
- group counseling complemented by participation in 12-step programs
- daily toxicology testing (urinalysis)

Recognizing that drug and alcohol addiction is often related to broader social issues, the program takes a whole person approach and includes several specialized components such as parenting classes, women's groups, trauma seminars, and groups for men on reducing violent behavior. Additionally, the center is in the process of obtaining funding to offer vocational training programs.

Approximately 500 client visits are conducted each week supported by a staff of two physicians, five counselors, and four clinical supervisors. Counselors and physicians have been trained and certified in ear acupuncture (auricular acupuncture) under the auspices of the National Acupuncture Detoxification Association (NADA), which provides close oversight and maintains rigorous standards for the model. Smith has developed a five-point formula, utilizing five acupuncture points in the ear to treat these patients. Treatment is provided in a group setting, allowing for, as Smith says, "less transference and greater patient empowerment" (M. Smith, oral communication).

A new patient typically receives an orientation to the program and a recommended plan of treatment. The patient then meets with a counselor and has an individual acupuncture session. The patient is expected to have daily acupuncture treatments until the urinalysis is drug-free for 10 days; the urinalysis is conducted on a purely voluntary basis. After this time, each patient continues counseling sessions, both individually and in group settings, and maintains a regular schedule of acupuncture for at least 4 months. The treatment protocol is based on self-responsibility, patient choice and empowerment, self-awareness and reflection, positive reinforcement, and group support.

Referrals to the clinic come primarily from city and state agencies, such as the Child Welfare, Probation and Parole, and Welfare departments, and interestingly, with few referrals from health care agencies. As a city-run hospital, Medicaid pays for the program. Since drug and alcohol abuse services are a carve-out of managed care, these services are covered irrespective of plan membership.

The Lincoln Center protocol is now being used in over 1,000 clinics worldwide. The crack cocaine addiction program alone is the largest in the world. Given the transitory and unsettled lives of people in this population, retention and success rates for the program are remarkably

high at 60%. A number of controlled studies conducted using this protocol undeniably show the high level of success of this model for the treatment of drug and alcohol addictions.

A CANCER CLINIC STAFFED BY VOLUNTEERS

Charlotte Maxwell Complementary Clinic
5691 Telegraph Avenue
Oakland, CA 94609
Beverly Burns, LAc
Board President
Phone: (510) 601-7660

The Charlotte Maxwell Complementary Clinic was founded by a group of volunteer acupuncturists, homeopaths, and massage therapists with a mission to provide alternative modalities of treatment to all irrespective of ability to pay. The audience targeted for these services were low-income women with cancer in the San Francisco Bay Area. Board President Beverly Burns strongly believes that by offering these services, the clinic is empowering women to take control over their lives and health care choices (B. Burns, oral communication). In fact, the clinic was named for a patient being treated for ovarian cancer, who subsequently died, but has been the inspiration for creating this important community resource.

The first step for the center was to obtain licensing as a primary care clinic in the state of California. This allowed the acupuncturists to serve as primary care providers and consolidate their malpractice insurance costs. This process began in 1989 and took 2 years, during which time they were actively fundraising. The clinic opened its doors in 1992 and has offered a range of services encompassing traditional Chinese medicine, massage therapy, homeopathy, visualization, and social services. Additionally, the clinic offers hospice services, an organic food bank, a support group, and occasional transportation services.

The clinic services are funded entirely through private fundraising, grant monies, and the pro bono contributions of services. "Financial pressures are one of the major challenges faced by the clinic," says Burns, "given the increasing demand and desire to expand services" (B. Burns, oral communication). The clinic is considering Medicare billing although the costs and time involved in collecting a modest reimbursement are high.

Each year, the clinic provides approximately 1,600 patient visits through an entirely volunteer staff of 16 acupuncturists, 4 homeopaths (one of whom is a physician), and 60 other active volunteers. Patients are seen in the evenings and on weekends since all practitioners are volunteers and have full-time practices. Three part-time paid staff manage the administrative and day-to-day operations of the clinic.

Most often, referrals are made by oncologists or social workers in the public hospitals. Following massive outreach to the three major public hospitals in the Bay Area to overcome their initial mistrust, interest in the clinic is high and referrals outnumber the capacity. Eligibility criteria to be seen at the clinic are fairly unrestricted as long as patients are Medi-Cal eligible or live within 300% of the poverty level. Many women, by virtue of becoming ill, have become poor; others are illegal immigrants who have not sought care due to fear of deportation.

Currently, Beverly Burns is working with Mt. Zion Hospital Breast Center on a small research project to study 15 women with Stage 4 terminal breast cancer. These women are not receiving chemotherapy and are on a regimen of Chinese herbs. Their health is being monitored through the study to measure any change in the progression of their disease. Burns believes that any increase in longevity and improvement in quality of life at this stage are particularly significant, given the late stage of the cancer.

The goal of Burns and her colleagues is to set an example for the health care community at large by developing a simple model of volunteerism and community service. The clinic is staffed through an ingenious system of volunteerism that requires only marginal commitment of time (just 6 hours a month) to provide much-needed services.

A COMMUNITY CLINIC THAT PROVIDES INTEGRATIVE MEDICINE

King County Natural Medicine Clinic
403 East Meeker Street
Kent, WA 98031
Tom Trompeter
Executive Director of Community Health
   Centers of King County
Phone: (425) 277-1311

The King County Natural Medicine Clinic is the nation's first publicly funded clinic in which patients receive an integrated, full spectrum of natural and alternative medicine services. This ground-breaking initiative is a collaborative effort between the Community Health Centers of King County (CHCKC), a private nonprofit system of community-based health centers with a primary mission to serve the underserved, and Bastyr University, internationally recognized as a pioneer in the study of natural healing and the leading university for naturopathic medicine in the United States, with funding from the Seattle/King County Department of Public Health. The clinic serves low-income, uninsured, Medicare or Medicaid recipients, as well as immigrants and refugees, and others who are medically underserved.

The development of the Natural Medicine Clinic has been driven by the needs of the clients of the health centers. In 1995, a survey of patients in CHCKC's clinics showed that 60% were interested in receiving natural and alternative medicine services. CHCKC is a consumer-driven and -directed organization focused on the needs of clients; 50% of the board of directors are former clinic patients. CHCKC management and staff made a commitment to ensure that they would find ways in which to provide access to these services to their clients, says Tom Trompeter, executive director (T. Trompeter, oral communication).

The clinic opened its doors as an integrative health care center in October 1996, offering primary health care services provided by clinicians in collaborative teams.

These integrated services include:

- family practice primary care
- health education and prevention
- prenatal and obstetrical services
- naturopathic medicine
- acupuncture
- massage therapy
- chiropractic care
- stress management
- nutrition counseling

Since nearly 20% of CHCKC patients are recent immigrants to the United States, translation services in over 10 languages are offered at no charge. Case management, mental health services, and patient advocacy with other social and government agencies are also offered by clinic staff.

In 1998, over 1,000 patients were seen for 4,400 visits at the Natural Medicine Clinic with a staff of one and one quarter FTE naturopaths and one full-time acupuncturist, who are both considered primary care providers. Other support staff include medical assistants and a triage nurse who also provides health education counseling. "The formal patient flow chart developed by the clinic to educate and appropriately direct patients about their options of natural/alternative medicine quickly became obsolete as patients are becoming more informed and selective of services they want," says Trompeter (T. Trompeter, oral communication).

CHCKC is funded by public grants and patient fees. Fees are based on a sliding scale and the patient's ability to pay. Medicare, Medicaid, and third-party reimbursement account for 60% of the funding, while county block grants compose another 15%. The remaining 25% consists of private donations, federal monies, and patient self-pay fees.

Trompeter, a 20-year veteran of community health centers in various parts of the country, finds the model at the Natural Medicine Clinic to be highly successful and of great value to patients and the community. This truly integrative model provides an opportunity for practitioners—both allopathic and alternative—to learn from each other, while creating the optimal environment to provide the best care both paradigms of medicine have to offer. The staff has learned the importance of training and communicating with each other, developing a comprehensive understanding of their styles of practice, and how these practices could be modified to meet the needs of their patients.

Trompeter's goal for the next year is to expand the availability of these services in King County to more clinics to allow for increased client access to integrative services. Additionally, he is interested in sharing this model with other institutions or agencies that are interested in integrating CAM therapies into their care delivery systems.

IMPLICATIONS

There are tremendous implications in the development of CAM, reflecting the largest grassroots movement in health care in the 20th century: a 1998 study conducted by the Health Forum, Arthur Andersen, and DYG Inc. polled consumers and providers in an attempt to understand leadership and consumer perceptions of the health care delivery system. In focus groups conducted nationwide, people of all income and education levels, with and without insurance, expressed nearly identical views on health and health care. In the resulting report, "Leadership for a Healthy 21st Century" (1999), one of the key findings was an extraordinary degree of experimentation with complementary and alternative modalities, particularly among women. The study found strong interest in these services among uninsured and underserved populations.

Complementary and alternative health care services fit the mission to improve the health of the population. CAM services are low-tech. Most of these modalities rely on minimal intervention and greater self-care, expanding the opportunities to increase the role of patients in managing aspects of their own health whenever possible.

A large percentage of the underserved or uninsured are immigrants or refugees. People from cultures with a strong tradition in herbal medicine, such as those of Latin America or Asia, are more likely to be comfortable with alternative therapies. In addition, people with chronic illness may be appropriate candidates for alternative therapies with proven efficacy. Chronic illness has been documented in a large proportion of the U.S. population, including the elderly. Opportunities to develop a new model of care incorporating alternative therapies have the potential to reduce the cost of providing care to these populations, without sacrificing quality of care.

Integrative medicine expands the range of reasonable, inexpensive, and effective options available for common ailments. For example, supplements and herbal remedies, when appropriate, are less expensive alternatives to costly prescription medications. Under the guidance of a knowledgeable integrative physician, these options can be made available to patients. Integrative medicine provides an opportunity to coordinate care and avoid potential contraindications or interactions between allopathic medications and alternative supplements that patients may be taking without informing their physicians (40% of patients do not share this information).

As communication and industry have expanded to span the globe, so has medicine. Medicine is no longer allopathic, Western, alternative, or complementary. It has taken on a global identity. As a result, the impact of information available on the Internet to the consumer and the increasing movement of immigrating populations have placed extraordinary demands on the American health care system. Consequently, many consumers are going outside the system and, in effect, this has created a parallel health care delivery system.

To meet the needs of the 44 million uninsured low-income and working poor in this country, there is an extraordinary opportunity to create a new model of care that would integrate the best that medicine has to offer, worldwide. The organizations showcased above are ready and willing to share their knowledge and expertise with the health care industry at large and would welcome the opportunity to be a part of this reinvention.

BIBLIOGRAPHY

Bernstein E, ed. *Medical and Health Annual.* Encyclopedia Britannica; 1998.

Eisenberg DM, Kessler RC, Foster C, et al. Unconventional medicine in the United States—prevalence, costs, and patterns of use. *N Engl J Med.* 1993;328:246–252.

Gallup JW. *Wellness Centers—A Guide for the Design Professional.* New York: John Wiley and Sons; 1999.

Leadership for a healthy 21st century. *Health Forum J.* 1999, Jan-Feb (suppl):1–27.

Smith M. *Hospital and Community Partnerships: Case Study 10.* Chicago, IL: American Hospital Association; 1991.

16.4   Pilot Program:
Providing Alternative Pain Management through Medicaid

David Bearman

Flexible Funding

The Santa Barbara Regional Health Authority (SBRHA) serves 41,000 Medi-Cal (California Medicaid) patients in Santa Barbara County. It has operated since 1983. Created by a special act of the California State Legislature, SBRHA has much more flexibility in its scope of benefits than the state-administered Medi-Cal program. The SBRHA board of directors has used that flexibility to approve experimental trials of various new modalities.

The Needs of Patients with Chronic Conditions

Patients with chronic pain tend to be demanding of their primary care providers and generally frustrated with their conditions. SBRHA's focus in this cohort of patients is on the treatment of chronic pain and on clients who have had limited or no response to conventional treatments for chronic physical pain from injuries, surgeries, or other conditions. Many of these members also have coexisting mental health problems, such as depression and anxiety. Several have exhausted conventional medical options. For most of these patients, pain relief typically consists of prescription medications or self-medication with alcohol or illicit drugs.

David Bearman, MD, is former Medical Director of the Santa Barbara Regional Health Authority.

Source: Adapted with permission from David Bearman, The Feldenkrais Method in the Treatment of Chronic Pain: A Study of Efficacy and Cost-Effectiveness, *American Journal of Pain Management*, Vol. 9, No. 1, pp. 22–27, © 1999, American Academy of Pain Management.

The Pilot Program

This information focuses on a pilot program for seven Medi-Cal clients with chronic pain using the Feldenkrais Method exclusively. The program was evaluated by using data processed by the National Pain Data Bank (NPDB) of the American Academy of Pain Management. Cost-effectiveness was assessed by comparing Medicaid costs for 1-year periods pre- and postintervention. The basic rationale for investigating CAM was one of economics and patient and conventional practitioner acceptance. Simply stated, traditional pain management programs are costly. Annual health care costs for chronic pain Medicaid patients in our area are $1,000 to $7,000.

The Intervention

The Feldenkrais Method has two forms: (1) group and (2) individual. In this pilot, the intervention involved an approach that systematically imitates the process through which children learn to walk. The practitioner uses verbal directions to guide people through specific sequences of relatively simple, comfortable movements. Most lessons take 45 to 60 minutes and are done while lying or sitting. Participants learn to eliminate excess effort or other inefficient habits of movement, while simultaneously discovering more comfortable and effective alternatives.

Seven participants were selected. All completed the program. The goals of treatment were to reduce complaints of pain, improve mobility and skill functioning, reduce use of licit and illicit analgesics, and reduce demand for health care services during the 1-year follow-up period.

The program began with a 2-week intensive phase, 4 to 5 hours each day, 4 days each week. This design was based on the immersion approach characteristic of conventional pain management programs. A secondary phase involved 6 more weeks with one meeting each week, 4 hours for the first two meetings, 2 hours for two meetings, and then just 1 hour for each of the final meetings. The participants met at Santa Barbara Cottage Hospital during August and September of 1995.

- *Efficacy.* Therapeutic efficacy and cost-effectiveness were evaluated by considering patient mobility and patient perception of pain, as well as total health care costs and pharmacy costs.
- *Test instrument.* The NPDB test instrument was administered before the program, immediately posttreatment, and (by telephone) at 1 year posttreatment.
- *Comparison of effectiveness.* The NPDB compared the Feldenkrais program with 12 other programs with 365 chronic pain patients in outpatient programs.
- *Cost.* SBRHA maintained historical cost data for all participants in the study. Medicaid costs were compared for the year preceding the Feldenkrais intervention and for 1 year following the end of the intervention. Costs were compared both before and after the intervention.

Results

Demographics

With regard to age, sex, race, marital status, and education, there were no major differences between participants in the Feldenkrais program and those in the comparison programs. SBRHA patients reported having pain in more areas than participants in the comparison programs and for longer periods of time (100% in pain for more than 24 months, compared with 47.2% in the comparison group). Prior to the program,

SBRHA patients had received more treatment for their pain than patients in comparison groups and a greater number of hospitalizations and prior surgeries.

Perception of Pain

Prior to the Feldenkrais program, 28% of SBRHA patients reported excruciating pain. Some of the methods they had tried to ease their pain were acupuncture, heat, manipulation, counseling, exercises, and medication. At the conclusion of the treatment phase, no participating SBRHA study patients reported excruciating pain.

Patients treated in the Feldenkrais program reported an increase in their ability to walk, bathe, dress, use the bathroom, drive a car, and engage in sex without the interference of pain. Prior to the program, 14.2% of the seven Feldenkrais program patients spent 9 or more hours each day lying down, and none posttreatment. Pretreatment, 74.2% of the SBRHA patients were experiencing pain all the time when they walked. At the conclusion, that number had decreased to 16.6%. At the start of the program, 71.2% experienced pain while driving, decreasing to 0% at the conclusion.

Patient Satisfaction

At the end of the Feldenkrais program, 100% of the patients reported some level of improvement. Feldenkrais clinician-perceived patient satisfaction was nearly 80% in the SBRHA group; in the comparison group, only 33.7% of patients were perceived by clinicians as satisfied.

Summary

Generally, the Feldenkrais participants showed dramatic improvements by the end of the program, with 80% stating that they were completely or almost completely satisfied with the overall treatment. Participants' health care visits decreased, and the cost of pain care was reduced. Furthermore, the cost of the study program to SBRHA was a small fraction of the cost of most standard pain treatment programs. Additionally, medication costs were reduced posttreatment.

An area of clear importance is the number of health care visits each patient had in a 12-month period. In the year prior to the Feldenkrais program, 71.4% had more than 20 appointments with a health care professional, and the rest had 8 to 10 appointments. In the year following the program, 100% had between 11 and 15 visits. Cost analysis of the Feldenkrais program documented pharmaceutical and outpatient medical costs of $141 per member per month (PMPM) during the 13 months prior to the intervention. For the 14 months following the program, costs were just $82 PMPM. This represents a 40% decrease. The $54 PMPM savings shows that with this group, the SBRHA recovered its direct cost of $700 per member within 13 months.

At the 1-year follow-up, while participants lost ground in most areas of pain control, function, and quality of life, they were judged generally healthier than at intake.

CONCLUSION

Initially, SBRHA patients were in worse precondition than patients in the NPDB comparison groups; they had more illnesses, had been in pain longer, and had been treated for longer periods of time. Additionally, this group had additional barriers associated with psychosocial factors, including less income, problematic employment status, and histories of abuse.

Following the program, SBRHA patients showed significant improvement in their levels of pain, decreased numbers of medications, and increased quality of life. Their total medical costs were lower. At the 1-year follow-up, SBRHA patients had lost some of the benefits they reported immediately after the program, but there was still significant progress overall.

The authors have concluded that the Feldenkrais Method shows promise in the treatment of patients with chronic pain secondary to headaches and/or musculoskeletal problems. This preliminary investigation has shown that the intervention needs more rigorous studies to confirm its apparent efficacy and cost-effectiveness suggested by the results.

PART IV

Credentialing and Staffing

CHAPTER 17

Credentialing Complementary Practitioners

17.1   Credentialing Demystified

Vickie S. Ina

Whenever an organization considers the development of a health care network, strategic analysis is essential to ensure the success of the program.

The critical steps are:

- Determine the budget for development and for ongoing operations.
- Identify liability for both the short term and the long term.

Vickie S. Ina, MBA, Former Senior Vice President, Product Development at Consensus Health dba OneBody.com, has over 15 years of senior management experience in managed care environments, including positions as Director of Network Management at OnCare Health, Director of Provider Relations at Foundation Health/Managed Health Network, and Director of Professional Relations at Blue Shield of California. Her responsibilities have encompassed negotiation of provider contracts, establishment of performance structures, management of credentialing, and involvement with regulatory and legal issues surrounding network management. She has directed a provider network of 4,000 practitioners serving more than 2 million clients and provided planning, development, and management of a capitated health plan. At Consensus Health dba OneBody.com, she has developed and managed the CAM networks and is now applying this experience to product development.

- Clarify the organization's willingness to assume risk for this endeavor.

THE CREDENTIALING PROCESS

In order to implement any health care program, the credentials of all potential practitioners must be verified through the credentialing process. There are several factors that will determine the level of simplicity or sophistication of the credentialing program, such as program design, liability, and marketing strategy. A good rule of thumb is, if the provider organization can afford to set high standards and there is a chance that the program and the risk exposure may be expanded, the qualification standards should be increased. It is always easier to relax the standards and allow more providers to enter the network at a later time. However, once standards have been established, it is more difficult, operationally and legally, to raise the standards and therefore eliminate some of the current providers and reduce the size of the network in the future.

Having defined program goals, a team of internal and/or external personnel must be created.

These individuals will be responsible for:

- operational design and the management of the credentialing program
- the development of an application and contract (This is usually done by an outside vendor or internally by legal counsel, or the health plan's network management staff. In any case, legal review is an integral part of this process.)
- creation of a database to manage and monitor practitioner information
- definition and implementation of peer-review activities, such as application review, quality review, and utilization management.

Credentialing Programs

The credentialing process provides an organization with the ability to objectively assess a practitioner's expertise (that is, his or her training, experience, and skill). Quality standards may incorporate both professional benchmarks and internally self-defined standards. Once the credentialing standards have been defined, the organization must adhere to these standards in order to avoid legal and financial penalties.

For the practitioner-managed organization, credentialing is an evaluation and screening tool that defines quality standards and the organization's exposure to professional and operational liability.

For the health plan, credentialing is an evaluation process that allows the health plan to determine its liability for "deep pocket" exposure. Completion of the process increases the assurance that compliance with quality standards such as National Committee on Quality Assurance (NCQA) and state regulatory agencies will be maintained. These compliance requirements are sometimes necessary to maintain a managed care license and to meet quality service requirements. If credentialing services are delegated by the health plan to an outside consultant, the health plan should develop a program to monitor these services in order to minimize its exposure

to liabilities, such as financial penalties, adverse public relations, and practitioner or member complaints.

For the consumer, credentialing or qualifying standards provide a level of comfort that the recommended practitioners can be trusted to provide quality service and that they have received a type of "Good Housekeeping Seal of Approval."

Credentialing Programs for Complementary Health Care Providers

The credentialing of complementary and alternative medicine (CAM) practitioners will vary from organization to organization. Credentialing is also defined by the nature of the service provided. For example, if the organization is simply offering a referral service, limited credentialing may be performed. If the organization intends to work with health plans, offering panels of practitioners or carve-out services, it should be held to the highest standards, comparable to traditional credentialing programs for physicians. Although organizations such as the NCQA do not yet have specific requirements for CAM providers, its standards can and should be mirrored in the screening process for CAM providers whenever the insurer is assuming risk for the practitioner's services.

It is important to establish standards clearly before beginning the credentialing process. Through the members of the credentialing committee, what constitutes quality training for all specialties and techniques offered should be determined. Before practitioners are solicited to join the network, the number of hours of training and the educational institutions whose programs will be considered acceptable should be determined. When assessing a complementary credentialing program or developing one, areas for practitioner selection found in Exhibit 17.1–1 should be reviewed.

When developing a comprehensive credentialing program, it is important to obtain essential information and documents; these typically include:

Exhibit 17.1–1 Basic Credentialing Records and Information

> A process to locate and verify all primary source documents listed below should be developed.
>
> - Comprehensive provider application and contract
> - Professional license or certification requirements
> - Records indicating satisfactory completion of specialty training
> - Required professional insurance standards
> - Required years of experience
> - Peer review of the practitioner's application and all related documents
> - Practitioner capabilities for data reporting and profiling
> - Thorough on-site review of provider offices, records, and operations

- a comprehensive application that provides information on personal demographics, training, and work experience, including malpractice and claims history. It is important that the practitioner sign and attest to the accuracy of this information
- a copy of the practitioner's current state license in the respective specialty with no restrictions. (Being as specific as possible avoids time lost searching through unnecessary certificates. Credentialers should ask for only those programs they plan to verify.)
- verification of the completion of required specialty training and programs
- copy of the appropriate insurance policies with address and phone number indicating current malpractice and general liability coverage at appropriate levels

- release form to verify insurance and claims history with malpractice insurance carriers
- an attestation statement by the practitioner, verifying his or her physical and mental capability to provide the required services
- satisfactory claims history from organizations such as the National Practitioner Data Bank (NPDB), insurance carriers, Medicare/Medicaid, or county business-licensing bureau
- provider contract that clearly outlines each party's responsibilities and obligations, terms and conditions, grievance and appeals process, and termination process (with or without cause)
- reimbursement programs and fee schedule (as appropriate).

In addition, in our organization, we also require:

- minimum number of years in practice
- current business license in the practicing county when available
- certificates of completion from various training programs that are verified by our organization
- interview (frequently conducted at the on-site visit) to determine the practitioner's ability to communicate health care protocols and educate clients about the contracted services.

After the necessary documents have been gathered, all provider information should be verified with great care. This means that certificates of training should be verified with the issuing institution or program. If a health plan is going to market a massage therapist as a "deep-tissue massage therapist," then that special training in deep tissue massage should be verified. The certification of an individual listed as a teacher of Alexander technique must be verified as having been completed through an accredited organization. In the case of acupuncture, although physicians can practice acupuncture under their medical degrees in most states, their training in acupuncture should also be verified.

LICENSING AND LEGAL REQUIREMENTS

Licensing and legal requirements vary from state to state. (See Section 17.4, State Law Defining the Practice of Acupuncture in Three States.) Each state has significantly different standards of practice and required or optional licenses, certificates, and registries for CAM health care providers. Information about state requirements is usually obtained through one of a number of sources.

The department of health (often called department of public health) is frequently the unit in state government that overseas licensure. If a particular specialty is regulated by the state, then the appropriate agency will usually exist under the auspices of the department of health. Some examples:

- office of professional regulation
- board of medical examiners
- division of quality medical assurance
- health professions bureau
- officc of health services

For information about specialties that are not regulated at the state level, it is also appropriate to inquire one of the above agencies. They will often have information and resources related to these disciplines. State certification may be available for specific specialties and subspecialties. In order to obtain information regarding certification and professional standards, organizations for practitioners within a specialty are excellent resources. The following are examples:

- National Certification Commission for Acupuncture and Oriental Medicine (NCCAOM)
- American Association of Oriental Medicine (AAOM)
- Council on Chiropractic Education (CCE)
- American Massage Therapy Association (AMTA)
- National Board of Certification for Therapeutic Massage and Bodywork (NBCTMB)

- American Association of Naturopathic Physicians (AANP)
- Naturopathic Physicians Acupuncture Academy (NPAA)

Licensure is an important form of professional recognition for alternative providers. Being licensed by a state instills a higher level of confidence in the practitioners and in the health plans offering their services. The license indicates that the profession and the practitioners have gone through a certain level of review and that the state is now involved in the liability exposure by licensing them. By issuing the license, the state board has taken a level of responsibility to verify the training and quality of service of these practitioners.

In states that regulate CAM practitioners, the issues around licensure are very straightforward. Either the practitioner has a license or he or she does not. If the practitioner is not licensed in the state, but holds some form of certification or registration, a peer-review committee should be involved in determining the appropriateness of the specific training. In either instance, it is essential to perform a primary source verification of licensure or certification and the completion of appropriate training. This information is confirmed by contacting the issuing institution.

When the state has no licensing procedure for the practitioners of a CAM specialty, the task of the credentialing body is to define the standards for competence and excellence within that field. This is best done by involving the participation of capable practitioners and membership organizations in that particular specialty. (See Exhibit 17.1–2.)

The following resources provide regulatory and legal information and statistics:

- *Acupuncture and Oriental Medicine Laws*, yearly edition by Barbara Mitchell and the American Association of Oriental Medicine (AAOM)
- *Official Directory of Chiropractic Licensure and Practice Statistics*, yearly edition by the Federation of Chiropractic Licensing Boards (FCLB)

Exhibit 17.1–2 Credentialing Alternative Specialties Not Defined by State Law

> To credential massage therapists in the state of California, we had to determine our own standards for experience and training because there is currently no state law that formally licenses massage. We have worked closely with associations and leading practitioners in the field. Our credentialing committee of practitioners in massage and bodywork assisted us in defining the level and nature of training and experience to be considered the basis for quality service provision. These credentialing standards were also reviewed by our medical advisory board to ensure quality and consistency.
>
> We determined that 500 hours of certified hands-on training would be the minimum standard. Although a national certification is available that requires 1,000 hours of training, we agreed that the additional 500 hours did not define a qualified practitioner versus an unqualified one. Most massage therapists are quite capable after 500 hours. Rather, it was concluded that the 1,000 hours were essentially a refinement of the specialty. In addition, setting the standard at 1,000 hours would have significantly limited the pool of quality practitioners. To ensure quality, both the training and also 3 years of experience are required. Years of experience provide a benchmark for identifying capable practitioners.

- *Acupuncture and Oriental Medicine Alliance* (AOMA) (primarily legislative activity)
- *American Association of Naturopathic Physicians* (AANP)
- *National Board of Homeopathic Examiners* (NBHE)

For examples of how state law defines the scope of practice, see Section 17.4.

ACCREDITATION AND PROFESSIONAL TRAINING

Every state has specific educational and training requirements for health care practitioners. A list of the programs and institutions recognized by state government can be obtained by contacting the specialty regulatory body directly. For listings of nationally recognized programs and institutions, contact the national association within the discipline that accredits or oversees professional training.

The following are examples of some helpful organizations:

- *Accreditation and Training Resources*
  - National Board of Certification for Therapeutic Massage and Bodywork (NBCTMB)
  - Accreditation Commission for Acupuncture and Oriental Medicine (ACAOM)
  - National Certification Commission for Acupuncture and Oriental Medicine (NCCAOM)
  - Council on Chiropractic Education (CCE) Commission on Accreditation
  - American Naturopathic Medical Certification and Accreditation Board (ANMCAB)

- *Professional Training*
  - American Massage Therapy Association (AMTA)
  - Associated Bodywork and Massage Practitioners (ABMP)
  - American Oriental Bodywork Therapy Association (AOBTA)
  - Council of Colleges of Acupuncture and Oriental Medicine (CCAOM)
  - American Chiropractic Association (ACA)
  - Federation of Chiropractic Licensing Boards (FCLB)
  - American Association of Naturopathic Physicians (AANP)
  - American Naturopathic Medical Association (ANME)
  - National Center for Homeopathy (NCH)

The standards for appropriate education in CAM therapies tend to be less clearly defined than those in medical education. Medical schools are listed with the medical licensing board, based on accreditation and review by independent evaluators. These institutions set standards for the determination of sufficient medical education, to enable a physician to apply for a state license. This is not the case in CAM services. There is a range of variability in the quality of different training programs. There are different levels of accreditation. Credentialers need to carefully evaluate the curriculum and the reputation of each program. Again, it becomes important to work through the credentialing process with actual practitioners and leaders knowledgeable within each specialty.

Information on professional training resources is provided in Section 17.3, Resources, including addresses, telephone numbers, and e-mail addresses.

MALPRACTICE AND SITE VISITS

There are several primary ways to determine whether there is malpractice history against a practitioner. It is essential to check the national data banks to rule out the possibility that a practitioner may have a pending or past malpractice suit. This information is relatively easy to check.

Due to the confidential nature of the information, only those organizations that have an appropriate reason to query the data bank are allowed access into the program. Access is restricted to organizations either holding risk for the care provided by the practitioner or for quality management. Such organizations typically include health maintenance organizations (HMOs), health plans, management services organizations, and medical groups. The data bank can be accessed and queried through a variety of ways including mail, fax, or Internet.

It is important to understand that the data bank does not cover everyone. For example, malpractice suits against massage and bodywork practitioners are not required to be reported to this data bank. However, practitioners who are not on file in the database can be tracked through information from their malpractice insurance companies, where there will be a record of any suits against them as part of their claims histories.

In summary, there are a number of different points for quality control checks:

- The National Practitioner Database (NPDB) can be researched by a qualified organization for claims history against a particular provider. Complaints about quality of care that have resulted in judgments against doctors are filed with the NPDB. Acupuncturists are also listed in this database, particularly physicians who provide acupuncture. Chiropractic claims are listed in this database as well.
- The Chiropractic Information Network—Board Action Database (CINBAD) is a database that records claims filed against chiropractors.
- Malpractice insurance policies typically require a statement of claims history. If the practitioner provides a release, it is possible to query the malpractice insurance carrier to determine whether there are pending, past, or current suits that have been filed against the practitioner. When a malpractice suit is filed, it must be listed with both the NPDB and also with the malpractice insurance company. Any existing claims are included in the insurer's background information on the practitioner. These claims can then be evaluated through the peer-review process of the credentialing committee. Although a practitioner may have had a malpractice claim filed against him or her, that fact alone does not automatically disqualify the practitioner nor necessarily reflect the quality of the practitioner.
- An attestation statement by the provider confirms his or her past history and physical and mental ability to provide service. Practitioners must attest to personal history in matters such as felony convictions, drug or alcohol abuse, and mental competence.

- Business license registration within the county may sometimes be included as part of credentialing because criminal checks are usually performed as a requirement for obtaining a business license.
- Some state licensing and medical boards also conduct criminal background checks.

In general, health plans have a much greater level of confidence in the entire credentialing process once they learn the level of safeguards and quality assurance that is built into the process.

Site Visits

A costly, but necessary step in credentialing is to visit each practitioner's office as a prerequisite for participation in the network. These visits can serve multiple purposes. They offer an opportunity to verify information on licensing and insurance coverage submitted by the practitioner, to provide the practitioner with information about the program and expectations, to answer questions and concerns on a personal level, and to learn about regional differences in practitioner operations. This information is critical to the credentialing committee's assessment of a practitioner.

The site visit provides an opportunity to actually see the office. Through the visit, credentialers gain firsthand knowledge of the quality of the practitioner's service provision. The visit also allows the credentialers a unique opportunity to observe hygiene and safety factors.

- Is the office environment professional?
- Is the office in compliance with basic health department and Occupational Safety and Health Administration regulations?
- Does the building have emergency exits that are properly marked?
- Does the staff know how to handle emergencies?
- Does the office have current fire extinguishers?
- Do staff use proper needle disposal procedures?
- Is the environment clean and free of hazards?

All these aspects of practice are important, not just to the health plan, but to the consumers who will be seen by these practitioners. Health plans want to be sure that a member of the credentialing staff has personally evaluated each facility, and that the standards for safety and professionalism have been met. The ultimate goal is to ensure a level of quality that will inspire consumers with the confidence that all providers on the panel meet a high standard.

Other issues in the review focus on aesthetics and the comfort of the client:

- Is there a waiting room?
- Is there sufficient space for the number of people who will be referred there?
- Is there adequate privacy for patient care?
- Is the environment comfortable and attractive?

The site visit provides an opportunity to verify that the practitioner has actually signed the contract, so that he or she is legally bound by it, and legal assurances are in place. Does the practitioner understand the terms and conditions of the contract? The contract has little value if the practitioner cannot comply with it. To address this need, organizations such as Consensus Health offer training to reinforce information on contractual obligations. Consensus provides training seminars twice a year for all practitioners.

The Credentialing Committee

After all these documents and processes are complete, each practitioner's file is submitted to a credentialing committee of peers (for example, licensed acupuncturists reviewing licensed acupuncturists). Including peer review in the credentialing process ensures that quality standards such as those of NCQA are satisfied and that the practitioner is seen by his or her peers as a quality provider.

Management Information Systems

All credentialing programs must be supported by an information system that will generate reports on provider data, track the expiration of practitioner license and insurance policies, and support directory and marketing requirements. These functions can be satisfied by using software programs that are sold by credentialing verification organizations and software vendors, or developed within the organization. Each organization's needs will vary and require different solutions.

CREDENTIALING COMPLEMENTARY SERVICES WITH AN OUTSIDE CONSULTANT OR VENDOR

Most large organizations have a standard operating procedure for credentialing. However, current research has found that 50% of the organizations surveyed used an outside vendor for credentialing complementary practitioners (National Market Measures, 1999). Why would a health plan or medical group be interested in using an outside vendor, particularly if the organization has its own credentialing committee in house? There can be a number of different reasons.

Expertise, Information, and Data

The process of credentialing complementary practitioners can differ significantly from that of traditional credentialing by physicians or hospitals. Verifying the qualifications of a practitioner within an alternative specialty (such as massage or bodywork) may involve unique resources and expertise.

Vendors may bring with them proprietary data resources on CAM utilization. Clients come to rely on the expertise and data of vendors because of the current lack of substantive quantitative information elsewhere in the field. Vendors may also provide data on appropriate utilization through their in-house resources. When a health plan decides to go forward in the integration process without traditional data such as clinical trials, the plan needs data that indicate how CAM therapies are currently being used, and what kinds of outcomes are typically achieved. Some vendors have the capacity to capture data, particularly utilization data. Proprietary databases of CAM evidence and experience have

been developed by a number of organizations, including Consensus Health. One of the goals of Consensus is to quantify and qualify the state of the existing research, through reliable information from a variety of sources, such as:

- claims information
- encounter information from practitioners
- client self-reports, using validated instruments such as the SF-36 and the SF-12
- member surveys.

Access to additional data on industry norms may be available through the experience and aggregate data gathering of the vendor. The consulting relationship allows the company buying the service to have access to comparative data. If a health plan credentials its own practitioners, it may be lacking the larger frame of reference of industry norms in terms of quality standards and credentials. An outside vendor who works with multiple health plans, numerous HMOs, and a variety of independent physician associations (IPAs) and hospitals will have a database that allows the client to feel comfortable that the norm of the group is the norm of the industry and not just a skewing.

Specialized information on provider education and standards within CAM specialties are often not part of the health care organization's knowledge base. In certain fields, credentialing may even involve the establishment of standards and guidelines for the first time. For example, Consensus was the first organization to credential massage therapists for a health plan. This process included the development of protocol and guidelines for credentialing. Consensus established initial standards, comparable to those of NCQA, for defining competence, sufficient training and experience, and good education within this CAM specialty.

Expense

The need for new credentialing resources may involve great expense. For example, the process of credentialing massage therapists might require contacting a variety of teaching institutions to verify educational certificates and malpractice insurance coverage through the massage therapists' associations. In this type of situation, an outside vendor may be able to provide the service more efficiently and cost-effectively for an HMO or a health plan since their systems often require modification to accommodate this process. The cost per unit for credentialing tends to be reduced when a service is provided in volume due to economies of scale.

Time Factors

The time required for a consultant to perform these kinds of services tends to be less than that of a health plan or an HMO because the focus is concentrated on the field of complementary medicine. Average credentialing preparation time for physicians is typically 90 to 120 days. Consensus currently averages 60 to 90 days in the credentialing of its network practitioners.

Avoiding Conflict of Interest

Vendor services may help clients avoid conflicts of interest. Consultants are in a position to be objective and neutral because they operate independently from the health plan. If, for example, the health plan has an affiliation or an established relationship with a medical group, reviewing the credentials of members of the medical group could create a conflict of interest. Credentialing decisions could impinge on the existing relationships. It is much easier for a vendor to reject a practitioner or to require that individual to obtain further training. These issues can be sidestepped by having the consultant thoroughly review all candidates and then make the decisions on the basis of objective standards.

Physician Training

Consultants can provide continuing medical education for health plan physicians. If the consultant/vendor has physicians on staff who are educated in both traditional medicine and CAM, the consulting physicians can translate the information into medical terms that can be evaluated intelligently by client physicians. Physicians with dual training can provide insight from a peer perspective, framed in terms that tend to bridge the disciplines.

It is important to involve doctors and to provide them with background information on alternative therapies, so that they can appropriately refer patients. For example, in 1997 the National Institutes of Health endorsed the use of acupuncture for nausea, vomiting, and pain management. Western pharmaceuticals are also used for these conditions. Now, more doctors and health plans are recognizing that an acupuncturist may also be an appropriate referral for these and other conditions. There are also cost benefits of utilizing CAM services and products in lieu of traditional services and pharmaceuticals. Consensus also provides the CAM practitioners with training that includes information on when to refer patients back to their physicians.

As the inclusion of complementary therapies increases, physicians will play an increasingly important role in the integration of services as the source of referrals to CAM networks in their health plans. The physician is ideally placed within the system to encourage appropriate utilization. A doctor's level of comfort with referrals to CAM practitioners will depend on his or her level of exposure, education, and knowledge of these specialties. Doctors with a genuine understanding of the applications of CAM are an asset to the health plan. They will find they can establish a valued niche within their profession. Consultants can provide the resources and information physicians want to become more highly knowledgeable about these therapies.

Program Design

Vendors can also assist with program design. For example, Consensus has developed a discounted program that offers consumers credentialed panels of highly qualified practitioners.

This enables its clients to make CAM services available without having to fully integrate them into their coverage. The discounted programs also offer Consensus the opportunity to continue to gather data on the levels of utilization and the health conditions for which people are seeing CAM practitioners.

The consultant can provide guidance in the development of practice guidelines. For example, in chiropractic care, the most frequently seen conditions are neuromuscular disorders. However, if acupuncture services are similarly limited to neuromuscular conditions, the therapy is not being used to maximum advantage. It is important to develop thorough in-depth guidelines, based on the expertise of leaders in the field who are actually working within these specialties.

A consultant can provide basic information on how to define and monitor appropriate care through treatment guidelines and care pathways. This provides a model in complementary health services that is comparable to the model utilized for other clinical services, and begins to create a convergence of perspectives within the health plan and their services. Ideally, consultants guide the development of clinical guidelines that define appropriate levels of care, appropriate utilization of services, and quality service provision.

Professional Assurances

Employers want the assurance that there is no exceptional risk involved in the use of CAM therapies. Employers and health plans want a safety net when introducing CAM services. They want to verify that all legal and program requirements have been met to ensure the well-being of their members. A good consultant will credential practitioners at a very extensive level to ensure that they are appropriately trained and qualified.

The utilization of an outside vendor for CAM credentialing is best evaluated on the basis of the organization's program goals, timeline, budget, and tolerance for risk, internal resources, and expertise.

REFERENCE

National Market Measures. *The Landmark Report II.* Sacramento, CA: Landmark Healthcare; 1999.

17.2   Vantage Point: Credentialing Naturopathy

Eileen Stretch

LICENSURE AND TRAINING

Naturopathic physicians are licensed in 11 states. Those who are licensed have had 4 years

---

Eileen Stretch, ND, is Associate Medical Director for American WholeHealth Networks, Inc, which assists health plans integrate CAM by providing networks nationwide.

of naturopathic medical school, which includes course work in basic science, pathophysiology, treatment, and 2 years of clinical experience in an outpatient setting. In states in which no licensure is available for naturopathic physicians, practitioners may call themselves naturopaths, but there is no standard of training associated with this title.

Untrained Naturopathic Practitioners

Many of the providers currently in practice are not formally trained and would not meet the credentialing standards of naturopathic medicine in states that provide licensure. Naturopathic practitioners in states that do not provide naturopathic licensure should not be credentialed into health plans unless there is primary source verification of graduation from an accredited naturopathic college or university. Some practitioners who call themselves naturopaths actually have mail-order degrees. They may have never seen a patient in a clinical setting, or they may be self-taught and may have never received formal clinical training. Without state regulation, these mail-order practitioners may mislead the public as to their training, whether intentional or not, and can create significant risk to the public's health.

Educational Standards for Credentialing

I recommend that credentialing standards for naturopathic physicians include graduation from a 4-year, full-time naturopathic medical program at an accredited college or at a college that is a candidate for accreditation. Currently, there are only three accredited schools in the United States: Bastyr University in Seattle, the National College of Naturopathic Medicine in Portland, Oregon, and Southwest College of Naturopathic Medicine in Scottsdale, Arizona. A new school in Bridgeport, Connecticut, is a candidate for accreditation.

School Entry Requirements and Training

The requirements for entry into a conventional medical program and a naturopathic medical school are the same. An undergraduate degree is required in either program. In comparing the training of a medical doctor and a naturopathic doctor, the 4 years of schooling are very comparable, but the clinical training of a naturopathic physician takes place in outpatient environments. In contrast, most clinical training for

physicians is provided through inpatient hospital settings.

Residency Programs

In allopathic medicine, there is a required residency program that typically lasts 2, 3, or 4 years. A cardiac surgeon might require 11 years of residency, but most programs are 2 to 3 years. In naturopathic medicine, there are no required residencies; at this point, they are optional. The leadership within the profession has proposed mandatory residencies in the future, but they will have to be developed. Some naturopathic physicians have chosen to do a residency as part of their training.

National Examination in Naturopathic Medicine

One can acquire a license and the right to practice after graduation from the accredited school by taking the Naturopathic Physician Licensing Examinations (NPLEX) including the basic science and clinical components and then a jurisprudence exam within the state.

State Laws

Note that each state has its own laws regarding licensure and scope of practice. Naturopathic physicians are trained as primary care physicians. They are licensed to work with patients in outpatient settings. They can diagnose and treat any nonemergent acute and chronic conditions. The scope of practice around treatment includes the therapeutic use of botanical medicine, nutritional medicine, homeopathy, physical medicine (for example, manipulation similar to the techniques used by chiropractors), massage and other forms of bodywork, hydrotherapy, counseling, stress reduction, and lifestyle management. Naturopathic physicians are all trained in each of those practices. Regarding diagnosis, naturopathic physicians use all of the conventional methods to diagnose disease. They are trained to interpret radiographs. They learn to interpret blood work, as any physician would. They are also trained to perform minor surgery, and in many jurisdictions, they are licensed to perform that service.

Scope of Practice

Naturopathic physicians are very well trained in terms of scope of practice, in the limitations of the discipline, and in knowing when it is necessary and appropriate to refer patients to conventional medicine. That is an important aspect of training. All practicing naturopathic physicians establish relationships with medical doctors, so that they can refer their patients when necessary. Most insurance companies require naturopathic physicians to indicate that they have established referral relationships.

Emergency Care

Currently, there is no state in which naturopathic physicians are granted full hospital privileges. In one location in Hawaii, naturopaths work in a hospital, but the role there is as adjunct providers. In general, naturopathic physicians do not provide emergency medical care. In my own practice, there are physicians in Seattle whom I can call on the rare occasions when I must have a patient hospitalized. I send my patient to the hospital, call the physician, and he or she has the patient admitted.

17.3   Resources

Vickie S. Ina

CONTACT INFORMATION FOR CREDENTIALING

Acupuncture

American of Association of Oriental Medicine (AAOM)
433 Front Street
Catasauqua, PA 18032
Phone: (610) 433-2448
E-mail: AAOM1@aol.com
Web site: http://www.AAOM.org
Source for acupuncture and Oriental medicine laws

Accreditation Commission of Acupuncture and Oriental Medicine (ACAOM)
1010 Wayne Avenue, Suite 1270
Silver Spring, MD 20910
Phone: (301) 608-9680
Recognized by U.S. Department of Education (formerly the NACSCAOM)

National Acupuncture and Oriental Medicine Alliance (NAOMA)
14637 Starr Road, SE
Olalla, WA 98359
Phone: (206) 851-6896 or (206) 524-3511
Web site: http://www.healthy.net/naoma
Public education and legislative activity

National Certification Commission for Acupuncture and Oriental Medicine (NCCAOM)
11 Canal Center Plaza, Suite 300
Alexandria, VA 22314
Phone: (703) 548-9004
NCCA written and practical exams; certification in acupuncture, Oriental medicine, Chinese herbology, and Oriental bodywork

Chiropractic

American Chiropractic Association (ACA)
1701 Clarendon Boulevard
Arlington, VA 22209
Phone: (800) 986-4636 or (703) 278-8800
Web site: http://www.amerchiro.org

Council on Chiropractic Education (CCE)
and Commission on Accreditation
8049 N. 85th Way
Scottsdale, AZ 85258
Phone: (480) 443-8877
E-mail: cce@cce-usa.org
Web site: http://www.cce-usa.org

Federation of Chiropractic Licensing Boards
(FCLB) (Western Office)
901 54th Avenue, Suite 101
Greeley, CO 80634
Phone: (970) 356-3500
Web site: http://www.fclb.org

Massage

American Massage Therapy Association
(AMTA)
820 Davis Street, Suite 100
Evanston, IL 60201-4444
Phone: (847) 864-3511
Web site: http://www.amtamassage.org
Minimum of 500 hours required for
membership

Associated Bodywork and Massage
Professionals (ABMP)
1271 Sugarbush Drive
Evergreen, CO 80439-9766
Phone: (800) 458-2267 or (303) 674-8478
Web site: http://www.abmp.com

National Certification Board for Therapeutic
Massage and Bodywork (NCBTMB)
8201 Greensboro Drive, Suite 300
McLean, VA 22102
Phone: (703) 610-9015
Web site: http://www.ncbtmb.com

Written exam for certification; only national
certifying organization for
massage/bodywork

Naturopathic Medicine and Homeopathy

American Association of Naturopathic
Physicians (AANP)
8201 Greensboro Drive, Suite 300
McLean, VA 22102
Phone: (877) 969-2267
Web site: http://www.naturopathic.org

American Naturopathic Medical Association
(ANMA)
PO Box 96273
Las Vegas, NV 89193
Phone: (702) 897-7053
Web site: http://www.anma.com

American Naturopathic Medical Certification
and Accreditation Board (ANMCAB)
8170 S. Eastern Avenue, Suite 4-133
Las Vegas, NV 89123
Phone: (702) 897-4915
Web site: http://www.anmcab.org

Council for Homeopathic Certification (CHC)
P.O. Box 460190
San Francisco, CA 94146
Phone: (415) 789-7677
Web site: http://www.homeopathy-council.org

National Board of Homeopathic Examiners
(NBHE)
5333 Franklin Road
Boise, ID 83705
Phone: (208) 426-0847
Awards diplomate certification to health care
professionals

For additional information on accreditation
and approved institutions, contact the U.S. Department of Education.

17.4   State Law Defining the Professions Licensed and Regulated by State

Laws for CAM vary state by state. The following examples provide a sense of regulatory definitions and requirements. See Table 17.4–1 for a list of health professions regulated by state. California is an example of a highly regulated state that sets high standards.

SELECTED INFORMATION FROM CALIFORNIA STATE LAW ON ACUPUNCTURE

4926. In its concern with the need to eliminate the fundamental causes of illness, not simply to remove symptoms, and with the need to treat the whole person, the Legislature intends to establish in this article, a framework for the practice of the art and science of oriental medicine through acupuncture . . .

Definitions
4927. (e) Acupuncture means the stimulation of a certain point or points on or near the surface of the body by the insertion of needles to prevent or modify the perception of pain or to normalize physiological functions, including pain control, for the treatment of certain diseases or dysfunctions of the body and includes the techniques of electroacupuncture, cupping, and moxibustion.

Practice of Acupuncture
4937. (b) To perform or prescribe the use of oriental massage, acupressure, breathing techniques, exercise or nutrition, including the incorporation of drugless substances and herbs as dietary supplements to promote health.

Qualifications Required
4938. (a) Is at least 18 years of age.
(b) Furnishes satisfactory evidence of completion of one of the following:
(1) An educational and training program approved by the committee . . .
(2) Satisfactory completion of a tutorial program in the practice of an acupuncturist which is approved by the committee

(3) . . . education and training outside the United States and Canada . . . which meets the standards established . . .
(c) Passes an examination administered by the committee.
(d) Is not subject to denial.
(e) Completes a clinical internship-training program approved by the committee.

Approval of Schools and Training Programs
4939. (2) The committee shall establish standards for the approval of schools and colleges offering education and training in the practice of an acupuncturist, including standards for the faculty. (Currently, the state of California accepts only master's level programs in acupuncture and not certificate programs.)

Continuing Education
4945. (b) The committee shall require each acupuncturist to complete 30 hours of continuing education every two years as a condition for the renewal of his or her certificate...

Acupuncture Tutorial
(d) The clinical training shall consist of a minimum of 2250 hours in the following areas:
(1) Practice observation
(2) History and physical examination
(3) Therapeutic treatment planning
(4) Preparation of the patient
(5) Sterilization, use and maintenance of equipment
(6) Moxibustion
(7) Electroacupuncture (AC and DC voltages)
(8) Body and auricular acupuncture
(9) Treatment of emergencies, including cardiopulmonary resuscitation
(10) Pre- and post-treatment instruction to the patient
(11) Contraindications and precautions

Training

(e) The theoretical and didactic training shall consist of a minimum of 600 hours (approximately 40 semester units) in the following areas:

(1) Traditional Oriental Medicine—a survey of the theory and practice of traditional diagnostic and therapeutic procedures.

(2) Acupuncture anatomy and physiology— fundamental of acupuncture, including the meridian system, special and extra loci, and auriculotherapy.

(3) Acupuncture techniques—instruction in the use of needling techniques, moxibustion, electroacupuncture, . . . precautions, . . . contraindications and complications.

(4) Clinical medicine—a survey of the clinical practice of medicine, osteopathy, dentistry, psychology, nursing, chiropractic, podiatry, and homeopathy . . .

(5) History of Medicine—a survey of medical history (and) transcultural healing practices.

(6) Medical terminology—fundamentals of English language medical terminology.

(7) General sciences—a survey of general biology, chemistry, and physics.

(8) Anatomy—a survey of microscopic and gross anatomy and neuroanatomy.

(9) Physiology— . . . basic physiology, . . . neurophysiology, endocrinology, neurochemistry.

(10) Pathology—a survey of the nature of disease and illness, including microbiology, immunology, psychopathology, and epidemiology.

(11) Clinical sciences—a review of internal medicine, pharmacology, neurology, surgery, obstetrics/gynecology, urology, radiology, nutrition, and public health.

THE LEGAL DEFINITION OF ACUPUNCTURE IN THE STATE OF HAWAII

Hawaii has one of the widest breadths of regulated CAM services, and therefore a description of some of the scope of practice and requirements in Hawaii has been included.

16-72-5 Scope of practice of acupuncture.

(1) Authorized treatment which consists of pain relief and analgesia; functional disorders, including functional components of diseases; and abnormal conditions; and

(2) Referred treatment of other areas when referred by a medical doctor licensed in the State under chapter 453, HRS, and dentists licensed under chapter 448, HRS. Similarly, the acupuncture practitioner may refer patients with ailments beyond the practitioner's scope of treatment to a medical doctor or dentist.

16-72-14 Formal education and training.

(a) An applicant shall submit satisfactory proof of graduation from a school or college, which includes in its curriculum educational courses and training established to qualify students to practice acupuncture or oriental traditional medicine. The course of study shall extend for a minimum duration of three academic years (one thousand five hundred hours) and shall consist of not less than two academic years (six hundred hours) of study of acupuncture or oriental traditional medicine and not less than twelve months (nine hundred hours) of supervised clinical internship program. The clinical practice shall be served under the direction of a licensed acupuncture practitioner. If a clinical internship program, as described herein, is not required to receive a certificate or diploma of graduation from the school or college, the applicant must complete at least twelve months of clinical practice consisting of at least nine hundred hours under the supervision of a licensed acupuncture practitioner who has been in practice for not less than five years.

(b) The acupuncture or oriental traditional medicine course curriculum shall cover, but not be limited to, subjects such as:

(1) History and philosophy of oriental traditional medicine (Nei-Ching, Taoism, Chi and Hsieh, Yin and Yang, and others);

(2) Traditional human anatomy, including location of acupuncture points;

(3) Traditional physiology, including the five elements organ theory;

(4) Traditional clinical diagnosis, including pulse diagnosis;

(5) Pathology, including the six Yin and seven Chin;

(6) Laws of acupuncture (mother and son, husband and wife, and five elements);

(7) Classification and function of points;

(8) Needle techniques;

(9) Complications;

(10) Forbidden points;

(11) Resuscitation;

(12) Safety and precautions;

(13) Use of electrical devices for diagnosis and treatment;

(14) Public health and welfare;

(15) Hygiene and sanitation; and

(16) Practical clinical acupuncture practice.

(Auth: HRS 436E-7) (Imp: HRS 436E-5)

THE LEGAL DEFINITION OF ACUPUNCTURE IN THE STATE OF NORTH CAROLINA

North Carolina has standards that are comparable to some of the other state regulations. They are not quite as stringent as California's, but clearly follow the same pattern of quality requirements.

.0101 Qualifications for Licensure

In addition to and for the purposes of meeting the requirements of G.S. 90-455 an applicant for licensure to practice acupuncture shall:

(1) Submit a completed application,

(2) Submit fees as required by Rule .0103 of this Section,

(3) Submit proof of a score of not less than 70% on the National Certification Commission for Acupuncture and Oriental Medicine (NCCAOM) acupuncture written & point location exams or a score of not less than 70% from any state utilizing the NCCAOM examination,

(4) Submit a certified copy, certified by the issuing institution, of a transcript including evidence of graduation from a three-year postgraduate college, accredited by, or in candidacy status by, the Accreditation Commission for Acupuncture and Oriental Medicine or, if outside of the U.S., the California Acupuncture Committee,

(5) Submit proof of successful completion of the Clean Needle Technique course offered by the Council of Colleges of Acupuncture and Oriental Medicine (CCAOM).

.0102 Requirements/Waiver/Qualifications/Licensure detailed in G.S. 90-455

(4)(b)(ii) Training: Accrue 15 points (a minimum of 5 points in both categories in Sub-items (4)(b)(ii)(A) and (B) of this Rule:

(A) Education:

(I) Structured—For each 100 hours of documented completion of a formal training program approved by Board: 1 point. A formal training program is an acupuncture college certified or approved by the state or country in which it operates.

(II) Apprenticeship—For each 150 hours of supervised apprenticeship training with an acupuncturist [and which is verified by such acupuncturist(s)]: 1 point.

(B) Experience:

An applicant must accrue a minimum of five points in any combination of Sub-items (4)(ii)(B)(I) and (II) of this Rule. Acupuncture must comprise at least 90% of the applicant's practice. Treatments for cessation of smoking and weight loss shall not be adequate to satisfy experience requirements if such therapies comprise more than 40% of the applicant's practice.

(I) Treatment of not fewer than 100 different patients for not less than 2000 patient hours within the last three years prior to application for licensure: 5 points.

(II) Treatment of not fewer than 100 patients for not less than 4000 patient hours within the last three years prior to application for licensure: 10 points.

.0104 Definitions

The following definitions shall apply throughout this Chapter:

(1) "Acupuncture adjunctive therapies" include but are not limited to auricular, nose, face, hand, foot, and scalp acupuncture therapy; and

Table 17.4–1 Health Professions Regulated by State/Jurisdiction

	Acupuncturists	Chiropractors	Dental Hygienists/Assistants	Dentists	Homeopaths	Medical Assistants	Naturopaths	Nurse Midwives	Nutritionists/Dieticians	Optometrists	Pharmacists	Physical Therapists	Physicians—MDs	Physicians—DOs	Physician Assistants	Podiatrists	Practical/Vocational Nurses	Psychologists/Behavioral Scientists	Registered Nurses	Respiratory/Inhalation Therapists	Social Workers	Speech Pathologists
AL	—	2	2	2	—	—	—	2	—	2	2	—	1	1	1	2	2	—	2	—	—	—
AK	3	2	2	2	—	—	3	2	—	2	2	2	1	1	1	1	2	2	2	—	2	—
AZ	—	2	2	2	2	—	2	1	—	2	2	2	1	2	2	2	1	2	1	—	2	—
AR	—	2	2	2	—	—	—	2	—	2	2	1	1	1	1	2	2	2	2	1	2	2
CA	1	2	2	2	—	1	—	2	—	2	2	1	1	2	1	1	2	2	2	1	2	1
CO	2	2	2	2	—	—	—	2	—	2	2	2	1	1	1	2	2	2	2	—	2	—
CT	—	2	1	1	2	—	2	3	3	2	2	2	1	2	2	2	2	2	2	3	3	3
DE	3	2	2	2	3	3	3	3	2	2	2	2	1	1	1	2	2	2	2	3	2	2
DC	1	2	2	2	—	—	3	2	2	2	2	2	1	1	1	2	2	2	2	2	2	—
FL	2	2	2	2	—	—	3	3	1	2	2	2	1	2	—	2	2	2	2	1	2	—
GA	1	1	2	2	—	—	—	3	2	2	2	2	1	1	1	2	2	2	2	1	2	2
GU	2	2	2	2	—	—	—	—	—	2	2	2	1	1	—	2	2	2	2	—	—	2
HI	2	2	1	1	—	—	2	2	—	2	2	2	1	2	2	2	2	2	2	—	—	2
ID	—	2	2	2	—	—	—	2	2	2	2	2	1	1	1	2	2	2	2	2	2	—
IL	—	2	—	2	—	—	—	—	—	2	2	2	1	1	1	2	2	—	2	—	2	—
IN	—	2	2	2	—	—	—	1	2	2	2	2	1	1	1	2	2	2	2	1	2	2
IA	1	2	2	2	—	—	—	2	2	2	2	1	1	1	—	2	2	2	2	2	2	2
KS	—	2	2	2	—	—	—	2	2	2	2	2	1	1	1	1	2	2	2	1	2	2
KY	—	2	—	2	—	—	—	3	—	2	2	1	1	1	1	2	2	—	2	—	—	—
LA	1	1	2	2	—	—	—	2	—	2	2	2	1	1	1	1	2	2	2	1	2	2
ME	2	2	1	1	—	—	2	2	2	2	2	1	2	2	2	2	2	2	2	2	2	2
MD	2	2	2	2	—	—	2	2	2	2	2	2	1	1	1	2	2	2	2	1	2	2
MA	1	2	2	2	—	—	—	2	—	2	2	2	1	1	2	2	2	2	2	—	2	2
MI	—	2	2	2	—	—	—	2	—	2	2	2	1	2	1	2	2	2	2	—	2	—
MN	1	2	2	2	—	—	—	2	2	2	2	1	1	1	1	2	2	2	2	1	2	3
MS	—	2	2	2	—	—	—	2	2	2	2	2	1	1	—	1	2	2	2	2	—	2
MO	—	2	2	2	—	—	—	—	—	2	2	2	1	1	—	2	2	2	2	—	—	2

continues

Source: Reprinted with permission from the *Federation of State Medical Boards, Table 51: Health Professions Regulated by States, 1999–2000 Exchange*, Vol. 3, pp. 86–87, © 1999, the Federation of State Medical Boards of the United States.

Table 17.4–1 continued

	Acupuncturists	Chiropractors	Dental Hygienists/Assistants	Dentists	Homeopaths	Medical Assistants	Naturopaths	Nurse Midwives	Nutritionists/Dieticians	Optometrists	Pharmacists	Physical Therapists	Physicians—MDs	Physicians—DOs	Physician Assistants	Podiatrists	Practical/Vocational Nurses	Psychologists/Behavioral Scientists	Registered Nurses	Respiratory/Inhalation Therapists	Social Workers	Speech Pathologists
MT	1	2	2	2	—	—	2	2	1	2	2	2	1	1	1	1	2	2	2	2	2	2
NE	—	2	2	2	—	—	—	2	2	2	2	2	1	1	1	2	2	2	2	2	2	2
NV	2	2	—	2	2	—	—	—	—	2	2	2	1	2	1	2	2	2	2	—	—	2
NH	2	2	2	2	3	3	2	2	3	2	2	1	1	1	1	1	2	2	2	2	2	2
NJ	2	2	1	2	—	—	—	2	—	2	2	2	1	1	—	2	2	2	2	—	—	2
NM	2	2	1	2	—	—	—	2	2	2	2	2	2	2	1	2	2	2	2	3	2	2
NY	1	1	1	1	—	—	—	1	1	1	1	1	1	1	1	1	1	1	1	1	1	1
NC	2	2	2	2	—	—	—	2	—	2	2	2	1	1	1	2	2	2	2	—	—	2
ND	—	2	—	2	—	—	—	2	—	2	2	2	1	1	1	2	2	2	2	2	2	—
OH	—	2	2	2	—	—	—	1	2	2	2	2	1	1	1	1	2	2	2	2	2	2
OK	—	2	2	2	—	—	—	2	1	2	2	1	2	2	1	2	2	2	2	—	2	2
OR	—	2	2	2	—	—	2	—	—	2	2	2	1	1	1	1	2	2	2	1	2	2
PA	1	2	2	2	—	—	—	1	—	2	2	2	1	2	1	2	2	2	2	1	2	2
PR	1	2	2	2	—	—	—	—	2	2	2	2	2	1	—	2	1	2	2	—	2	1
RI	3	2	2	2	—	—	—	2	—	2	2	2	2	2	2	2	2	2	2	3	2	2
SC	1	2	2	2	—	—	—	2	2	2	2	2	2	1	1	2	2	2	2	1	2	2
SD	—	2	—	2	—	—	—	1	2	2	2	1	1	1	1	2	2	2	2	—	—	—
TN	—	2	2	2	—	—	—	2	2	2	2	2	1	2	1	2	2	2	2	2	2	2
TX	2	2	2	2	—	—	—	—	—	2	2	2	1	1	2	2	2	2	2	—	—	—
UT	2	2	1	1	—	—	2	2	2	2	2	2	1	2	1	2	2	2	2	2	2	2
VT	2	2	2	2	—	—	2	2	2	2	2	2	1	2	1	1	2	2	2	—	2	—
VA	1	1	2	2	—	—	1	1	—	2	2	1	1	1	1	1	2	1	2	1	2	2
VI	—	—	—	—	—	—	—	—	—	—	—	—	—	—	—	—	—	—	—	—	—	—
WA	2	2	2	2	—	3	2	2	3	2	2	2	1	2	1	2	2	2	2	3	3	2
WV	2	2	2	2	—	—	—	2	2	2	2	2	1	2	1	1	2	2	2	2	2	2
WI	2	2	2	2	—	—	—	2	2	2	2	1	1	1	1	1	2	2	2	—	—	2
WY	—	2	—	2	—	—	—	—	—	2	2	2	1	1	1	2	2	2	2	—	—	—

Note: 1 = regulated by state medical board, 2 = regulated by separate/other board, 3 = regulated but under no board.
Source: Reprinted with permission from the *Federation of State Medical Boards, Table 51: Health professions regulated by States, 1999–2000 Exchange*, Vol. 3, pp. 86–87, © 1999, the Federation of State Medical Boards of the United States.

stimulation to acupuncture points and channels by any of the following: needles, cupping, thermal methods, magnets, gwa-sha scraping techniques.

(2) "Acupuncture diagnostic techniques" include but are not limited to the use of observation, listening, smelling, inquiring, palpation, pulse diagnosis, tongue diagnosis, hara diagnosis, physiognomy, five element correspondence, ryodoraku, akabani, and electroacupuncture.

(3) "Acupuncture needles" mean solid filiform needles and include but are not limited to intradermal, plum blossom, press tacks, and prismatic needles.

(4) "Dietary guidelines" include but are not limited to nutritional counseling and the recommendations of food and supplemental substances.

(5) "Electrical stimulation" includes but is not limited to the treatment or diagnosis of energetic imbalances using TENS, Piezo electrical stimulation, acuscope therapy, auricular therapy devices, and percutaneous and transcutaneous electrical nerve stimulation.

(6) "Herbal medicine" includes but is not limited to tinctures, patent remedies, decoction, powders, diluted herbal remedies, freeze dried herbs, salves, poultices, medicated oils, and liniments.

(7) "Massage and manual techniques" include but are not limited to acupressure, shiatsu, Tui-Na, qi healing, and medical qi gong.

(8) "Therapeutic exercise" includes but is not limited to qi gong, Taoist self-cultivation exercises, dao yin, tai qi chuan, ba gua, and meditative exercises.

(9) "Thermal methods" include but are not limited to moxibustion, hot and cold packs and laser acupuncture. All acupuncture devices shall be administered in accordance with Federal Drug Administration guidelines.

.0401 Practice Parameters

The following are the practice parameters for acupuncturists in North Carolina:

(1) A licensed acupuncturist shall practice within the scope of training offered by a college accredited, or in candidacy status, by the National Accreditation for Schools and Colleges of Acupuncture and Oriental Medicine.

(2) A licensed acupuncturist must practice within the confines of his training. Parameters for diagnosis and treatment of patients include: Five Elements, Eight Principles, Yin Yang Theory, Channel Theory, Zang Fu Organ Theory, Six Stages and Four Aspects of Disease Progressions.

.0402 Acupuncture Procedures

(5) Diagnosis:

(a) Diagnosis shall be made utilizing methods connected with the traditions represented in Oriental medicine as listed in Rule .0104 of this Chapter. Examples of diagnostic measures include the Eight Principles, Five Elements, Pulse diagnosis, and Tongue diagnosis.

(b) The diagnostic procedures shall be recorded at each visit . . .

(8) Failure to Progress:

(a) If a patient fails to respond to treatments, discussion about other forms of treatment or referral to another health care professional shall be made.

(b) In the case of persistent, unexplained pain, or the unexplained worsening of any condition in the face of ongoing treatment, referral or consultation shall be made. In choosing a referral source, priority shall be given to previously seen practitioners.

(c) Requests by the patient for information about other forms of treatment or referral shall always be honored.

CHAPTER 18

Human Resources

18.1 Human Resources in Integrative Medicine

Leah Kliger

KEY CHALLENGES FOR HUMAN RESOURCES IN INTEGRATIVE MEDICINE

The importance of human resources in integrative medicine cannot be overstressed. The greatest expenditures in health care delivery are the salaries and benefits paid to staff and providers. Yet there is a tendency in the development and implementation phases of complementary and alternative medicine services to concentrate on program development, financial considerations, reimbursement, and facility design and neglect the human capital side. When attention is given to human resource issues, organizations often focus only on programmatic details while other critical aspects of personnel selection and human resources may get neglected.

Initially, a plan must be elaborated that outlines how the workforce can be recruited, de-

veloped, and utilized to its fullest potential. It is crucial to provide a common philosophy as a foundation for any people-centered system. How will human resources align with the organization's mission, vision, values, and critical success factors?

Challenges include:

- Attracting, motivating, and retaining quality staff.
- Forging staff into a unique organization—one that takes a holistic approach to health and healing.
- Creating a culture that allows individuals and teams within the organization to be as dynamic as the organization itself.
- Developing an environment that encourages personal, professional, and team growth. Hallmarks of such cultures include shared decision making, partnering with patients, and impeccable communication.
- Constructing a shared philosophy of diversity that celebrates commonalities and differences.
- Assimilating a variety of disparate approaches and philosophies that have dem-

Leah Kliger, MHA, CH, is Director, Integrative Medicine, Evergreen Healthcare, Kirkland, Washington; a health care consultant with The Lakes Group, Kirkland, Washington; and assistant clinical professor at University of Washington Graduate Program in Health Services, Seattle.

onstrated success in other settings yet preserve the autonomy so critical to success in an integrated setting.

- Balancing the need for internal controls, structure, and compliance with local, state, and federal laws and requirements with the need to be flexible and responsive to individual needs and philosophies.
- Designing a compensation system for both the conventionally trained doctors and the complementary medicine providers that aligns the values of the organization with individual skills and team competencies.

PLANNING

Developing a prototype for the human resources system is vital to success. The ideal model is defined by the program's purpose, vision, values, and other critical success factors that define the integrative center, program, or service lines. The organization's phase of development will to some degree define and drive the set of skills and competencies that will be required of its staff. Those competencies may be quite different during the planning stage compared with the implementation and operations phases. Obtaining feedback from patients that describes what they seek from providers is an important component.

CREATING THE ORGANIZATIONAL CULTURE

A holistic organizational culture needs to be created when the service is initially established. Culture change will be more difficult to forge later. In centers that exist within a hospital or health system, or work in close cooperation with a mainstream institution, the challenge is to mesh the culture of the new unit with that of the existing system. For example, establishing an integrative component in an existing cancer program could be problematic. Attitudes and beliefs have already been established; divestiture of these values during a time of transition can be difficult. Clearly, it is easier to define the

organizational culture in a freestanding integrative medicine center that has its own distinct identity and organizational boundaries.

In addition, CAM practitioners may be relatively unfamiliar with bureaucracy, policies, procedures, and the management practices of a larger organization. Sometimes, a great deal of adjustment may be required. Alternative practitioners who create an integrative center may be at a disadvantage when the need arises to develop reciprocal working relationships with the local hospital as they may lack the experience required to successfully interact in a mainstream environment. How can the human resources function support these organizational needs?

Key questions to answer when creating the organizational culture include:

- How can an organizational culture be created within the program that reflects a holistic orientation? How will these values be fostered within the framework of this particular program?
- Will the staff of the merged integrative medicine center develop a new culture and identity or retain their own?
- How is a service orientation established and what rewards are offered?
- What is the nature of the culture in the larger organization and how will the center fit within that organizational framework? In many cases, the majority of CAM practitioners may have never worked for a large organization and can find the interface frustrating.
- How is a service orientation motivated and rewarded throughout the organization?

If the service will be part of a larger health system, it is vital that it provides the staff of the mainstream system opportunities to understand CAM to the greatest extent possible by offering ongoing staff education on a number of levels through a variety of programs. Good communication coupled with participation will increase receptivity to the new service within the larger system.

Staff can be offered therapies to increase their experiential understanding of complementary medicine. Modalities such as acupuncture, mindfulness meditation, or music therapy that are designed to reduce stress are particularly relevant. CAM services should also be made available to staff in departments, such as oncology, surgery, and critical care, where the nature of the work is high pressure. Staff members who experience the benefits of CAM will become the best marketers, and this can increase buy-in from other employees in the health system. Services could be offered free or at a reduced fee to staff.

Provide staff with a vision of how the organization will build and maintain an environment conducive to performance excellence, full participation, a commitment to mind-body-spirit ideals, and personal and organizational growth. The core human resources values need to be developed by staff. These values will underpin the way people work together and treat each other and patients. Employees and providers should be encouraged to respect the perspectives and contributions of all team members. Responsiveness to staff needs, including sensitivity to personal and family life, is also important.

RECRUITMENT POLICIES, PRACTICES, AND REALITIES

Deciding exactly how the organization will recruit staff is a crucial step. Should the hiring be performed in-house or should it be outsourced to a vendor or consultant that specializes in this type of recruiting and credentialing? If recruiting will be performed in-house, identify those individuals who will recruit and make job offers and those who will lead and manage each position.

The Recruitment and Retention Process

These important steps should be followed before the first person is hired:

1. *Assess the job market.* Are there particular shortages for the skilled clinical professionals needed? Recruiting can be performed with the assistance of local schools of acupuncture, massage, and naturopathic medicine. The national associations that serve alternative practitioners should be contacted; they may have local and state chapters with job banks. These organizations include the American Massage Therapy Association, the American Association of Naturopathic Physicians, the American Holistic Medical Association, American Association of Oriental Medicine, and the American Music Therapy Association.

2. *Define the program in greater depth.* Will it involve self-directed teams or a more formal hierarchical system? Certain categories of staff may be more familiar working in a one- or two-person office or as solo practitioners and relatively unfamiliar with the management practices of a larger organization. The person conducting interviews needs to develop a list of situational questions in order to ascertain whether the applicants understand the different realities they will encounter.

3. *Estimate the number and type of positions required:*
   - Will all of the staff be employees, or will some have a contractual relationship?
   - Will the service begin with part-time staff, gradually increasing hours as service volumes grow?
   - Will the service employ only licensed practitioners, or will it employ nonlicensed professionals as well? For example, a state may have licensure for massage practitioners and acupuncturists, but not for naturopathic doctors. Some integrated clinics or service lines decide to hire only licensed physician acupuncturists or licensed registered nurses trained as massage practitioners, particularly in states where licensure is not yet available.

4. *Write a job description for each and every position.* The description should include a summary of the job, a list of

usual activities performed, reporting responsibilities, educational requirements, and the minimum experience required.

How Will the Service Attract and Retain Quality Staff Members? It is encouraging to know that job seekers are often highly motivated by the prospect of participating in the development of an integrative medicine center or CAM research. Consequently, the recruitment process is not as difficult as it can become later when financial realities and job pressures intrude.

PERSONNEL COMPETENCIES

Customer Service

Everyone on staff must have excellent customer service skills. These abilities extend beyond written communication. Good verbal communication is essential to ensure that the level of customer service is impeccable. Active listening is an important component. All staff must also demonstrate emotional maturity, which involves the ability to provide constructive feedback and resolve conflict. These are all teachable skills.

Considerations for Leadership

In an integrative center, a different skill set is required for leadership and director-level staff. Leaders must have a passion for integrative medicine, but also have strong business and health care delivery skills. They should be collaborators and team builders who will enhance the group dynamic by empowering other staff members to make decisions. *Leaders in this emerging field ideally demonstrate a range of professional capabilities:*

- political astuteness
- skill in communication and motivation
- marketing savvy
- demonstrated proficiency in financial planning and accounting
- high tolerance for ambiguity
- emotional maturity
- collaboration and team building

- the capability to undertake needs assessments and conduct research
- strong organizational and program development skills.

Clinical Leadership

Identify a champion among the clinicians of the organization. It is essential that the clinical leadership have demonstrated impeccable clinical competencies and be held in high regard in the allopathic medical community. A clinical leader must be able to communicate with a wide range of providers, including physicians at the local hospitals, practitioners in the CAM community, and patients. He or she must be able to relate to all stakeholders and be an advocate for body-mind-spirit medicine.

It can be difficult to find leaders with dual credentials, but they do exist. A capable integrative physician is genuinely immersed in both approaches to medicine; and leaders in a number of areas can be found:

- physicians who are also highly trained in science
- administrators who have a background in integrative medicine
- researchers who have also become deeply knowledgeable regarding complementary medicine.

Clinical Skills

One of the hallmarks of a successful integrative center is that all clinicians must have outstanding clinical skills. Clinical excellence provides the basis for referrals. Practitioners must have an enthusiasm for lifelong learning so that they keep their knowledge and credentials current. This will also accrue respect for the center. Competence is the best form of advertising. Patients who do well will tell others.

Clinicians in an integrative center must also be team players, with a collaborative work style. Cohesive functioning of the multidisciplinary team, building relationships throughout the system, and developing reciprocal referrals depends on cooperation.

COMPENSATION AND BENEFITS

The service must establish a sound compensation benefits system based on market and financial realities, yet one that is aligned with the organization's holistic vision:

- Will the compensation and benefits system include a combination of pay for individual and/or team performance?
- Will it be based on productivity measures? By design, CAM practitioners usually spend much more time with each client or patient than a conventionally trained physician.
- How much will be based on customer satisfaction?
- How will the compensation plan be tied to productivity goals? Compensation tied only to production targets may alienate CAM providers, cause ill will, and lead to conflict. Conversely, using no incentives can often lead to low volumes, disgruntled physicians, and financial disaster. Implementing quality improvement targets and team goals can be coupled with the necessary internal measures to mitigate the inherent tension yet achieve success.
- Will there be other forms of compensation or perks as motivators?

Receptionists and medical assistants should be paid what they are worth to the organization. Often, the front office staff make only slightly above the minimum wage rate. However, as the first point of contact for both new and returning clients, their customer service skills and work ethic can do more to build the client base than a marketing campaign with a budget twice that of a receptionist's annual salary. These are the people who can make or break the encounter, both on the telephone and in person. If they are caring, concerned, and understanding, the experience for new clients will be positive because that initial contact sets the tone.

A consultant may help design the compensation system, particularly one who has worked on the development of such a system for other integrated centers. A compensation system designed for conventional medical or hospital-based practice frequently does not work well for a holistic model of care delivery.

EDUCATION AND TRAINING

Patients will be attracted to the service if it is a reliable and credible source of care and service, yet one that is somehow unique. A strong commitment to staff development and education promotes a positive climate. Ultimately, these efforts enrich the well-being and satisfaction of patients and staff alike.

Training Initiatives

Develop an ongoing training program. Allocate time at each staff meeting for learning. This can take the form of brief case reviews by individual practitioners, or an all-provider dialogue about a particular patient. Everyone should be included since all staff must have some basic knowledge of CAM in order to respond intelligently to questions, regardless of position.

To increase staff empathy, role-playing various scenarios is an excellent way of appreciably improving the quality of client services. Staff need a great deal of tact when discussing personal health matters that require privacy and confidentiality. Identify a separate consultation area for sensitive discussions or suggest these discussions be conducted in a treatment room.

Administrative aspects of training should not be overlooked. For example, receptionists should have a laminated card with appropriate phone numbers and hours of operation. Flyers, postcards, or marketing materials should be distributed internally prior to the initiation of any external marketing campaigns. Staff and providers should not be surprised or underinformed.

Design an Evaluation Component into the Training Program. How effective are the training efforts? How is effectiveness measured?

Consider Training an Important Tool for Achieving Good Customer Service. It is not a matter of luck. Customer service training is vital for patient satisfaction and financial success.

Customer Service Can Also Be a Form of Marketing. Discuss ways in which the organization's brand can be established and reinforced. At staff meetings, ask those who have handled a complaint or difficult situation positively to describe it and the outcome. Staff will not only be providing patient care; they will be selling information, credibility, and image.

Employees must know what is expected of them, increasing their confidence in their ability to deliver on expectations. Realistic volume standards should be set that enable practitioners time to return phone calls and keep waiting times to a minimum. Otherwise, those answering the phone and greeting patients are left with a huge, unmanageable dilemma.

Teach the Importance of Time Management. In an integrative setting, practitioners take more time with patients than in other settings. The staff need to learn to set priorities. Staff need to communicate in a friendly manner that keeps the process moving, yet is not perceived as abrupt. An organized process should be developed for conducting patient exams and providing treatments so that they are thorough. The center administration should regularly review diagnosis, intervention, and patient education requirements.

Develop Mechanisms To Support Provider and Staff Development and Career Opportunities. An annual dollar amount should be budgeted for off-site training and continuing education. Leave policies must reinforce this commitment.

PROVIDER AND EMPLOYEE SATISFACTION

How are employee and practitioner satisfaction addressed? How are health and healing fostered among staff? To what degree can the same quality of trust, health, and well-being be achieved with staff as one would like to achieve with clients?

Conduct not only patient satisfaction studies, but employee satisfaction surveys as well. Everyone in the organization must know that he or she is valued and important, from leadership to the people who answer the telephone.

Create a safe, healthful physical environment. Be sensitive to subtle aspects of the environment such as acoustics, temperature, and humidity levels. Noise can be reduced with acoustic panels, fabric, or carpets. Appropriate music or natural sounds (for example, water falling) can enhance the environment. Natural aromas can enhance specific moods or activities. Use natural light whenever possible. When not possible, substitute full-spectrum light filters or bulbs. Select healing colors such as greens and purples for the decor. Develop ergonomically correct work areas, free from hazardous materials.

CONCLUSION

Developing a human resources and staffing function in any health care organization is a complex endeavor. Crafting one that works—and works well for all stakeholders—in an integrative setting requires persistence, replacing self-interest with respect for all people at all levels, and a commitment to continuous improvement of the "human capital" side of the organization. Providers and staff in integrative services have, in the words of author Peter Block, "Chosen service over self." Establishing a human resources plan and forging a culture that supports the values of body, mind, and spirit health care can create a different kind of workplace. While not a total guarantee of success, it provides the common framework that offers sustainability, adds value, and launches prosperity.

18.2   Mind-Body Medicine Programs in Hospital Systems

Adrianne Mohr

At the Institute for Health and Healing of the California Pacific Medical Center, one of the goals is to provide palliative bodywork and psychospiritual support to patients. In order to offer these services at an affordable cost, a program has been developed that draws on the skills of interns training as bodyworkers and massage therapists. This program has proven to be of great benefit to both patients and integrative bodywork interns.

THE RELEVANCE OF STRESS REDUCTION

When patients come into the hospital, they may find the experience overwhelming. They frequently have a very high level of stress on both the physical and emotional level. Physically, their health is in crisis, and typically they are receiving diagnostic procedures, surgery, or other forms of intensive interventions. Emotionally, their daily lives have been disordered by being away from home and in the hospital. The bodywork program is designed to reduce this sense of stress.

The program's role is to create a psychospiritual environment that facilitates healing. However, the objective of the bodyworkers is not to be curative; that is the work of the physicians.

Client services in this program include massage, bodywork, and meditation. The intern may train the patient in meditative practices that can be used independently to help him or her relax during surgery or other procedures, to bring peace of mind, and to promote healing. The patient and intern may choose to sit together in

silent meditation for 5 to 10 minutes. The interns have the luxury of being able to provide patients with extended healing sessions of up to 40 to 45 minutes. (Interns are encouraged to develop an instinctive understanding of how to decrease the stress of their clients.) Each of the practitioners approaches patients differently, in support of the unique psychological and spiritual aspects of the individual patients.

The program also wants to provide a sense of grounding to practitioners. Therefore, the center point of this internship is a meditation practice to enhance and sustain the practitioners' ability to be supportive of their clients. Meditation and other self-sustaining practices such as yoga, T'ai chi, or Qigong provide interns with an awareness of self-renewal and self-healing. Given the extent and intensity of the work, it is vital that they have some form of self-sustainment in place in their lives. Every week, each of the students sees at least 5 patients in addition to his or her private practice of approximately 20 clients. Meditation and other self-nurturing practices enable them to address their own spiritual and emotional needs.

The practice of Mindfulness Meditation has been incorporated into the program, as taught by Jon Kabat-Zinn from the University of Massachusetts. Within the bodywork program, all interns take this course in its entirety. The course is also offered each semester at the hospital as part of the wellness program. Mindfulness meditation is becoming more broadly recognized as a valuable tool for physicians, nurses, and other hospital staff whose jobs entail high stress. Many corporations and human resources departments also provide training in these techniques for staff in high-pressure jobs such as attorneys—evidence that the benefits of this approach are becoming more widely acknowledged.

Adrianne Mohr, CMT, is Coordinator of the Integrative Bodyworks Program of the Institute for Health and Healing, California Pacific Medical Center in San Francisco.

This type of practice is relevant to the needs of many of the professionals and staff in the hospital environment. Frequently, almost all of the primary hospital staff experience situations of high stress, in part as a result of the life-and-death nature of their work. The social workers and discharge planners also deal with frequent crises. The bodyworkers provide support to both patients and staff.

WHAT MAKES SOMEONE A HEALER?

It is possible that being a healer is a gift. Like many other skills, it may be one that can be cultivated and enhanced but that cannot be taught. Consequently, the people hired for the internship are not necessarily classically trained Swedish massage therapists. Many are actually overqualified for the job. Yet their qualifications are not ultimately the basis on which they are selected.

They are chosen based on the sense of who will provide the greatest therapeutic benefit to patients. Among candidates who are equally well trained, it is the sparkle in someone's eye or their core integrity rather than the knowledge of a specific technique that distinguishes one candidate from another. Managers endeavor to intuitively sense those who will be healers in the hospital. These individuals often have extraordinary abilities as listeners. They tend to be very nurturing. There is also a willingness to deal with situations that are very tough, such as the unpleasantness of disease and the challenges of death and dying. This is a different type of practice than one in which the practitioner deals with essentially healthy people. It is a more intense form of service that clearly brings with it great rewards. A kind of enrichment grows out of pairing medicine with the mind-body approach to bodywork.

18.3   Developing the Integrative Team

Lon Hatfield

TEAMWORK

One of the challenging aspects of developing an alternative medicine center is that CAM practitioners are accustomed to independent practice with a great deal of autonomy. Many become very good at what they do, but they lack practice in integrating what they do with the work of

Lon Hatfield, MD, PhD, is a family practice physician and biochemist now specializing in integrative medicine. He is founding medical director of the Healing Arts Center in Colville, Washington, an alternative medicine center with ten practitioners, and also cofounder in 1979 of the nationally recognized Northeast Washington Medical Group, an allopathic medical center, which now has 25 physicians.

others. Practitioners who do well in an organizational environment and are accustomed to being team players are typically trained in biomedicine. These practitioners may not emphasize the creative side of medicine, and they may find it difficult to genuinely change the conceptual frameworks and paradigms that are the basis for their practices.

At this point in time, creating an integrative center means bringing together practitioners who are already trained in different disciplines and enabling them to work collaboratively in a creative, nonthreatening environment. Until integrative medicine becomes codified, the integration will tend to occur through this type of group practice. As CAM becomes more fully integrated into medical training, specialized practitioners may emerge who have in-depth training in both biomedicine and an alternative discipline.

At the Healing Arts Center, a great deal of effort has been made to maximize the cohesion of the team by bringing the right people together. This can be difficult to second-guess. There have been a few practitioners who found they could not integrate both mainstream and alternative perspectives in their thinking. It is important to recognize when there is not a good fit. The center continues to encourage the right blend of people who work well together.

DEVELOPING A KNOWLEDGE BASE IN INTEGRATIVE MEDICINE

There are also people who are conceptually drawn to integrative practice but have not yet developed the knowledge base necessary for genuine integrative practice. That is a challenge for most practitioners because they cannot spend their entire lives training—going to medical school and then chiropractic school or a naturopathic college and on and on. Although there are individuals who have that type of interest and dedication, they are rare and will be highly sought after as the integrative movement contin-ues to grow. An example of this kind of dilemma involves the physicians who want to study acupuncture but only have time for a brief training course. The programs that are available are very good and provide an enhanced understanding of acupuncture, but in a brief several week training course, a practitioner cannot be made a skilled acupuncturist. There is a general tendency to underestimate the depth and breadth of knowledge involved in the substantive alternative disciplines.

Physicians often opt for this approach to acupuncture training because it is a way they can study and continue to do everything else they currently do. Over time, they come to realize that they have only skimmed the surface and that there is an enormous body of information and practice wisdom to be mastered. One of the best ways to learn these skills is by pairing an introductory course with follow-up mentoring. When providers with different skills practice together in an integrative program, working side by side can facilitate more rapid learning. Perhaps an ideal combination would be the use of periodic brief training programs, paired with ongoing mentoring opportunities in the daily clinical environment.

PART V

Regulations

State Law Regulation of the Practice of Medicine: Implications for the Practice of Complementary and Alternative Medicine

Michael H. Cohen

Physicians, health care executives, insurers, and risk managers involved in the delivery of complementary and alternative medicine (CAM) and in referrals to CAM practitioners must understand the implications of the way state law regulates the practice of medicine. In fact, laws governing the practice of medicine also regulate the integration of CAM practices into the mainstream health care system. It is helpful to look at both representative statutes and cases to get a broad overview of these legal rules.

STATE MEDICAL PRACTICE ACTS

Each state has enacted a medical licensing statute (or medical practice act) pursuant to the police power. Although the definitions of "prac-

Michael H. Cohen, JD, MBA, MFA, is Director of Legal Programs at the Center for Alternative Medicine Research and Education, Beth Israel Deaconess Medical Center, and the Harvard Medical School Division for Research and Education in Complementary and Integrative Medical Therapies, and is Lecturer in the Department of Medicine, Harvard Medical School. He received his J.D. from Boalt Hall School of Law, University of California, Berkeley, his M.B.A. from the Haas School of Management, University of California, Berkeley, his M.F.A. from the Iowa Writers' Workshop, University of Iowa, and his B.A. from Columbia University. He is the author of *Complementary and Alternative Medicine: Legal Boundaries and Regulatory Perspectives* (Johns Hopkins University Press, 1998), and *Beyond Complementary Medicine: Legal and Ethical Perspectives on Health and Human Evolution* (University of Michigan Press, 2000).

Source: Cohen, Michael H. *Complementary and Alternative Medicine: Legal Boundaries and Regulatory Perspectives.* pp. 24–38, 56–72. © 1998, The Johns Hopkins University Press. Reprinted with permission of The Johns Hopkins University Press.

tice of medicine" vary by state, all state statutes include a combination of some of the following: (1) diagnosing, preventing, treating, and curing disease; (2) holding oneself out to the public as able to perform the above; (3) intending to receive a gift, fee, or compensation for the above; (4) attaching such titles as "M.D." to one's name; (5) maintaining an office for reception, examination, and treatment; (6) performing surgery; and (7) using, administering, or prescribing drugs or medicinal preparations. The sections below briefly describe some of the permutations.

Diagnosis, Treatment, Prevention, and Cure

All states define the "practice of medicine," in part, by using such words as "diagnosis," "treatment," "prevention," "cure," "advise," and "prescribe." These words are usually used in conjunction with "disease," "injury," "deformity," "mental condition," or "physical condition." For example, New York defines the "practice of medicine" as "diagnosing, treating, operating, or prescribing for any human disease, pain, injury, deformity or physical condition."[1] Similarly, Michigan includes "diagnosis, treatment, prevention, cure, or relieving of a human disease, ailment, defect, complaint or other physical or mental condition, by attendance, advice, device, diagnostic test, or other means."[2] If Michigan's statute is read literally, "relieving . . . a . . . complaint . . . by . . . advice" constitutes practicing medicine. Similarly, under the Arkansas statute, "suggesting . . . any form of . . . healing for the intended palliation" constitutes the "practice of medicine."[3]

Holding Oneself Out to the Public

Most states also include holding oneself out to the public as a medical practitioner in defining the "practice of medicine." Some states describe this as "publicly professing" to assume duties incident to the practice of medicine, such as diagnosing, healing, and treating,[4] or "publicly professing" to be a physician or surgeon.[5] Other states, such as Hawaii, Minnesota, New Mexico, Oregon, Vermont, and Wyoming, also include "advertising" that one is a physician or otherwise authorized to practice medicine in the state.[6]

In Florida, New York, and North Carolina, the courts have included holding oneself out as a physician in the definition of "practicing medicine."[7] In Louisiana, an appellate court has interpreted the medical practice act to mean that "practice of medicine" does not mean actually diagnosing and treating diseases, but rather, holding one's self out to the public as being engaged in the business of diagnosis and treatment.[8] By finding that "holding one's self out to the public" can suffice as "practicing medicine," irrespective of actual diagnosis or treatment, legislatures and courts have further broadened the definition's sweep.

Intending To Receive a Fee, Gift, or Compensation

A number of states define the "practice of medicine" as diagnosing and treating disease "with the intention of receiving compensation, or a fee or gift." In some of these states, the courts have incorporated the requirement of a fee within the definition of the "practice of medicine."[9] By way of comparison, the Hawaii, Louisiana, and Utah statutes specifically state that one can be held to practice medicine irrespective of compensation.[10]

Attaching a Title

In about one half of the states, attaching to one's name one or more of the following constitutes the "practice of medicine": "doctor," "doctor of medicine," "doctor of osteopathy," "physician," "surgeon," "physician and surgeon," "Dr.," "M.D.," "D.O.," or other words or abbreviations to indicate or induce others to believe that one is licensed to practice medicine and engaged in the duties characteristic of the "practice of medicine."

Delaware also includes using the word "healer" in connection with one's name.[11] In Nebraska, Christian Science healing has been held to constitute the "practice of medicine."[12] Ohio, Oklahoma, Oregon, and Vermont include using the word "professor" in connection with the person's name.[13] In Maine and Ohio, the use of any such words or letters is prima facie evidence of intent to represent one's self as engaged in the "practice of medicine or surgery."[14] For example, one is guilty of practicing medicine without a license if one uses "M.D." in a manner that induces a belief that the individual is engaged in medical practice.[15]

Maintaining an Office

In many states, maintaining an office to receive, examine, and treat patients constitutes practicing medicine. In Indiana, maintaining a "place of business for the reception . . . of persons suffering from . . . conditions of the body or mind" suffices.[16] In Texas, maintaining an office to treat people was held to constitute the practice of medicine, whether or not defendant claimed to be a physician or medical practitioner.[17] In Utah, maintaining an office or place of business for the purpose of attempting to "diagnose, treat, correct, advise . . . for any human . . . condition . . . real or imaginary" constitutes practicing medicine.[18]

Performing Surgery

Approximately one half of the states include performing surgery or operation in the definition of practicing medicine. Although the Massachusetts medical practice act does not mention surgery or operation, the Supreme Judicial Court has held that the "practice of medicine in any of its branches" includes the practice of surgery and the art of setting fractured bones.[19] Of the various statutory definitions, performing surgery is the narrowest and most tailored to prohibiting untrained practitioners.

Using, Administering, or Prescribing Drugs

More than one half of the states include the use, administration, or prescription of drugs or medicine in the "practice of medicine." However, only a few define "drug."[20] Indiana, for example, adopts a broad and inclusive definition: "any medicine, compound, or chemical or biological preparation intended for internal or external use of humans, and all substances intended to be used for the diagnosis, cure, mitigation, or prevention of diseases or abnormalities of humans, which are recognized in the latest editions published of the United States pharmacopoeia or national formulary, or otherwise established as a drug or medicine."[21] New Mexico's statute includes not only prescribing any drug or medicine but also "offering or undertaking to give or administer any dangerous drug or medicine for the use of any other person, except as directed by a licensed physician."[22] Such broad definitions of the word "drug" pose problems for nonmedical providers that offer herbal and nutritional therapies as part of professional practice.

Miscellaneous Definitional Provisions

Maryland includes ending a human pregnancy in its definition of the "practice of medicine."[23] Delaware's statute and New York's case law include diagnosing of diseases of any person, including dead persons.[24] Treatments such as manipulation expressly constitute the "practice of medicine" in Arkansas, Maine, and South Carolina.[25] In Hawaii, the practice of medicine includes "hypnotism," as well as "the use of . . . any means or method . . . either tangible or intangible."[26] Although it is relatively unusual for medical practice acts to expressly include such modalities as manipulative therapy and hypnosis

within the definition of "medicine," such broad language reflects the medical profession's view in the late nineteenth century that healing must come from legislatively authorized biomedical practice.

UNAUTHORIZED PROFESSIONAL PRACTICE

The breadth of medical practice acts puts three groups at risk of prosecution for practicing medicine unlawfully. The first consists of providers who lack licensure. State prosecutors can argue that these nonlicensed practitioners are "diagnosing" and "treating" patients under the medical practice acts, and thus are practicing medicine unlawfully.

The second group consists of licensed providers (including physicians) and group practices, insurance companies and managed care organizations who hire or refer patients to providers practicing medicine unlawfully. This group may be liable for aiding and abetting unlicensed medical practice.[27]

The third group consists of licensed providers, such as chiropractors and, in many states, licensed naturopaths, massage therapists, and others, who are deemed to violate their statutory authorized scope of practice by engaging in diagnosis and treatment of disease.*

The Nonlicensed Provider

In some states, modalities such as naturopathy, massage therapy, hypnosis, and energy healing are not specifically addressed by statute, and thus may be viewed as encompassed by the prohibition on unlicensed medical practice. For example, *People v. Amber*[28] involved an acupuncturist indicted for practicing medicine without a license. At the time, New York had no acupuncture licensure. The defendant acupuncturist argued that the statutory prohibition on the

---

*The third group is discussed further in Chapter 4 of *Complementary and Alternative Medicine: Legal Boundaries and Regulatory Perspectives.*

unlicensed "practice of medicine" referred to "Western allopathic medicine," and did not encompass systems such as Chinese acupuncture, which differs in its "philosophy, practice and technique."

The court disagreed, holding that diagnosis constitutes any "sizing up or a comprehending of the physical or mental status of a patient." The court added that whether certain actions constitute the practice of medicine depends on facts, and not on "the name of the procedure, its origins or the legislative lack of clairvoyance." The court stated, "A statute intended to regulate, limit or control the diagnosis and treatment of ailments must necessarily be broad enough to include the gamut of those known, whether or not recognized and even those not yet conjured."

The court emphasized that "the patient seeks treatment, not out of curiosity but only because he is suffering pain . . . [and] can expect the anticipated relief from the healing methodology." In the court's view, even determining "the existence of a disharmony brought about by the disequilibrium of Yin and Yang" constituted a "diagnosis" under the statute. Such a determination required expertise, specifically, "palpating the twelve pulses to read the condition of the twelve organs and thus determine which of the twelve meridians must be used . . . to restore the vital essence of 'ch'i' or vital energy." The court also noted that a practitioner need not use any particular language or mention a specific disease to make a diagnosis under the statute.[29]

Under the court's ruling, any healing modality, present or future, comes within the ambit of medicine, including "[e]very means and method . . . to relieve . . . infirmity." By defining "diagnosis" as any sizing up of a client's condition, including the relative balance of yin and yang, the court includes nutritional, psychological, spiritual, and other nonmedical assessments of health under the statute's rubric.

Stetina v. State[30] involved another nonmedical provider of health care lacking independent licensure. Defendant Stetina was a nutritionist who practiced iridology. Stetina determined from examining the state investigator's eyes that he had, among other things, nutritional and abdominal problems and poor circulation. The defendant recommended that the investigator receive colonic irrigation, mineral water, kelp, amelade, progestine, and more raw food.

Stetina sought to distinguish her conduct, which aimed at helping individuals follow proper nutritional advice, from the medical practice act, which aimed at "protect[ing] people from their own credulity" in medical matters. Stetina argued that medical doctors frequently give inadequate attention to the patient's diet and nutrition, making her work a necessary complement to medical care. Stetina presented an expert witness who agreed with this assessment, as well as two witnesses who testified to their overall physical and mental improvement after a consultation.

The Indiana Court of Appeals upheld the lower court's permanent injunction, forbidding Stetina from practicing medicine without a license. The court observed that the medical practice act was not solely designed to protect patients from their own gullibility and from fraudulent practitioners. Rather, the act intended to protect against "the well-intentioned but unskilled practices of health care professionals, as well as against those well-intentioned and skilled practices which simply exceed the scope of acceptable health care." The court concluded that whether Stetina's services had social and medical value was not susceptible to judicial determination, but required legislative determination.

The lower court's injunction, however, permitted Stetina to engage in "lecturing to or educating members of the public on her view of the value of nutrition or . . . selling products to members of the public." The appellate court agreed that Stetina could "disseminate information concerning the value of good nutrition" and sell nutrition-related products to the public. The line between merely disseminating information on one hand, and making a diagnosis on the other, may be difficult to draw, particularly if the provider suggests specific remedies for particular ailments.

Although providers such as acupuncturists now are licensed in many states, cases such as *Amber* and *Stetina* retain precedential value and express judicial attitudes toward nonlicensed providers. In jurisdictions where acupuncture, naturopathy, massage therapy, hypnosis, energy healing, colon hydrotherapy, and other practices are neither licensed nor specifically prohibited, providers of these services risk prosecution under state medical practice acts. In fact, courts have interpreted the medical practice acts broadly against providers where state legislatures have failed to create separate licensure. The list includes midwives, naturopaths, homeopaths, hypnotherapists, providers of colonic irrigation, nutritionists, and iridologists.[31] In addition, individuals offering ear piercing, tattooing, and massage have been indicted for unlawfully practicing medicine.[32] Courts have justified such broad interpretation of medical practice acts as facilitating the protection and preservation of public health.

Independent Holistic Practice

The broad language of some medical practice acts, and of judicial opinions upholding convictions of nonlicensed practitioners under these laws, expresses biomedical dominance and the conceptual narrowing of professional healing practice to biomedical diagnosis and treatment. Such narrowing is unnecessary. Many lawmakers view diagnosis and treatment as solely within the purview of biomedical doctors simply because biomedical doctors, until recently, succeeded in pushing alternative providers out of professional health care. Others acknowledge that such professional healing practice can exist outside the scope of the definition of "medicine." For example, Massachusetts's medical practice act, enacted in 1894, specifies that the prohibition on unlicensed medical practice does not apply to "clairvoyants or persons practicing hypnotism, magnetic healing, mind cure, massage, Christian science cosmopathic method of healing."[33] Similarly, modern licensing statutes acknowledge that providers from chiropractors

to acupuncturists do engage in sizing up conditions (or diagnosis) and treatment within the providers' training.

For example, various acupuncture licensing statutes permit pulse diagnosis according to traditional Chinese medicine to determine the flow of ch'i along the various meridians. Such diagnostic activities differ from medical diagnosis and treatment. They do not utilize biomedical principles; they rely on the provider's unique training, and purport to address vital energy rather than pathology.[34]

While some medical practice acts are drafted more broadly than others, the case can be made for interpreting these statutes as prohibiting the nonlicensed provider only from engaging in *medical* diagnosis and treatment (that is, the diagnosis and treatment of pathology). In other words, the prohibition is against furnishing or purporting to furnish disease care within the biomedical model, but not wellness care within the holistic healing model. For example, somatic (body awareness) practice provided by an Alexander technique instructor seeks not to repair the client's broken arm, but to increase the flow of vital energy through the arm by teaching the client awareness of breath, posture, and movement.[35] Similarly, a client with asthma may see a nonlicensed hypnotherapist to increase awareness of imbalance and tension associated with breathing.[36] Such services constitute treatment only in the sense that any intervention ultimately affects healing. In this view, lay naturopaths, homeopaths, iridologists, nutritionists, energy healers, and other providers are not criminally liable under medical practice acts because they are not practicing *biomedicine*.[37]

This view is consistent with the maxim that courts should construe criminal statutes narrowly. It respects biomedical licensure within a larger universe of holistic health care[38] and is consistent both with nondiscrimination clauses[39] and with the modern resurgence of holistic practice, as expressed in contemporary licensure of holistic providers. Moreover, such interpretation accords with the policy goal of protecting patients from nonmedical providers who purport to cure a pathological condition using biomedical methodologies.

Further, healers, nutritionists, iridologists, reflexologists, lay homeopaths, and others frequently practice in states without professional licensure. Yoga and meditation teachers, Feldenkrais and Alexander instructors and other somatic practitioners, health food store proprietors, purveyors of nutritional supplements, and others routinely offer suggestions about client wellness that could, in the broad view of diagnosis and treatment articulated in *Amber*, be viewed as unlicensed medical practice. The view that independent holistic practice does not violate medical practice acts finds expression in the fact that such nonlicensed providers generally remain free from prosecutorial attention.[40]

Finally, interpreting medical practice narrowly is consistent with the carve-out in *Stetina* for dissemination of nutritional information. This suggests a potential delineation between furnishing information, products, and/or services to encourage health (by nourishing, stimulating, and balancing vital energy) and purporting to cure disease (biomedical practice).[41]

A Texas statute similarly protects dissemination of information for self-care, by providing that nothing in its medical practice act "shall be construed to prohibit or discourage any person from providing or seeking advice or information pertaining to that person's own self-treatment or self-care, nor . . . to prohibit the dissemination of information pertaining to self-care."[42] The statute clarifies that it "confers no authority to practice medicine,"[43] thus distinguishing dissemination of advice or information relating to self-care from diagnosing and treating pathology. Lay homeopaths, herbalists, and others have offered professional services under the protection of this statute, without violating the state's medical practice act. Such legal protection may become a future model for healing professionals who presently remain without licensure.

REFERENCES

1. New York Educ. L. § 6521.

2. Mich. Comp. Laws Ann. § 333.17001(d).

3. Ark. Code Ann. § 17-93-202(2)(B).

4. See Ill. Ann. Stat. ch. 111, para. 4459; Iowa Code Ann. § 148.1; Kan. Stat. Ann. § 65-2869; Neb. Rev. Stat. § 71-1,102; N.C. Gen. Stat. § 90-18; R.I. Gen. Laws § 5-37-1(i); S.C. Code Ann. § 40-47-40; Tenn. Code Ann. § 63-6-204.

5. See Iowa Code Ann. § 148.1; Neb. Rev. Stat. § 71-1,102; Kan. Stat. Ann. § 65-2869; S.D. Codified Laws Ann. § 36-4-9; Tex. Rev. Civ. Stat. Ann. art. 4510a.

6. Haw. Rev. Stat. Ann. § 453-2; Minn. Stat. Ann. § 147.081; N.M. Stat. Ann. § 61-6-6; Or. Rev. Stat. Ann. § 677.085; Vt. Stat. Ann. tit. 26, § 1311; Wyo. Stat. § 33-26-102(a)(x)(A).

7. Reams v. State, 279 So.2d 839 (Fla. 1973) (providing that defendant was deemed to be practicing medicine if he held himself out as being able to diagnose disease or physical conditions); People v. Mastromarino, 265 N.Y.S. 864, 864-5 (N.Y. Sup. Ct. 1933) (holding that one who held himself out as being able and offered to diagnose, treat, operate or prescribe for any human disease, practiced medicine within meaning of Section 6521); State v. Nelson, 317 S.E.2d 711, 714 (N.C. App. 1984) (finding intent of statute to protect public against those who would hold themselves out as medical doctors).

8. Louisiana State Bd. of Med. Examiners v. Craft, 93 So.2d 298, 300-01 (La. Ct. App. 1957).

9. See State v. Ghadiali, 175 A. 315, 318 (Del. Gen. Sess. 1933) (holding defendant guilty of practicing medicine where he recommended the use of an appliance to cure an ailment with the intention of receiving, either directly or indirectly, money or some other form of compensation); *Nelson*, 317 S.E.2d at 714 (declaring the intent of the statute to protect the public against those who would hold themselves out as medical doctors who would expect compensation in return for those services); State v. Griener, 114 P. 897, 899 (Wash. 1911) (sustaining conviction where defendant diagnosed ailments using vibrator, used manual manipulations, prescribed dietary advice and collected fee); 10 Op. Att'y Gen. 1003 (Wis. 1921) (finding that one who advised, prescribed methods of treatment, diet and exercise and charged substantial sums was practicing medicine and should have procured a certificate to do so).

10. Haw. Rev. Stat. Ann. § 453-2 ("either gratuitously or for compensation"); La. Rev. Stat. Ann. § 1262 (same); Utah Code Ann. § 58-12-28.

11. Del. Code Ann., tit. 24, § 1703.

12. State v. Buswell, 58 N.W. 728 (Neb. 1894).

13. Ohio Rev. Code Ann. § 4731.34; Okla. Stat. Ann. tit. 59, § 492; Or. Rev. Stat. Ann. § 677.085; Vt. Stat. Ann. tit. 26, § 1311.

14. Me. Rev. Stat. Ann. tit. 32, § 3270; Ohio Rev. Code Ann. § 4731.34.

15. State v. Baylor, 439 N.E.2d 461, 462-3 (Ohio App. 1981).

16. Ind. Code Ann. § 25-22.5-1-1.1(a)(2).

17. Black v. State, 216 S.W. 181 (Tx. Crim. App. 1919).

18. Utah Code Ann. § 58-12-28(4)(a).

19. Commonwealth v. Dragon, 132 N.E. 356, 357 (Mass. 1921).

20. See Ind. Code Ann. § 25-22.5-1-1.1; N.C. Gen. Stat. § 90-18; Utah Code Ann. § 58-12-28.

21. Ind. Code Ann. § 25-22.5-1-1.1. Utah defines "drugs or medicine" using similar terminology in Utah Code Ann. § 58-12-28. Oklahoma also uses a similar definition to define "drugs" in Okla. Stat. Ann. tit. 59, § 353.1, but specifically excludes food from the definition.

22. N.M. Stat. Ann. § 61-6-6. The North Carolina Supreme Court has defined "drug" as "any substance used as a medicine or in the composition of medicines for internal or external use" and defined "medicine" as "any substance or preparation used in treating disease." State v. Baker, 48 S.E.2d 61, 66 (N.C. 1948) (holding that patent or proprietary remedies that may be purchased without a prescription constitute drugs).

23. Md. Health Occ. Code Ann. § 14-101(k)(2)(ii) (1991).

24. Del. Code Ann., tit. 24, § 1703(b)(2) (1987); Gross v. Amback, 71 N.Y.2d 859 (1988) (practice of medicine includes performing an autopsy).

25. Ark. Code Ann. § 17-93-202 ("whether by the use of drugs, surgery, manipulation, electricity, or any physical, mechanical, or other means whatsoever"); Me. Rev. Stat. Ann. tit. 32, § 3270 (manipulation); S.C. Code Ann. § 40-47-40(c) ("manipulation, adjustment or method . . . by any therapeutic agent whatsoever").

26. Haw Rev. Stat. § 453-1.

27. Most statutes list aiding and abetting the unlawful practice of medicine as grounds for professional discipline. See, e.g., Ariz. Rev. Stat. § 32-1401(cc) ("[m]aintaining a professional connection with or lending one's name to enhance or continue the activities of an illegal practitioner or medicine"); Col. Rev. Stat. Ann. § 12-36-117(k) ("aiding or abetting, in the practice of medicine, of any person not licensed to practice medicine").

28. 349 N.Y.S. 2d 605 (Sup.Ct. 1973). All quotations below are taken from the *Amber* decision.

29. Thus, the court denied defendant's motion to dismiss the indictment. Id. at 613.

30. 513 N.E.2d 1234 (Ct.App.Ind. 1987). All quotations below are from the *Stetina* opinion.

31. See State v. MountJoy et al., 891 P.2d 376, 384 (Kan. 1995) (midwives, holding that conviction of the unauthorized practice of the healing arts does not require proof of criminal intent); State v. Howard, 337 S.E.2d 598 (Ct.App.N.C. 1985) (naturopaths); Sabastier v. State, 504 So.2d 45 (Dist.Ct.App.Fla. 1987) (homeopaths); People v. Cantor, 18 Cal.Rptr. 363 (Sup.Ct. 1961) (hypnotherapists); Williams v. State of Ala., ex rel. Med. Licensure Commission, 453 So.2d 1051, 1053 (Ala.Civ.App. 1984) (colonic irrigation providers); Stetina v. State ex rel. Med. Licensing Bd. of Indiana, 513 N.E.2d 1234 (Ind.Ct.App. 1987) (nutritionists; iridologists).

32. Hicks v. Ark. State Med. Bd., 537 S.W.2d 794, 796 (Ark. 1976) (ear piercing); State v. Brady, 492 N.E.2d 34 (Ct. App. Ind. 1986) (tattooing); People v. Burroughs, 285 Cal.Rptr. 622 (1991) (massage).

33. Mass. Ann. Laws ch. 112, § 7. Most states exempt healers, practicing in a religious context as part of a recognized spiritual tradition and practice. See, e.g., D.C. Code Ann. § 2—3301.4(d)(1).

34. Cf. Sermchief v. Conzales, 660 S.W.2d 683, 689-90 (Mo. 1983) (reversing conviction of nurses for practicing medicine, citing legislative authorization for the "nursing diagnosis, as opposed to a medical diagnosis," when the nurse "finds or fails to find symptoms described by physicians in standing orders and protocols for the purpose of administering courses of treatment prescribed by the physician in such orders and protocols"); Parma v. Wolff, 635 N.E.2d 76, 78-79 (Ohio Mun.Ct. 1993) (nonlicensed defendant's use of machine to determine imbalances of hips and shoulders did not constitute a chiropractic diagnosis in violating of the chiropractic licensing statute, particularly since defendant told patient: "This is only a preliminary screening, this is not an examination, and that any examination must be done by a licensed chiropractor.").

35. "Somatics is the study of the body: working with the expression, discovery, and mapping of the body's relation to learning, cognition, and emotional and physical well-being." Jocelyn Oliver, *Conscious Evolution Through Somatic Education*, AHP Perspective 8 (Jan./Feb. 1996) (available from the Association for Humanistic Psychology, 45 Franklin Street, Suite 315, San Francisco, CA 94102, 415-864-8850).

36. "Somatic practices enable us to develop a conversation with our body and its systems that results in higher and higher levels of conscious self-regulation. What results is a more conscious body, one which responds easily to positive stimuli and which is easy to rebalance, one in which conscious attention and intention can be felt

to have immediate and dramatic effect on tissue quality and state." Id.

37. At the same time, many certificates offered by holistic providers and schools have no legal value. See Jack Raso, *Alternative Health Education and Pseudocredentialing*, Skeptical Inquirer 39 (July/Aug. 1996).

38. Such an interpretation finds expression in a 1977 settlement involving a criminal case against Dana Ullman, a Berkeley homeopath. Ullman had a practice of contracting with clients to provide information concerning homeopathic remedies for particular conditions. Ullman referred his clients to licensed physicians for the diagnosis and treatment of pathology. The municipal court judge, with the district attorney's consent, dismissed the action provided Ullman agreed to not "engag[e] in the diagnosis and treatment of pathology as prescribed by the charging statute." People v. Ullman, No. 98158, *Settled Statement* (Mun. Ct. Ca. 1977); Katy Butler, *Pioneer Health Care Accord*, San Francisco Chronicle 5 (Mar. 30, 1977).

39. A number of states have provisions prohibiting discrimination against a particular school or system of medicine. For example, California provides that the medical practice act "shall not be construed so as to discriminate against any particular school of medicine or surgery . . . or any other treatment, nor shall it regulate, prohibit, or apply to any kind of treatment by prayer . . . ." Cal. Bus. & Prof. Code § 2063. Similarly, Massachusetts and Rhode Island prohibit construing the medical practice act "to discriminate against any particular school or system of medicine." Mass. Ann. Laws. ch. 112, § 7; R. I. Gen. Laws. § 5-37-14. These statutes arguably prohibit discrimination against independent holistic providers, who are practicing systems of medicine not recognized by biomedicine. The statutes above are broader than Indiana's, which prohibit discrimination against "practitioners of any school of medicine holding unlimited licenses to practice medicine recognized in Indiana." Ind. Code Ann. § 16-22-8-39(c). For an interesting interpretation of Texas's constitutional nondiscrimination provision, see Ex Parte Halsted, 182 S.W.2d 479 (Tex.Ct.Crim.App. 1944) (finding chiropractic statute unconstitutional because it established lower requirements for chiropractor treatment of human disease than required in medical licensure).

40. For a case contrary, and consistent with *Amber*, see State v. Kellogg, 568 P.2d 514 (Idaho 1977) (naturopaths who have not graduated from medical school may not take the medical licensing exam and practice medicine). Curiously, although lay naturopaths may not practice in Idaho, licensed veterinarians are permitted the veterinary practice of "acupuncture, chiropractic, magnetic field therapy, holistic medicine, homeopathy, herbology/naturopathy, massage and physical therapy." Idaho Code § 54-2103.

41. See Heidi Rian, *An Alternative Contractual Approach to Holistic Health Care*, 44 Ohio L.J. 185 (1983) ("When practitioner and client are concerned with maintaining health rather than with treating disease, when the therapy carries a low potential for harm, and when the nature of the agreement and distribution of responsibilities can be made reasonably clear, a contract can protect the interests of both client and practitioners . . . and provide needed flexibility in the developing field of holistic health care.")

42. Tex. Rev. Civ. Stat. art. 4495b(e). The provision is similar to exceptions from medical practice acts for the domestic administration of family remedies. See, e.g., Mass. Ann. Laws. ch. 112, § 7.

43. Id.

CHAPTER 20

Malpractice in Complementary and Alternative Medicine: Practical Implications for Risk Managers

Michael H. Cohen

This chapter defines the application of malpractice law to the use of complementary and alternative medicine (CAM) practices by physicians; reviews potential malpractice defenses and ways in which physicians, medical institutions, risk managers, and insurers might utilize such defenses; and describes legal rules relevant to malpractice lawsuits against CAM providers.

APPLYING MALPRACTICE LAW TO CAM

Malpractice is defined as unskillful practice that fails to conform to a standard of care in the profession, and results in patient injury. If one definition of complementary and alternative medicine suggests treatments not commonly taught in medical education or used in U.S. hospitals, such as chelation therapy, ozone therapy, homeopathy, and nutritional and herbal treatments, then physicians integrating these treatments into conventional care depart from biomedical norms of practice—almost by definition—and thus risk malpractice liability. Moreover, legislatures and courts frequently look to lack of general medical acceptance or lack of Food and Drug Administration (FDA) approval as indicative of failure to follow the standard of care.

In a civil malpractice action, the patient will claim that the applicable conventional care is the standard procedure for the patient's condition, and that providing the CAM treatment falls below the standard of care. The court may be tempted to equate nonstandard care, which involves a different therapeutic choice than generally used for the condition in question (for example, chelation therapy over bypass surgery), with substandard care, which falls below the standard in the community and constitutes malpractice. Even if significant scientific evidence exists to show that the CAM therapy has efficacy or results in positive outcomes for patients, courts may view the very selection of a nonstandard therapy as failing to meet the requisite level of professional care.[1] For example, at least one state has provided by statute that using chelation therapy to treat arteriosclerosis or any other condition (except heavy metal poisoning) without FDA approval constitutes unprofessional conduct,[2] which in turn can become a basis for a civil malpractice action.

Michael H. Cohen, JD, MBA, MFA, is Director of Legal Programs at the Center for Alternative Medicine Research and Education, Beth Israel Deaconess Medical Center, and the Harvard Medical School Division for Research and Education in Complementary and Integrative Medical Therapies. He is also a Lecturer in the Department of Medicine, Harvard Medical School.

Source: Cohen, Michael H. *Complementary and Alternative Medicine: Legal Boundaries and Regulatory Perspectives.* pp. 24–38, 56–72. © 1998, The Johns Hopkins University Press. Reprinted with permission of The Johns Hopkins University Press.

POTENTIAL DEFENSES AVAILABLE TO PHYSICIANS INTEGRATING CAM THERAPIES INTO CLINICAL PRACTICE

Physicians offering such treatments could benefit from several malpractice defenses that have been applied to conventional medicine.

The Respectable Minority

First, the respectable minority, or "two schools of thought," defense, provides that a physician who undertakes a mode of treatment which a respectable minority within the profession would undertake under similar circumstances does not incur malpractice liability. In other words, physicians may choose between alternative approaches to diagnosis and treatment, so long as the alternative approach is accepted by a respectable minority in the medical community.

The respectable minority defense suggests that use of therapies such as homeopathy, chelation therapy, and nutritional treatment should not be judged as negligent per se, simply because such treatments deviate from the conventional standard of care. However, courts differ as to what constitutes a respectable minority.[3] The question is complicated with CAM, because data as to efficacy currently are found in nontraditional publications or use more subjective research methodologies, both of which could be deemed by a court to indicate lack of "reasonableness" and "prudence." At least in a disciplinary proceeding, one court has found that a physician failed to follow even a respectable minority in the medical profession, in offering metabolic therapy, using laetrile, in conjunction with chemotherapy.[4]

Clinical Innovation

The defense of clinical innovation shields from malpractice liability those physicians who choose innovative therapeutic procedures to help particular patients or alleviate desperate situations.[5] The defense is available so long as the physician has not violated applicable legal rules, such as Institutional Review Board approval, for experimental or research-oriented therapeutic procedures. However, the defense of clinical innovation is limited to innovative therapeutic procedures to help particular patients or alleviate desperate situations, and may not extend to treatments outside the biomedical model or for regular patient populations.

Providers' best defense to malpractice is rigorous research to establish the treatment as part of the standard of care for the condition in question. For example, if chelation therapy became the standard of care for certain cardiac problems, or at least an acceptable treatment modality to assist in the prevention and amelioration of cardiac disease, the physician's malpractice exposure for using chelation therapy would diminish. Similarly, if homeopathic remedies became the first treatment of choice for certain conditions, such as insomnia or anxiety, then suggesting homeopathic medicine rather than prescription medication will fall within the standard of care. In fact, to the extent biomedical education and practice lag behind alternative therapies that improve patient outcomes, utilizing such therapies may be considered to be *above*, rather than below, the standard of care.

As medical schools incorporate complementary and alternative therapies into the curriculum, and as conventional physicians increasingly use CAM or refer patients to providers for complementary care, malpractice standards of care will incorporate various holistic modalities. Physicians will rely on expert testimony to demonstrate that the therapy in question has, in fact, become the standard of care in the community for the disease in question. Paradoxically, this shift will increase the liability of conventional physicians for failure to incorporate CAM modalities. For example, the interesting suggestion has been raised that if prayer is shown to be efficacious in treating disease, a physician will be negligent for failing to pray for the patient (or meditate on the patient's health) as part of standard treatment. Similarly, biomedical physicians who dismiss all alternative therapies as quackery and ignore nonbiomedical options may find themselves liable for malpractice when their patients present information and research that is publicly available (eg, on the Internet) regarding alternatives or holistic complements to their conventional care.

Utilizing the Defense of Assumption of Risk

The doctrine of assumption of risk, by recognizing the patient's responsibility for some treatment choices, also could mitigate malpractice liability for use of CAM. The leading case from which this principle emerges is *Schneider v. Revici*.[6]

The patient, Edith Schneider, learned that a lump was found in her breast, refused a biopsy, and told her physician she would seek a doctor who would treat her nonsurgically. The physician referred her to two general surgeons, each of whom advised her to undergo a biopsy and possibly a partial mastectomy. Mrs. Schneider instead consulted Dr. Emanuel Revici for unconventional treatment.

Mrs. Schneider signed a detailed consent form, acknowledging that Dr. Revici's treatments lacked FDA approval and that no guaranties were being made as to treatment results, and releasing Dr. Revici from liability. Dr. Revici commenced treatment with selenium and dietary restrictions. He also recommended that Mrs. Schneider have the tumor surgically removed. After 14 months, the tumor had increased in size, and cancer had spread to Mrs. Schneider's lymph system and left breast. She finally underwent a bilateral mastectomy elsewhere, followed by 16 months of conventional chemotherapy. She sued Dr. Revici, alleging common law fraud, medical malpractice, and lack of informed consent.

The jury returned a verdict solely on the medical malpractice claim, but found that Mrs. Schneider was 50% comparatively negligent; based on this finding, the jury halved the award. On appeal, the Second Circuit reversed and remanded for a new trial, holding that because express assumption of risk was available as an

affirmative defense to medical malpractice and, if proved, would totally bar Mrs. Schneider's claim, the lower court had erred in refusing to instruct the jury on assumption of risk. The court noted: "[W]e see no reason why a patient should not be allowed to make an informed decision to go outside currently approved medical methods in search of an unconventional treatment. While a patient should be encouraged to exercise care for his own safety, we believe that an informed decision to avoid surgery and conventional chemotherapy is within the patient's right to 'determine what shall be done with his own body.'"[7] The court concluded that there existed sufficient evidence that Mrs. Schneider assumed "the risk of refusing conventional to undergo the Revici method," to allow the jury to consider assumption of risk as a *complete* defense to any malpractice on the part of Dr. Revici.[8]

The *Revici* court also held that evidence as to the effectiveness of Dr. Revici's treatment was improperly excluded by the district judge. The court rejected the plaintiff's argument that the issue in medical malpractice is not treatment effectiveness, "but whether that treatment is a deviation from accepted medical practice in the community."[9] In a later case, *Boyle v. Revici*,[10] the Second Circuit held that the patient's failure to sign a consent form did not preclude the jury from considering the assumption of risk defense. Thus, the jury could consider evidence that the patient "consciously decided not to accept conventional cancer treatment and instead sought Dr. Revici's care, despite known risks of which she was aware."[11]

The court in *Shorter v. Drury*[12] similarly found assumption of risk a significant barrier to malpractice liability. In *Shorter* the patient, a Jehovah's Witness, bled to death after refusing a blood transfusion when a medical procedure perforated her uterus. Shorter had signed a document releasing the hospital "from any responsibility whatsoever for unfavorable reactions or any untoward results due to my refusal to permit the use of blood or its derivatives."[13] The jury found the physician negligent, but reduced damages by 75% based on Shorter's assumption of the risk that she would die from bleeding. The court upheld the release, reasoning that the form did not exculpate the physician from his own negligence, but only from risks created by the patient's refusal to accept blood transfusions.

Both the two *Revici* decisions and *Shorter* frame the patient's decision to pursue unconventional treatment in terms of assumption of risk. This shifts the focus from physician decision making to patient choice. In this way, assumption of risk provides a basis for the patient's right to select unconventional treatment modalities over the objections of the physician or of prevailing medical norms. The doctrine could serve to shield from malpractice liability the physician who, in consultation with the patient, chooses CAM to treat a condition.

Legal rules regarding assumption of risk vary by jurisdiction. Risk managers should investigate the law in their respective jurisdictions regarding the acceptability of assumption of risk as a defense to medical malpractice, and its likely adaptation to therapies involving CAM.*

CAM PROVIDER MALPRACTICE

Professional Standards of Care

A CAM provider is held to a standard of care appropriate to the profession. For instance, in a malpractice action against a licensed chiropractor, the plaintiff has the burden of proving "the degree of knowledge and skill possessed or the degree of care ordinarily exercised" by practicing chiropractors in similar communities and under similar circumstances.[14] Thus, a chiropractor is held to a chiropractic standard of care, a naturopath to the standard of care of the naturopathic profession, an acupuncturist to the same standard as other acupuncturists, and so on.

Typically, reference to the individual profession's standard of care to evaluate malpractice

---

*This point is discussed further in Chapters 2, 4, and 5. Michael H. Cohen's *Beyond Complementary Medicine: Legal and Ethical Perspectives on Health Care and Human Evolution* (University of Michigan Press, 2000).

is a matter of common law. In some states, the legislature provides a statutory definition for the standard of care to be applied. For example, Nevada defines homeopathic malpractice as "failure on the part of a homeopathic physician to exercise the degree of care, diligence and skill ordinarily exercised by homeopathic physicians in good standing in the community in which he practices."[15]

It is often difficult to determine exactly what protocols or procedures are within the standard of care for CAM. Standards of care are more diffuse and fluid than in biomedicine because holistic treatments involve widely varying schools of thought, treatment philosophies, and techniques, and offer highly individualized or nonstandardized treatments. Many treatments, such as massage therapy, draw on the provider's intuitive or subjective faculties rather than on uniform, professionally prescribed practices.

Despite the less formalized agreement around standards of care, some professions have established guidelines for practice which could serve as the basis for standards of care in malpractice actions. For example, the American Association of Naturopathic Physicians has issued guidelines of naturopathic medical practice to provide general criteria for practice.[16] The guidelines list a range of therapeutics from which a naturopathic physician may choose, consistent with the legislatively authorized scope of practice in the naturopath's particular state. The therapeutics include acupuncture, homeopathy, natural childbirth, massage therapy, and other therapies. Among other things, the naturopathic physician is obligated to keep up with changes in professional practice, to make appropriate referrals, to conform with the professional code of ethics, to take thorough histories, to keep clear records, and to take appropriate physical and mental exams. The guidelines establish criteria for patient diagnosis using conventional and other diagnostic methods (such as those of Ayurvedic and Oriental medicine).

Similar professional standards exist in the chiropractic profession.[17] Both chiropractic practice and naturopathy are less removed in theory and practice from the biomedical model than therapies such as acupuncture, which has even less formalized consensus around standards of care. Nonetheless, even in acupuncture, the National Commission for the Certification of Acupuncturists (NCCA), with assistance from the Centers for Disease Control and Prevention, has developed procedures such as the Clean Needle Technique (CNT) as part of its national certification program. The purpose of CNT is to ensure that patients receive safe and sterile needles. The NCCA National Board Examination requires that applicants demonstrate adequate knowledge of CNT to maintain safe clinical procedures. Thus, although the acupuncture community has not established written guidelines setting forth standards of care for the profession, most courts probably would view CNT as part of the standard of care because the community as a whole accepts CNT as a common baseline for safe clinical practice. A patient injured through unsterilized or contaminated acupuncture needles likely will succeed in a malpractice claim if the patient proves that the acupuncturist violated CNT.

Acupuncturists currently lack the consensus necessary to develop many formal standards of care. Because acupuncturists treat imbalance and ch'i, rather than conditions or diseases, they do not rely on standardized treatments for treating particular ailments. Individual acupuncturists may treat colitis or anxiety differently, for example, varying the number of sessions, the placement of acupuncture needles, and the way in which herbal or other Oriental treatment will be used. Standards of care may vary from school to school, community to community, or even among acupuncturists within the same school or community.

There is little case law on malpractice claims against alternative providers, not only because standards of care are so diffuse,[18] but also because patient expectations are different than with biomedical doctors. Naturopaths, chiropractors, acupuncturists, massage therapists and other providers on the whole render individualized and personalized health services, leading to a lower incidence of malpractice litigation.[19] Holistic

providers take detailed physical and emotional histories and thus tend to spend more personal time with patients or have more emotional contact with them.[20] Providers have patients take responsibility for supporting the healing process through appropriate nutrition, exercise and movement, meditation/breathing/stress reduction, lifestyle changes, counseling, and emotional nourishment, and thus reduce malpractice exposure by structuring the provider-patient relationship as a collaborative venture to health. Providers offer treatments, such as acupuncture, that carry risks that are low and can easily be managed (for example, learning to maintain patient safety through proper needling technique).[21] On the whole, claims rates against CAM providers are far lower than for physicians.[22]

Heightened Standard of Care

Whereas ordinarily, physicians may not testify against a nonmedical provider regarding the provider's professional standard of care, such testimony is permitted where there is an overlap in an area of knowledge or treatment.[23] Thus, when an overlap exists between the holistic provider's expertise and training and that of the biomedical provider, the holistic provider may be held to a heightened or biomedical standard of care, rather than a standard of care appropriate to the provider's profession. For example, where chiropractors, pursuant to their legislative authorization, ordinarily take x-rays, conduct urine analysis, take or order blood and other routine laboratory tests, or perform physical examinations, failure to perform the enumerated procedure may be judged against a biomedical standard of care, and constitute malpractice.[24] Similarly, if a chiropractor purports to use spinal manipulation to cure the patient's diabetes, the chiropractor will be held to a biomedical standard of care; the jury will judge the chiropractor's conduct against that of a reasonable biomedical doctor under similar circumstances.[25]

As CAM providers' legislatively authorized scope of practice expands to include additional areas within biomedical practice, providers may face increased, expanded, or heightened malpractice liability. Recently, for example, Oregon has permitted acupuncturists the right to use Western diagnostic tests.[26] Once authorized to take x-rays, the acupuncturist who fails to do so, instead preferring to rely on diagnostic techniques of Oriental medicine (such as pulse and tongue diagnosis), may have violated the standard of care. Acupuncturists who feel Western tests "have no place in Oriental medicine" will be held liable for failing to order such tests, and will be forced to order Western tests "defensively which is the very behavior for which we criticize our Western practitioner cousins."[27] The same applies to providers such as chiropractors whose legislative authority includes taking x-rays, conducting physical exams, and other functions within the biomedical model.

Duty To Refer and Misrepresentation

CAM providers are vulnerable to malpractice actions when they assume too much responsibility for the patient's biomedical condition and fail to refer the patient to an appropriate conventional professional. The duty in fact is necessary to prevent patients from overrelying on nonmedical providers, when they need biomedical attention. The duty to refer facilitates safe integration of holistic healing modalities with biomedicine since, like scope of practice boundaries, it forces nonphysicians to recognize the limits of their skill and training.

For example, in chiropractic care, courts impose a duty of reasonable care in the analysis and treatment of patients which includes the duty to (1) determine whether the patient presents a problem treatable through chiropractic, (2) refrain from further chiropractic treatment when a reasonable chiropractor should be aware that the patient's condition will not be responsive to further treatment, and (3) if the problem is outside the chiropractor's skill, training, and expertise, inform the patient that the condition is not treatable through chiropractic.[28] In some states, this entails a duty to refer the patient to biomedical care when the condition is not amenable to chiropractic treatment.[29]

A chiropractor who negligently fails to inform the patient that the condition is not one amenable to chiropractic treatment (or, in some states, to refer the patient in such cases to a medical doctor) has committed malpractice. For example, a chiropractor's negligent failure to inform the patient of a possible herniated disk and to refer the patient to a physician has been held to constitute malpractice.[30] Likewise, a chiropractor who takes an x-ray pursuant to statutory authorization and finds a fracture and fails to refer the case to a medical doctor is liable for malpractice.[31]

In many states, the oath administered to chiropractors by the state licensing board requires referral to medical doctors where the patient's problem exceeds the limits of chiropractic care.[32] Such an oath may be admitted into evidence to show the standard of chiropractic care and violation.[33] The duty to refer also exists, at least by statute, in some form for other providers such as acupuncturists.[34]

In addition to liability for failure to refer, providers are liable for misrepresentation when they make claims exceeding their training and ability. For example, in claiming that chiropractic adjustment can cure diabetes, a chiropractor is liable for misrepresentation as well as malpractice.[35] To show misrepresentation, a plaintiff must introduce evidence of intent to defraud, deceive, and/or misrepresent. Plaintiff may prove the statements were misrepresentation by introducing expert testimony. If the statements made by the provider were "within a generally accepted view of the science" of the relevant modality, then there is no misrepresentation.[36] On the other hand, if the professional community does not accept the view espoused by the provider, then the provider may be liable for misrepresentation. Making clear statements about practice parameters and referring patients to biomedical care where necessary not only minimizes liability, but also maintains boundaries appropriate to the professional care in question.

MALPRACTICE LIABILITY IN MANAGED CARE ORGANIZATIONS

Health care institutions, including hospitals, nursing homes, clinics, and managed care organizations (MCOs), face at least two kinds of malpractice exposure when utilizing CAM treatments: (1) direct liability (for an act or omission of the organization) and (2) vicarious liability (for an act or omission of the provider).[37]

Under the doctrine of corporate negligence, courts can impose direct liability on MCOs that negligently hire or negligently supervise health care professionals. The landmark case is *Darling v. Charlston Community Memorial Hospital*.[38] The plaintiff had broken his leg in a college football game. Negligent care in the emergency room resulted in amputation of the leg. The Supreme Court of Illinois held the hospital liable for failure to take due care in selecting and supervising the negligent treatment offered by its medical staff.

Similarly, in *Thompson v. The Nason Hospital*,[39] the Pennsylvania Supreme Court held that a hospital owes the patient a nondelegable duty to ensure the patient's safety and well-being at the hospital, a duty the court classified into four general areas: (1) a duty to use reasonable care in the maintenance of safe and adequate facilities and equipment; (2) a duty to select and retain only competent physicians; (3) a duty to oversee all persons who practice medicine within its walls; and (4) a duty to formulate, adopt, and enforce adequate rules and policies to ensure quality care.

Ideally, CAM providers linked to health care institutions should have levels of training, skill, and professionalism commensurate with that of peers practicing within the biomedical model. Professional organizations can mitigate health care institutions' liability concerns by developing programs and criteria to ensure high standards in provider credentialing and care. Conversely, health care institutions that have CAM providers on staff, contractually engaged or within a referral network, can mitigate the risk of direct liability by ensuring that such health care providers are properly licensed, certified, or registered and have achieved the highest level of professional certification available. Health care institutions further should keep accurate records of the selection and review process for such providers and should investigate whether the selected provider has a history of being sanctioned or liable for negligent practice.

Further, health care institutions can attempt to meet their duty to nonnegligently retain and supervise individual providers through periodic review and monitoring of CAM providers, and internal risk management programs. The institutions also must ensure that providers are delivering services within their legally authorized scope of practice. For instance, massage therapists should not be engaged in spinal manipulation, and chiropractors (absent specific legislative authorization) should not be recommending homeopathic remedies. Institutions need to develop recognized protocols for collaborative practice between providers and to clarify providers' specific roles within such collaborative or integrated health care. Due care further requires peer review of services and practices and utilization review, to ensure that CAM services are appropriate, cost-effective, and beneficial to patients.

Even if health care institutions manage to avoid direct liability, they must address the risk of vicarious liability for the negligent acts of CAM providers within their domain. The doctrine of vicarious liability (or respondeat superior) considers individual providers to be agents of the health care institution rather than independent contractors. In vicarious liability, negligent acts of the agent are attributable to, and considered to be acts of, the principal. Courts frequently support the imposition of vicarious liability by finding "ostensible agency" or "apparent authority," in which the organization's structure gives the appearance that the provider is an agent of the institution.[40] Ostensible agency purports to protect the patient's expectation that the organization is responsible for the injurious conduct.

The ostensible agency theory has eroded the defense that individual physicians are independent contractors, rather than agents of the health care institution. The independent contractor defense is most likely to succeed where the patient directly contracts with the health care provider for a specific treatment, and the provider arranges for admission to a particular hospital, if necessary. Independent contractors usually are responsible for their own income tax and method of receiving payment from patients, own their instrumentalities of practice, make their own clinical judgments, and do not submit such judgments to the medical authority of supervisors in the clinic.

Conversely, the independent contractor defense will likely fail, irrespective of any contractual provision between institution and health care provider disclaiming responsibility for the provider's negligence, when the institution, among other things, exercises control over providers through rules relating to staff privileges, requires providers to meet institutional quality of care standards, requires consultation with appropriate staff physicians where appropriate, has exclusive control of patient billing and fees, and provides clerical and medical support personnel, as well as instruments and supplies, to providers at no cost.

However, if a health care institution loosens its supervisory control over its providers to reduce the risk of vicarious liability, the organization also increases the risk of direct liability for the negligent acts of its providers. Further, the institution may be liable to patients under additional theories such as breach of contract for failure to deliver the level of care promised in its agreement. Institutions must balance the risks of direct and vicarious liability.

Institutions probably will find it advisable to err on the side of greater control, supervision, and standards, as the legal rules governing malpractice liability for CAM providers and treatments continue to unfold.

REFERENCES

1. An unpublished opinion upheld a jury verdict for the defendant doctor in a malpractice case, where plaintiff alleged that seizures were due to chelation treatment, defendant's expert testified there was no relation between treatment and seizures, and there was no evidence that defendant used fraud or deception in prescribing the chelation treatment or adversely affected the public interest. Ireland v. Eckerly, 1989 Minn. App. LEXIS 13, *3.

2. Ariz. Rev. Stat. § 32-1401(gg)(iii). The medical board's charge of unprofessional conduct then may be a basis for the patient's civil malpractice action.

3. See, e.g., Chumbler v. McClure, 505 F.2d 489 (6th Cir. 1974) (permitting defense where there was a division in medical profession regarding use of drug for treatment of cerebral vascular insufficiency, even though only one neurosurgeon in the community followed the minority school); Downer v. Veilleux, 322 A.2d 82, 87 (Me. 1974) (permitting defense when physicians are "merely electing to pursue one of several recognized courses of treatment"); Henderson v. Heyer-Schulte Corp., 600 S.W.2d 844 (1980) (restating test as "reasonable and prudent" physician test); Hutchinson v. Broadlawns Med. Ctr., 459 N.W.2d 273 (Iowa 1990) (in action for failure to properly diagnose, and issue was whether plaintiff had a localized or generalized infection, defense was inappropriate where there was only one agreed approach to each type of injection); D'Angelis v. Zakuto, 556 A.3d 431, 433 (Pa. 1989) (allowing defense for procedure following school of thought involving a "considerable number of physicians," but disallowing defense where the "symptoms of a disease or the effects of an injury are so well known that a reasonable and competent and skillful physician or surgeon ought to be able to diagnose the disease or injury").

4. Clark v. Dep't of Prof. Reg., Bd. of Med. Examiners, 463 So.2d 328 (Fla.Dist.Ct.App. 1985).

5. See, e.g., Brook v. St. John's Hickey Mem. Hosp., 380 N.E.2d 72 (Ind. 1978).

6. 817 F.2d 987, 992 (2d Cir. 1987).

7. Id. at 995 (citing Schloendorff v. Society of New York Hospital, 105 N.E. 92, 93 (1914)); see also Maxwell Mehlman, *Fiduciary Contracting: Limitations on Bargaining Between Patients and Health Care Providers,* 51 U. Pitt. L. Rev. 365 (1990).

8. 817 F.2d at 996.

9. Id. at 990.

10. 961 F.2d 1060 (2d. Cir. 1992).

11. Id. at 1063.

12. 695 P.2d 116 (Wash. 1985).

13. Id. at 119.

14. Louisiana Rev. Stat. § 9:2794 (quoted in Piazza v. Behrman Chiropractic Clinic, 601 So.2d 1378, 1379 (La. 1992)).

15. Nev. Stat. § 630A.060.

16. These are available from the AANP, 2366 Eastlake Avenue East, Suite 322, Seattle, Washington 98102 (206-328-8510).

17. See, e.g., *Oregon Chiropractic Practice and Utilization Guidelines* (available from the Oregon Board of Chiropractic Examiners) [hereinafter "*Chiropractic Practice Guidelines*"].

18. One court has declined to include as part of the standard of care the standard within a particular *school* of chiropractic. Kerman v. Hintz, 406 N.W.2d 156, 161 n. 8 (Ct.App. Wisc. 1987).

19. For example, in Virginia, chiropractors had .5 percent incidence of malpractice, as compared to 19 percent for hospitals and MCOs, 11 percent for obstetrics and gynecology, 8 percent for internal medicine, 6 percent for nursing, and 5 percent for dentistry. See *Judiciary Year in Review* (Virginia 1995). Less than one percent of naturopathic physicians nationwide have been sued for malpractice, according to the American Association of Naturopathic Physicians, *Safety, Effectiveness, and Cost Effectiveness in Naturopathic Medicine* 5 (1991) (citing insurance company data).

20. Alan Dumoff, *Including Alternative Providers in Managed Care—Managing the Malpractice Risk: Part 2*, Medical Interface 127 (June 1995).

21. *Response to Arizona Sunrise Committee*, in Mitchell BM, *Legislative Handbook*, at 47, 49. Most lawsuits stem from failure of acupuncture to cure (breach of warranty rather than malpractice). Id. (Letter from insurance carrier).

22. Studdert DM, Eisenberg MD, Miller FH, Curto DA, Kaptchuk TJ, Brennan TA. Medical malpractice implications of alternative medicine. *JAMA.* 1998;280:18; 1610–1615.

23. See Susan M. Hobson, *The Standard of Admissibility of a Physician's Expert Testimony in a Chiropractic Malpractice Action*, 64 Ind. L.J. 737, 741-2 (1989) (citing cases). In addition, even where prohibited from testifying regarding the chiropractic standard of care, a physician may testify as to the *cause* of an injury (for example, that a ruptured disc was caused by chiropractic manipulation). Morgan v. Hill, 663 S.W.2d 232 (Ct. App. Ky. 1984).

24. Cf. Salazar v. Ehmann, 505 P.2d 387, 389 (Colo. Ct. App. 1972) (chiropractor's failure to take x-rays may constitute chiropractic malpractice).

25. Wengel v. Herfert, 473 N.W.2d 741, 744 (Mich. Ct. App. 1991).

26. See Paul Rosen, *Issues Surrounding Primary Care Status and Incorporation of Western Modalities*, in *Acupuncture Laws*, at 133, 133 [hereinafter "Rosen, *Issues*"]. See also Or. Rev. Stat. §§ 677.757(1)(b)(A) (authorizing acupuncturists to engage in "[t]raditional and modern techniques of diagnosis") and 677.762(3) (providing that legislation does not prohibit dispensing vitamins or minerals or dietary advice).

27. Rosen, *Issues*, at 134.

28. Kerman v. Hintz, 418 N.W.2d 795, 802-03 (Wis. 1988).

29. See, e.g., Mostrom v. Pettibon, 607 P.2d 864 (Wash. App. Ct. 1980).

30. Tschirhart v. Pethel, 233 N.W.2d 93, 94 (Mich. Ct. App. 1975).

31. Id.

32. Salazar v. Ehmann, 505 P.2d 387, 389 (Colo. Ct. App. 1972).

33. Id.

34. See, e.g., Minn. Stat. § 147B.06.1(a) (before treating a patient, the acupuncturist must ask whether the patient has been examined by a licensed physician and must review the diagnosis); Rev. Code Wash. § 18.060.140 (requiring every licensed acupuncturist to develop a written plan for consultation, emergency transfer, and referral to other providers).

35. Wengel v. Herfert, 473 N.W.2d 741, 744 (Mich. Ct. App. 1991).

36. Id.

37. See generally Diana Bearden & Bryan Maedgen, *Emerging Theories of Liability in the Managed Health Care Industry*, 47 Baylor L. Rev. 285 (1995).

38. 211 N.E.2d 253 (1965).

39. 591 A.2d 703 (1991).

40. See Boyd v. Albert Einstein Med. Center, 547 A.2d 1229 (Pa. Superior Ct. 1988); McClellan v. Health Maint. Org. of Penn., 604 A.2d 1053 (Pa. Superior Ct. 1992).

CHAPTER 21

The Role of Informed Consent in the Delivery of Complementary and Alternative Medical Therapies

Michael H. Cohen

This chapter evaluates physicians' legal obligation to disclose the availability of complementary and alternative medicine (CAM) modalities in clinical practice. The chapter specifically addresses when and what physicians must disclose to their patients regarding therapeutic options involving CAM.

THE REQUIREMENT OF INFORMED CONSENT

Informed consent presents one of the major unresolved areas in the integration of CAM therapies into the health care system.[1] Legal requirements of informed consent aim to protect the patient against nonconsensual interference with his or her body in medical matters. Informed consent requires the physician to disclose and ensure that patients (or authorized surrogates) comprehend all information material to the patient's decision to undergo or reject a specific medical procedure.[2] Inclusion of CAM in any

Michael H. Cohen, JD, MBA, MFA, is Director of Legal Programs at the Center for Alternative Medicine Research and Education, Beth Israel Deaconess Medical Center, and the Harvard Medical School Division for Research and Education in Complementary and Integrative Medical Therapies. He is also a Lecturer in the Department of Medicine, Harvard Medical School.

Source: Cohen, Michael H. *Complementary and Alternative Medicine: Legal Boundaries and Regulatory Perspective.* pp. 24–38, 56–72. © 1998, The Johns Hopkins University Press. Reprinted with permission of The Johns Hopkins University Press, and *Beyond Complementary Medicine: Legal and Ethical Perspectives on Health Care and Human Evolution,* © 2000, University of Michigan Press.

such requirement is likely to have a significant impact on clinical practice.

In attempting to determine whether and when such an obligation exists—or should exist, this chapter first examines whether disclosure would be:

1. consistent with informed consent ideals generally
2. appropriate for paradigmatically foreign therapies
3. of benefit to the physician-patient relationship.

This chapter then analyzes cases framing disclosure.

Disclosure and Informed Consent Ideals

To satisfy informed consent, physicians must disclose the nature of the problem, the purpose of the proposed treatment, and the probability of its benefits and risks, as well as the probability of benefits and risks of alternative treatments or doing nothing.[3] Whether such disclosure must, or should, encompass CAM modalities has not yet been addressed in the literature. The question of appropriate disclosure becomes especially troubling where treatments are supported by results of studies published in medical literature, but are not generally accepted or adopted by physicians nationwide.

For example, is a surgeon obligated to advise the patient that there are reports that chiropractic care may be more effective, and less invasive, than surgery for certain cases of low-back pain?[4] Is a gynecologist obligated to inform patients about the possible effect of acupuncture on reduction of pain medication in dysmenorrhea?[5] Should neurologists afford patients the opportunity of taking ginkgo biloba for improving dementia due to circulation problems,[6] and possibly Alzheimer's?[7] To what extent must primary care physicians disclose information about the possible benefits of nutritional therapies, such as treatment of benign prostatic hypertrophy with saw palmetto and other herbal preparations,[8] and treatment of depression with *Hypericum* (St. John's Wort)?[9] Should they inform patients with irritable bowel syndrome that Chinese herbal formulations may in some cases offer improvement in symptoms?[10] Such questions likely will multiply as studies are conducted with increasing rigor by research centers, including those funded by the National Center for Complementary and Alternative Medicine.[11]

The argument against disclosure of the risks and benefits of such therapies stems from the lack of satisfactory scientific evidence and medical consensus to support regular use of such therapies. Since CAM treatments normally fall outside conventional medical education and clinical practice, these treatments by definition are not within the therapeutic armamentarium of the conventional physician, and therefore are unlikely to be considered or raised. Moreover, the physician's promise to "do no harm" militates against giving the patient false hope based on irresponsible or incomplete information. Prevalent also are concerns about presenting therapies with uncertain benefits and unknown risks, creating false expectations, or diverting patients from needed conventional care to inefficacious or dangerous therapies.[12]

Arguments favoring disclosure of such therapies stem primarily from deep respect for patient autonomy interests.[13] The premise of informed consent—that patients have the right to *all* information material to their medical decision making—arises from the notion of bodily integrity: the patient's "right to determine what shall be done with his [or her] own body."[14] One could

argue that this right should transcend majoritarian medical views of certain therapies, and should include the right to receive information about nonconventional therapies that are not fully accepted, yet are supported by a material and credible body of evidence.[15]

It may be relevant in this regard that historically, medicine has expressed opposition or outright hostility toward "irregular" practitioners and nonconventional therapies. It also may be relevant that many of these therapies challenge dominant medical paradigms or methodologies. To demand that such therapies receive general medical acceptance before requiring their inclusion in informed consent disclosure might effectively cut off many patients from access to information about their risks and benefits. To broaden the disclosure obligation, in contrast, would counter the historical medical parochialism toward CAM therapies, and enhance patient access to the information being filtered through their physicians about such therapies.

Consumer demand has led to the recommendation that physicians routinely ask their patients about use of such therapies.[16] This recommendation has included therapies such as imagery and spiritual healing, which are foreign to conventional paradigms, supported largely by anecdotal reports, or not yet amenable to generally accepted methods of validation.[17] Beyond asking what patients use, the above arguments suggest that physicians should initiate discussion of available evidence regarding various therapies. In this way, the informed consent doctrine can offer a potential bridge to integrative care—an arena in which physicians are obligated to satisfy patient demand for information about CAM therapies.[18]

Disclosure of Paradigmatically Foreign Therapies

Assuming informed consent disclosure of CAM becomes appropriate in any given situation, such disclosure may require an evolutionary synthesis in the way physicians discuss the benefits and risks of integrative treatment plans.

One of the trademarks of holistic health care is its emphasis on factors outside biochemical, pharmacological, and other scientifically accessible explanations, and its reliance on different paradigms concerning health and the disease process.[19] Examples include the manipulation of *chi* in acupuncture, and the use of highly diluted homeopathic remedies for constitution and disposition. As noted, informed consent requirements are framed in terms of what a reasonable patient (or, in some jurisdictions, reasonable physician) would find material to a treatment decision. Under conventional scientific methodologies, the therapeutic vagueness of many CAM therapies makes it difficult to determine precisely what risks and benefits require disclosure. For example, although one can describe a series of physical risks involved in using acupuncture needles (eg, the risk of inserting an unsterile needle), as a practical matter, risks relating to such traditional Oriental medicine concepts as altering the flow of *chi* lend themselves less easily to disclosure. Similarly, while homeopaths insist that low dilutions have subtle effects on disease and healing,[20] and that it is disadvantageous to take too many remedies or the wrong remedy, it may be difficult to describe the risks of doing so.

More significantly, it is difficult to conceive what kind of disclosure would be appropriate for a system of health care that has not yet emerged—eg, integrative care, in which homeopathy, acupuncture, and other such modalities are appropriately blended with conventional medical practices. The pharmacological interactions between Western drugs and Chinese or Tibetan herbs, for example, have not been studied—let alone interactions within the paradigm of traditional Oriental medicine. While future studies might quantify some risks in Western medical terms, other risks might have to be expressed in terms of Chinese medicine. Similarly, what kind of comprehensible disclosure is material to a patient's decision to accept acupuncture and hypnotherapy to reduce postoperative pain? Should a physician warn patients not to do yogic headstands following open-heart surgery?[21] What risks are foreseeable and describable?

Such questions suggest that informed consent doctrine may not, at first, find an easy adaptation to therapies that rely on concepts foreign to conventional medicine. In this respect, the informed consent issue differs from situations in which physicians use a therapy approved by the Food and Drug Administration (FDA) for an off-label use, or engage in clinical innovation using conventional modalities. In these situations, physicians at least have the benefit of existing foundational assumptions about the therapies and conventionally accepted uses. Ultimately, integrative health care may require still deeper collaboration between physicians and alternative healers to create comprehensible disclosure, capable of maximizing patient understanding of the therapeutic routes presented, yet also of capturing paradigmatically foreign ideas about disease processes and health management.

Disclosure and the Physician-Patient Relationship

Whether the CAM therapy in question fits within existing medical guidelines or challenges current paradigms, appropriate disclosure of the risks and benefits of such a therapy may serve an additional role, beyond satisfying patient autonomy interests: that of improving the physician-patient relationship. Such disclosure ideally would protect physicians by satisfying patient interest in information, broadening patient choice, and enhancing patient confidence in the physician's knowledge. Such disclosure also may loosen medical intolerance for therapies outside of orthodoxy, increase medical innovation (or at least patient perception of openness), reduce misunderstanding, and thus lower malpractice risk. Indeed, one court has suggested that adequate informed consent could shield a physician from malpractice liability for providing a CAM therapy.[22]

Informed consent has received praise for respecting patient autonomy and equalizing the balance of power in the physician-patient relationship. Yet scholars have urged a shift from the authoritarian, formulaic, and inflexible disclosure of informed consent to a partnership between physician and patient in an atmosphere of conversation and shared exploration.[23] This shift suits CAM's emphasis on patient responsibility for self-care. Such increased responsibility can enhance shared insights into the therapeutic possibilities—and limits—of procedures in each domain of knowledge.

As suggested in surveys of patient usage of CAM therapies, many patients are demanding treatments and modalities beyond the training, education, and therapeutic inclination of many primary care physicians. Patients will continue to challenge extending the boundaries of the therapeutic arsenal, while physicians, faithful to good science, will challenge therapies through conventional knowledge. In the process, informed consent can move further from doctrinal rigidity toward its ideal of dialogue.

PRECEDENTS GOVERNING DISCLOSURE

While no court to date has expressly ruled that a physician must disclose the availability of CAM alongside conventional medical care, existing cases provide ground for the evolution of legal authority in this area. Typically, courts have required disclosure only of less invasive alternatives within conventional medicine. Within these parameters, courts have shown reluctance to expand the limits of what must be disclosed. For example, in *Thornton v. Annest*, a Washington appellate court held that informed consent did not require the physician to disclose the possibility of an x-ray and consultation with a gynecologist as alternatives to removing the patient's fallopian tubes during an exploratory surgery.[24]

Some courts have held nonconventional alternatives to be outside the realm of required disclosure. For example, in *Madsen v. Park Nicollet Medical Center*, the Minnesota Supreme Court held that disclosure of an in-home birth as an alternative to managing pregnancy in the hospi-

tal was not required.[25] Similarly, in *Plumber v. State Dept of Health & Human Resources*, a Louisiana appellate court held that disclosure of cancer treatments alternative to chemotherapy was not required.[26] The court reasoned that in "conventional medical wisdom, the alternative to chemotherapy in this situation would be simply to not undergo chemotherapy."[27] Commentators have criticized such reasoning as being unduly dismissive of the patient's right of bodily self-determination,[28] overly protective of biomedical dominance, and inadequately attentive to patient interests outside a narrow range of orthodox choices.[29]

In *Moore v. Baker*, a patient sued for malpractice based on the physician's failure to disclose the possibility of EDTA chelation therapy as an alleged safer, equally effective alternative to a carotid endarterectomy.[30] The U.S. District Court for Southern District of Georgia held that plaintiff failed to show that reasonably prudent physicians generally recognized and accepted the treatment. The U.S. Court of Appeals for the Eleventh Circuit affirmed, based on a finding that the mainstream medical community did not recognize the claimed alternative in treating coronary blockages.[31] The Eleventh Circuit suggested that it would have decided the case differently had medical education and testimony been more favorable toward the therapy in question.

The Eleventh Circuit in *Moore* did not delineate exactly what would qualify as sufficient validation of a CAM modality to justify required inclusion in informed consent disclosure. One wonders whether one randomized controlled trial would suffice; or whether several studies in nontraditional or foreign medical journals would satisfy the requirement. One strategy is to look to the current tests for informed consent: What kind of disclosure would a reasonable patient (or in some jurisdictions, reasonable physician) find material to a decision to undergo or forgo treatment?

For example, the Ornish program, which incorporates yoga, meditation, and lifestyle changes, is being widely adopted by medical centers and reimbursed by insurance companies for the prevention and treatment of cardiac disease.[32] A cardiologist's failure to disclose the possibility of such a treatment approach, therefore, could conceivably serve as a basis for a malpractice claim when the patient is injured by a conventional therapy that is more invasive or more toxic than such a program. Similarly, some studies have shown that social support could play a meaningful role in recovery from breast cancer and other medical problems.[33] Presumably, this is the kind of information that both a reasonable patient and a reasonable physician would want to see disclosed. Failure to disclose the availability of such therapies (together with potential risks and benefits) could give rise to a malpractice claim based on lack of adequate informed consent—provided that the patient can show causative injury (eg, that the patient would have declined the conventional treatment had he or she received full information about the risks as compared with nonconventional alternatives).

The described expansion in informed consent in no way would substitute for the obligation to disclose and discuss all material treatments available through conventional medicine. A thorough discussion of conventional choices would be necessary as usual. Nor would disclosure of CAM treatments material to patient decision making relieve the physician of liability if the physician induced patient overreliance on the alternative therapy in lieu of necessary conventional care and failed to exercise due care, as a result of which the patient suffered injury or died. Further, even jurisdictions accepting an express assumption of risk defense will tend to look toward a full and fair disclosure of risks and benefits by the physician, and thus to find liability if such disclosure has been incomplete.

To avoid such legal risk, physicians may be tempted in their informed consent disclosure to heighten warnings regarding particular therapies or concerning their use in lieu of conventional treatment. Such warnings might include, for example, the physician's own beliefs about a particular therapy or course of treatment, or the fact that the therapy challenges conventional

scientific models. Presumably, such warnings would reflect available research and change as new information becomes available. Warnings may or may not make sense under prevailing models—for example, the possibility of a "kundalini awakening" or spiritual crisis for patients who are especially sensitive to energy healing may not presently find explanation in contemporary medical and scientific terms.[34]

Whether such heightened warnings make legal and ethical sense in any given situation requires deeper consideration of the balance between autonomy, beneficence, nonmaleficence, and the physician's interest in medical innovation on one hand, and professional integrity and standards on the other. While, as noted, some of the boundaries for informed consent disclosure governing CAM follow the parameters of existing law, others must await more specific unfoldment of integrative care and energy medicine.

CONCLUSION

Informed consent rules to date have failed to address the medical profession's growing exploration of CAM. Yet, as specific therapies garner credible levels of scientific validation, physicians' duty to obtain informed consent will evolve. In light of existing malpractice rules, such disclosure has the potential to manifest increased respect for patient autonomy and the physician-patient relationship, without encouraging inappropriate reliance on, or the forgoing of, appropriate conventional care. Such disclosure thus has the potential to increase clinicians' awareness of possible patient benefit from CAM approaches, and to advance and diversify integrative methods of managing disease and maintaining health.

In sum, although no court yet has articulated a duty to disclose the risks and benefits of CAM therapies as part of the informed consent obligation, such a duty well may arise as well-designed and well-executed trials furnish sufficient evidence of efficacy such that a reasonable patient or reasonable physician would find the information material to a treatment decision.

REFERENCES

1. The need to address these issues has become more urgent with congressional creation of a National Center on Complementary and Alternative Medicine within the National Institutes of Health, S. 2440, sec. 601 (1998) (amending 42 U.S.C. § 281 et seq.), passage of the Dietary Supplement Health and Education Act (which authorizes widespread consumer access to dietary supplements), Pub. L. No. 103-417, 108 Stat. 4325, codified at 21 U.S.C. §§ 301 et seq., introduction of the federal Access to Medical Treatment Act (which would authorize patient access to non-FDA-approved treatments, under certain conditions) S. 578 and H.R. 756 (1997), and state statutes relieving physicians from discipline solely based on using complementary and alternative medicine, The Federation of State Medical Boards, Federation Bulletin: The Journal of Medical Licensure and Discipline. 84;3;1–289,182 (1997).

2. Canterbury v. Spence, 464 F.2d 772 (D.C. Cir. 1972).

3. Barry R. Furrow, Timothy L. Greaney, Sandra H. Johnson, Timothy S. Jost, & Robert L. Schwartz, Health Law 243–247, 268–280 (Minneapolis: West Publishing, 1995).

4. S. Bigos, Acute Low Back Problems in Adults, Clinical Practice Guidelines (Rockville, Maryland: U.S. Dept. of Health and Human Services, Public Health Service, Agency for Health Care Policy and Research), 1994; AHCPR Pub. 95-0643.

5. J. Helms, Acupuncture for the Management of Primary Dysmenorrhea, 69 Obstet. Gynecol. 51–56 (1987).

6. J. Kleijnen & P. Knipschild, Ginkgo Biloba for Cerebral Insufficiency, 34 Br. J. Clin. Pharm. 352–358 (1992).

7. P.L. Le Bars, M.M. Katz, N. Berman, T.M. Itil, A.M. Freedman, & A.F. Schatzberg, A Placebo-Controlled, Double-Blind, Randomized Trial of an Extract of Ginkgo Biloba for Dementia, 278(8) JAMA 1327–1332 (1997).

8. F. Di Silverio, G.P. Flammia, A. Sciarra, M. Caponera, M. Mauro, M. Buscarini, et al., Plant Extracts in BPH, 45 Minerva Urologica e Nefrologica 143–149 (1993).

9. K. Linde, G. Ramirez, C.D. Mulrow, A. Pauls, W. Weidenhammer, D. Melchart, St. John's Wort for Depression—An Overview and Meta-Analysis of Randomized Clinical Trials, 313(7052) Brit. Med. J. 253–258 (1996).

10. A. Bensoussan, N.J. Talley, M. Hing, R. Menzies, A. Guo, and M. Ngu, Treatment of Irritable Bowel Syndrome with Chinese Herbal Medicine: A Randomized Controlled Trial, 280(18) JAMA1585–1589 (1998).

11. Charles Marwick, Alterations Are Ahead at the OAM, 280(18) JAMA 1553–1554 (1998).

12. L.A. Vincler & M.F. Nicol, When Ignorance Isn't Bliss: What Healthcare Practitioners and Facilities Should Know about Complementary and Alternative Medicine, 30(3) J. Health & Hosp. L. 160, 163 (1998).

13. Jay Katz, The Silent World of Doctor and Patient (New York: Free Press, 1994).

14. Schloendorff v. Society of N. Y. Hosp., 105 N.E. 92, 93 (N.Y. 1914).

15. Michael H. Cohen, A Fixed Star in Health Care Reform: The Emerging Paradigm of Holistic Healing, 1:27 Ariz. State L. J. 79, 137–141 (1995).

16. David M. Eisenberg et al., Unconventional Medicine in the United States: Prevalence, Costs, and Patterns of Use, 328:4 N. Engl. J. Med. 256 (1993).

17. Id.

18. While the physician may feel ethically prohibited from providing a therapy he or she personally feels lacks safety or efficacy, the physician also should be alert to potential claims such as patient abandonment or even malpractice if the therapy has efficacy and he or she refuses to provide it. If a physician does choose to provide rather than refer for the therapy, the physician should be aware of any legal rules or professional regulations requiring credentialing or training in the therapy (for example, physician use of acupuncture), statutory and FDA rules governing the use of herbs and other dietary supplements, and any applicable medical board decisions; insurance reimbursement implications also must be considered, as well as legal rules governing health care fraud.

19. Stephen Schwartz, Holistic Health: Seeking a Link between Medicine and Metaphysics, 266(21) JAMA 21 (1991).

20. David Reilly, M.A. Taylor, N.G. Beattie, J.H. Campbell, C. McSharry, T.C. Aitchison, et al., Is Evidence for Homeopathy Reproducible?, 344(8937) Lancet 1601 (1994).

21. J.H. Lin, Evaluating the Alternatives, 279(19) JAMA 706 (1998).

22. Charell v. Gonzales, 660 N.Y.S.2d 665, 668 (S.Ct., N.Y. County, 1997), affirmed and modified to vacate punitive damages award, 673 N.Y.S.2d 685 (App Div., 1st Dept., 1998), reargument denied, appeal denied, 1998 N.Y. App. Div. LEXIS 10711 (App. Div., 1st Dept., 1998), appeal denied, 706 N.E.2d 1211 (1998).

23. Robert M. Veatch, The Patient-Physician Relation: The Patient As Partner (Bloomington: Indiana University Press, 1991).

24. 574 P.2d 1199, 1203 (Wash. Ct. App. 1978).

25. 431 N.W.2d 855, 861 (Minn. 1988).

26. 634 So. 2d 1347, 1351 (La. Ct. App. 1994).

27. Id.

28. Lynn Payer, Medicine and Culture: Varieties of Treatment in the United States, England, West Germany, and France 22 (New York: Henry Holt & Co., 1998).

29. Marjorie Shultz, From Informed Consent to Patient Choice: A New Protected Interest, 95 Yale L. J. 219, 229–233 (1985).

30. 1991 U.S. Dist. LEXIS 14712 (S.D. Ga., Sept. 5, 1991).

31. 989 F.2d 1129, 1132 (11th Cir. 1993).

32. Dean Ornish, L.W. Scherwitz, R.S. Doody, D. Kesten, S.M. McLanahan, S.E. Brown, et al., Effects of Stress Management Training and Dietary Changes in Treating Ischemic Heart Disease, 24(1) JAMA 54 (1983).

33. See David Spiegel, J.R. Bloom, H.C. Kraemer, & E. Gottheil, Effect of Psychosocial Treatment on Survival of Patients with Metastatic Breast Cancer, 2(8668) Lancet 888 (1989).

34. See Christina and Stanislav Grof, The Stormy Search for the Self (Los Angeles: Jeremy P. Tarcher, 1990); Lee Sannella, The Kundalini Experience (Lower Lake, California: Integral Publishing, 1976).

Part **VI**

Clinical Operations

243

CHAPTER 22

Two Perspectives in Complementary Care

22.1 Expanding the Continuum of Care in Medical Practice
Wayne B. Jonas with Nancy Faass
22.2 Integrative Medicine and the Future of Medical Education
Andrew Weil

22.1 Expanding the Continuum of Care in Medical Practice

Wayne B. Jonas with Nancy Faass

DISEASE MANAGEMENT

The primary therapeutics of modern medicine were developed to treat acute conditions. One hundred years ago, infectious disease was one of the primary causes of morbidity and mortality. The other major challenges in medicine were the consequences of trauma and of keeping people alive under those circumstances. We have found very effective ways to treat such conditions and have developed a model of health care that has been extremely successful. That model is now acknowledged all over the world.

One of the consequences of the success of that model is that we are no longer dying from those acute conditions. We were so successful that we have actually shifted the epidemiology of human illness. Consequently, the focus of medicine has also shifted to conditions for which the model has been less successful. As a result of the changes in disease and population characteristics, we now have more people who live for longer periods of time with multiple chronic conditions. The acute care model does not work as well for the management of chronic illness. The treatment of chronic illness involves a fundamentally different perspective. Thus, we must develop new approaches to the types of illnesses that now predominate. It is not that we should abandon the technological model, but rather that we should focus the technologies and range of treatments that we have available to address the majority of conditions now facing our health care system.

Wayne B. Jonas, MD, is an Associate Professor in the Departments of Family Medicine and of Preventive Medicine/Biometrics at the Uniformed Sciences University of the Health Sciences (USUHS) in Bethesda, Maryland, and a family practice physician. He has served as director of the Office of Alternative Medicine at the National Institutes of Health and the director of Medical Research Fellowship at Walter Reed Army Institute of Research. He has also participated as chair of the Program Advisory Council for the NIH office of Alternative Medicine, as director of a WHO Collaborating Center for Traditional Medicine, and as a member of the Cochrane Collaboration. Dr. Jonas has authored more than 60 publications and books, made hundreds of presentations around the world, is on the editorial board of 6 peer-reviewed journals, and is a member of the White House Commission on Complementary Medicine.

This chapter is based on interviews with Dr. Jonas.

We currently have additional resources available that we could apply to the management of chronic disease. In behavioral medicine, we actually know quite a bit about what motivates and discourages people, and we know how to bring about behavioral changes. That is a foundation that we could build into the management of chronic disease. The marketing and advertising industries have done a great deal of research on what actually affects human behavior. We have not yet fully incorporated this knowledge into health care delivery.

We have gained a good sense of the basic elements involved in prevention, but it appears to be fairly difficult for individuals to implement in actuality. Most people tend not to do the healthy things they know they should be doing. Solving this piece of the puzzle seems to have been one of the elements of success for the Ornish programs. These programs use a group support model as a way of helping people stay on track. The group dynamic sustains people through the process of change.

At the present time, there are limitations in our ability to implement Ornish-style programs broadly. One of the reasons that an Ornish program cannot be provided in most health systems is that the resources are not yet in place to offer comprehensive lifestyle interventions. In contemporary medicine, we do have some resources available: For example, we are trained in certain areas of nutrition. However, if I send patients to the nutritionist, they will be covered for only two or three visits. In terms of the exercise component of the program, as a doctor, I can prescribe the services of an exercise therapist to work with my patients and get them started on a therapeutic exercise program. However, at most hospitals, that type of program is not yet available.

In addition, patients need not only a new diet or an exercise program—they also need a better understanding of how to manage their lives in a way that promotes health and stimulates the body to heal itself. They need support to make new habits part of their daily lives in order to maintain the benefits. Although there are support groups available, they are typically not targeted toward the needs of individuals in a lifestyle program. Thus, there is not currently an infrastructure generally in place to support these types of programs on a broad scale.

LIFESTYLE MEDICINE

All of the major alternative systems of healing have lifestyle management as their foundation, including Chinese medicine, Ayurveda, and naturopathic medicine. Each system achieves this in its own unique cultural way, but they all have a focus on lifestyle as the very starting point. They ask, What is this person's life about, and how is his or her lifestyle causing health problems? What can be done to manage lifestyle in a way that promotes health, and how does that management fit into his or her behavior?

These traditional health systems all have components that focus on therapeutic diet, exercise, social support, and spiritual connections. Only on that foundation does the physician add supportive treatment with herbs, acupuncture, or some other form of intervention. The therapies are used against specific, targeted problems in the context of a healthy lifestyle.

Consequently, we are well served by expanding the continuum of our chronic disease management systems to include lifestyle programs and health promotion. If lifestyle interventions are effective in correcting advanced disease states, it is likely that they are also effective in preventing the development of the underlying problem, in many cases. However, prevention is very difficult to measure. If we can collect the data showing that lifestyle programs can make a difference for people who are ill, we will have data that are also likely to apply to prevention. In both populations, the focus is on self-healing and the correction of underlying problems.

EXPANDING THE CONTINUUM

Employers could potentially have a very important motivating role in expanding the continuum of health care to include prevention and wellness. Employers who have the greatest stake in this approach are those who have permanent employees. For companies with a great deal of turnover in staffing, it is less attractive to invest in long-term health. For some of the larger corporations, this approach could be beneficial. To the extent that health affects performance and health care costs, employers may be motivated to explore preventive programs.

The first step in this process is to develop a clear understanding of the model on which chronic disease management must be based and how it is different from the specific cause model on which acute disease management has been so successfully built. We must also initiate more programs that support the development of health. This could include a range of options, such as core lifestyle programs that are offered to everyone with chronic disease. The challenge is to determine how to do this in a cost-efficient way and to engage the stakeholders' and consumers' commitment in the process.

22.2   Integrative Medicine and the Future of Medical Education

Andrew Weil

INTRODUCTION

By rolling back infectious disease, the major killer in the early twentieth century, scientific medicine is left to deal with a more stubborn and costly problem—chronic degenerative disease. The success of medicine has also contributed to the successful aging of the population, and, as the number of elderly citizens increases, so do medical expenses. The "baby boomers," who will soon constitute a gigantic demographic bulge of older people, have not yet reached the ages when their medical costs will skyrocket.

Andrew Weil, MD, is founder and Director of the Program in Integrative Medicine at the University of Arizona School of Medicine. He is a graduate of Harvard Medical School, has worked for the National Institute of Mental Health, and served as a researcher in ethnopharmacology with the Institute of Current World Affairs and the Harvard Botanical Museum. Dr. Weil is author of numerous highly successful books on health and medicine.

Source: Reprinted from *American Journal of Medicine*, Vol. 108, Andrew Weil, The Significance of Integrative Medicine for the Future of Medical Education, pp. 441–443, Copyright 2000 with permission from Excerpta Medica, Inc.

Another reason for the expense of conventional medicine is its extreme dependence on technology. Medical technology is inherently costly, and, unless we change that dependence, there is little hope of cutting costs. Moreover, another powerful economic force impacting medicine is a still-growing consumer movement that is demanding low-tech options for preventing and treating illness. Consumers are very clear about their desire for natural, complementary, and alternative therapies. This is not a passing fad, but rather a worldwide sociocultural trend with deep roots and great economic significance.

THE CHALLENGE OF INTEGRATIVE MEDICINE

What do patients want? They want greater empowerment in medical interactions. Patients want physicians who have time to sit down with them, help them understand the nature of their problems, and will not promote drugs and surgery as the only ways of doing things. They want physicians who are aware of nutritional influences on health and who can answer intelligently questions about the bewildering array of dietary supplements and natural therapeutic agents in health food stores. They want physicians who are sensitive to mind–body interactions and who are willing to look at patients as mental and emotional beings, spiritual entities, and community members, as well as physical bodies. Patients want physicians with whom they can discuss options such as Chinese medicine.

It is possible to teach both patients and practitioners about the strengths and indications of standard medicine without in any way rejecting its real achievements. Alternative medicine is a rich mixture of wisdom and folly. A few alternative therapies are dangerous, more are ineffective, and still more are unproven. However, many conventional practices are also unproven.

The challenge is to sort through all the evidence about all healing systems and to try to extract those ideas and practices that are useful, safe, and cost-effective. Then we must try to merge them into a new, comprehensive system of practice that has an evidence base and that also addresses consumer demands. The most appropriate term for this new system is *integrative medicine*. It is neutral, accurate, and acceptable in academic discourse, and avoids the misleading connotations of alternative medicine (which suggest replacement of the standard system).

EDUCATING PHYSICIANS OF THE FUTURE

At the Program in Integrative Medicine at the University of Arizona, postdoctoral fellows receive didactic instruction in such fields as nutritional medicine, mind/body medicine, lifestyle medicine, and spirituality and medicine. To term these fields *alternative* would be a great mistake. They are relevant to the training of all physicians of the future. The curriculum that we are developing for these didactic modules will be ready to be moved into undergraduate medical education as soon as schools begin to request it. Other foundational courses include the philoso-

phy of science, the art of medicine, and healing-oriented medicine, as well as information about the theory, practice, strengths, and weaknesses of the major alternative therapies.

The fellows also receive practical instruction in such modalities as osteopathic manipulative therapy, traditional Chinese medicine, and guided imagery. The aim here is not to make them experts in other forms of medicine but to train them to know when other approaches may be useful and how to refer patients to them.

Effecting such change will require an initiative by leaders in medical education. Again, there is cause for optimism. First, Congress has now mandated the teaching of integrative medicine, both in postgraduate fellowships and in medical school, and has authorized the director of the National Center for Complementary and Alternative Medicine (NCCAM) to make this a priority. Second, numerous schools are starting programs in integrative medicine and have indicated willingness to participate in conversations about curriculum development.

In July 1999, a consortium of deans and their representatives from schools interested in integrative medicine convened at the Fetzer Institute in Kalamazoo, Michigan. The schools represented were Duke University; Stanford University; University of Arizona; University of California, San Francisco; University of Maryland; University of Massachusetts; and University of Minnesota.

There was a consensus at this historic meeting that integrative medicine is a direction of medicine of the future. In addition, there was further consensus that integrative medicine is not simply about giving physicians alternative or complementary modalities to add to their black bags, but rather is concerned with the transformation of medicine. Aspects of that transformation include the restoration of the centrality of the physician–patient relationship, a realignment of medicine with the natural healing process, and an expanded scientific paradigm. The group affirmed the importance of scientific method and the need for evidence-based treatments. Subcommittees were formed to address issues related to curriculum, research, and clinical practice; and plans were made for future meetings and efforts to bring other schools to the table.

Integrative medicine offers the promise of restoring values that were prominent in medicine of the recent past and also offers the potential for cutting health care costs, improving health, renewing consumer confidence and satisfaction, and reducing the unhappiness of physicians. It can develop in a planned, thoughtful way, consistent with good science and ethics, or it can develop haphazardly and recklessly. Designing a new kind of medical education for the new millennium is an urgent priority.

CHAPTER 23

The Development of Care Management: Systems To Achieve Clinical Integration

Maria Hill

As managed care markets continue to evolve, so too does clinical integration with the development of more tightly knit integrated delivery systems. These systems integrate physician services, administrative and organizational functions across agencies, and health care delivery sites over the continuum of care. With advancing stages of managed care, integrated delivery networks, with affiliated or employed providers, are expected to assume financial and clinical risk. To succeed financially, these networks must operationalize exceptional care management principles and strategies over the continuum of care. The goals for an integrated delivery system are demonstration of the best practice or outcome for a case type or population and coordination of a patient's wellness or illness treatment plan of care, both across all geographic sites as well as over a member's lifetime.

Conrad (1993) identified the following five mechanisms for clinical integration:

1. *information provision* and exchange among providers regarding system and patient care issues
2. *care management strategies* including clinical pathways, integration of clinical and financial information to manage care, and case management systems
3. *common clinical culture* through establishment of a corporate vice president of clinical integration, systemwide per-

formance improvement, and continuous quality improvement processes within a matrix system
4. *common educational programming* for clinicians and patients
5. *payment incentives* for clinical integration through capitation for covered lives and bundled pricing

Capitation reverses the logic of successful performance measures. The shift in mindset is to:

1. Reduce inpatient admissions and lengths of stay (LOS) through micromanagement of each hour of the patient's plan of care against preestablished cost and clinical outcomes.
2. Establish a system for primary health promotion to prevent disease.
3. Create a secondary prevention program with early recognition and detection to prevent long-term illness and disability.
4. Develop a high-risk case management system.

The focus of this chapter is care management strategies, including the operational tools, roles, and systems to establish clinical integration.

REQUIREMENTS FOR CLINICAL INTEGRATION

Care management is a sophisticated, interdependent process that plays a central role in clinical integration. It combines clinical, fiscal, and information science to manage the continuum of

Source: Adapted from M. Hill, The Development of Care Management Systems, *Advanced Practice Nursing Quarterly*, Vol. 4, No. 1, pp. 33–39, © 1998, Aspen Publishers, Inc.

health care to achieve best practice. It represents a system of organizing care that is efficient, effective, and timely. For each case type or patient population, best practice is defined as the achievement of optimal clinical outcomes at the best price, with the highest degree of patient satisfaction (Jacobsen and Hill, 1998).

The four core components integrated within the care management process include:

1. clinical pathway/CareMap tools with a concomitant variance management system
2. collaborative group practices that report to a care center or service and assume accountability for fiscal and clinical outcomes for a defined group of patients
3. case management and other newly developed roles that function in a matrix model within the health system to promote clinical coordination and integration of care for complex patient populations over the continuum
4. a shared, integrated information system with clinical documentation of the plan of care, variance management, monitoring of clinical and cost performance measures across the episode and continuum, and provision of programmatic data management with a decision support capability

A CONCEPTUAL FRAMEWORK FOR CARE MANAGEMENT

The Clinical Pathway System

Because patient care is so complex and variable from patient to patient, practitioner to practitioner, and institution to institution, it can be a challenge to guide the care delivery process. The goal of the CareMap system is to manage care delivered and outcomes achieved through a collaborative care process. The clinical pathway is the central tool used to organize and manage patient care. Pathway use is emerging from the

inpatient setting and being employed in ambulatory, subacute, home, and long-term care settings. Adaptations to the general tool layout and format are being created to reflect the needs of patient care in each of these care environments (Hill, 1997). In this way, care needs across the episode and continuum are captured and used by the multidisciplinary team to guide, document, and manage care delivered and received.

The CareMap is a multidisciplinary plan and record of care designed for a case type/population of patients. The key components of the CareMap/clinical pathway include a timeline, problem list, intervention statements for all disciplines intimately involved with the care delivery process for the identified case type, and affiliated outcome statements. The tool format is flexible to accommodate management of care across the health/illness episode. Pathways are being created as plans of care to promote primary wellness, health maintenance, and disease prevention; to manage inpatient and outpatient procedures; and to coordinate acute care episodes, manage chronic diseases, and oversee terminal care. In each of these settings, the tool is evolving as an integrated document of care delivered and outcomes achieved. Select interventions from preestablished guidelines, protocols, and algorithms are combined and added to the pathway to create a unique hybrid tool.

Clinical Pathway Development

The clinical pathway represents a collaborative effort of its authors: clinicians from the relevant disciplines, departments, and agencies. Successful teams are often cochaired by a physician and team facilitator. The team reviews current care and establishes the timeline (LOS/visits), issues/problem list, clinical and cost outcomes to be achieved, and the essential interventions to be considered for every patient within the population or case type. The team reviews current data from within the system including LOS, cost, practice patterns by individual physician and physician groups, and external data sources for benchmarking. The group evaluates these data, determines the scope of practice for the pathway, develops inclusion and exclusion criteria for patients placed on the tool, and brainstorms system issues that prevent efficient management of patient care.

The components of the pathway are created following a review of:

- population-/case type-specific literature
- practice guidelines and algorithms from appropriate professional societies
- standards of care from each discipline and agency
- clinical pathways from other facilities (including those in the integrated delivery system)
- discussion regarding best practice following chart review in each facility and evaluation of care by the expert clinicians in the group
- LOS, cost-to-charge ratios or cost data, resource use by account profile, emergency department (ED) visits, and readmission rate
- managed case requirements for LOS and cost including Milliman & Robertson (1999) and InterQual criteria (McKesson HBOC, 2000)
- outpatient pharmaceutical data, claims data, immunization rates, and so forth
- national, regional, and local LOS; cost; and quality indicator data

The team is responsible for examining care delivery in a new way. This examination consists of three tasks. The first task is to challenge traditional practice patterns in all settings performed by all disciplines. Are the interventions evidence-based or based on tradition, preference, or convenience? The second task is to anticipate potential complications, while strategizing creative interventions to prevent occurrence. These interventions are to be built into the pathway system and measured to ensure success. An illustration would be to perform a nutritional risk screen on all frail patients admitted with pneumonia to include a diet history, serum albu-

min, and skin turgor test. The third task is to identify the key variance (the subset of variance indicators for the case type or product line) to be tracked and monitored over time.

Establishing Collaborative Practice Groups

Collaboration is the act of working together as an interdisciplinary, interagency team to manage the health of a select group of patients efficiently and effectively. The key factors for team success are commitment to identify and continually improve performance measures; physician participation and leadership from each agency; focused, collaborative communication and patient care management; the ability to interpret, analyze, and act on data; and creative problem solving. Clinical pathway system development creates the need for the clinically expert team to meet on an ongoing basis to develop action plans to analyze and respond to trends in data.

In maturing systems, this team evolves into a collaborative practice group. The charge of this group is to oversee clinical, financial, and administrative management of the patient population. For example, due to community need, a group may come together to develop and promote orthopedic/musculoskeletal programming for older persons. During the subsequent meetings the group may come together to establish focused, measurable annual goals; implement and monitor pathway systems; review, analyze, and act on cost, clinical, functional, and patient satisfaction data; redesign clinical systems to process patient care; update the pathway, as necessary; and determine whether the annual group goals have been met.

Sample goals and performance measures for the joint replacement practice group may include decrease case type cost by 10%, decrease deep-vein thrombosis complication by 5%, achieve 0% readmission rate within 30 days postoperatively, decrease readmission to subacute level of care by 30%, keep patient satisfaction scores stable, and attain statistical improvement in Short Form 36 scores between the presurgical and 1-year postoperative intervention period.

The Significance of Clinical and Fiscal Outcomes

The shift from task to outcomes management is a fundamental component of the pathway system. The clinical outcomes being monitored in all health settings have changed significantly over the past several years. Managed care and capitation financial arrangements have assisted in shifting the focus from the categories of morbidity, mortality, infection rates, fall rates, and medication errors to clinical outcomes. The clinical outcome categories include physiologic, functional, behavioral, knowledge, and self-management skills. The focus is on short, intermediate, and long-term health outcomes. Intermediate goals indicating progress toward outcomes are developed, tracked, and monitored by the collaborative group on an ongoing basis. The goal is for the group to create a balance scorecard in all four performance categories including fiscal, clinical, functional, and patient satisfaction.

Physiologic outcomes include parameters for laboratory values and parameters for vital signs and weight. Examples of functional outcomes are to bathe and dress independently, ambulate 25 feet with an assistive device, prepare meals, and obtain transportation. Behavioral outcomes may include the ability to reach and maintain a target weight, ability to identify and avoid triggers for asthma, and ability to take the dosage of medication prescribed on time. Knowledge or performance outcomes include performing adequate return demonstration of pick line care, obtaining a blood sugar reading on a glucometer, and administering an insulin injection. Self-management skills are demonstrated through the patient's and the family's ability to manage health. Patient and family perceptions of quality and satisfaction with care received are obtained through administration of commercial questionnaires available in written or oral formats.

In the pathway system, these data are managed currently on an individual patient and retrospectively with an aggregate group of patients. The individual patient is managed in the context of a pathway. If the criteria are not met on time,

an alternate plan is established. Aggregate data provide information on the management of a patient population over time. For example, pathways to manage asthma are created and used in the outpatient, home, and inpatient settings. Data elements to be monitored are identified. Sample data collected on asthmatic patients may include number of clinic visits with concomitant current procedure terminology code, incidence of respiratory infections, ED visits, inpatient admissions and LOS, knowledge of asthma triggers, appropriate treatment regimens, and ability to self-manage. This information is then compiled with variance, financial, patient satisfaction, and a health status survey to create performance measures for the case type. These measures are tracked, trended, and analyzed; action plans are drawn up to improve care as necessary; and results are reported by the collaborative practice group to the appropriate central quality committees.

The Definition of Variance and Variance Management

Variances from the clinical pathway are the exceptions or the unexpected events that occur while following this multidisciplinary plan of care. Variances can occur from the problem list, interventions, or outcomes statements. Variances can be positive or negative. Positive variances occur when select interventions are not necessary for a patient or, for example, when a newly diagnosed diabetic patient progresses ahead of the outlined educational schedule. Negative variances occur when an intervention cannot be completed or an outcome is not met within the identified timeline. Negative variance depicts lack of patient progress.

Variance formalizes the evaluation phase of the individual patient plan of care and structures the scientific analysis for the aggregate case type. Variance analysis provides caregivers with a mechanism to study variations in care and to improve continually the care delivery process and outcomes of care realized by patients and families. This system becomes the core of the continuous quality improvement/performance improvement initiative.

To establish a variance management system, the institution must invest the resources and define the individuals responsible for each step in the process, from recording the occurrence to compiling reports and analyzing data. In addition, the variance tracking system must be streamlined. It must focus on data collection for a select subset of variances that the collaboratory practice group believes is imperative to monitor from a cost and a quality perspective. Variance information should be analyzed in quick cycle times (2 to 4 weeks depending on volume), with rapid turnaround and analysis of data. Immediate actions such as clinical practice changes or system redesign based on the results of the data are enacted. Successful teams working with coronary bypass surgical patients are completing this entire cycle within 6 to 8 weeks (Anderson and Henry, 1988).

Integration of Clinical Pathways over the Continuum

Clinical integration of patient care occurs at three levels. The first is at the direct patient level with coordination and integration of care over the health system. The goal is to provide a seamless experience for the patient and family. Smooth transitions from one level of care to another are the expectation. Clinical pathways that cross the episode assist in creating an organized, cohesive, and outcome-oriented plan of care across settings and disciplines. The second level is within the service line or institution. An organizational standard of care is employed and no matter what physician service the patient is admitted to or which group of therapists, nurses, or social workers cares for a group of patients, the care is the same. The third is the integrated delivery system. At this level, a standard of care exists for all entities within the entire health system.

When merging organizations into an integrated system, it is imperative to create an infrastructure that supports pathway development and use at all levels. To be successful, the executive leadership at each agency within the integrated delivery system must support and participate in development and evaluation of these systems. A corporate executive steering committee must be charged with assessing each agency's pathway system and work plan, evaluating program success within each of these agencies, and examining the similarities and differences between the agencies. The committee must then create and oversee the work plan for system-wide implementation. The ultimate committee goal is to create a central, organizing system acknowledging which factors must be standardized across the entire integrated system. Standardized elements may include case type, LOS, critical variance indicators, and clinical outcomes statements. It also involves creating a corporate clinical variance management system through the quality improvement structure with a reporting process, selecting performance measurement staff composed of data analysts and biostatisticians responsible for designing reports, interpreting information for the collaborative practice groups, and suggesting follow-up studies to the practice changes identified (Robertson, 1997).

CASE MANAGEMENT

Case management is a very complex phenomenon. Simply stated, case management is the coordination of services for complex patients and their families. The role of the case manager should be reserved for the case types or cases demonstrating risk for high cost, poor health care outcomes, and poor coordination of services in a complex integrated delivery system. Case management is often confused with care management. Clinical pathway tools and utilization management are used with both care coordination strategies; however, care management is a unit- or setting-based model. All patients require care management, but less than 10% of patients cared for within an integrated system should require case management services. The case manager expedites services across the episode or continuum of care, managing the transitions of care across settings.

Although many models of case management have emerged, coordination of care is the central component of the role. *The key defining characteristics of the role include:*

- coordinating care over an episode or across the health continuum
- ensuring and facilitating the achievement of clinical and cost outcomes
- negotiating, procuring, and coordinating needed services and resources
- intervening at key intervals along the health continuum
- working with a collaborative practice group to address performance measures
- creating opportunities and systems to enhance outcomes

It is essential that the integrated delivery system establish the goals for case management and the details of the case manager role. Management of systemwide clinical and financial risk contributes to the growth of this program and role. To manage risk, the focus of case management programs can be disease/population management at the level of the integrated system (heart failure, asthma, and acquired immunodeficiency syndrome [AIDS]), episodic management for a subset of patients within a specific scope of services (hip fracture, high-risk pregnancy, and coronary artery bypass graft surgery), and site specific within a specified level of care (stroke patients within acute care setting). All three levels of case management may exist within the system. Clarifying and coordinating the differences in roles, role expectations, and outcomes are paramount as the case management program grows in sophistication.

The goal of the case manager within any role in the organization is to be the integrator or manager of care for identified patient outliers. Better managed care is accomplished by timely prediction of the needs of the high-risk patients, early intervention to prevent or decrease the number of acute exacerbations of the condition, proactive prevention of advancement of the disease, and continual surveillance of role performance for the caseload of patients with identified changes in practice and concomitant outcomes achieved.

The case manager role is multidimensional; expert clinical, administrative, managerial, and interpersonal skills are required. *The role of the case manager includes a range of functions:*

- Triage patients into the caseload via screening tools, specified data, and referrals.
- Develop a network of services within which to operate to achieve outcomes.
- Establish a system for care coordination across each geographic location within the episode or continuum of care.
- Establish communication systems with physicians, team members, payers, vendors, patients and families, and community resources.
- Develop a therapeutic, inclusive relationship with patients and families, fostering self-management skills.
- Provide service and benefit coordination and assess and coordinate noncovered services.
- Create methods to track patient care outcomes and cost through the health system.
- Evaluate the impact of case management services on a patient population.
- Discharge patients from the caseload, as appropriate.

Case management is a powerful strategy to manage the care of complex patients and patient populations. To design a successful system, clear, measurable program goals must be established; clear case-level objectives must be outlined; and tools to objectify data must be employed (eg, Barthel Exam, Mini Mental Status Exam, and Living with Heart Failure Questionnaire). Careful scrutiny must be employed when looking for nurses with the skills required for successful case management of a caseload of patients.

The role of the continuum-based case manager requires the highest of skills. The goal is to provide the right care, at the right cost, at the right time, at the right place, and by the right provider. This position requires expert clinical knowledge, well-established professional relationships within a network of services, innovative thinking regarding patient placement, delivery of the same quality of services at the lowest cost for the entire episode of care, and continual demonstration and justification of the cost impact of the case management role. For example, the case manager may perform a case benefit analysis and act on her or his authority to authorize patient referral to a specialist for care, direct nursing home placement from the ED, and pay for uncovered home care services. The aforementioned actions require the authority to act with system savvy, clinical expertise, creativity, and risk-taking behavior; to have a good working relationship with the patient and family; and to demonstrate business acumen.

AUTOMATION

The development of software to automate the clinical pathway and variance management system could rectify the struggles with documentation. Automation allows information to be captured in real time, prevents duplication of effort with variance tracking, and enhances the integrity and accuracy of data. Automation also facilitates retrieval of relevant clinical information for review. Last, automation makes data abstraction across the continuum feasible.

A major component of care management is the management of information. As the institution commits to clinical integration, managing patient information, case management plans, and system performance measures are imperative. Information technology must be in place that gathers, processes, reports, and allows for access of information at all points of care delivery along the continuum. Data must be available at the level of the individual patient, case type, product line, institution, and integrated delivery system. Clinicians are begging for systems that support documentation of the plan over the continuum, clinical decision-making capabilities at the individual and aggregate patient population levels, and data and outcomes management capabilities. Because these technologies are integral to survival as providers take on clinical and financial risk, a strategic information system plan that defines the functional and technologic requirements for support is needed. The ability to create a robust plan is highly dependent on clear articulation of clinically based goals for the information system, analysis of continuum-based reengineering efforts, and knowledge of care management strategies (Jacobsen and Hill, 1998). Once this is accomplished, a group can be identified to create the functional requirements necessary for the hardware and software solutions, develop a request for proposal for submission to the vendors, and embark on a selection process.

CONCLUSION

The essence of clinical integration is the coordination of care of an individual patient and group of patients over time. Successful care management in an environment of increasing clinical and financial risk requires new and better strategies. Clinical pathways, collaborative practice groups, and case management systems provide the tools, roles, and systems necessary to integrate care at the level of the individual patient, the patient population, institution, and integrated delivery system. Continual advancement and evolution of these tools, roles, and systems, along with the marriage of information system strategies, are essential for survival.

REFERENCES

Anderson B, Henry S. Collaborative review of multivariate data to produce rapid change in practice. Paper presented at Third Leadership Conference, Variance from Clinical Paths: Optimizing Care and Cost. Sponsored by The Center for Care Management; January 30, 1988; Atlanta, GA.

Conrad D. Coordinating patient care services in regional health systems: the challenge of clinical integration. *Hospitals Health Serv Adm.* 1993;38(4):491–508.

Hill M. Managing quality through outcome-based practice: CareMaps, case management and variance analysis. In: Meisenheimer CG, ed. *Improving Quality: A Guide to Effective Programs.* Gaithersburg, MD: Aspen Publishers, Inc; 1997.

Jacobsen T, Hill M. Achieving information system support for clinical integration. In: Tonges M, ed. *Clinical Integration: Strategies and Practices for Organized Delivery Systems.* San Francisco: Jossey-Bass; 1998.

McKesson HBOC. InterQual Products. <http://www.interqual.com>.

Milliman & Robertson. Case management: recovery facility care. In: Schibanoff J, ed. *Healthcare Management Guidelines.* Vol 6. Seattle, WA: Milliman & Robertson, Inc; 1999.

Robertson S. North Shore Health System used CareMaps as a clinical integration tool. *Issues Outcomes.* 1997;3(5):1–2.

CHAPTER 24

Clinical Strategies in Integrative Medicine

24.1   A Group Model for the Management of Chronic Illness

Christopher Foley

THE ROLE OF PATIENT EDUCATION

Time is one of the commodities in shortest supply for physicians. Consequently, any strategy that allows us to reproduce our efforts effectively is worthy of consideration. There is need for a style of medicine that transfers the knowledge base with greater reproducibility. Excellent medical practice cannot be based on just the skills, experience, and wisdom of the individual clinician. We need to reengineer our current delivery methods to maximize our effectiveness.

Christopher Foley, MD, completed his medical education at the University of Minnesota and has practiced internal medicine in St. Paul for 18 years. In 1995, he left his private practice to direct the HealthEast Healing Center in St. Paul/Minneapolis—one of the first clinics in the country designed to provide alternative therapies in conjunction with mainstream medicine. HealthEast's integrative health initiatives have been relocated to HealthEast's new 21st century hospital, Woodwinds in Woodbury, a suburb of St. Paul. Dr. Foley is also a clinical assistant professor at the University of Minnesota.

Currently, the major burden on the system involves the management of chronic illness. As we redesign delivery, I believe that health care can be managed through a combination of private consultation and group services in a series of teams, just as most other organizations function today. However, in this case, the teams would be made up of clients—teams of clients receiving education about their medical condition, group support, and some generalized guidance about how to manage their conditions. This approach has already been found to be very useful, for example, in the management of heart disease (in the Ornish model) and diabetes.

This is not to deny in any way the importance and the necessity of the doctor–patient relationship, with its very confidential and personal nature. The group form of delivery is not to be provided to the exclusion of private dialogue. However, the power of the facilitated sharing of experience, paired with patient education, is a tremendous resource to be included when we design health care delivery.

Background

My perspective on the value of patient groups results from a very specific experience that occurred several years ago. At the time, I was seeing a great many patients with chronic conditions, particularly women with silicone gel breast implants suffering from an ill-defined connective tissue disease. One morning, we began running quite late. These appointments always seemed to take longer, because there were no neat problems or clean diagnoses. I decided to meet with several patients at the same time, and I asked each one whether we could meet together as a group. This experience made a lasting impression on me. The role of the physician appeared to have changed, and the effect on the participants was therapeutic.

The Group Experience

• *Shared experience:* These women were all meeting each other for the first time in a venue that was sanctioned by the doctor (in the role of facilitator). The experience of the group created what can be called "the shared experience." Since that time, I have come to believe that one of the great ties that binds people together is shared experience. Shared experience is one of the major aspects of family cohesion. It is also one of the sources of emotional bonding in a disaster or emergency situation. Shared experience is a common theme in group support that probably continues to be undervalued.

• *Democratic group process:* At that shared visit, the entire power grid was completely flattened. Patient autonomy in the group was significantly increased. The group was my first experience of what can occur when patients are empowered in an educational support group environment.

• *The development of mutual support:* Rather than a group of individuals—patients—we suddenly had a team. Information was shared across the group, including information on complementary and alternative medicine. The shared experience and group dynamic provided the basis for a dynamic energy.

• *Access to new information:* New information was exchanged across the group and across all relationships: patient-to-patient, doctor-to-patient, and also patient-to-doctor. In the process, I learned that there is an entire parallel universe of complementary medicine that I had personally known little about. The new resources that I encountered as a result of that group ultimately changed my view of medicine.

I developed an interest in complementary medicine and began studying—buying textbooks, subscribing to journals, and meeting people who were innovative thinkers in the field. Some of them were from overseas; I went to their conferences and later became a speaker at these conferences. I found myself exposed to an entirely new learning discipline, one that expanded the options I could offer my patients—not only new tools, but also a different set of lenses for viewing health and disease.

I became the director of the HealthEast Healing Center in Minneapolis and saw patients not only in my capacity as a conventional physician, but also as advisor and facilitator. I saw patients individually and in the group model. In the first year, we initiated small group sessions focused on fibromyalgia, chronic pain, women's health, and men's health.

Large Groups: The Community Forum

At the Center, we also began offering drop-in educational sessions free of charge on Wednesdays at lunchtime. The room was designed to hold about 75 people. Initially, the forum attracted about 10 or 12 people. It soon grew to a group of 20, and eventually to standing room only.

I began educating my patients about functional medicine, explaining ways in which we can understand and improve our health at the earliest sign of dysfunction. Our topics included cellular function, gut ecology, gut–brain axis, detoxification, energetics, and homeopathy.

Patients (and potential patients) were enriched by the shared experience. Periodically, people would speak from the audience who had educated themselves extensively, and many were people with chronic illness. They would offer interesting pieces of new information that expanded the dialogue. My willingness to be honest about the limits of my knowledge probably did more to bond me to that community than anything else I did. There was so much cross-pollination at these talks that they became alive with energy.

Small Groups: Disease Management

The small group sessions are essentially different from the large drop-in groups. A small group typically involves five or six patients being seen for a particular diagnosis or diagnostic category. The ideal group number is from four to ten people, depending on the disorder and the focus of the discussion. The more advanced and serious the condition, the smaller the group. For intensive illness, such as multiple sclerosis and ulcerative colitis, the groups should be quite small. When we are focusing on very general issues, such as aging or women's health, the groups may be as large as a dozen.

The purpose of the small group is to facilitate disease management—the management of chronic conditions. The key is that people with chronic illness do best when they receive monitoring, feedback, and support on a periodic, ongoing basis.

Applications of the Group Model

The group practice model is also ideal for physician education: A resident or physician can join the group with much less obtrusiveness than if he or she sat in on private, one-to-one office visits. When there is one patient, the addition of a second physician can change the power dynamic significantly by creating a ratio of two professionals to one client. However, if there are four or five patients attending with a goal of patient education, the addition of a second physi-

cian or resident does not impinge on the balance of power in the group. This is one of the great ways that we will be able to educate physicians who want to practice integrative medicine.

The practice of integrative medicine will not suit everyone. The majority of physicians are best suited to the acute management system, but others are looking for a practice style that best suits the way they conceptualize and practice. Integrative medicine has a great deal to offer them. For example, recently trained female physicians tend to be attracted to a style of practice that includes patient education, and many of them will bond with this model.

All physicians learn the same basic medical and biochemical information. The paradigms of functional medicine mesh nicely with mainstream medical concepts. They are meaningful but not difficult to grasp. The group delivery allows a vehicle at no cost, rather than physician time, for medical training.

This model must be costed out and analyzed from an economic standpoint. Like any other endeavor, I and my insurers cannot provide this type of care if it loses money, either for the health care system or for the insurer. At this point, the data are not yet in as to the cost-effectiveness of group services, for example, to patients with diabetes. Insurers are concerned that this will be an add-on service—that they will be responsible for group costs in addition to acute care costs. People who monitor chronic conditions sense intuitively that, if this method is allowed to develop, it will ultimately become an effective way to manage demand and provide quality care.

A group-delivered service, used in tandem with a functional medicine model, could allow us to practice demand management. These approaches provide early intervention and problem-solving on a level that enables and enhances the management of chronic illness and medical demand.

24.2   A Group Model of Patient Services in Women's Health

Tracy W. Gaudet

BENEFITS TO PATIENTS, PHYSICIANS, AND HEALTH PLANS

In the process of disease management, physicians frequently spend a great deal of their time educating patients in the important basics of managing their conditions. For patients with chronic disorders, education is an important strategy. Patients with complex chronic illness want to understand their conditions and typically want to know all of the treatment options available to them, including those in integrative medicine. Group education addresses this need in a way that maximizes the physician's time, empowers the patient, and adds the element of group support.

In my own practice in obstetrics and gynecology, I saw many patients who were perimenopausal and menopausal. In the process of patient education, I found myself basically saying the same thing to each of them, one-to-one, over and over again, even on the first visit. It occurred to me that this was not the most effective use of my time or their money, so I began to hold group sessions for patients. I also hoped that my clients would find the group helpful as a forum for the exchange of information. Patients were highly enthusiastic.

Not only did participants in my group sessions get the information they sought, they also benefited from the support of other women who were dealing with the same type of health concerns. I

developed a number of groups focused on meeting the needs of women with conditions such as menopause syndrome, rheumatoid arthritis, and cancer.

Providing patient information in a group setting can be very effective. It is valuable to physicians because it significantly expands the amount of time spent with patients, and a great deal can be accomplished in the group setting. When researchers in northern California (Sadur et al, 1999) looked at group education in diabetes and other chronic illness, they found that the patients who participated in the groups were healthier and happier. Participants achieved better control of their diabetes. The physicians who initially developed the groups had been concerned that they would be overwhelmed by individual medical questions or patients who might monopolize the group. They found that this was not a problem. Although patients were hungry for information, they were able to have most of their questions answered in the context of the group. Subsequent one-to-one visits were much easier and went faster. In addition, patient satisfaction improved. Models of group education and support for patients definitely merit further research and development.

Patient groups seem to be particularly relevant to individuals with chronic illness who are seeking information and treatment options. Most patients respect their physicians. They do not want to go behind their doctor's back. However, they also want to know all of their options, including alternative medicine. Patients value having their physicians' acknowledgment and guidance in exploring the range of safe treatments available.

It is the opinion of many of us in the profession of health care that the group model tends to decrease cost and utilization, particularly for

Tracy W. Gaudet, MD, is Associate Director of The Duke Center for Integrative Medicine and former Executive Director and Medical Director of the University of Arizona, Program in Integrative Medicine.

Courtesy of Tracy Gaudet, MD, Duke University Department of Obstetrics and Gynecology, Durham, North Carolina.

those with chronic disorders whose complex needs are not easily met. These seem to be the people who tend to overuse the system, reappearing in emergency departments or changing from doctor to doctor in their search for relief. They may also incur high expenditures for diagnostic testing.

The group encourages greater patient autonomy. Patients begin to learn techniques and approaches that can be used at home to manage their conditions and, as a result, they tend not to utilize the system as frequently. This model has the potential to save the system money and to increase patient satisfaction as well.

REFERENCE

Sadur CN, Moline N, Casta M, et al. Diabetes management in a health maintenance organization. Efficacy of care management using cluster visits. *Diabetes Care.* 1999;22(12):2011–2017.

24.3   Evolution of an Integrative Practice

Brian Bouch

Hospital-based emergency medicine and family practice medicine were the primary focuses of my medical practice from 1973 until 1984, and I am board-certified in emergency medicine. In 1985, I began the formal study of acupuncture, then opened a small practice, initially providing family medicine and acupuncture. Gradually, the practice expanded into other areas of complementary medicine as I brought in practitioners with various kinds of training. A skilled osteopath joined me, enabling us to offer osteopathic manipulation. I also associated with a licensed acupuncturist, who has been active in the practice for the past 12 years.

Once I had gained the initial formal training, my own skills in the use of complementary ther-

apies developed as I continued to learn from my colleagues. Through working with the acupuncturist, who is highly knowledgeable in Chinese herbal therapy, I expanded my knowledge of botanicals. I have also learned the use of herbal therapies from extensive reading, workshops, and other practitioners. My knowledge of homeopathy is focused on a practical level—not through a formal study of classical homeopathy, but rather by learning how to use first-aid homeopathic remedies for acute conditions. Massage and bodywork have become another part of my knowledge base. Having a massage practitioner in the office who provides deep-tissue work has given me the opportunity to learn the subtleties of that discipline.

Nutritional therapy is the other area in which I have spent time in intensive study and have gained additional training. The use of nutrition in my practice includes not only diet recommendations, but also the focused use of supplements and megavitamin therapy. Functional medicine is a related field, which includes an emphasis on digestive ecology and the prevention of leaky gut syndrome, based on the work of Jeffrey Bland, PhD (see Chapter 62). These perspectives grow out of the Western paradigm and can be found

Brian Bouch, MD, a graduate of Dickinson College, summa cum laude, Phi Beta Kappa, and University of Pennsylvania School of Medicine, has had careers in family practice, public health medicine, emergency medicine (board certified), and complementary and alternative medicine practice. He divides his time between CAM practice in northern California, teaching acupuncture to physicians, and providing medical oversight to the OneBody.com Internet Web site.

in mainstream literature but are addressed in functional practice through diet and nutrient therapy, rather than the use of medication.

The development of my practice as a complementary provider has entailed a great deal of self-education through workshops, in-depth reading, and conversations with colleagues about what is effective and what works. Everything I learn brings me back to the question of what will have the greatest impact on patient care problems with the least potential for doing harm. Complementary therapies have provided me with a skill set of low-risk approaches to many of the chronic problems that constantly surface in my clinical practice.

Over the past 15 years, my medical practice has evolved into an integrative complementary medicine clinic, typically with four to six practitioners: myself and another physician (who also provides acupuncture), a licensed acupuncturist, an osteopathic physician who does manipulation, a massage therapist, and, usually, a nutritionist.

In addition, I participate in an integrative medicine committee in Sonoma County, California, a subcommittee of Primary Care Associates, a group of over 60 primary care physicians and a dozen specialists. It is a large, exceptionally active group. Meeting with the committee provides me with an opportunity to learn the interests and concerns of a wide range of physicians.

Teaching and consulting are other meaningful aspects of my work in integrative medicine. Since 1987, I have taught in UCLA's course, "Medical Acupuncture for Physicians," serving as one of the primary instructors. For the past 4 years, I have also been the medical director of Consensus Health, dba OneBody.com. Our mission has been to increase the availability of complementary medicine to consumers nationwide. We have done this by creating networks of CAM practitioners, which we carefully screen and credential. The networks are contracted with major health insurers, such as Blue Shield of California and Blue Cross Blue Shield of North Carolina, to promote access to CAM at a discount as a value-added benefit for their subscribers. We are also developing and negotiating contracts with insurers in other states, which reflects the prevalence of this trend. Another major focus has been participation in OneBody.com, a comprehensive Web site on CAM, featuring extensive clinical information, on-line community, and CAM practitioner referrals.

24.4   Building Bridges between the Disciplines

Tori Hudson

As a naturopathic physician, it has always been important to me to work with physicians in mainstream medicine and to learn from them. While I was still in medical school studying naturopathic medicine, I sought opportunities early in my education to preceptor with medical doctors. At that time, I chose two placements with family practice physicians because, as a student,

Tori Hudson, ND, is a graduate of the National College of Naturopathic Medicine and has served the college as medical director, associate academic dean, interim academic dean, and professor of gynocology. She maintains a private practice at two locations in the Portland area and in 1999 was named "Physician of the Year" by the American Association of Naturopathic Physicians. As a researcher, she has performed studies in a number of areas of women's health, including cervical dyslasia, menopause, and breast cancer. She is author of a textbook, *Gynecology and Naturopathic Medicine*, and also of *Women's Encyclopedia of Natural Medicine* (Keats, 1999).

I knew that the foundations I most needed were in basic science and diagnosis.

When I graduated and became a resident and a teacher, I was a young doctor eager to learn. I wanted to continue my education through exposure to professionals who had high levels of expertise. When I wanted to learn gynecology more intensely, I knew that I should be spending time with gynecologists, not just naturopaths or simply my own case load. If I wanted to learn cardiology, I knew that I should be with the cardiologists. Once I began teaching, I continued to welcome opportunities to observe medical doctors in practice and made it a point to have them come speak in my classes.

In regard to patient care, I consider it my professional responsibility to work collaboratively with other health care professionals. If the patient has a serious condition, it becomes even more important to communicate about treatment and to coordinate care.

BUILDING BRIDGES IN MEDICAL PRACTICE

There are physicians with whom I have had collegial communication for more than 16 years. I have sent many patients to them, and they have sent patients to me. They are guest lecturers in my classes each year, and I have visited their practices. I am also able to send my naturopathic students to preceptor with them, and a number of them participate in our integrative medicine residency rotation.

There are many ways in which physicians in the mainstream can be integrative in their approach. One is to be open-minded about questions that patients raise. Another is to call an alternative practitioner when responding to pa-

---

*Editor's note: In 1996, the MEDLINE database of the National Library of Medicine, NIH, was significantly expanded to include more citations from the medical literature regarding botanicals, nutrients, and alternative therapies. Physicians now also have access to resources such as *The PDR for Herbal Medicine*, published by Medical Economics.

tients' questions, such as, Can I take ginkgo (*Ginkgo biloba*)? Periodically, doctors contact me with questions, wanting to know whether a particular herb has a history of toxicity and how it interacts with various medications. When I began these preceptorships more than 16 years ago, there was very little information available to physicians about alternatives in medicine.*

Patients Are a Source of Mutual Referrals

When a number of patients praise a particular physician highly, I make it a point to call their doctor and exchange pertinent information or discuss their case. If this communication goes well, as it almost always does, I begin referring patients to that physician. Likewise, the doctors with whom I have established rapport have a better sense of who I am and how I practice. Often, we find that there are other patients for whom we both provide care, so the exchange of information continues. These physicians eventually serve as experts from whom I can seek advice and vice versa.

There have also been many times when I needed a competent second opinion. The doctors I call are usually those I know. Ultimately, the doctors with whom I have had the best communication have been those who see me as a colleague and someone with whom they want to share information. This has provided the basis for exchanging expertise. Over the years, an integrative network of health care professionals has evolved in our community.

Coeducation Expands Professional Opportunities

I have continued to expand my practice experience through preceptorships that developed out of professional contact. Typically, I would ask whether I could spend a few hours a week in the office with a physician, observe some protocols and surgeries, or learn from them in their practice. I would usually visit once a week, at a set time, for a specific period of time. For example, the gynecological preceptorship initially lasted a year, then evolved into an opportunity for me to establish a practice in that office, seeing my own patients. Based on my experience at the gynecologist's office, I decided to specialize in women's health. In that practice, the doctor would bring me in with her during patient visits. As we became more comfortable and she developed more trust in me, she would ask for my opinion, particularly if it was a condition that lent itself to a range of options. Eight years later, I still have a practice there one day a week, although I now also have my own main clinic.

Integrative Medicine As a Market Niche

In the preceptorships, patients have been highly enthusiastic about my participation. The fact that their doctor was open to an alternative medical perspective seemed to be very meaningful to them. Over time, the inclusion of integrative medicine created a unique marketing niche for these physicians. Their patients were delighted and told their friends. It became an exceptionally positive experience.

At another level of integrative practice, physicians in biomedicine may find that they want to become more knowledgeable about complementary therapies. Through conferences or patient referrals, they may become acquainted with practitioners of complementary medicine. Meaningful integrative practice evolves out of knowledge, training, and practice wisdom. There are many ways to become involved in this integration. The same is true for alternative practitioners.

Practice Experience in Complementary Therapies

I have described ways in which alternative practitioners can observe in mainstream medical practices. Mainstream practitioners can do the same. I have hosted preceptorships many times over the years, and I notice that the frequency of these mutual exchanges has increased significantly. A medical doctor will phone me to ask

to observe in my office, typically, for a day, or a week, or once a week for a period of time. Not long ago, the president-elect of the Oregon Medical Association sat in with me for one day. He just wanted to see what we do and was pleasantly surprised.

Physicians sometimes come from out of town and spend the entire week with me. They sit in on all of my cases. I always ask the patients' permissions first. Most often, patients say yes. Typically, patients express enthusiasm about the exchange—they are happy to see this kind of collegial exchange develop. Research shows that most patients do use integrative medicine, rather than simply alternative therapies (see Chapter 2).

I regularly have an internal medicine resident with me one day per week from a local hospital. We see patients together, and I often consult with them to provide a second opinion. It becomes quite easy to build this type of preceptorship into your practice.

In the context of my teaching, I have become accustomed to structuring mentoring programs, and it has worked well. I have had several family physicians spend one morning a week with me for three months. In that length of time, it is very possible to gain a sense of how I practice. In the ideal situation, professionals who are sitting in have the opportunity to see the follow-up visits, as well as the initial visit. Then physicians can hear the patients report on how they are responding to treatment, and it is possible to observe the outcomes of different interventions, rather than just hear about them abstractly. This allows the observer to develop a knowledge base from which to assess the effects of the therapy. In tandem with their review of research and other resources, such observers begin to decide for themselves.

An Integrative Medicine Residency

In conjunction with my work as a professor of naturopathic medicine, I have developed an integrative medicine residency. I have drawn on professional relationships with physicians in the community, arranging placements for naturopathic residents to work with them in their offices. This type of communication can link both disciplines. For example, in one preceptorship, the oncologists wanted to know about the use of St. John's wort for patients with brain tumors and asked for the research. They put my student to work searching the literature.

The residents will also accompany the doctors on rounds in the hospital and have an opportunity to observe surgery. This is not a big step for the physicians because they are accustomed to hosting residents. The residents are provided with outstanding opportunities for learning and expanded understanding. When this kind of exchange occurs, we all benefit.

24.5   Interprofessional Referral Protocols

Robert D. Mootz

Over the past decade, there has been a significant increase in awareness of alternative medicine therapies and documented growth in utilization (Eisenberg et al, 1998). However, due perhaps to strained political relations between alternative care providers and organized medicine, many patients have avoided communicating their use of such service to physicians. As a result of more research and exchange of information, the opportunity for better communication among all providers has never been better (Triano and Raley, 1994). Consequently, there is the need to establish clear ground rules for interdisciplinary communication and referral (Barnett, 1998). Although there is a culture of patient referral and reporting within mainstream medicine, similar protocols and written communication have often been less common in alternative care disciplines.

It is in the best interest of the patient to have a clinician of record who tracks and coordinates activity with other providers and specialists (Triano, Rashbaum, and Hansen, 1998). Additionally, the provider who refers courteously and appropriately may be more likely to engender future referral activity from others (Mootz, 1990; Mootz, 1987; Mootz and Meeker, 1990). By following a few basic protocols, a provider can interface with other specialists in a professional manner that can contribute to a positive practice experience while maintaining appropriate input in the management of complex cases. In this way, both the patient and other providers can be confident that everyone working on a case will be in communication and that each provider's goals and methodology for care will be understood.

REFERRAL DIRECTION

Referral can originate from the complementary practitioner to other specialists or from other practitioners to the complementary provider. The protocols are different, depending on the direction of the flow. When a practitioner sends a patient to another specialist, it is important to communicate the nature of the referral. Because most specialists are very busy, a brief written report letter is most useful. A short, explicit report is more likely to be read by the

Robert D. Mootz, DC, is Associate Medical Director for Chiropractic at the Department of Labor and Industries in Washington state and editor of the journal *Topics in Clinical Chiropractic*. He has coauthored and edited several texts and monographs on chiropractic care of special populations and chiropractic technologies, as well as an Agency for Health Care Policy and Research monograph on the chiropractic profession and a report by RAND on the appropriateness of manipulation of the cervical spine. His current research includes an inventory of procedures in use by alternative care providers, disability prevention, and occupational health services delivery.

specialist. However, when a patient referral is received, the optimal response following evaluation is a more detailed report of findings and recommendations.

Since the advent of managed care, increasing time pressure has been placed on all providers. Although thoroughness is an important component, particularly when a referral has been received, it is essential that concise and efficient written communication occur. Although a phone call or verbal explanation to the patient is sometimes easier and more personal than report writing, the need to have a permanent record of interventions and recommendations for the chart of the other provider is essential for both clinical management and medicolegal considerations. It will also make other providers feel more comfortable with the work of that practitioner.

REFERRAL PURPOSE

There are several reasons for making a referral (Mootz, 1990). The referring provider may want a second opinion about a case, help in the management of a case, or the transfer of complete management of a case to another practitioner. It is important that the referring provider make the purpose for the referral clear. If referrals are made without a clear understanding of the purpose, it is possible that future problems between the clinicians could develop. For example, without a letter of introduction explaining what has been done previously for the patient and the reason for the referral, the specialist may recommend a course of care that has already proven ineffective. This can usually be prevented through communication with the specialist in advance regarding case response and management approaches to date (including what has been attempted by others seeing the patient earlier).

When a practitioner wants another doctor to evaluate a patient (review the case, update the history, or perform an examination) and report observations and recommendations, that practitioner should request a consultation and evaluation. If the referring practitioner requires that the other doctor provide treatment, he or she should request a consultation, evaluation, and treatment. By being clear about this in advance, there is little doubt as to the purpose of the referral, thereby minimizing potential misunderstandings. For the same reasons, it is important that the referring practitioner be clear about the continuing role that he or she will have in the management of the case. It is the responsibility of the primary treating practitioner to ensure that all care being provided is coordinated and that no clinician counteract the efforts of other clinicians involved in the case. In addition to actual treatment, this includes recommendations for home care, such as exercises, work restrictions, applications of hot/cold packs, or nutritional advice.

If the doctor accepting the referral understands the referring practitioner's rationale for care, any differences of opinion can be worked out, preventing frustration for the patient when conflicting advice is given. Although it is typical for specialists to report back, it is a good idea to request that the doctor report back on his or her findings at the time the referral is made. These days, unpaid time for written reporting is harder to come by, and follow-up with other doctors may sometimes be needed, particularly if there is some uncertainty regarding care planning.

OUTGOING REFERRAL PROTOCOL

The following steps should be taken when making a referral to another clinician. Any provider can follow these guidelines when referring to another, as well as to practitioners in another discipline. Chiropractors tend to refer patients to other practitioners regularly, and some studies have suggested that those who also send written reports receive more direct referrals from others (Mootz and Meeker, 1990).

In the referral process, the role of the practitioner is to:

1. **Identify the services that the patient needs and clarify the need for referral**

with the patient. This can help to prevent apprehension on the part of the patient.

2. **Identify a clinician who can provide these services.** If the practitioner has not established an interreferral relationship previously, he or she should personally telephone the clinician and very briefly describe what is needed, and ask whether the clinician would be willing to accept the referral. If the other clinician agrees, the practitioner should proceed with the next step. Should a doctor be unable to accept (for example, too busy or outside of his or her area of expertise), the practitioner should request the name of someone the other specialist would recommend and proceed to make contact with that person or with the referring practitioner's next choice.

3. **Have the office staff contact the other clinician's office and arrange for scheduling the patient.** It is extremely helpful, as well as professional, to provide the other office with the patient's entrance data (name, address, phone, insurance information, and other essential information). Often, it is most convenient for the other office to call the patient directly to schedule exact appointment times.

4. **Write a letter briefly describing the reason for the referral and provide a short summary of the history, findings, and past treatment.** As previously mentioned, the referring practitioner should be sure to indicate what role, if any, he or she intends to play in the continuing care and further management of the patient.

5. **Follow up on the progress of the patient with the other provider.** Even if the specialist fails to report back to the referring practitioner, politely following up with a letter or a phone call conveys genuine interest that engenders respect.

As the primary provider of record, the referring practitioner should play an important role in overall management and follow-up of the pa-tient, especially when two or more providers are directly involved in the ongoing care of a patient (Mootz, 1987).

INCOMING REFERRAL PROTOCOL

When referrals come to a practitioner, the procedures and expectations differ somewhat. Receiving a complete and timely report back from a specialist is a satisfying experience and makes a practitioner feel comfortable to refer patients again. Therefore, when that same practitioner receives patients from others, he or she should respond in the same way. Doing so communicates the practitioner's expertise in a professional manner and increases the comfort level of the referring physician. This can be particularly true of traditional medical providers who receive very little training or exposure in alternative therapies.

The following steps summarize the procedures for reporting back on patients referred to a practitioner.

1. When a referred patient has been scheduled, a brief letter on letterhead stationery thanking the doctor should be sent, confirming the date and time of the appointment. A form letter or preformatted postcard will suffice, but generally, correspondence on professional letterhead regarding patients is more likely to be read and even kept in the patient chart. Although various thank-you cards may be nice for referrals from nonprofessionals, these are inappropriate to send to referring physicians. The practitioner should indicate that he or she will report back after the evaluation. Before beginning the case, the practitioner should determine whether the patient is being sent for evaluation only or for evaluation and treatment. If it is unclear what the referring physician wants when the patient is initially referred, the practitioner should call the doctor, briefly summarize his or her findings and recommendations, and

ask whether the referring physician is in agreement with the planned course of action.

2. Upon completion of the evaluation, a fairly detailed report should be sent, summarizing the practitioner's findings (history, examination, and any special studies, such as laboratory and radiographs), clinical impressions, and recommendations. This should be done even if the practitioner has verbally outlined the findings, as described in the previous step. It is common courtesy to close by thanking the referring physician for the opportunity to assist in the evaluation and/or care of the patient. I recommend that this initial report be sent in the form of a narrative on letterhead—but again, clearly organized and concise. The use of a form specifically designed for this purpose may be adequate, as well. These typically have sections for notations about findings and recommendations. However, handwritten entries need to be legible, and details such as abbreviations or the names of tests must be clear because they may not be meaningful to anyone outside of that discipline.

3. If it is determined that the practitioner will be providing treatment, a very brief letter indicating progress should be sent to the referring physician at periodic intervals (for example, following a reexamination). It is perfectly acceptable for a progress report to be brief, for example, a one-page letter or preformatted form.

4. When care is complete, a brief final report should be sent, summarizing progress and indicating that the patient has been discharged. Any recommendations given to the patient for future self-care or follow-up should also be noted.

Just as the practitioner is the primary provider of record when referring a patient out, a doctor who refers a patient to that practitioner is the primary physician of record. Therefore, professional courtesy dictates that the referring doctor's concerns be addressed. The patient should never be involved in a difference of opinion between the two practitioners. Every effort should be made to articulate the contribution to care in a manner that is competent and appropriate to the physician of record. By following the previous steps, this can be readily accomplished. Undoubtedly, there will be times when not all recommendations will be followed by the physician of record. However, in the long run, it is most important to develop a foundation of trust and cooperation with other practitioners, always in a context of maximizing benefit for the patient. These interdisciplinary linkages provide the opportunity to work collegially, bringing expanded resources to bear on complex conditions.

Although wellness care, holistic perspectives, and preventive lifestyles are valued in principle, the application of a wellness paradigm in the complementary community tends to be much more extensive. Therefore, it is important to recognize this difference in practice philosophy. When referrals are received, it is wise to determine and communicate recommendations for both immediate and long-term care. The treatment should include recommendations for the specific situation (such as acute low-back pain) as well as any relevant discussion of a more lasting lifestyle intervention. It is important for practitioners in both complementary and mainstream disciplines to remember how frustrating it is when another provider manages the case without communicating clearly. Referral protocol is most effectively aimed at setting the stage for clear and comfortable collaboration to increase the number of therapeutic options available.

CONCLUSION

The clinician who refers the patient out is considered the provider of record (Mootz, 1990). By communicating and coordinating approaches, the patient will receive consistent care, and the referring provider will not have the sense that patients are being coopted. Although these referral protocols require some extra work, developing an office routine that consistently and efficiently allows for smooth inter- and intraprofessional interaction fosters more respect from patients and colleagues alike (Mootz, 1987). Most importantly, when practitioners coordinate and cooperate with one another, patients benefit the most.

Proper referral protocol may not be followed by all providers. This, however, should not deter practitioners from behaving professionally.

Many allied health professionals and general practitioners tend to treat referrals in a very casual manner. The provider who functions with timely, thorough, and consistent communication to peers is identified in the community as competent, qualified, and concerned. This communication provides the basis for contacts and procedures that may facilitate involvement with other health care modalities, medical specialties, or institutions (Tiano, Rashbaum, and Hansen, 1998). Successful interaction with other providers can contribute ultimately to better understanding and cooperation between the disciplines.

REFERENCES

Barnett PB. Clinical communication and managed care. *Med Group Manage J.* 1998;45(4):60–66.

Eisenberg DM, Davis RB, Ettner SL, et al. Trends in alternative medicine use in the United States, 1990–1997: results of a follow-up survey. *JAMA.* 1998;280(18): 1569–1575.

Mootz RD. Interprofessional referral protocol: how to make referrals that benefit all parties. *Today's Chiropract.* September/October 1987;37–40.

Mootz RD. Interprofessional relations: appropriate referral protocols. *Am Back Soc Newsletter.* 1990;6(4).

Mootz RD, Meeker WC. Referral patterns of California Chiropractic Association members. *Am Back Soc Newsletter.* 1990;6(3):17.

Triano JJ, Raley B. Chiropractic in the interdisciplinary team practice. *Top Clin Chiropract.* 1994;1(4):58–66.

Triano JJ, Rashbaum RF, Hansen DT. Opening access to spine care in the evolving market: integration and communication. *Top Clin Chiropract.* 1998;5(4):44–52.

CHAPTER 25

Clinical Perspectives in Risk Management

David C. Kailin

INTRODUCTION

This chapter is primarily intended to encourage managers and practitioners to assess the dimensions of risk, and to implement practical strategies for the prevention of harm. Within each discipline, technique-specific best practices and risk management strategies must be developed and implemented. The discipline of acupuncture provides a relevant model for risk management that can be adapted to other complementary and alternative medicine (CAM) services.

Standard acupuncture textbooks, which are often translations or adaptations of Oriental reference works, present the student with the conceptual and technical bases for the practice of traditional Oriental medicine. These texts contain the essence of the traditional technical art, including certain aspects of safety (for example, maximum needle insertion depths). However, defining safe techniques requires broader frames of reference than traditional Oriental medicine offers.

With the introduction of acupuncture to America, several key elements of praxis have been left understated (if not entirely unstated). Among these are issues of how to proceed in the contexts of American medicine and culture. Failure to grasp prevailing health care, legal, and personal expectations could lead to adverse outcomes.

David C. Kailin, medical futurist and Chief Executive Officer of Convergent Medical Systems, Inc, in Corvallis, Oregon, assists organizations in the development of preferable health care futures.

Source: Adapted with permission from *Clinical Dimensions of Risk Management, Acupuncture Risk Management,* © 1997, CMS Press.

Risk management extends beyond technical safety; it involves cultural and social contexts.

Acupuncturists are accountable to prevailing local standards of medical practice and judgment. Yet were acupuncturists to hold nothing but local standards, they would have naught to offer. The clinical value of acupuncture derives from its practitioners' distinctive perspectives, extensive knowledge base, and unique therapeutic techniques. Integrated practice must achieve a delicate balance, distinguishing greater from lesser medicolegal risks in the meshing of Oriental and American practice standards. The task involves subtle levels of judgment, perhaps acquired with some difficulty by those individuals who lack prior biomedical professional experience in this culture. Issues of helping, harming, safety, and liability are deeply intertwined; they span technical, legal, medical, ethical, and social domains. Effective risk management requires educated discernment.

Until recently there seemed little need to attend to such issues since acupuncture occupied a liminal place in America, marginalized enough to be ignored. Acupuncture's profile has risen, with the mainstreaming of alternative therapies into medical institutions and reimbursement plans. Regulatory bodies have discovered the need to make accommodations to assimilate acupuncture. Acupuncturists find themselves increasingly answerable to surrounding medical and regulatory communities. The transition from alternative to orthodox is a challenge for all involved.

The essence of that challenge is to retain the integrity of acupuncture while adapting it to the contexts of American medicine. Acupuncturists must be responsive to biomedical standards of practice and to legal, regulatory, and institutional frameworks. Standards of practice are evolving to reflect these exigencies throughout the profession (Kailin, 1997). Integrative practice administrators must be responsive to the unique aspects of acupuncture that generate clinical utility and effectiveness. Otherwise, the clinical capabilities of acupuncture (or any CAM modality) may be greatly limited. Cursory integration can leave only the appearance of providing acupuncture services. The potentials of integration—to transform the core tasks of medicine in ways that are more humane, effective, and sustainable—could rapidly devolve to a shallow veneer of marketing. Conscientious integration requires balanced judgment to retain the integrity of the original discipline.

CONCEPTS OF RISK MANAGEMENT

In large corporations, the functions of risk management are divided among specialized professionals. In private practice, acupuncturists usually manage all aspects of risk in concert with their other duties. Effective risk management requires a working knowledge of risk management functions. Several basic terms are defined below.

Risk avoidance is the creation of conditions for the total absence of a risk. The exclusive use of presterilized disposable needles, used once and then immediately discarded into a sharps container, entirely prevents the potentials for patient-to-patient disease transmission associated with reusable needles. This is an example of risk avoidance that simultaneously induces few other risks.

Risk control means decreasing the frequency or severity of potential harm. Risk control strategies are applied in instances where risk avoidance is not possible or practical. Gloving the hand that holds the cotton ball just prior to needle removal decreases, but does not entirely prevent, the practitioner's blood contact infection risk. Risk of infection via accidental needle stick, among other events, remains possible.

Risk selection involves the linked choices of "which risks to incur" and "which risks not to incur." One must choose preferable sets of risks. For example, installing a smoke detector decreases the risk of damage to property and life from undetected fires. Yet it simultaneously increases risk of damage from false alarms. As is frequently the case, the control of one risk induces other risks. When risks cannot be avoided altogether, preferable sets of risks are selected. With each risk control selection, the set of resultant risk reductions and risk inductions must be evaluated anew. A brief discussion of risk management functions (Head, 1989) is given below.

- **Risk assessment concerns** identifying the nature and location of risks, establishing (when possible) their causes, frequency, potential severity, and costs.
- **Risk control planning** involves analyzing and selecting risk avoidance and risk control strategies for assessed risks, and developing an implementation plan to reduce risks.
- **Risk control implementation** means putting a risk control plan into action. This may involve some or all of the following interventions:
  — safety-related administrative policies
  — reengineering of the work environment
  — redesign of tools
  — redesign of work practices
  — use of personal protective equipment
  — provision of immunizations
  — use of safety devices
  — employee risk control education programs
  — risk monitoring
  — risk financing
- **Risk control communication** concerns the initial and periodic training of employees in risk control rationales, policies, and procedures. It includes communicating with employees about actual and potential adverse events that occur in their workplace.
- **Risk monitoring** involves recording the occurrence of adverse events and high-risk situations, particularly after implementa-

tion of a risk control plan. Employee compliance with risk control efforts may be monitored. Risk monitoring provides informational feedback for a continuing process of risk control planning.

- **Risk financing** typically involves the transfer of certain risks through insurance. Acupuncture professional liability policies often contain exclusions for specified techniques or conditions. It is important to read the policy carefully, to be certain that coverage includes the techniques that alternative providers will be using.

- **Crisis response** involves preparations for effective response to specific types of emergencies. Common emergency preparations might include fire, burglary, earthquake, electric power loss, computer failure, computer security breaches, and medical emergencies.

INCIDENCE AND NATURE OF MATERIAL HARM

Many dimensions of clinical risk are difficult to quantify. For example, one senses, but cannot easily measure, the ebb and flow of communication and trust with patients. The incidence and nature of material harms to patients are particularly difficult to establish. Malpractice insurance claims constitute the primary data relevant to the question of incidence of harm: how often material harms occur. Claims and medical journal articles also inform about what kinds of material harms occur. Precise estimates of the incidence and severity of harms cannot be made from available data.

An insurance executive estimated that claims arose involving 2% of approximately 1,200 acupuncturist policyholders in 1996. Average payout for settled claims between 1993 and 1999 amounted to $8,597 (M. Shaw of Acupuncture Insurance Services, oral communication, 6/00). This figure is roughly one-twentieth the amount for primary care medicine (Studdert et al, 1998), twice the average indemnity per paid claim for massage therapists, and one sixth the amount for chiropractors (see Table 25–1).

It is important to place the risks of acupuncture in the context of relative risk. When compared with the performance of standard biomedical practices, acupuncture has a record of extraordinary safety. One has to search the archives to find the rare record of an acupuncture-related death occurring anywhere in the world. By comparison, biomedical errors alone are estimated to cause between 44,000 and 98,000 deaths per year in America (Institute of Med-

Table 25–1 Malpractice Claims, CAM and Primary Care Medicine, 1995

Discipline	Number of Claims in 1995 per 100 Policy Holders	Average Payment in 1995, per Paid Claim (in dollars)
Acupuncture[1]	2.0	$8,597
Chiropractic[2]	2.6	$52,385
Massage therapy[3]	0.2	$4,864
Primary care medicine[4]	9.0	$179,732

[1]Acupuncture data from Acupuncture Insurance Services, Elmhurst, Illinois, which insures more than 17% of acupuncturists in the U.S.; figure represents the average cost of claims paid, 1993 to 1999, M. Shaw, written communication, 6/00.

[2]Chiropractic data from NCMIC, West Des Moines, Iowa, which insures more than 50% of chiropractic providers in the United States, in Studdert et al, Medical malpractice and alternative medicine. *JAMA.* 1998;280(18):1611.

[3]Massage data from Altert H. Wohlers & Co., Park Ridge, Illinois (Studdert et al, 1998).

[4]Data on primary care medicine from Gonzales M, ed. *Socioeconomic Characteristics of Medical Practice 1997.* American Medical Association; 1997:39–44.

icine, 1999). A study of New York hospitals found the occurrence of adverse events in 3.7% of hospitalizations, with 13.6% of those events leading to death (Brennan et al, 1991).

What sorts of material harms have happened to acupuncture patients? A review of malpractice insurance claims, medical journal reports, and clinical narratives suggests the following events occur, some of which are minor, but may be perceived as adverse by viewers who have not received sufficient information about the nature of these therapies. Minor bruising at acupuncture points is an occasional occurrence and is generally insignificant. The techniques of cupping and coining produce dermal marks that usually resolve in 2 to 5 days. Direct moxibustion can generate a small (approximately 3-mm) burn, and can leave a scar (while indirect moxibustion creates only mild local warming). Accidental burns have occurred from direct moxibustion, indirect moxibustion, and cupping. Most acupuncturists have had patients faint or nearly faint, an outcome that can be largely avoided by positioning the patient supine, prone, or reclined during treatment. Infections, nerve damage, and pneumothorax are very rare outcomes. Readers are encouraged to consult and periodically monitor the medical literature for acupuncture adverse events using resources such as MEDLINE.

Herbal medicine presents another set of risks, including the potential for herb-drug interactions. An occasional gastritis is related to ingestion of herbs. There have been cases of misidentified herbs and adulterated or misbranded herbal formulas, some resulting in serious consequences.

Acupuncturists, like nurses and physicians, are at risk of contracting hepatitis B and C, HIV, and other bloodborne infections. Occupational Safety and Health Administration Bloodborne Pathogen Standards, when properly applied to the practice of acupuncture, provide a significant measure of prevention.

When encountering CAM therapies, fear of the unfamiliar can magnify the sense of potential risk. Practitioners should take steps to minimize

preventable harm, while taking care not to overestimate potential risk. Relative safety is one of the substantive virtues of acupuncture.

CONTEXTS OF RISK

The concepts and functions of risk management can be applied to 10 distinct contexts of risk in acupuncture practices. These contexts are relevant to the majority of medical disciplines, and further commentary will serve to highlight a few acupuncture-specific issues:

- physical plant
- employers and employees
- records and billing
- medical advice
- medical emergencies
- interpersonal aspects of treatment
- legal aspects of treatment
- Food and Drug Administration (FDA) regulations
- bloodborne pathogens
- technical aspects of treatment, specific to the discipline

For records, a basic Subjective Objective Assessment and Plan (SOAP) notes format (with notes in English) is adequate for the medical record. Billing codes should not obscure the provision of acupuncture if acupuncture treatment was the primary purpose of the visit.

Legal aspects of treatment include several scope of practice issues. Acupuncturists must be circumspect with respect to charting biomedical diagnoses if making such diagnoses is not within their legal scope. Each state defines the technical scope of practice for acupuncture in its own ways.

FDA regulations pertain to acupuncture devices and dietary supplements including herbs. Acupuncture needles have been transitioned from Class III experimental devices to Class II devices marketable for clinical practice. Several electroacupuncture units are also available as Class II devices.

Technical aspects of treatment include technical and clinical guidelines, best practices, equipment sterilization and disinfection protocols, and other basic hygienic and safety practices. For example, in the practice of acupuncture, technical risk control strategies relate to the use of acupuncture needles, moxibustion, cupping, coining, herbs and dietary supplements, acupressure, electroacupuncture, laser devices, and magnetic devices. Best practice protocols have been developed, and are included in a text that serves as a reference for the acupuncture board examinations of the National Certification Commission for Acupuncture and Oriental Medicine (Kailin, 1997).

Acupuncture and other CAM therapies are not risk-free, but the relative risks in terms of frequency and severity of harm are substantially lower than those encountered in general practice medicine. Most significant risks related to CAM can be identified and mitigated. Given well-informed clinical risk management, CAM can continue to demonstrate a most remarkable record of safety.

REFERENCES

Brennan TA, Leape LL, Laird NM, et al. Incidence of adverse events and negligence in hospitalized patients: results of the Harvard medical practice study I. *N Engl J Med.* 1991;324:370–376.

Head GL. *Essentials of Risk Control.* Vol 1. 2nd ed. Malvern, PA: Insurance Institute of America; 1989.

Institute of Medicine. *To Err Is Human—Building a Safer Health System.* Washington, DC: National Academy Press; 1999.

Kailin D. *Acupuncture Risk Management.* Corvallis, OR: CMS Press; 1997.

Studdert DM, Eisenberg DM, Miller FH, Curto DA, Kaptchuk TJ, Brennan TA. Medical malpractice and alternative medicine. *JAMA.* 1998;280(18):1610–1615.

PART VII

Assessment and Research

CHAPTER 26

Criteria for Assessing Successful Integration

Charles A. Simpson and Nancy Faass

INTRODUCTION

Assessing the integration of complementary and alternative medicine (CAM) services into health care systems always involves an evaluation of relationships to the larger system. This is true whether the assessment is focused on administrative functions, clinical functions, or the relationship of the practitioner to the system. A systems perspective provides the general framework, whether that system is an insurance company, a health maintenance organization (HMO), a hospital system, an integrative medicine center, or some other type of organization. The systems perspective is also relevant whether the provider unit is seen in terms of individual practitioners, complementary disciplines, or networks of CAM practitioners. The role CAM services play in the larger system is continuously being evaluated. The potential impact and success of these services on health system performance and on member health may well hinge on the depth and quality of integration into the larger system.

The Value of Assessment to All Stakeholders

The ability to assess the degree of integration can be of value to health plan managers in reviewing current programs and planning for the future. Practitioners can benefit by knowing the degree to which prospective managed care arrangements potentiate integration. Purchasers and patients can compare and evaluate CAM offerings in light of the depth and quality of integration presented by a potential health system partner. Assessment of integration can define more clearly the relationship of CAM to the mainstream. Periodic evaluations can clarify how CAM services are valued and what the expectations are for performance within a particular setting.

The actual organization may be large or small. The model is as relevant to a freestanding integrative medical center as it is to a large network. Any model can be evaluated through the matrix of measurement, assessing each specific function in the context of the degree to which CAM and CAM practitioners are integrated into the larger system. From the perspectives of administrative, clinical, or practitioner-system integration, each dimension reflects a different point of view and has unique aspects that are relevant to the CAM-system interface.

ASSESSING ADMINISTRATIVE INTEGRATION

Administrative integration is the extent to which administrative functions support all aspects of care delivered, CAM and mainstream alike. To the degree that administrative functions also provide support for the complementary medicine unit, CAM will be as much a part of the system as any other of the more traditionally integrated medical services.

Charles A. Simpson, DC, has been a practicing chiropractor for over 20 years. He is a founder and currently the Chief Medical Officer of Complementary Healthcare Plans of Portland, Oregon.

Key functions that can reflect the measure of administrative integration include:

- organizational mission and strategic planning
- information management
- continuous quality improvement and total quality management
- staff education

Additional parameters include:

- financial management
- human resources
- other administrative services that support clinical functions

Organizational Mission and Strategic Planning

Mission

Currently, many hospitals, physician groups, HMOs, and other types of health care delivery organizations are interested in the addition of CAM services.

- Within the context of the organization's vision, goals, and plan of action, to what extent is CAM viewed as an integral part of the enterprise?
- How open is the corporate position to expanding the continuum of care and including programming for wellness and new options for treating chronic illness?
- Is CAM seen strategically primarily for its marketing appeal, or is it seen for the value it can contribute?

Planning

Administrative integration is frequently reflected in strategic planning functions:

- How does a CAM offering fit into the strategic plan of the organization?
- Which strategic planning activities incorporate consideration of CAM, CAM practitioners, and users of CAM?

- If CAM programming has been developed, do the program initiatives reflect a fully integrated, multidisciplinary approach to health care?

Leadership

- What is the level of commitment to this type of programming throughout the organization?
- Do administrative and clinical leaders indicate a commitment to CAM inclusion?
- Or does the leadership view CAM as a necessary evil to compete in a new market?
- How does the organization view uncertainty and innovation?
- Are the values of the organizational culture such that potential risks and benefits must be completely defined before proceeding? (This is not a matter of judgment, but rather a reflection of perspective.)

Stakeholder Input

- How does the organization obtain information from its stakeholder communities?
- Is information about CAM coming strictly from the marketing department?
- Are member preferences and clinician champions of CAM sought out to offer ideas and information about CAM inclusion?

Information Systems

The integration of information flow is a key dimension in the assessment of integration. Health care systems at all levels rise or fall on the competency of the system's information management.

- Is the organization's strategic vision supported and operationalized by the ability to capture and use meaningful information, and is that information relevant in meeting the strategic objectives?
- Are available information systems able to support other key administrative functions as well, such as CAM utilization management and quality management?

- Are systems in place that are able to retrieve encounter data and related administrative information as a platform for measuring CAM performance?
- Is there the ability to look at patient-centered data across the continuum of care, including CAM care?
- Is the level of information and data sufficient to enable the organization to develop pricing and resource allocation models that can leverage the efficiencies and cost savings of CAM interventions?

Quality Management

From a strategic point of view, the CAM effort should be held to explicit performance criteria. As with any other business operation, the CAM unit must fulfill the basic objectives of the organization's business goals.

- Do systemwide quality management processes unify activity by focusing on common outcomes, targets, and goals?
- To what extent do quality improvement programs measure CAM clinical activities?
- To what extent are quality measures and evaluations relevant to CAM practitioners, practice, and patients?
- Are CAM interventions being evaluated to the same extent as mainstream interventions using all the same strategies to assess outcomes?
- Is patient satisfaction assessed across the entire span of all patients throughout the system, including those who are being seen in a CAM setting?

Professional and Staff Education

The extent to which time and resources are devoted to educational opportunities for clinicians, administrators, and marketing people on the one hand, and purchasers and consumers on the other, can be a measure of the degree of integration.

- Is the integration of patient care being fostered through systemwide efforts to educate mainstream clinicians about appropriate CAM referrals?
- Are CAM practitioners being trained about practice and procedures in health systems, population-based health care, mainstream clinical protocols, and referral protocols?
- Have resources been devoted to educating the marketing staff about the value of CAM services?
- Has this education been done in a way that translates into better understanding of CAM by purchasers?
- Are educational efforts being made to help members and patients use CAM more effectively and appropriately?
- Does in-service training support the efficient use of CAM services in the system and promote more complete and seamless integration?

EVALUATING PRACTITIONER-SYSTEM INTEGRATION

Practitioner-system integration is the extent to which practitioners are linked to the system economically; use the facilities and services of the system; and take part in planning, management, and governance of the system. Leveraging these relationships further deepens integration.

Key measures of practitioner-system integration include:

- financial integration
- marketing support
- access to facilities and services
- participation in planning management and governance

Financial Integration

In health care organizations, a fundamental dimension of the practitioner-system relationship is based on and defined by the economic relationship. Economic involvement is the key dimension of practitioner-system integration.

- How are the various elements of financial relationships structured?

- Are economic arrangements essentially similar to those in the uninsured realm, with costs paid out of pocket by the patient?

Within managed care organizations:

- Does financial integration occur through the use of fee schedules and discounted unit prices for service?
- Are risk-sharing arrangements in place to motivate practitioners to provide services efficiently?

Throughout health care:

- Do the incentives in place tend to increase or decrease utilization inappropriately?
- Are incentives present that reward patients for using services wisely?
- What is the effect on short-term utilization? On long-term utilization?
- Do fee schedules honor professional compensation and equitable discounts?
- Are they balanced by sufficient patient volume to motivate practitioners appropriately?

In terms of discounts and fee schedules, it is both the extent to which practitioners are party to decision making on economic issues and the resultant favorableness of pricing that determine the attitude of the practitioner and drive economic incentives in practice. In the fullest measure of integration, financial incentives ideally engage CAM practitioners and align them with the system. This has the potential to produce the greatest value, the highest quality, and the most cost-effective outcomes.

Marketing Support

A reflection of economic involvement is seen in the amount of marketing promotion directed toward CAM services and the volume of patient referrals and revenue that the practitioner actually experiences through the system.

- What volume of referrals to practitioners occurs as a result of their relationship to the system?

- Is there vigorous marketing that promotes CAM interventions and the value of an integrated approach to health care?
- Does marketing promote practitioners individually as well as in tandem with the larger health system or center?
- Is the marketing implemented in a fashion that builds strong loyalty on the part of patients?

Access to Facilities and Services

The extent to which CAM practitioners have access to and make use of facilities and services within the health care system reflects another dimension of practitioner-system integration.

- In the integrative medicine center, is the program structured so that practitioners have cost-effective access to office space?
- Is use of the system's facilities by CAM practitioners defined through contractual obligation?
- Do contracted practitioners refer patients to facilities of the health plan for diagnostics such as radiographs or laboratory testing?

Practice Management Services

Management of the practice also reflects the degree of integration and occurs across a continuum. In a highly integrated system, these services are shared by different practitioners, whether in a network model or a more fully integrated multispecialty clinic.

- Does each practitioner have his or her own administrative staff conduct the billing even though the practitioners share the same building?
- Or do practitioners employ the services of a single administrative and billing service?
- In a third model, is the organization comparable to a medical group in which all practitioners work together and share revenues, profits, and losses, as well as an administrative support staff?

Participation in Governance and Policy Making

Participation is important in maintaining quality service provision. If the organization has respected clinical leaders from the CAM professions who have an effective impact on policy and oversight, then on a structural level, there is some assurance that the integrity of clinical services remains intact. This participation functions as a safeguard to prevent the system from drifting away from quality service if practitioners lose the ability to provide service effectively and maintain patient satisfaction. To the degree that the organization is responsive, there is the ability to restore that integrity. However, if the system is making all decisions based only on system needs, then patient and practitioner needs and identity are more likely to be overlooked. The value of the clinical intervention could decline, and the integrity of the service would be lost. This is a profound reason for the importance of effective provider-system integration. If practitioners do not have the ability to advocate appropriately for quality patient care, it becomes very difficult to maintain quality.

MEASURING CLINICAL INTEGRATION

The scope of clinical integration focuses on providing the most appropriate treatment and approach to care for the patient. Complementary therapies are provided within the system through clinical practice guidelines and algorithms for medical decision making. This aspect of integration reflects the extent to which patient care is coordinated across all disciplines and sites, to maximize the quality and value of services.

The extent of CAM integration is also reflected in the various parameters used to measure clinical services within a number of domains:

- clinical protocols
- clinical outcomes
- patient satisfaction
- cost-effectiveness
- quality of service provision

Clinical Protocols

The use of explicit and carefully developed clinical protocols has gained currency throughout health care. Protocols that reflect state-of-the art clinical expertise are evidence-based, developed through the collaborative efforts of the clinicians who deliver the care, and formulated through explicit processes of evidence selection and consensus development. Reducing variation through the use of protocols can improve quality and, frequently, reduces cost. However, the best interventions are not always the least expensive. Yet, if the intent of health care is to maximize value for purchasers and consumers, a case can be made that less expensive care is not always preferable to good care.

- Is clinical thought focused on those interventions that have evidence supporting their use regardless of whether they may be considered mainstream or alternative?
- Do practitioners have ready access to MEDLINE or other electronic databases, outcomes data, and a variety of clinical information resources for the care of patients?
- Is evidence accumulated and made available to practitioners regarding the most effective use of CAM interventions?
- Is a consensus process used as appropriate in the development of clinical protocols and care pathways?
- To what extent are CAM interventions included in protocols, guidelines, pathways, and other means by which systems attempt to guide clinical practices?
- Are protocols in place that utilize CAM for a range of patient needs, including preventive care, early intervention, and alternative approaches to chronic conditions?
- Or is CAM considered appropriate only "when standard medical treatment has failed"?
- Is the clinical environment conducive to integrative perspectives and teamwork?

Outcomes Measurement

Increased levels of integration are reflected when an alternative practitioner has input into general measures of health. The ability to be included in outcomes data suggests that the managed care organization or health system views the practitioner as an active participant in the overall function of the organization and in attempts to keep its members healthy. If CAM practitioners are omitted from the data set, the data will ultimately be skewed.

An evaluation of this domain includes a range of considerations.

- To what extent is the potential impact of CAM services included in the measurement of clinical outcomes?
- To what degree are CAM practitioners engaged in data collection to track the health of the plan's insured population? (This can also be considered a true measure of practitioner-system integration.)
- Are CAM practitioners participating in data gathering for national outcomes databases such as Health Employers Data Information Set, a National Committee on Quality Assurance standard?
- Are instruments identified and in use that focus on dimensions relevant to CAM?
- Do evaluations include the assessment of preventive care and early interventions?
- When outcomes measures are developed by the organization, do CAM practitioners participate in that design?

Patient Satisfaction

It has always been extremely important for managed care organizations to collect data on patient satisfaction. CAM providers typically have very satisfied patients. If the focus of a managed care enterprise is to promote patient satisfaction, then obviously these services are appropriate to evaluate. It is possible that the greater the level of successful integration, the more likely that patients will be satisfied with their experiences in the health system. For example, a patient is much more likely to use and to be satisfied with an insured benefit than with an uninsured benefit.

Assessment must be relevant to the discipline being evaluated. For example, chiropractic treatment focuses on musculoskeletal problems of various kinds. The obvious issue is that people do not die from back pain, but they frequently experience chronic pain. They may be unable to work. Using a measure of increased life expectancy, there will be no perceived value in chiropractic. However, in evaluating productivity (the ability to work) or the capacity to perform basic activities of daily living, the majority of the research indicates that there is measurable value in chiropractic treatment for musculoskeletal conditions.

- How rapidly was the patient able to return to work?
- Did the patient regain his or her full functional capacity in performing his or her job?
- What was the patient's ability to perform activities of daily living? What was the level at the initial assessment, midpoint, and discharge evaluation?
- What was the patient's status regarding functional activities (mental or practical activities such as paying bills, cooking, or making a telephone call)?

Outcomes measurement focused on patient satisfaction also ideally include the subjective appraisal of how patients feel about their clinical encounters over and above whether they get better.

This means finding ways to measure the patient's perception of value:

- To what degree did patients find encounters positive on a range of different parameters?
- Was it easy to get an appointment?
- Did their practitioners listen to them?
- Were their questions answered?
- What was the outcome in terms of their health?

Cost-Effectiveness

Organizations that have the ability to collect data on patient satisfaction also have the capacity to move to the next level of analysis, which is cost-effectiveness. An assessment of the balance of cost and effectiveness is developed through outcomes data collection.

For example, the key question in terms of cost-effectiveness and CAM is whether complementary services are additive:

- Do CAM services add extra costs?
- Or do they replace routine medical costs? Which costs were replaced and approximately how much was saved?
- What has been the impact of CAM treatment on the outcome and cost of treating various chronic disorders?
- Do we have a measure of how much improvement was actually achieved?
- Is baseline information on severity available to make a true determination of cost-effectiveness?
- How much health care would have been used in another approach to treatment?

Quality of Service Provision

Well-Trained and Experienced Practitioners

Another concern is that service may be provided in name only. If practitioners lack the depth of training and clinical experience essential to provide skilled CAM services, the benefit of the therapy will be lost. To maintain quality provision of complementary health care, the supervision of a medical director with training and clinical experience in the field is vital. Having quality assurance initiatives in place that are relevant to CAM is also important. Although a managed care organization or health system can market an array of alternative health care for its members, if the members are not finding the services effective, ultimately the benefits that attract consumers to CAM will be lost. Quality can also be tracked by continuing to measure patient satisfaction as an important outcome.

Evaluating Services Using the Benchmarks of the Discipline

As the integration continues, there will be situations in which the parent organization may not realize that the CAM services it offers do not totally reflect the state-of-the-art of the discipline and that its practitioners do not have the in-depth training possessed by practitioners in the field. If the organization is using the benchmarks of biomedicine rather than the benchmarks of that discipline, these shortcomings will not be recognized until customer complaints surface. CAM disciplines would become sham benefits and lose their popularity.

Credentialing is one way to monitor benchmarks of professional quality, but it remains to be seen how that will be monitored from inside the organization. Again, one safeguard is quality medical oversight by well-trained practitioners or by physicians with dual training who are immersed in the CAM field and recognize competence and quality care within that discipline.

CONCLUSION

The primary focus of an integrated health care delivery system is maximizing value for the customer. In the current market, health plans serve two primary customers:

1. purchasers—employers and government
2. consumers of health care—patients and health plan members

From the *customer's* perspective, an assessment of the degree of CAM integration in a health plan suggests that plan's potential to deliver value. From a *plan manager's* point of view, it is imperative to understand how effective integration of CAM health care into mainstream medical care can contribute more than simple market advantage. The potential of effective CAM integration is to increase the value of the plan's product.

CHAPTER 27

Technology Assessment

27.1 Technology Assessment and Potential Applications to Complementary Medicine

Daniel T. Hansen and Robert D. Mootz

Imagine that you are the chief executive officer of a Fortune 500 company. Your company employs more than 8,000 people nationwide, and you are accountable for their livelihoods and their health benefits. You are also accountable to the stockholders and the company's board of directors. New competitors have emerged offshore that can pay lower wages and provide minimal health benefits. They are thus able to deliver a rival, quality product for far less. This past year your organization responded by lowering prices, maximizing efficiency, and reducing overhead costs. Still, sales are down, and three of the last four quarters have been in the red. You

have reduced and stabilized your fixed expenses and optimized inventory and raw materials expenditures.

One cost has not remained fixed, however. Health care expenditures went up 74% in the current year, and you have just received word that just to maintain the same level of benefits for your employees in the coming year, costs are going to increase another 124%. A significant portion of your total health care dollars goes to medical pension benefits for retired workers who are no longer a productive part of the company. Your employee demographics have remained relatively constant for the past 5 years, and the rate of inflation has not exceeded 4% for 4 years running. What are you going to do?

Daniel T. Hansen, DC, is Assistant Medical Director for Quality and Outcomes Management, Texas Back Institute.

Robert D. Mootz, DC, is Associate Medical Director for Chiropractic at the Department of Labor and Industries in Washington state, and editor of the journal *Topics in Clinical Chiropractic*.

Adapted from Daniel T. Hansen and Robert D. Mootz, Formal processes in health care technology assessment, *Topics in Clinical Chiropractic*, Vol. 3, No. 1, pp. 71–83, Aspen Publishers, Inc. © 1996.

A CONTEMPORARY DILEMMA: HEALTH CARE COSTS

If you were to react like most health care purchasers and other consumers, you might start trying to contain and stabilize the escalating costs. What are your options? Letting employees go? Moving offshore? Or, what about seeking new "suppliers" for health care services? Have you ever changed your automobile policy when suddenly faced with a large rate increase? Have you ever stopped buying office supplies from the local stationery store when a new discount store opened up?

In the past, when individuals paid most of their own health care out of pocket, cost containment was very much in the hands of the patient. Today, many patients do not even see bills for services or, when they do, they sigh with relief that most of the cost is dealt with by third parties. In an age of instant information and rapidly increasing technology, patient demand for access to the latest and greatest test procedures, the best specialists, and multiple clinical opinions and options has been high. This demand remained high until employers started to offer employees a range of health plans, with a variety of cost-sharing options. Although free choice and unrestricted access plans are still available, patients and purchasers alike are opting for programs that have small or no copayment requirements and that restrict access to a group of selected providers in exchange for lower premiums.

Similar scenarios are confronting American businesses, employees, and consumers on a daily basis. Many of the fundamental, underlying problems that have contributed to escalating and unpredictable health care costs are only beginning to be addressed. *Health care purchasers and policy makers are asking tougher questions of providers and the health care system at large.*

- Are there any health care services being paid for that are unnecessary or redundant?
- Are any ineffective?
- Are there procedures or techniques that help people heal more quickly or for less money than others?
- If a test or procedure is paid for, will it ensure a better outcome than cheaper alternatives or natural progression alone?
- If a cheaper alternative is found, are the quality and outcome of the service comparable?

- What are the important elements related to quality of health care?
- Which doctors, clinics, and interventions do patients want to meet their needs?

The health care demands on contemporary society require careful, systematic assessment of complex problems along with thorough, reasoned, and coordinated responses from a variety of key constituents in private and public sectors.

Constants exist within all attempts to find solutions. Any potential solution must address cost control and predictability; quality and appropriateness of care; and integration of the needs of patients, purchasers, and physicians into workable delivery and reimbursement systems. The issues are emotionally and politically charged, and everyone from consumer groups, labor unions, physician trade associations, the insurance industry, and taxpayer groups can find special interest organizations that support their perspectives.

There is a clear need for strategies to appraise and incorporate systematically the needs of all stakeholders in the identification and development of solutions. One of the emerging fields in the critical appraisal of complex health care issues is technology assessment. Complementary and alternative medicine practitioners are often in a position of advocating for the needs of an individual patient and for fair practice rights. Both are legitimate needs of a functional health care system. A number of recently developed and evolving technology assessment strategies can serve as tools to help the complementary medicine community navigate some of the issues in the modern health care system.

There is value in reviewing important issues confronting individual practitioners, licensing and oversight bodies, and professional trade associations.

With increased development and application of health care technology, health care costs have risen. Innovations that extend the capabilities of existing technologies are generally more expensive to operate than those they replace. For example, computed tomography (CT) scans are replacing radiographs, and magnetic resonance imaging is replacing CT scans, both at substantially increased costs. General consensus exists that technological innovation is cost-increasing, although theoretically it can be cost-decreasing or cost-saving if a less expensive technology is substituted for a more expensive one, or if the new procedure replaces a variety of procedures. Simple survival is no longer the only important outcome; rather, quality of life and associated costs have become important issues for both consumers and providers (Patrick and Erickson, 1993).

For example, in the field of chiropractic, vendors of technology (devices, procedures, and so forth) have tended to promote their products in the chiropractic marketplace without sufficient testing for efficacy, reliability, validity, and so on. The result has been waves of popularity for devices that claim that they objectify the need for chiropractic care (eg, Moire photography, thermography, surface electrode electromyography, special radiographic studies, and spinal ultrasound). The claims for their objectivity are often accompanied by promises of increased revenues and reimbursement by insurance company. These "constructs" of their applications are typically doctor-centered, in that the applications and outcomes have clear benefit only to the practitioner. They typically do not address the patient's perspective; that is, they do not respond to the question of whether the device or procedure will help the patient get better faster, be more functional, or have an improved quality of life.

METHODS OF TECHNOLOGY ASSESSMENT

Current use of medical technology assessment can be found in government-based organizations and efforts undertaken by various health care purchasers and policy makers. Assessments of technology are an important administrative segment of most health care purchasers, especially managed care organizations. Recently, quality standards developed by National Commission on Quality Assurance have included language mandating that managed care organizations have a process in place to assess health care technologies using formal appraisal methods (O'Kane, 1994).

There are four basic components of a scientific, defensible process for both clinical and coverage decision making. These components are:

1. Outcomes data are preferably derived from controlled clinical trials that support the safety and effectiveness of a specific indication.
2. There is evidence of acceptance by the practicing medical community of specific applications of a technology.
3. There is a rigorous, evaluative process that synthesizes and analyzes outcomes data and expert opinion.
4. There is consistency in the use of terminology, as it is translated from the technology assessment process to coverage policy.

The process must be designed to ensure scientific and methodologic defensibility. Also, it must be designed to facilitate and substantiate the medical and coverage decision-making processes. Last, the process must be designed to enable and expedite the implementation of the managed care philosophy (ie, outcomes-based decision making) within a particular health plan (McGivney, 1994).

Ferrara and associates (1994) state that various methodologies exist for technology assessment. These methodologies are not mutually exclusive. Many organizations have attempted to combine the strengths of several techniques to improve their results.

The randomized controlled clinical trial is the method most familiar to the scientific and health care community. These trials are rigorous and challenging to conduct and involve considerable time and expense because they depend on well-designed research protocols and large numbers of patients assigned in a randomized fashion.

Performance analysis is an examination of the technical performance of a technology with regard to the criteria of reproducibility, safety, and reliability, which are expressed in terms of sensitivity and specificity. From this analysis, a receiver-operator curve can be generated that graphically displays the sensitivity of a technology as it is applied to a specific diagnostic task.

A *case series* is a collection of studies that describes the use of a particular technology for a specific patient condition, longitudinally added over time that includes all eligible patients regardless of outcome. A series may project forward or backward in time. However, a prospective study, especially if a control group is included, is considered to be more reliable even if subjects are not randomly assigned.

Case studies are comprehensive reviews of the medical applications of a particular technology. They include economic, legal, and ethical implications as well as clinical indications. Case studies are often presented as state-of-the-art documents that reflect both a synthesis of the literature as well as the expert, clinical experience of the authors.

Meta-analysis is increasingly being used as a means to combine studies of similar construction to answer questions that have been inadequately or equivocally addressed by a single study. This technique depends on the comparability of studies and requires careful attention to the issue of selection bias due to inadequate sampling and due to the fact that studies with negative results are often not published.

Consensus development is a process whereby a panel of experts arrives at a collective opinion by using group interaction, mailings, or both. In the Delphi technique, opinions regarding a particular technology are collected, and a summary is produced after each round of opinion until a consensus report can be written. A methodology referred to as the forum method (short for the technology assessment and practice guidelines forum) was recently developed in response to some of the shortcomings of the consensus process. It includes some features of the Delphi technique and group process. RAND has pioneered a modified Delphi process to rate appropriateness of a large number of indications for the use of health care procedures. This process involves individual initial ratings of appropriateness, a discussion among panelists, and a revision of rating with the goal of reaching an agreement, when possible, without forced consensus.

An *opinion survey* is a technique in which participants do not interact with each other and a report is generated that reflects the collective judgment of those experts involved. There is no revision of initial opinion.

The importance of proper process has been stressed throughout health care literature, including popular and referred chiropractic literature (Hansen et al, 1992; Clum, 1995; Brook et al, 1986; Audet et al, 1990; Coulter and Adams, 1992). They suggest that responsibility for technology assessment and the associated processes and attributes resides with all stakeholders of health care, especially the practitioners or providers that use the technologies (Goodman, 1994). Thus, to ensure that awareness of technology assessment is broadened and that reports of technology assessment exercises are disseminated and implemented, payers, managed care organizations, device developers, colleges, administrative boards, and trade associations must contribute to practitioner knowledge and understanding. Moreover, consistent with the trend toward continuous quality management, the affected parties must measure outcomes of technology assessment as they regard public health, health care economics, and the inherent resources found in the chiropractic profession.

Health care providers have some obvious responsibility to obtain knowledge through self-learning opportunities. Likewise, professional associations, licensing boards, and chiropractic colleges need to provide focused learning opportunities that enhance learning and understanding. Furthermore, payer groups and managed care organizations have a strong financial interest to see that there is a proper compliance with and favorable outcomes from technology assessment implementation. Thus, they, too, need to offer learning opportunities. Device developers also have an important role to play because they can provide background information on the attributes of the assessment of their respective technology. A number of resources and organizations exist and are readily accessible to doctors, physician organizations, and other interested groups by telephone, mail, and Internet.

Common Misconceptions and/or Faulty Assumptions in Technology Assessment

- *Ignoring the literature.* Consideration of only studies favorable to one's position will undermine the integrity of any formal technology assessment process.
- *Strength of personalities.* Consensus efforts can be overwhelmed by well-informed, articulate, or assertive individuals who may or may not have a good and unbiased grasp of the real issues. Balancing personalities and knowledge bases on both sides of an issue is a must.
- *Preconceived conviction approach.* "If you know you are right, no amount of evidence to the contrary will ever convince you otherwise." While this posture may be helpful for political ascendancy within a trade association, it is bad for the science and explicit process required in technology assessment.
- *"All evidence is created equal" approach.* Studies can be of varying quality and type. The methodologic strength of any given study must be weighed appropriately. Thus, a methodologically good study with dissenting results cannot be thrown out. Likewise, a weak methodologic study with good outcomes must be discarded.
- *Experts-R-Us.* Bringing individuals on board who have impressive degrees or credentials (provided they agree with you) is a strategy that can only backfire in the long term. Often, someone unfamiliar with the ins and outs of a particular field may be bamboozled into supporting something that looks good on the surface, but has no understanding of the substan-

tive underlying weaknesses or issues. Ultimate credibility of a technology assessment endeavor will rest on the process and content, not on who poses for a picture or writes a foreword in the proceedings.
- *Consensus of true believers.* Perhaps the most common error among clinical disciplines is to assume that a fair result cannot be attained unless all parties are unequivocal supporters of the cause. For example, surgical guidelines for spinal fusion developed only by spinal fusion surgeon in isolation might meet with a serious credibility problem. Why should it be any different for practitioners of complementary medicine?
- *Being misled by a good salesperson.* Medical device developers, however well intentioned, must tend to the marketplace, recoup development costs, and show a profit. Often the concern with side effects, scientific investigation criteria, or patient outcomes can be secondary to the need to market a product. Consider the government regulations on new pharmaceuticals that have had to be put in place as a result of past eagerness to bring a drug to market before good independent safety and efficacy research is available.
- *Remaining uninformed.* Technology assessment is not something just for intellectuals. Table 27–1 presents inventories of technology assessment attributes and indicates some of the constituencies that have roles to play. Good information is relevant to all stakeholders.

CONCLUSION

The competitive nature of the indemnification industry in the United States and the need for careful use of limited health care resources require that we carefully evaluate which health services should be available in a given community. Health care system reform requires that systematic processes be applied to ensure cost-effectiveness, safety, and efficiency of proce-

Table 27–1 Role of Various Groups in Increasing Practitioner Knowledge Regarding TA

Assessment/Attributes of Practitioner Knowledge of TA	Individual Providers	Health Purchasers	MCOs	Device/Procedure Developers	Chiropractic Colleges	Licensing Boards	Professional Associations
Education and training							
Level of training	X			X	X	X	X
Critical appraisal skills	X				X		X
Decision-making/analysis skills	X				X		X
Skills displacement	X		X	X	X		
Legal—regulatory							
FDA, NIH, OSHA, NIOSH	X		X	X	X	X	X
Patent law/intellectual	X			X			
Property rights	X			X			
Legal—malpractice							
Malpractice	X		X	X	X	X	X
Informed consent	X					X	X
Risk	X			X			
Strict liability	X			X			
Patient competency	X				X		X
Standard of care	X			X	X	X	X
Organizational							
MCO/facility accreditation (NCQA, Joint Commission)	X	X	X	X	X		X
Ethical							
Informed consent	X				X	X	X
Right to life/death	X						
Access to technology	X	X	X	X	X	X	X
Norms/standards of care	X		X	X	X	X	X
Allocation of community resources	X	X	X	X	X		X
Risks	X		X	X	X	X	X

continues

Table 27–1 continued

Assessment/Attributes of Practitioner Knowledge of TA	Individual Providers	Health Purchasers	MCOs	Device/ Procedure Developers	Chiropractic Colleges	Licensing Boards	Professional Associations
Economic							
Cost benefit	X	X	X	X	X	X	X
Cost-effectiveness	X	X	X	X	X	X	X
Third-party payers		X	X	X			X
Allocation of economic resources	X	X	X		X		X
Personnel displacement	X		X		X		X
Safety							
Risks	X		X	X	X	X	X
Efficacy							
Risks	X		X	X	X	X	X
Cost benefit	X	X	X	X	X	X	X
Cost-effectiveness	X	X	X	X	X	X	X
Dissemination							
Adoption of technology	X	X	X	X	X	X	X
Use of technology	X	X	X	X	X	X	X
Distribution of technology	X	X	X	X	X		X
Educational/scientific constraints	X		X	X	X	X	X

FDA, Food and Drug Administration; NIH, National Institutes of Health; OSHA, Occupational Safety and Health Administration; NIOSH, National Institute of Occupational Safety and Health; MCO, managed care organization; IRB, Institutional Review Board; NCQA, National Commission on Quality Assurance; Joint Commission, Joint Commission on Accreditation of Healthcare Organizations.

Source: Reprinted with permission from G.R. Goodman, Increasing Physician Acceptance of Technology Assessment through a Focused Training Program, *International Journal of Technology Assessment,* Vol. 10, No. 2, pp. 312–316, © 1994, Cambridge University Press. Reprinted with the permission of Cambridge University Press.

dures and devices used on patients. Technology assessment affords a means to critically review available information, as well as to extrapolate from the consensus of representative experts and users. Some of the key issues identified in this chapter relative to proper application of technology assessment include interpretation of evidence, consensus building, dissemination and implementation of technology assessment results, and measurement of effect of the technology assessment on health practice and on society as a whole. There is a risk of misapplying technology assessment that can range from inappropriate use in policy and reimbursement settings to biased efforts employing a facade to disguise a marketer's special interest.

Today's health care system is moving toward a patient-centered, value-driven industry (Elwood, 1988). To navigate through this new paradigm, practitioners, academics, scientists, administrators, policy makers, patients, payers, and device developers will be watching the compass, knowing that the process is open, documented, dynamic, retrievable, and reproducible as new information and opinion yield modification and revision.

The "choice of ages" for the chiropractic discipline appears to be whether to pursue status in the mainstream of health care or to stay entrenched as a segment of alternative health care. The public is beginning to appreciate that manipulation, the principal mode of treatment by chiropractors, replaces other treatment approaches that have long served as the mainstream medical alternatives in mechanical spinal problems. Most insurance and reimbursement systems are evolving to include chiropractic services as a carve-out, replacing what would have been allocated for drugs, surgery, or even hospitalization. In order for other chiropractic methods to gain similar acceptance, and for manipulation and adjusting to be embraced as reasonable alternatives in nonmechanical conditions, rigorous scrutiny through formalized technology assessment process will be a prerequisite. Perhaps the greatest value of these efforts will lie in their ability to focus on meaningful clinical and social outcomes, thereby offering the chiropractic profession an important tool for clinical refinements that focus on quality patient care.

The tasks of the chiropractic professional in the assessment of technologies should be clearer. There should be a heightened realization that chiropractors are not in this situation alone and that their partners include patients, purchasers, managed care organizations, device developers, colleges, licensing boards, trade associations, and other community resources. The tough questions now being asked by the consuming public need to be answered. Awareness and action on public expectations, use of proper methodologies and processes to answer the tough questions, and broad efforts on focused learning opportunities on technology assessment are all agenda items for a responsible place in health care.

REFERENCES

Audet AM, Greenfield S, Field M. Medical practice guidelines: Current activities and future directions. *Ann Intern Med.* 1990;113:709–714.

Brook RH, Chassin MR, Fink A, Solomon DH, Kosecoff J, Park RE. A method for the detailed assessment of the appropriateness of medical technologies. *Int J Technology Assessment Health Care.* 1986;2:53–63.

Clum GW, ed. AHCPR clinical guideline 14: An ICA analysis. In: *Acute Low Back Problems in Adults: An Abridged Version with Analysis and Commentary.* San Lorenzo, CA: Life Chiropractic College of Chiropractic–West; 1995.

Coulter ID, Adams AH. Consensus methods, clinical guidelines, and the RAND study of chiropractic. *J Chiro.* December 1992;29(12):52–61.

Elwood PM. Shattuck lecture—outcomes management: A technology of patient experience. *N Engl J Med.* 1988;318(23):153–155.

Ferrara EP, Servis KW. *State Task Force on Clinical Guidelines and Medical Technology Assessment.* Albany, NY: New York State Department of Health; 1994.

Goodman GR. Increasing physician acceptance of technology assessment through a focused training program. *Int J Tech Assessment.* 1994;10(2):312–316.

Hansen DT, Adams AH, Meeker WC, Phillips RB. Proposal for establishing structure and process in the development of implicit chiropractic standards of care and practice guidelines. *J Manipulative Physiol Ther.* 1992;15(2):430–438.

McGivney WT. Technology assessment and coverage decision making. *J Am Assoc Pref Provider Org.* Sept/Oct 1994:11–17.

O'Kane M. *1994 Standards for the Accreditation of Managed Care Organizations.* Washington, DC: National Commission on Quality Assurance; 1994.

Patrick DL, Erickson P. *Health Status and Health Policy.* New York, NY: Oxford University Press; 1993.

27.2   Resources for Technology Assessment in Health Care

Daniel T. Hansen

FEDERAL INFORMATION RESOURCES

Agency for Health Care Policy and Research (AHCPR)
5600 Fishers Lane
Rockville, MD 20852
Phone: (301) 594-1364

AHCPR Publications Clearinghouse
PO Box 8547
Silver Spring, MD 20907
Phone: (800) 358-9295

AHCPR supports and conducts research on health services, clinical practice guideline development, and technology assessment. The agency also disseminates information.

Institute of Medicine (IOM)
National Research Council
National Academy of Sciences (NAS)
2101 Constitution Avenue, NW
Washington, DC 20001
Phone: (202) 334-2352

National Academy Press
Washington, DC 20055
Phone: (202) 334-3313; (800) 624-6242

This is an organization chartered by the NAS to enlist distinguished health professionals to examine policy matters pertaining to public health.

National Center for Health Statistics (NCHS)
Centers for Disease Control
6525 Belcrest Road, Room 1064
Hyattsville, MD 20782
Phone: (301) 458-4636

This agency collects, analyzes, and disseminates health statistics on vital events and health activities and an annual compilation of U.S. health trends entitled *Health United States*.

National Technical Information Service (NTIS)
U.S. Department of Commerce
5285 Port Royal Road
Springfield, VA 22030
Document Sales, phone: (800) 553-6847

This is a central source for publicly funded scientific and technical information.

JOURNALS

American Journal of Public Health
APHA Publication Sales
Washington, DC
Phone: (202) 789-5600; fax: (202) 789-5661

Business and Health/Medical Economics
Subscriber Services
Montclair, NJ
Phone: (800) 432-4570; fax: (201) 358-2795

Health Affairs Journal
Bethesda, MD 20814-6133
Phone: (301) 656-7401

Health Care Financing Review
Health Care Financing Administration
Subscriptions, Government Printing Office
Phone: (202) 512-1800

Quality Management in Health Care (QMHC)
Aspen Publishers, Inc
Frederick, MD 21701
(800) 234-1660

Report on Medical Guidelines and Outcomes Research
Capitol Publications/Aspen Publishers, Inc.
Alexandria, VA 22314
Phone: (800) 799-0207

WEB SITES

Centers for Disease Control and Prevention
http://www.cdc.gov

Cochrane Collaboration
http://hiru.mcmaster.ca/cochrane/default.htm

Health Care Financing Administration (HCFA)
http://hcfa.gov

Health Services/Technology Assessment Text (HSTAT)
http://text.nlm.nih.gov

National Commission on Quality Assurance (NCQA)
http://www.ncqa.org

National Library of Medicine
http://nlm.nih.gov

PubMed in the National Library of Medicine
http://www.ncbi.nlm.nih.gov

Office of Technology Assessment
http://www.ota.nap.edu/pubs.html

RAND Corporation
http://www.rand.org

Robert Wood Johnson Foundation
http://www2.umdnj.edu/shpp/homepage.html

CHAPTER 28

Research in Complementary and Alternative Medicine

28.1 Methods in Research on Complementary and Alternative Medicine
Jeffrey S. Levin, Thomas A. Glass, Lawrence H. Kushi, John R. Schuck, Lea Steele, and Wayne B. Jonas
28.2 Profile: Research in a Teaching Hospital Integrative Medicine Center
Debra Canfield
28.3 NCCAM Centers and Their Specialties
28.4 The Cochrane Collaboration: Complementary Medicine Field
The Complementary Medicine Program, University of Maryland School of Medicine

28.1 Methods in Research on Complementary and Alternative Medicine

*Jeffrey S. Levin, Thomas A. Glass, Lawrence H. Kushi, John R. Schuck,
Lea Steele, and Wayne B. Jonas*

In 1993, a widely cited study in the *New England Journal of Medicine* noted the "enormous presence in the U.S. health care system" of alternative therapies (Eisenberg et al, 1993). These were defined simply as unconventional medical practices not widely taught in U.S. medical schools or generally available at U.S. hospitals. Such practices increasingly are referred to as "complementary" to emphasize that they may be used adjunctive to or integrated with, and not merely in lieu of, more conventional medical therapies. Concomitantly, the field as a whole is becoming referred to as *complementary and alternative medicine* (CAM).

The authors called on physicians to obtain clinical data on the use of such therapies during patient encounters and looked forward to the promotion of scholarly research on CAM by the National Institutes of Health (NIH) through its newly formed Office for the Study of Unconventional Medical Practices, now known as the National Center for Complementary and Alternative Medicine (NCCAM). Other statements

Jeffrey S. Levin, PhD, MPH, is Senior Research Fellow, National Institute for Healthcare Research, Rockville, MD.

Thomas A. Glass, PhD, is Assistant Professor, Department of Epidemiology, Johns Hopkins University School of Hygiene and Public Health, Baltimore, MD.

Lawrence H. Kushi, ScD, is Ella McCullum Valteich Professor of Human Nutrition, Department of Health and Behavior Studies, Columbia University Teachers College, New York, NY.

John R. Schuck, PhD, is the (late) Emeritus Professor, Department of Psychology, Bowling Green State University, Bowling Green, OH.

Lea Steele, PhD, is the Director, Persian Gulf War Veterans Health Initiative, Kansas Commission on Veterans Affairs, Topeka, KS.

Wayne B. Jonas, MD, is Associate Professor, Department of Family Medicine, Uniformed Services University for the Health Sciences, Bethesda, MD.

Source: Adapted with permission from Jeffrey S. Levin et al., *Quantitative Methods in Research Medical Care*, Vol. 35, No. 11, pp. 1079–1094, © 1997, Lippincott-Raven.

attesting to the importance of additional research on the use and therapeutic effectiveness of alternative therapies followed in mainstream journals, such as *The Journal of NIH Research* (Jonas, 1993) and *Journal of the Royal Society of Medicine* (Ernst, 1995). Original research and reviews of existing work have appeared in other prominent journals, such as *Annals of Internal Medicine* (Cassileth et al, 1984) and the *British Medical Journal* (Kleijnen et al, 1991), and a published NIH report has outlined priorities for research in this area (Berman and Larson, 1995).

Still unresolved, however, is whether conventional research methods can be or ought to be used to evaluate alternative therapies. The editor of a peer-reviewed scientific journal for this field, *Alternative Therapies in Health and Medicine*, has encouraged a reexamination of the fundamental ways in which alternative therapies are studied (Dossey, 1995), and, by its second issue, the journal already had published an article rethinking standard research methods in psychoneuroimmunology (Moyé et al, 1995). Another journal in this field, *Subtle Energies and Energy Medicine*, published a critical review of issues involved in measuring the efficacy of alternative therapies (Schneider and Jonas, 1994). According to an article in *Science* (Marshall, 1994), ongoing controversy and tensions about how research in this area should be designed and conducted were partly instrumental in the resignation of a former director of the NIH Office of Alternative Medicine (OAM) and his replacement by an expert on research methodology (Steinberg, 1995).

A key issue seems to be whether or not the randomized controlled trial (RCT) design ought to represent the "gold standard" for evaluating the efficacy of therapies. There does not yet appear to be either consensus or clarity among scientists and practitioners in this field. Many alternative practitioners feel that their therapies are so unlike conventional therapies and so complex or esoteric that they require different or even brand-new research methodologies and statistical procedures to capture their benefits ad-

equately. Many scientists disagree (Ernst, 1995) and hold to the RCT as the ultimate standard in studying CAM, exemplified by the evolving Cochrane Collaboration on Complementary and Alternative Medicine (NIH Cochrane Collaboration: Minutes of Meeting, Bethesda, MD: unpublished, 1995) (see Chapter 28.4). Other scientists also disagree with the assertion that alternative therapies are too unusual to study with existing methods, but are more guarded in their enthusiasm for the RCT and would prefer less "reductionistic evaluative approaches" (Patel, 1987). An edited British volume (Lewith and Aldridge, 1993) was devoted entirely to scholarly discussions rethinking clinical research methodology in the evaluation of alternative therapies. It is worth noting that debate on this issue is not limited to alternative therapies. An article in the *Journal of Clinical Epidemiology* (Herman, 1995) heralded "the demise of the randomized controlled trial" in conventional medical research. The relevance of and rationale for the RCT have been debated since it was first introduced to clinical medicine.

The vital importance of other types of empirical research on CAM may have become obscured in the debate about how to evaluate alternative therapies. Although evaluation of the efficacy of alternative therapies is a critical and central issue for alternative practitioners and for health policy, the narrowing of the research agenda has served to marginalize other issues that are yet to be addressed satisfactorily in relation to CAM (St. George, 1994). These include medical care utilization, health promotion and disease prevention, and basic science research. Addressing these research issues may require methodologic and analytic approaches perhaps less familiar to researchers whose work has been limited to conducting clinical trials.

Some research studies of these types have been conducted already, and their results have been significant and far-reaching. For example, the *New England Journal of Medicine* (Eisenberg et al, 1993) report on patterns of alternative medical care utilization has been one of the most influential studies of CAM to appear. It has done much to encourage scientific evaluation of alternative therapies and investigation of CAM in general. This study demonstrated the potential contribution of and need for accurate health services information, especially based on national probability data. In general, though, there has been little systematic health services research on CAM in the United States.

Other methodologic approaches also may be gainfully applied to the study of CAM. Epidemiologic studies could serve to document the effects on morbidity and mortality of specific alternative therapies and component health-related practices of complementary medical systems. Social research methods also could be used to test multifactorial models of etiologic or recovery mechanisms proposed by particular complementary systems. For these types of studies to occur, scientists and clinical researchers with substantive interests in CAM first need to be made aware of the variety of methodologic and analytic options available to them, many of which are better known in fields outside of medicine.

This chapter reports on the findings of the 1995 NIH Conference on Complementary and Alternative Medicine Research Methodology. The Quantitative Methods Working Group, convened by NIH for this meeting, consisted of experienced scientists and research methodologists working in academic and government settings. Members were selected for their considerable expertise in the conduct of large-scale programs of health-related research, including the directing of NIH-funded studies, and their knowledge of particular alternative therapies or complementary medical systems. The composition of the working group was diverse, with members representing the fields of social epidemiology, medical sociology, chronic disease epidemiology, psychology, human ecology, and family practice.

It is the intention of both the authors and the NIH that this "methodological manifesto" serve as a nontechnical outline of general principles to frame and guide the design and conduct of empirical research on the efficacy of alternative therapies, on the basic science underlying complementary systems of medicine, and on other issues related to prevention, recovery, and utilization of care.

ANTICIPATED METHODOLOGIC CHALLENGES

The working group began by summarizing anticipated methodologic challenges drawn from the concerns of experts who believe that evaluation of alternative therapies and investigation of mechanisms posited by complementary medical systems cannot be easily accomplished using mainstream research methods. These potential challenges are not unique to CAM, but, on the surface, appear to be problematic for research in this area. They are summarized here to illustrate the issues often raised by alternative practitioners who assert that their therapies or proposed mechanisms are too unusual to be evaluated or investigated through normal or existing means. These potential methodologic challenges include:

- Complex individualized interventions
- Individualization of therapeutic effects
- Focalized effects versus systemic pertubations
- Systemic correspondences and correlations
- Long-term effects
- Reconceptualization of the human body
- Multifactorial etiologies

Complex Individualized Interventions

Many complementary medical systems use multiple intervention strategies that vary considerably in substantive content and/or in application to particular individuals. Such complex and individualized protocols typically are composed of elements that are considered essential to the overall efficacy of the treatment or intervention plan. For example, conventional treatment for AIDS prescribes fairly standard protocols emphasizing zidovudine (formerly called azidothymidine [AZT]) therapy, whereas an eclectic complementary medical practitioner might recommend any of a variety of treatments (eg, dietary change, herbal medicine, acupuncture, hyperthermia, oxygen therapy, counseling and stress reduction, massage therapy), perhaps in conjunction with AZT, whose combination might differ across patients (The Burton Goldberg Group, 1994). It commonly is thought that standard study approaches are inadequate to generate data that allow comparisons between such complex approaches and more standardized therapeutic protocols.

Individualization of Therapeutic Effects

Corollary to the previous point, it is recognized that many alternative therapies assume distinctions among individuals, such that delivery of a single intervention will elicit different responses if administered to different people, to the same person at different times, or at different stages in the natural history of a disease. For example, a specific massage and dietary regimen prescribed for the treatment of rheumatoid arthritis might produce enhanced energy and reduced pain levels in some recipients but a temporary exacerbation of symptoms in others. Such differences in the effects of an intervention also may affect individuals' responses to other, more standard treatments (Inglis, 1965). Again, it is commonly thought that existing research methods are not adapted easily to situations that require assessments of different outcomes in different people.

Focalized Effects versus Systemic Pertubations

Interventions with small direct impacts or effect sizes, when delivered singly or specifically, may produce massive systemic changes (examples: a specific homeopathic remedy, a single acupuncture needle). The direction and magnitude of specific effects on individual markers may not be clinically important to identify or compare, because the intent of the application is

to precipitate systemic response and autoregulatory reorganization (Waldrop, 1992). For example, according to the literature on Bach Flower Remedies, treatment with the water violet formula is said to restore serenity (Howard, 1990). To assess change in serum levels of violet extract, therefore, would not be considered a meaningful evaluation of the efficacy of the treatment.

Systemic Correspondences and Correlations

Pathologic phenomena may be expressed simultaneously on multiple levels of a biopsychosocial system. This is in contrast with the perspective even of systems-oriented thinkers who view the pathogenic process as a chain-like causal sequence or cascade of effects whereby, for example, socioenvironmental stressors lead, in domino fashion, to behavioral, psychophysiologic, immunologic, and histologic changes. According to some complementary systems, equivalently positive outcomes may be obtained by intervening at different levels of the human system. For example, according to naturopathic medicine, mood disorders such as depression may be seen as amenable to treatment through altering dietary practices, drug and substance use, brain biochemistry, hormonal levels, or lifestyle behaviors (Murray and Pizzorno, 1991). After treatment targeting one of these factors (eg, dietary practices), the other factors may correspondingly each revert back or change to nonpathologic levels without further intervention as the person readjusts to a healthy equilibrium.

Long-Term Effects

Alternative therapies are often intended for prevention of illness or management of chronic medical problems whose natural history suggests gradual resolution or long-term maintenance. Interventions may be delivered over an extended period of time, and the duration between the initiation of treatment and the eventual resolution may vary among individuals. There may be other intervening confounders, such as interim changes (eg, in disease status), that may vary among individuals or be undefined by mainstream medicine or too subtle for conventional testing and instrumentation. It is commonly believed that these factors necessarily undermine efforts to analyze data for treatment effects.

Reconceptualization of the Human Body

Many complementary medical systems hold to an integrated view of human beings as unitary wholes whose medical problems cannot be understood in terms of the isolated organs and systems defined by conventional biomedicine (Stambolovic, 1996). Further, many complementary medical systems also have operant beliefs about anatomy, physiology, and pathophysiology that specify a role in pathogenesis or healing for certain phenomena (*chakras*, meridians, *chi*, orgone, auras, "nonlocal" effects) that are not believed to exist by mainstream biomedical science. For example, the assessment of a "subtle energy" such as *chi* may involve unusual instrumentation (Motoyama, 1977) whose operation invokes explanations that apparently contravene currently held physical laws (as in the case of radionics machines) but purports to measure biomarkers of physiologic processes that impact on medical outcomes (Braud and Schlitz, 1991).

Multifactorial Etiologies

Underlying world views in complementary medicine may involve more complex and multifactorial etiologies than are typically acknowledged, even among social epidemiologists and human ecologists, with their "web of causation" concept (MacMahon et al, 1960). Exposure variables or mechanisms that are posited as providing protection or increasing risk may interact with other physiologic, psychologic, and socioenvironmental factors. This situation is complicated further for complementary medical systems that postulate specific effects of phenomena, such as disruption of bioenergy homeostasis, spiritual disturbances, repressed memories, character armoring, *chakra* imbalances, impeded

flow of *chi*, or other unorthodox concepts. In addition, commonly accepted factors may exert nonuniform effects when stratified by levels of these more esoteric variables (Sadler and Hulgus, 1990; Kaptchuk and Croucher, 1987).

Several other issues have been identified in the NIH report on CAM (Cassileth et al, 1995). These included potential challenges related to measuring patients' subjective perceptions of quality of life, investigators' potential disbelief in particular alternative therapies, testing of therapies requiring systematic therapeutic learning, standardization of manual healing methods, use of new or unusual biochemical substances, and investigation of mechanisms that mix physics and biology or are proposed by systems with unconventional paradigms.

Once the working group began its deliberations, two conclusions quickly became apparent. The first conclusion reached was that all of the anticipated challenges basically reduce to two main themes:

1. A "multiplicity" issue—that is, how to study interventions whose particular component parts or treatment effects might vary across individual patients or subjects for reasons inherent to the complementary medical system being evaluated; and

2. A "world view" issue—that is, how to study either efficacy or mechanisms when the constructs, independent variables, outcome measures, and/or proposed pathways represent phenomena that differentiate from current scientific consensus and, thus, may not be believed by mainstream biomedicine to exist.

The second conclusion was that the current methods of testing therapeutic efficacy are believed to be robust in the face of these challenges and that the multiplicity and world view issues can be addressed and resolved in relatively straightforward fashion if a few broad methodologic principles are observed.

The types of problems generally considered to pose barriers to scientific inquiry actually may be the product of attempts to address both types of issues at once—that is, by mistakenly trying to design a single study to demonstrate the efficacy of a complex intervention within the context of or by validating the paradigm that gave rise to the treatment approach. In studies of treatment efficacy, for example, the primary goal is to investigate whether or not the intervention works better than a control treatment. Adding the objective of validating the mechanism purportedly underlying a beneficial effect might serve only to complicate the study design and obfuscate results that would be more visible with a simpler design. It is imperative, especially for researchers in this emerging field, that a particular study question be conceptualized in a way that can be answered clearly, using an approach that can be operationalized and understood by those who do not necessarily share the world view of the investigator. Studies that seek to substantiate a paradigm or mechanism of effects might best be conducted separately and, in any case, will be supported by associations between interventions and outcomes that have been demonstrated independently. Meeting the challenges posed by any study question, however, requires familiarity with options in study design, outcomes measurement, and analytic procedures.

A METHODOLOGIC MANIFESTO

The following recommendations represent general principles intended to inform the work of clinical and basic science researchers who plan to design and conduct empirical research studies that evaluate the efficacy of alternative therapies, investigate the basic science of complementary medical systems, or study epidemiologic, health services, or other issues related to CAM. These recommendations are just that—suggested guidelines, not concrete rules of absolutes. The points are meant primarily to broaden the perspective of researchers in this area and to increase their options and encourage flexibility. A principal impediment to research on CAM has been a narrow casting of what constitutes meaningful research questions and, consequently, an overemphasis on a few particular types of studies. These guidelines are suggestions, not dogma.

The main points of the methodologic manifesto are as follows:

1. Different study questions require different methodologic and analytic approaches.
2. Researchers should use the strongest possible design and most appropriate statistical procedures for a given study question.
3. Clinical trials are not the "only game in town."
4. Results of observational studies can inform the design of intervention trials.
5. Alternative therapies, yes; alternative outcomes, no.
6. Existing quantitative procedures are generally robust for researching alternative therapies and complementary medical systems.
7. Complex complementary medical systems can be studied as "gestalts."

1. Different Study Questions Require Different Methodologic and Analytic Approaches

Any research project involves three distinct and important phases: study design, data collection, and data analysis. The study design that a researcher selects should be very strongly and carefully contingent on the research questions posed—not vice versa, as is so often the case. The study question, therefore, should be stated clearly before proceeding with selection of a study design. The importance of a clear statement of the purpose and specific objectives of any research project cannot be overstated, because it will drive the collection of usable interpretable data.

Studies of therapeutic efficacy, medical care utilization, disease prevention, and pathogenic mechanisms differ in terms of goals, study questions, and outcome variables and, thus, require different methodologic and analytic approaches.

The efficacy of treatment is typically evaluated through clinical trials. Medical care utilization is studied most by health services researchers using survey sampling methods. The associated risk or protective effects of particular factors on rates of subsequent disease are usually determined through intervention studies or observational epidemiologic designs. These include descriptive and analytic study designs, such as case-control, cohort, and case series studies, and encompass prospective, retrospective, and ambidirectional designs. Finally, mechanisms of etiology, pathogenesis, and recovery are investigated by a variety of methods, including surveys, laboratory experiments, and pharmaco-epidemiology. Choosing a method or approach that cannot answer a given question will prevent that question from being meaningfully addressed.

2. Researchers Should Use the Strongest Possible Design and Most Appropriate Statistical Procedures for a Given Study Question

Researchers should endeavor not to settle for less than the best design and statistical procedures possible for a given study question, while acknowledging the financial or institutional constraints of a particular project. A specific intervention may not lend itself to conventions usually considered to be the gold standards of medical research (for example, the double-blind, placebo-controlled randomized clinical trial), but other study designs and statistical approaches still may be appropriate for answering a respective study question. In the case of intervention trials, it may be impossible to blind a practitioner to, for example, the type of massage therapy or bodywork administered to a research subject or to provide a true placebo for an alternative therapy not delivered in pill form. A strong study design still can be achieved in such cases that will produce valid and interpretable comparisons between treatment groups. When in doubt, researchers are encouraged to seek out consultation or collaboration with experts

experienced in designing and conducting health-related studies, such as epidemiologists, biostatisticians, health services researchers, medical sociologists, and health psychologists. Scientists from these fields are more likely to be familiar with the range of study design, methodologic, and statistical options available and appropriate for particular study questions, as well as their proper use.

This is important because different types of study questions are answered by information elicited from different knowledge domains associated with respective study designs and quantitative methodologies (for example, addressing attribution, mechanism, association, confidence, or generalizability) (Jonas, 1996). Questions related to the issue of attribution—a link between an intervention and an outcome—are typically investigated through clinical research on treatment efficacy, using methods such as a randomized controlled trial (for example, a stratified controlled trial of chiropractic spinal manipulation as adjunctive therapy for acute low-back pain) (Hadler et al, 1987). This methodology, however, may not be appropriate for other study questions that are best answered through research using other methods. Well-executed published studies can be identified in the CAM field that exemplify this point.

For example, questions related to mechanisms and associated biologic, biochemical, or biophysical actions or effects are typically investigated by basic scientists using laboratory procedures, as in a study by the Institute of HeartMath on electrophysiologic correlates of intentional emotional focus on the heart in 20 adults subjects (McCraty et al, 1993). Questions related to probabilistic associations between human or socioenvironmental phenomena or characteristics and particular medical or health outcomes—especially where experimental designs are unethical, impractical, or impossible—typically are addressed through observational study designs, such as epidemiologic or medical outcomes research or through empirical social research methods commonly used in medical sociology and health psychology. This was done in an Australian prevalence study comparing systolic and diastolic blood pressures in vegetarian and non-vegetarian Seventh-Day Adventists (Armstrong et al, 1977). Questions related to the confidence merited by existing scientific evidence or knowledge typically are addressed in the findings of consensus conferences, in practice guidelines, or in published literature reviews, through methods such as systemic reviews or metanalyses. A Dutch metanalysis of 107 controlled trials of homeopathy is an example of this approach (Kleijnen et al, 1991). Finally, questions related to the generalizability or extent of use of a particular intervention—and associated issues such as access, cost, feasibility, and patient satisfaction—are the province of health services research and typically are addressed through statistical modeling of outcomes such as rates of health care utilization (for example, a report in *Medical Care* of prospective survey findings detailing differences in rates of utilization of several alternative therapies among respondents with chronic fatigue or diagnosed with chronic fatigue syndrome or fibromyalgia or both [Bombardier and Buchwald, 1996]).

3. Clinical Trials Are Not the "Only Game in Town"

Existing epidemiologic and social research methods are appropriate, robust, and extremely valuable for observational research on CAM, where use of the experimental designs familiar to those who conduct clinical trials would be inappropriate. Many of the problems that face researchers in the CAM field are familiar to researchers in social epidemiology and other sociomedical fields. These fields entail the study of concepts with complex conceptual and measurement challenges equal to or exceeding those in areas of CAM. Examples include the rich epidemiologic literature on health effects of social relationships, personal behavior, and religious involvement (House et al, 1988; Hamburg et al, 1982; Levin, 1996). The tools of epidemiologic and social research also offer a cornucopia of options for scientists posing clinical and basic

science research questions related to the efficacy of alternative therapies or the mechanisms of complementary medical systems. These methods include observational research, systematic survey strategies of various types, probability sampling, multiwave panel studies, and a host of multivariate approaches. The variety of available methods also includes large randomized clinical trials, small randomized clinical trials, nonrandomized trials with contemporaneous controls, nonrandomized trials with historical controls, cohort studies, case-control studies, cross-sectional studies, surveillance studies, consecutive case series, and single case reports. In sum, there are numerous options for researchers seeking to investigate the efficacy of particular alternative therapies or health care interventions (Bollen, 1989; Bentler and Stein, 1992; Moses, 1995; D'Agostino and Kwen, 1995).

4. Results of Observational Studies Can Inform the Design of Intervention Trials

The evaluation of multifactorial etiologic models through observational research designs has been an important source of medical knowledge during the past several decades. This approach is particularly valuable when experimental designs are unethical, unfeasible, or impossible. Such research has helped to identify important factors instrumental in disease prevention, pathogenesis, or recovery that have then been verified experimentally in the laboratory or the community (for example, the relationship between cigarette smoking and lung cancer). In fact, new medical knowledge most often is obtained through observational means, whether through a complex prospective cohort study or through a simple care series. This is typically an important first step in understanding the effect of a previously unconsidered factor on a particular outcome (Hennekens and Buring, 1987).

In CAM research, epidemiologic studies demonstrating the effects of particular exposures or utilization patterns on health outcomes can provide data that will inform the formulation of testable hypotheses and the design of subsequent interventions and studies. Similarly, social survey research studies that use multivariate analysis can identify direct and indirect associations among a multifactorial set of variables and one or more health outcomes. This approach can be invaluable in the identification of covariate factors important to the design of subsequent interventions.

5. Alternative Therapies, Yes; Alternative Outcomes, No

Any type of unconventional therapy—and any type of unorthodox mechanism—can be researched productively, provided that it can be operationalized reliably and validly with appropriately standardized instrumentation. Assessment can be conducted through interview or the use of an evaluation instrument, whether it is electronic, paper-and-pencil, or some other format. It is also necessary that the research design include conventional outcome measures. Independent variables, their measurement, and their demonstrations of reliability can be expressed either in terms associated with conventional biomedical research or with the complementary medical system or paradigm studied. If one can reliably measure an independent variable whose validity can be verified by experts, then indicators can be incorporated into standard research designs. Reliability can be determined, regardless of the unconventionality of the phenomenon being assessed, if the complementary medical system has an identifiable, consistent set of rules for assigning values to quantify attributes of the intervention. This is the standard definition of measurement (Nunnally, 1978). In other words, existing conventional research strategies are robust and appropriate, even when the therapeutics of an intervention are said to be based on unknown or novel mechanisms of action. The unorthodoxy of a construct, conceptually speaking, is not a particular barrier to its psychometric validation and use in subsequent analyses.

CAM researchers are discouraged from using outcome measures unique to the paradigm being studied. Although they may provide useful information to practitioners within the CAM system, they tend to be less useful in communicating findings on the efficacy of a treatment to the wider biomedical community. This is especially true during this early stage of empirical research on CAM. For example, a study designed only to demonstrate that the flow of *chi* is enhanced by a particular therapy would be much less useful than an investigation that also demonstrated a decrease in physical symptoms or an enhancement of psychological well-being—in other words, conventional outcomes associated with the same therapy. We urge consideration of the need for both practicality and credibility in CAM research. Existing outcome measurement already offers a wide range of choices. These include clinical and laboratory indices; rates and ratios measuring morbidity, mortality, risk, and survival; and multidimensional indices of pain, overall health status, physical functioning, symptomatology, psychological well-being, and quality of life.

6. Existing Quantitative Procedures Are Generally Robust for Researching Alternative Therapies and Complementary Medical Systems

One of the most common assertions among alternative medical practitioners is that their therapies or therapeutic systems cannot be studied using existing research designs or analytic approaches. This assertion is usually based on either or both of two arguments—one methodologic and the other more related to the philosophy of science. The first argument is that existing methodologic procedures are incapable of solving particular technical challenges posed by characteristics inherent in CAM. There is little evidence for this view, which may be resolved by the use of any of a wide variety of designs and statistical techniques commonly used in many areas of health-related research. The second argument is that the rules of positivism (that science can deal only with observable phenomena) cannot be applied to the study of CAM because it represents "an alternative paradigm with its own standards, one that cannot be understood or assessed by practitioners of orthodox medicine" (Glymour and Stalker, 1983, p. 963). Therefore, it is argued, existing methods are categorically inappropriate. It is our contention, however, that the phenomena of interest to alternative practitioners are indeed amenable to documentation and measurement and, therefore, qualify as "observable phenomena."

The application of standard research methodologies and statistical procedures is not challenged or compromised *solely* by the unconventionality of the topics being studied. Many seeming challenges to standard methodologies may be addressed through existing procedures. Further, many commonly used but quite complex statistical procedures may be unfamiliar to mainstream and alternative medical practitioners but well known to social scientists and epidemiologists (examples include multiple logistic regression parameters expressed as adjusted risk ratios, structural invariance of latent means in CSM models, and multivariate pooled time-series analysis). New methodologies and statistical procedures are emerging continually, for example, approaches based on nonlinear dynamic modeling that can address complex scenarios when the robustness of current procedures is questioned. Next-generation methods have already shown promise for medical research (for example, chaos theory, neural net theory, graded membership theory, and fuzzy sets theory [Philippe, 1993]). In the context of a rich array of research tools and methodologies, there is a wealth of existing research methods and statistical procedures that can be appropriately applied to the study of CAM.

7. Complex Complementary Medical Systems Can Be Studied As "Gestalts"

Entire complementary systems of medicine can be conceptualized as integrated wholes, or "gestalts," for the purpose of evaluation. Intervention strategies can be designed to study the effects of a multifaceted complementary system as a system, rather than simply evaluating the effects of a single component part of the system. Otherwise, researchers risk imposing a reductionist bias as to what constitutes a whole, evaluable treatment. Isolating a particular element of a complementary system of treatment may distort the effects of both that element and the treatment system as a whole by decontextualizing the element and, as a result, may not provide a meaningful test of the therapy or intervention.

For example, macrobiotics is a Japanese complementary system that considers seasons, climate, farming methods, traditional customs, activity levels, and especially diet as key factors that impact on health (Rector-Page, 1994). The use of macrobiotics in the treatment of prostate cancer conceivably might involve a full regimen of dietary and cooking adjustments; massage; exercise; meditation; and changes in general attitude, clothing, and sleeping patterns. Further, the prescription of these particular elements might vary among individuals, according to criteria grounded in the professional judgment of macrobiotics practitioners. A study of the efficacy of this therapeutic system could consider "macrobiotic therapy" as the treatment, rather than any particular element of the overall intervention.

Several other key points are worthy of inclusion:

- Randomization is a more critical issue than blinding for studies of therapeutic efficacy because of the principal importance of ensuring sample representativeness and generalizability of findings.
- There is merit in defining exactly what constitutes "field investigation." A best-case series design, as encouraged by the National Cancer Institute, might prove useful in the conduct of such studies.
- Conceptualization and measurement of "subtle" mechanisms may or may not be an issue in given situations, because different designs create different requirements in the need to measure variables or mechanisms underlying therapeutic effects.

CONCLUSION

The majority of the health care–consuming public and mainstream practitioners are reserving some judgment on CAM until they have more information. Patients who seek treatment with alternative therapies deserve to know what is safe and effective. If alternative therapies are shown to meet these criteria, they deserve to be supported and reimbursed to the same extent as conventional medical interventions and to have legal restrictions surrounding

their practice relaxed. This can best be accomplished by expanding and improving research in this field. Studies of alternative therapies also would help to clarify for practitioners the specific circumstances and particular patients for which such treatments are appropriate and offer the greatest promise. Progress in the development and improvement of medical practices that do not fall under the rubric of conventional medicine depend on the emergence of reliable methods of evaluation for alternative therapies.

REFERENCES

Armstrong B, Van Merwyk AJ, Coates H. Blood pressure in Seventh-day Adventist vegetarians. *Am J Epidemiol.* 1977;105:444.

Bentler PM, Stein JA. Structural equation models in medical research. *Stat Methods Med Res.* 1992;1:159.

Berman BM, Larson DB, eds. *Alternative Medicine: Expanding Medical Horizons.* A report to the National Institutes of Health on alternative medical systems and practices in the United States. Washington, DC: Government Printing Office; 1995. NIH publication no. 94-066.

Bollen KA. *Structural Equations with Latent Variables.* New York: John Wiley & Sons; 1989.

Bombardier CH, Buchwald D. Chronic fatigue, chronic fatigue syndrome, and fibromyalgia: Disability and health-care use. *Med Care.* 1996;34:924.

Braud WG, Schlitz MJ. Consciousness interactions with remote biological systems: Anomalous intentionality effects. *Subtle Energies.* 1991;2:1.

Cassileth B, Jonas W, Cassidy CM. Research methodologies. In: Berman BM, Larson DB, eds. *Alternative Medicine: Expanding Medical Horizons.* A report to the National Institutes of Health (NIH) on alternative medical systems and practices in the United States. Washington, DC: Government Printing Office; 1995:289. NIH Publication No. 94–066.

Cassileth BR, Lusk EF, Strouse TB, Bodenheimer BJ. Contemporary unorthodox treatments in cancer medicine: A study of patients, treatments, and practitioners. *Ann Intern Med.* 1984;101:105.

D'Agostino RB, Kwen H. Measuring effectiveness: What to expect without randomized control group. *Med Care.* 1995;33(4):AS95.

Dossey L. How should alternative therapies be evaluated? An examination of fundamentals. *Alt Ther Hlth Med.* 1995;1:6.

Eisenberg DM, Kessler RC, Foster C, Norlock FE, Calkins DR, Delbanco TL. Unconventional medicine in the United States: Prevalence, costs and patterns of use. *N Engl J Med.* 1993;328:246.

Ernst E. Complementary medicine: Common misconceptions. *J Royal Soc Med.* 1995;88:244.

Glymour C, Stalker D. Engineers, cranks, physicians, magicians. *N Engl J Med.* 1983;308:960.

Hadler NM, Curtis P, Gillings DB, Stinnett S. A benefit of spinal manipulation as adjunctive therapy for acute low back pain: A stratified controlled trial. *Spine.* 1987;12:702.

Hamburg DA, Elliot GR, Parron DL, eds. *Health and Behavior: Frontiers of Research in the Biobehavioral Sciences.* Washington, DC: National Academy Press; 1982.

Hennekens CH, Buring JE. *Epidemiology in Medicine.* Boston: Little, Brown & Co; 1987:101.

Herman J. The demise of the randomized controlled trial. *J Clin Epidemiol.* 1995;48:985.

House JS, Landis KR, Umberson D. Social relationships and health. *Science.* 1988;241:540.

Howard J. *The Bach Flower Remedies Step by Step: A Complete Guide to Prescribing.* Saffron Walden, England: CW Daniel Company; 1990:29.

Inglis B. *The Case for Unorthodox Medicine.* New York: G.P. Putnam's Sons; 1965.

Jonas WB. Evaluating unconventional medical preferences. *J NIH Res.* 1993;5:64.

Jonas WB. *Medicine and the Mind: Does Methodology Matter?* Paper presented at Evolution of a New Paradigm: Science and Inner Experience, Sixth Annual Conference of the International Society for the Study of Subtle Energies and Energy Medicine (ISSEEM); June 22, 1996; Boulder, CO.

Kaptchuk T, Croucher M. *The Healing Arts.* New York: Summit Books; 1987.

Kleijnen J, Knipschild P, Riet G. Clinical trials of homeopathy. *Br Med J.* 1991;302:316.

Levin JS. How religion influences morbidity and health: Reflections on natural history, salutogenesis and host resistance. *Soc Sci Med.* 1996;43:849.

Lewith GT, Aldridge D, eds. *Clinical Research Methodology for Complementary Therapies.* London: Hodder & Stoughton, 1993.

MacMahon B, Pugh TF, Ipsen J. *Epidemiologic Methods.* Boston: Little, Brown & Co.; 1960.

Marshall E. The politics of alternative medicine. *Science.* 1994;265:2000.

McCraty R, Atkinson M, Tiller WA. New electrophysiological correlates associated with intentional heart focus. *Subtle Energies.* 1993;4:251.

Motoyama H. Physiological measurements and new instrumentation. In: Meek GW, ed. *Healers and the Healing Process.* Wheaton, IL: Quest; 1977:147.

Moses LE. Measuring effects without randomized trials? Options, problems, challenges. *Med Care.* 1995;33(4): AS8.

Moyé LA, Richardson MA, Post-White J, Justice B. Research methodology in psychoneuroimmunology: Rationale and design of the IMAGES-P clinical trial. *Alt Ther Health Med.* 1995;1:34.

Murray M, Pizzorno J. *Encyclopedia of Natural Medicine.* Rocklin, CA: Prima Publishing; 1991:260.

Nunnally JC. *Psychometric Theory.* 2nd ed. New York: McGraw-Hill; 1978.

Patel MH. Evaluation of holistic medicine. *Soc Sci Med.* 1987;24:169.

Philippe P. Chaos, population biology, and epidemiology: Some research implications. *Human Biol.* 1993;65:525.

Rector-Page LG. *Healthy Healing: An Alternative Healing Reference.* 9th ed. Sonora, CA: Healthy Healing Publications; 1994:52.

Sadler JZ, Hulgus YD. Knowing, valuing, acting: Clues to revising biopsychosocial model. *Compr Psychiatry.* 1990;31:185.

Schneider CJ, Jonas WB. Are alternative treatments effective? Issues and methods involved in measuring effectiveness of alternative treatments. *Subtle Energies.* 1994;5:69.

St. George D. Research into complementary medicine: Going beyond the limits of clinical trials. *Advances.* 1994;10(3):59.

Stambolovic V. Medical heresy: The view of a heretic. *Soc Sci Med.* 1996;43:601.

Steinberg J. Alternative-medicine office: A time to heal. *J NIH Res.* 1995;7:34.

The Burton Goldberg Group. *Alternative Medicine: The Definitive Guide.* Puyallup, WA: Future Medicine Publishing; 1994:494.

Waldrop MM. *Complexity: The Emerging Science at the Edge of Order and Chaos.* New York: Simon & Schuster; 1992.

28.2   Profile: Research in a Teaching Hospital Integrative Medicine Center

Debra Canfield

The Hennepin Alternative Medical Division and Clinic are located in a large, multistory ambulatory care center, the Hennepin County Medical Center, associated with one of the teaching hospitals of the University of Minnesota Medical School. Like most academic settings, research is ongoing throughout the institution, and the research component was the first program initiated in the Alternative Medicine Division, which has participated in a wide variety of successful studies. Some of the first research programs in addictions and acupuncture were conducted here and published in the early 1980s. Within the past three years, the Alternative Medicine Clinic also

Debra Canfield has been Operations Coordinator since 1996 for the Alternative Medicine Division at Hennepin County Medical Center in Minneapolis and has also served as public information specialist for the NIH-funded Center for Addictions and Alternative Medicine Research.

has published research focused on short-term outcomes and patient demographics.

Research services relate to a number of major functions:

- National Institutes of Health (NIH) research
- clinical outcomes research
- protocol development
- epidemiological studies
- academic research

RESEARCH CONDUCTED WITH NIH

- *A national center for the treatment of addictions.* The National Center for Complementary and Alternative Medicine (NCCAM) at NIH has recently re-funded the Addictions Research Center at Hennepin County Medical Center, which serves as one of the 11 NCCAM clinical-research centers. The director of the Alternative Medicine Division, Patricia Culliton, is a co-founder of this Center and was the co-director on the original project, one of the two first NIH CAM research centers in the country. Some of the staff in the Alternative Medicine Division and Clinic participate in the research and a percentage of their salaries are paid throught the grant.
- *Participation in government-funded research protocols.* The NIAAA (the National Institute on Alcohol Abuse and Alcoholism) and NIDA (the National Institute on Drug Abuse) are sponsors of addictions-related research in which the Alternative Medicine Center is also active. Current research projects include a study involving Chinese herbs for the treatment of symptomatic hepatitis C and another study evaluating a botanical compound used in the treatment of alcoholism.

CLINICAL OUTCOMES RESEARCH

The Clinic of the Alternative Medicine Division collects outcomes data on all patients. The goal of the program from the inception has been to provide outstanding care and to track the outcomes of our interventions. Every patient who is seen in the Clinic receives medical history forms and the SF-36, which provide the basis for outcomes research and follow-up data gathering.

The availability of good data has aided the development of the Clinic in a number of areas:

- *Demonstrating safety and efficacy.* As an alternative medicine center in an academic setting, we are under the scrutiny of colleagues who are skeptical of our program. If we are to persuade them of its value, we must demonstrate that it is safe and that it works.
- *Providing data as the basis for consensus.* Having quantitative outcomes information can provide the basis for obtaining the buy-in of the medical staff in the context of an alternative model. Data will provide some indication of the value of a range of treatment options. New therapies will eventually be included as options in conventional treatment plans as the data on safety and efficacy accumulate.

PROTOCOL DEVELOPMENT

- *The development of new treatment protocols.* When a patient is seen with a condition that may not respond to traditional treatment, for example fibromyalgia, our clinicians research information regarding the potential effectiveness of an alternative approach such as acupuncture or chiropractic. Recommendations to the patient may be based on internal outcomes data, as well as the medical literature and the staff's consensus.
- *The refinement of existing protocols.* Over time we will be able to determine if one approach is better than another and under what circumstances. This type of research could have a profound effect on the future of complementary medicine.

• *Data aggregation.* Outcomes data focused on the treatment of a specific condition can provide the basis for a range of findings. The data can be analyzed to determine if a particular treatment such as acupuncture is beneficial for that condition. As data accumulate from the treatment of numerous patients with a specific diagnosis such as carpal tunnel syndrome, the research can track the condition, identify utilization patterns, and define the optimal schedule of treatments. The data can be used to answer questions such as, Are treatments to be provided twice a week or three times a week? Will treatments be offered over a three-week period or over six weeks? Treatment protocols can be tracked specifically and in aggregates through information available in the database. As additional data are obtained in follow-up, it becomes possible to determine which approach has been most helpful.

EPIDEMIOLOGIC STUDIES

The research of the Alternative Medicine Clinic and the Hennepin County Medical Center includes data collection that provides the basis for epidemiological analysis:

• Developing in-depth data, including epidemological trends and treatment response
• Gathering data that provide information for future research directions
• Tracking epidemiological patterns that emerge from the data on service delivery, which can be sorted by diagnosis using ICD-9 codes

ACADEMIC RESEARCH

The Division is also considered an appropriate site for participation in academic research because of the diverse client base of patients served from both the inner city and the suburbs. Currently, this Clinic is one of the participants in a multisite federally funded study conducted by Yale University on alternative therapies for cocaine addiction.

• *Research in partnership with other departments.* The Division also works with other departments within the Medical Center, which provides access to a wide range of experts in various fields of medicine. For example, the Brain Institute is another research unit located within the Hennepin County Medical Center. It focuses on the treatment of brain injury and performs research that also encompasses alternative medicine and addictions. Work with the Institute provides an additional venue for our involvement in research.

A RESOURCE TO RESEARCH INSTITUTIONS

The Division's participation in research is based in part on resources that have been developed within the program that we make available to collaborating programs and organizations. As a result, when there is a major research project that involves alternative medicine elsewhere in the hospital, it is often provided through our unit.

Recruitment and credentialing. The Division can recruit well-trained practitioners to participate in the research projects. The credentials of these practitioners have already been verified to confirm that they have the requisite education, experience, and licensure. The Clinic also has the experience to credential new providers, to write research protocols, and to design consent forms.

All of these programs and resources increase the viability of an integrative medicine program, particularly one working within a Western medical setting.

28.3   NCCAM Centers and Their Specialties

Institution/University	Specialty and Principal Investigator (PI)
Center for Addiction and Alternative Medicine Research (CAAMR) Minneapolis Medical Research Foundation 914 South Eighth Street, Suite D917 Minneapolis, MN 55404 Phone: (612) 347-7670 Fax: (612) 337-7367 <http://www.mmrfweb.org/caamrpages/caamrcover.html>	Specialty: Addictions Principal Investigator: Thomas J. Kiresuk, PhD
Center for CAM Research in Aging and Women's Health Columbia University College of Physicians & Surgeons 630 West 168th Street New York, NY 10032 Phone: (212) 305-2009 Fax: (212) 543-2845 <http://cpmcnet.columbia.edu/dept/rosenthal/>	Specialty: Aging & Women's Health Principal Investigator: Fredi Kronenberg, PhD
Center for Alternative Medicine Research on Arthritis University of Maryland School of Medicine Division of Complementary Medicine 2200 Kernan Drive Baltimore, MD 21207-6693 <http://www.compmed.ummc.umaryland.edu/>	Specialty: Arthritis Principal Investigator: Brian M. Berman, MD
Johns Hopkins Center for Cancer Complementary Medicine Johns Hopkins University 720 Rutland Avenue Baltimore, MD 21205 Phone: (410) 516-8000	Specialty: Cancer Principal Investigator: Adrian S. Dobs, MD
Specialized Center of Research in Hyperbaric Oxygen Therapy University of Pennsylvania 133 South 36th Street (6463801) Research Services, Mezzanine Philadelphia, PA 19104-3246 Phone: (215) 898-7005	Specialty: Cancer Principal Investigator: Stephen R. Thom, MD, PhD

Source: The National Center for Complementary and Alternative Medicine, National Institutes of Health, Bethesda, Maryland.

Center for Complementary and Alternative Medicine
Research in CVD
Adult Cardiac Surgery/Thoracic Transplantation
The University of Michigan
Taubman Health Care Center
2120, Box 0344
Ann Arbor, MI 48109
Phone: (734) 936-4984
FAX: (734) 764-2255

Specialty: Cardiovascular Diseases
Principal Investigator:
Steven F. Bolling, MD

Center for Natural Medicine and Prevention
Maharishi University of Management
Fairfield, IA 52557
Phone: (641) 472-7000

Specialty: Cardiovascular Disease and
Aging in African Americans
Principal Investigator:
Robert H. Schneider, MD

Consortial Center for Chiropractic Research
Palmer Center for Chiropractic Research
741 Brady Street
Davenport, IA 52803
E-mail: info@c3r.org
<http://www.palmer.edu>

Specialty: Chiropractic
Principal Investigator:
William C. Meeker, DC, MPH

Center for Health Research
Kaiser Foundation Hospitals
3800 N. Interstate Avenue
Portland, OR 97227-1110
Phone: (503) 335-2400

Specialty: Craniofacial Disorders
Principal Investigator:
B. Alexander White, DDS, DrPH

Oregon Center for Complementary and Alternative
Medicine in Neurological Disorders
Oregon Health Sciences University
3181 SW Sam Jackson Park Road
Portland, OR 97201
Phone: (503) 494-8311; 503-494-4707

Specialty: Neurological Disorders
Principal Investigator:
Barry S. Oken, MD

University of Arizona Health Sciences Center
Department of Pediatrics
1501 N. Campbell Avenue
P.O. Box 245073
Tucson, AZ 85724-5073
Phone: (520) 626-5170
FAX: (520) 626-3636

Specialty: Pediatrics
Principal Investigator:
Fayez K. Ghishan, MD, DCH

28.4 The Cochrane Collaboration: Complementary Medicine Field

The Complementary Medicine Program,
University of Maryland School of Medicine

OVERVIEW

The Cochrane Collaboration is an international group focused on research, whose aims are to prepare and maintain systematic reviews of randomized controlled trials on the effects of health care, and to make this information readily available to decision makers at all levels of health, including administrators, payers of health care, researchers, clinicians, and consumers. The organization began in the United Kingdom in 1993 at Oxford, England, and now has twelve centers, primarily based in academic institutions.

COCHRANE WORK GROUPS

There are three types of work groups within the Collaboration: Collaborative Review Groups, Cochrane Fields, and Cochrane Centers.

Collaborative Review Groups. Review Groups are responsible for performing systematic reviews on specific diseases and diagnoses; currently, there are close to 50 groups, representing disease conditions such as diabetes, depression, upper respiratory tract infections, and musculoskeletal disorders.

Cochrane Fields. Fields reflect the interest of a particular patient population (such as infants) or a specific approach to treatment (such as alternative therapies or physical therapy).

Fields work in collaboration with Review Groups to produce systematic reviews. The Review Group involved is determined by the research question. For example, a review of whether massage is effective in increasing the weight of low-birth-weight infants is performed by researchers working in collaboration with the Neonatal Group. The collaboration between Review Groups and Fields ensures that every systematic review receives input from practitioners who perform that type of treatment, scientists who are experts in research methodology, and specialists in the disease under study.

Cochrane Centers. The work of the Cochrane groupings described above is facilitated in a variety of ways by the work of Cochrane centers. The characteristics of each Cochrane center reflect the interests of the individuals associated with it and the resources made available to them, but all centers share a responsibility for helping to coordinate and support the Cochrane Collaboration. The responsibilities include:

- Maintaining a directory of people contributing to the Collaboration, with information about their individual responsibilities and interests
- Coordinating the Collaboration's contributions to the creation and maintenance of an international register of completed and ongoing randomized controlled clinical trials, thus facilitating the first phase of data collection for reviewers
- Developing successive editions of the Collaboration's guidelines and software to sys-

---

Mac Beckner is the Trial Registry Coordinator for the University of Maryland School of Medicine's Complementary Medicine Program. He coordinates the Cochrane Collaboration registry of randomized controlled trials in the Complementary Medicine Field, as well as the NIH NCCAM databases on CAM in Pain and Arthritis.

tematize and facilitate the preparation and updating of systematic reviews

- Exploring ways of assisting the public, health service providers and purchasers, policy makers, and the press to make full use of Cochrane reviews

THE COCHRANE COMPLEMENTARY MEDICINE FIELD

To meet the growing need for evidence-based documentation in the field of complementary medicine, researchers and practitioners from around the world came together in 1995 to discuss the possibility of joining the Cochrane Collaboration. This effort was headed by Wayne Jonas, then the director of the NIH Office of Alternative Medicine; Andrew Vickers, research director for the Research Council of Complementary Medicine, London; Brian Berman, director of the Program for Complementary Medicine at the University of Maryland; and Klaus Linde, research associate from Technical University in Munich. This effort resulted in the registration of the Complementary Medicine (CM) Field as an official work group within the Cochrane Collaboration by October 1996. Funding of the Cochrane CM Field was awarded through a supplemental grant to the University of Maryland Complementary Medicine Program.

The Complementary Medicine Field at the University of Maryland

The Complementary Medicine Program at the University of Maryland was initiated in 1991 and now has 4 divisions: informatics, clinical care, research, and education/training, with 11 full-time faculty members. This program is one of the NCCAM research centers and a portion of its funding has been devoted to the coordination of the Cochrane Collaboration Complementary Medicine Field. The Field encompasses a field coordinator, a registry coordinator whose role includes database management, a consumer rep-

resentative (one of the points of emphasis of the Collaboration is the inclusion of consumers), and an internationally-based advisory board. Its primary functions are:

- to develop a specialized database/registry of randomized controlled trials in complementary medicine
- to conduct systematic reviews of the literature in all areas of complementary medicine
- to disseminate this information to interested parties, including health care professionals and administrators, as well as consumers

Access

The Complementary Medicine Field can be accessed through the Cochrane Library or through the Web site of the University of Maryland. Resources include databases and the registry of controlled trials for all areas of complementary medicine, as well as a listing of the systematic reviews in this field, plus the CAMPAIN and ARCAM databases. A newsletter on the Web site provides updates on the reviews, as well as recent developments in the Collaboration and the Field.

Information aggregated through the CM Field is available on the Web through the Field's home page under Bibliographic Databases. This provides access to the Cochrane Complementary Medicine Field Registry of randomized controlled trials and controlled clinical trials, which contains more than 5,000 CAM research trials and 1,900 articles. In addition, the CMP registry can be searched on the Cochrane Controlled Trials Register by searching under the keyword "COMPMED."

Additional Databases

The Complementary Medicine Program (CMP) site also includes the Complementary and Alternative Therapies in Pain (CAMPAIN) database and the Arthritis and Complementary and Alternative Medicine (ARCAM) database. All three of these databases can be accessed through the CMP Web site at: <http://www.compmed.ummc.umaryland.edu>.

Cochrane Complementary Medicine Field

William Mac Beckner, Trial Registry
  Coordinator
Complementary Medicine Program
University of Maryland School of Medicine
220 Kernan Drive
Baltimore, MD 21207-6697
Phone: (410) 448-6997
Fax: (410) 448-6875
Email:
  <Mac@compmed.ummc.umaryland.edu>

THE COCHRANE LIBRARY

To provide both an organizational and analytical framework for assembling Cochrane reviews in electronic format, software has been developed by the Collaboration. Several databases are included in the Cochrane Library. One of them, the Cochrane Database of Systematic Reviews, contains Cochrane reviews, and another, the Cochrane Controlled Trials Register, is a bibliographic database of controlled trials. The Database of Abstracts of Reviews of Effectiveness (DARE) includes abstracts of systematic reviews that have been critically appraised by reviewers at the NHS Center for Reviews and Dissemination.

The Cochrane Library is published quarterly on CD-ROM and the Internet <http://www.update-software.com/cochrane/cochrane-frame.html> and is distributed on a subscription basis. The Web site for Update Software is the simplest way to 1) view abstracts for free, 2) purchase the CD-ROM, or 3) subscribe to an Internet-searchable version of the Cochrane Library. Additionally, ordering and price information for the CD-ROM can be obtained by calling Update Software in Vista, California, at (760) 631-5844.

CHAPTER 29

Practical Perspectives on Research in Complementary Medicine

Wayne B. Jonas with Nancy Faass

STAKEHOLDERS IN CAM RESEARCH

Research Supported by the Federal Government

Expanded interest from the federal government has provided funding increases for complementary medicine research, primarily through the National Institutes of Health (NIH). This has stimulated efforts in other sectors as well. The greatest impact of this research is conceptual. The research from the government tends to look at many CAM topics on clinical research and focuses primarily on randomized controlled trials. The NIH most excels at multicenter, randomized controlled trials that can be captured within the networks available to them. They are well positioned to do research in topical areas, such as drug or procedure studies, in which patient samples are available through these existing networks.

Other groups within the NIH are also working collaboratively with the National Center for Complementary and Alternative Medicine (NCCAM) on specific CAM research projects. However, these programs typically function under certain constraints. Most of the NIH Centers have budgets that are already allocated, in conjunction with long-term strategic plans. Typically, more than 90% of their budgets are committed to ongoing research grants. As a result, only to the extent that earlier programs are cut or completed, or that budgets are increased, does the NIH have the money for new projects. Consequently, despite the large overall budget, there is not a great deal of new money going into programs that NIH has not already planned out for a number of years. For more than a decade, the budgets were flat-lined, which caused a sizable backlog of pending projects. Recently, major budget increases have occurred that can partially offset this backlog.

How are we going to capture the data that we need so we will know what works and what does not? This depends on which data we want and how we define what works. The hope is that some of the stakeholders and groups that are profiting or will profit from projects in the field of complementary medicine will also be responsible for collecting data on benefit and harm.

U.S. Pharmaceutical Research

One source of potential research is through the pharmaceutical and herbal companies that benefit from the current labeling regulations for dietary supplements that allow botanicals to be put on the market in a nondrug status. The hope

Wayne B. Jonas, MD, a member of the White House Commission on Complementary and Alternative Medicine, has served as director of the Office of Alternative Medicine at the National Institutes of Health and director of the World Health Organization Collaborating Center for Traditional Medicine.

This chapter is based on interviews with Dr. Jonas.

is that some of these manufacturers will collect research data. However, extensive research is not likely to occur because the profit potential for botanical products is much less than that of patented drugs. As a result, the scope of resources that are committed to drug development is generally not available for botanicals. Rather, the majority of the studies will probably be linked to research and development in conjunction with use patents.

Currently, it is unclear whether manufacturers have any form of enforceable patent protection for botanical products. For example, if a company has a patent on a production process, that does not prevent others from claiming that they produce the same product in the same way and with the same standards, even though it is not necessarily the same product or may not have been produced at the same level of quality. Legal protections in this area are limited, and, consequently, other companies can build on the research of a company that has made an extensive investment.

In the pharmaceutical industry, hundreds of millions of dollars are spent per product. To bring a new drug to market, the current investment can be as high as $350 million, representing as much as 12 years of research and development. Given such an enormous investment, why would a manufacturer spend $350 million on an unpatentable herb, such as yohimbe, when it can develop and patent a drug such as Viagra, particularly if both substances are effective. In the end, the public pays because the unpatented products, such as botanicals and nutrients, are never developed, even though they may ultimately be as effective or have fewer side effects. Currently, an increasing volume of data is being generated on these products because there is some potential for profit, but under the current laws, the level of profit will never be comparable to that of drugs.

European Botanical Research

This raises the question of using European research. In Germany, for example, more research on herbal therapies has been performed. Herbal products have a status somewhat comparable to U.S. over-the-counter drugs, so there is greater profit to fund private research. However, in the past, European research has not been widely applied in the United States, where there tends to be a general bias against foreign research that has been documented in the medical literature. American researchers also tend to favor English-language studies.

There is currently more botanical research available from Europe than from the United States, but those data are not of the same scale or quality as that to which we are accustomed in drug development. For example, even though an herb may be a prescription item under German government regulation, the level of evidence that is required by the Commission E (the equivalent of the Food and Drug Administration) approval is not as extensive as that required for a new drug application in the United States.

Research issues include smaller sample size and issues of quality. In many studies, for example, the outcome measures may not have been the measures that were of greatest interest. They may not have been verified with objective measures. Commission E may perform decision making based on a considered judgment of risk. The FDA and scientists in this country have expressed concern about research issues, such as the reliability of the outcome measures. Another consideration is that Commission E uses information from traditional and historical sources, which tends to be more acceptable in Germany than in the United States.

Clinical Outcomes Research

The third group of stakeholders in research includes those organizations in managed care that are most likely to be able to provide quality monitoring and quality management in practice. They are the entities that are currently performing research, with ongoing quality monitoring as a basis for decision making about which services to provide, what not to provide, and how to modify services. This data gathering is accomplished almost entirely through outcomes research or quality monitoring that evaluates what happens when various kinds of technologies and therapies are applied. The hope is that these groups will be motivated to establish a baseline of data on complementary medicine.

However, outcomes research can be challenging. In outcomes research, it is generally not possible to overcome the confounding factors that are controlled for in random and controlled trials. It is possible to approximate a valid comparison, but without a well-controlled trial, these factors cannot be eliminated.

As managed care organizations begin to implement complementary medicine programs, it will be important if they establish quality monitoring or evaluation programs in tandem with new clinical services. There is a need for various forms of research that can capture and compare benefits across all technologies and clinical interventions.

There is also a need to define the criteria for data used in making medical decisions. Quality assessment systems can be enhanced so that they capture essential information for making clinical decisions, but that means that efforts to capture data must be designed into the program from the very beginning. Evaluation programs must be intentionally developed and prospectively designed to capture the information needed for programmatic considerations and decision making in benefit selection.

When a benefit program is to be evaluated, data can be collected, but it is not true research unless baseline health status has been determined for all clients and the major confounders have been identified. The data cannot simply be extrapolated. For example, data collected to provide a basis for clinical decision making for individual physicians cannot automatically be applied to other types of decision making, such as group benefits, overall statistical benefit, or the potential harm of a therapy. The data may not indicate, for example, the seriousness of the patients' illnesses or how long they have actually been ill. There is no way to determine whether the patients have had other comorbid factors that could have caused or influenced the outcome. To obtain meaningful data, the study must be designed to allow the comparison of groups. In addition, a separate independent evaluation of the outcomes must be performed to capture this type of information.

Epidemiological Studies

If the research involves a large sample size and data are captured on a consistent basis, useful comparisons can be performed through epidemiological or observational research. In these studies, differences between subgroups are evaluated because many of the primary confounding variables have been measured. We can make comparisons and perform statistical evaluations to determine the validity of the comparisons. In this type of research, it is necessary to have a large number of participants and the capability to track data on a large scale.

If the research finds dramatic differences— large effect sizes—a study can be performed with a smaller number of participants. If the effect sizes are small and may be obscured by other factors and variables, very large numbers are required (or the data will be washed out among the noise of everything else occurring). Consider the detection of adverse effects, particularly if they are fairly rare. To detect an adverse event that occurs one in a thousand, you must collect data on several thousand patients over a period of time. This is why we have recently seen drugs removed from the market after they have been approved, because even in a population of 3,000 patients in a randomized controlled trial, a rare but potentially fatal reaction may not be detected. In such a case, it is only when tens of thousands of patients have taken the medication that the problems become evident. Consequently, the reliability of the research depends on the frequency of the event, the magnitude of the difference, and the number and intensity of other confounding factors. All of these issues make detection difficult.

Epidemiological data can be obtained through a number of sources. For example, information from hospital records can be followed up, using the normal types of monitoring systems in place in hospitals. These studies can yield good information. This type of research can also be adapted to complementary medicine. Bastyr University performed a relatively large outcomes study that was funded by the NIH on complementary treatments for HIV conditions. The design involved at least 1,000 patients, who were followed over 2 years. Researchers were able to identify some interesting trends. For example, they found that a number of complementary interventions that practitioners had claimed were very useful in AIDS treatment did not seem to live up to the claims when they were actually tracked through objective outcomes. We need to know what really works for which conditions and for what types of patients.

OBTAINING VALID AND RELEVANT CAM DATA

Biased Data

It is common to find that practitioners have a biased perspective, particularly if they are conscientious, capable practitioners. This is due to the many confounding factors obscuring the cause of results. For example, skilled clinicians typically provide multiple therapies. In addition, if they are gifted and caring practitioners, their patients *will* feel better and get better. Further, capable clinicians are seeing a self-selected audience, which consists of those who have benefited the most from the therapies they provide and, therefore, continue treatment. Those who do not benefit typically terminate care and are lost to follow-up, so the practitioner is seeing primarily the positive results. Consequently, it is difficult for the practitioner to have an accurate perspective on the potential effectiveness of a particular therapy. A physician may believe that he or she is a good doctor because patients come back and say that they are feeling better and getting better, but that does not mean that a particular therapy is an average benefited. Rather, their improvement may be the result of the many factors that go into good and skilled care provided by a physician.

Sufficient Data

The challenge of distinguishing good therapies from good medical practice is something we have learned in conventional medicine over the past 50 years. This is not an issue unique to complementary medicine—it has to do with the nature of data. Conventional medicine has often been disappointed by therapies that were enthusiastically adopted and delivered, only to be shown later that the data were incorrect. That is one of the reasons the medical community now takes such a conservative stance—its practitioners do not want to repeat those mistakes. We have learned the value of science and the difficulties of separating out the effects of particular therapies.

As a result, medicine has learned what type of information we need to make decisions properly. The issue in research is not so much a matter of asking *what* the ideal data are as it is a matter of asking what *kind* of data is *sufficient*. How much data do we need to understand exactly what works and what is contributing to a particular outcome through cause and effect? This issue has an impact not only on study design but also on cost, because the stricter the scientific criteria, the more difficult the research becomes and the higher the cost. As the research becomes more rigorous, there is a diminishing return per unit cost.

How much data will it take for us to know that an alternative therapy is a reasonable approach, for example, for poststroke rehabilitation? That involves value judgments. How can we move forward? When I hear about a new "miracle cure," I find myself asking what kind of data my insurance company would need to say that they should provide this treatment, that they should reimburse for it, and that they should accept it (or not). I also wonder about what kind of proof of effectiveness members of my family would want to make fundamental medical decisions. The answer to that question is different for different groups. Sometimes, it is different for different people.

We should consider whether we can set reasonable standards that are at least useful for different types of groups. We know that these criteria do not meet everyone's standards for all purposes, but that they meet the standards of a particular population.

RESEARCH IN COMPLEMENTARY MEDICINE

It is possible to build a baseline data collection into both new and existing programs. Many hospitals and HMOs now collect baseline information as part of their standard procedures, as well as providing quality assessment. The same approach to record keeping and data gathering should be provided for complementary medicine as these programs are brought into the mainstream. It is possible that the larger hospitals will track the data, but smaller hospitals may not. Some of the larger health care plans will also probably participate in this type of data capture. It would be useful if this research and data gathering could be encouraged by the provision of government incentives.

Currently, the NIH has funded some studies through NCCAM. David Riley, a practitioner in Santa Fe, has collected outcomes data comparing treatment by several thousand homeopathic patients with those of conventional medicine to evaluate the outcomes for various conditions. At the King County Clinic in the Seattle area, comparative data are being gathered on naturopathic and biomedical treatments. This center is a public health clinic that provides naturopathic medicine and acupuncture. The outcomes collection and monitoring that are occurring there are specifically focused on CAM. The goal is to learn what kinds of data can be obtained, how it can be used, and whether it is sufficient

to provide a basis for making various kinds of medical decisions.

Numerous groups in Europe are also performing this type of research. At the University of Munich, a research team led by Dieter Melchart is gathering outcomes data from spa hospitals and Chinese hospitals in Germany. They have collected systematic data on thousands of patients. Another group at the University of Freiberg, under the direction of Harald Walach, has been working with German insurance companies. The insurers are willing to fund alternative treatments if data collection is performed to document the outcomes.

We now have outcomes measures that are to be quite reliable. The SF-36 is disease-independent and therefore relevant to a range of applications in tracking treatment programs, but does not track prevention. There are many other instruments that look at quality of life and health outcomes. Some of them have been well validated and collected on very large numbers of patients; others have not. Their reliability determines their utility as a basis for comparisons with findings between interventions. In Scotland, Reilly has developed a measure, the Glasgow Homeopathic Outcomes Scale, through which he collects ongoing outcomes data on quality of life, changes in symptoms, and other variables in groups of patients undergoing complementary treatment. This is an example of a scale that attempts to capture a broad perspective, making it more useful for complementary medicine. This instrument is now being used by some researchers in Europe and a few in the United States.

It is anticipated that, in the United States, some of the larger health plans will begin to collect data on some of the services they provide. However, their data will capture and reflect only a small portion of the larger CAM market. Reimbursement is also predicted to increase on a limited scale. Funders may expand their benefits packages to include a certain number of acupuncture or chiropractic visits or massage sessions. They may or may not include herbal supplements, and they may or may not include homeopathic care. Different limited packages are likely to be provided by insurers. This variability may ultimately result in outcomes data from different types of therapeutic packages.

Currently, all of the offerings are primarily focused on disease treatment. It will be of interest to see how the current endeavors develop and whether they will begin to provide data on health promotion.

ORGANIZATIONAL STRUCTURES

PART VIII

Networks

CHAPTER 30

An Overview of Network Structures and Functions

30.1 Network Structures and Functions
    Charles A. Simpson
30.2 Checklist: Evaluating Specialty Plans, PPOs, and Other Types of Networks
    Marla Jane Orth

30.1   Network Structures and Functions

Charles A. Simpson

INTRODUCTION

Beginning after World War II, the increasing prevalence of third-party reimbursement for health care changed the landscape of medical practice forever. Recent reforms of the market by managed care have further altered fundamental relationships among patients, their practitioners, and those who pay the bills. One aspect of these transformations has been the consolidation of individual solo-practitioner practices into physician groups and a diversity of combinations of physicians and physician groups into still larger organizations.

As mainstream medical physicians have come to be organized in order to participate in managed care, so, too, have CAM practitioners begun to develop organizations that can integrate effectively into the variety of managed care arrangements. Many of these organizations are modeled on their medical predecessors. They display a breadth and diversity of structure,

function, and financial relationships that are sometimes difficult to characterize.

CAM Practice and CAM Insurance Coverage

CAM providers historically have been in a financial relationship with their patients that is reminiscent of health care before the advent of third-party reimbursement. Cash-based practice has been, and continues to be, the rule in financing CAM services. A survey of Eisenberg et al (1993) revealed that 75% of CAM services were paid for out of pocket, without the benefit of insurance reimbursement.

Insurance coverage is a relatively new innovation for most CAM providers. Some CAM disciplines, such as chiropractic, have enjoyed increasingly respectable levels of recognition and reimbursement over the years. Other CAM disciplines, such as massage therapy, naturopathic medicine, and homeopathy, however, have yet to gain a foothold at the insurance payment threshold.

Opportunities and challenges have developed for CAM practitioners as the market moves from this history of cash-based reimbursement

---

Charles A. Simpson, DC, is a founder and Chief Medical Officer of Complementary Healthcare Plans of Portland, Oregon.

toward increasing measures of financial integration within health systems as they play out in managed care. Many practitioners do not have the technical resources to develop an effective billing system. Having grown up in a cash-based economy, not all CAM practitioners understand the fundamentals of communicating with institutional payers or may be unfamiliar with appropriate use of Current Procedural Terminology (CPT) coding systems and the International Classification of Diseases (ICD-9). Limitations in the communication of clinical and financial information that health systems depend on for routine operation can be a significant barrier to participation in organized systems. To be effective partners in managed care arrangements, networks devote significant resources to educating CAM practitioners in these fundamental communication techniques.

MANAGING FINANCIAL RISK

The fundamental innovation of all managed care strategies is to make providers and consumers of health care more sensitive to the costs of that care. Cost accountability has been approached in a variety of ways, each with its own characteristics of financial risk to the participants: payers, practitioners, and patients. The structuring of health care benefits incorporates the drive to accountability and hoped-for efficiency and cost savings. Various designs have been implemented in CAM benefit offerings by health plans. Each represents differing degrees of financial integration and financial risk management. Each has different implications for payers, practitioners, and patients with respect to their financial obligations.

DISCOUNT (AFFINITY) BENEFITS

Discount benefits can be considered an initial level of financial integration of CAM providers into managed care systems. This approach uses negotiated fee schedules to provide discounted services to plan members but not as an actual insurance benefit. This allows health plans to offer CAM services but experience no financial risk for CAM utilization. Members seek services from practitioners who may be prescreened and credentialed providers, thus assuring some measure of quality. Payment for services is directly from the patient in cash. The patient experiences the benefit of a negotiated discount. The health plan carries no risk for the use of CAM services by their members.

In discount/affinity arrangements, CAM practitioners experience financial incentives essentially similar to those that operate in cash-based, fee-for-service health care. However, practitioners who participate in the panels accept a cut in payment in exchange for the benefit of marketing to plan members and for driving increased patient volume. In that transactions are strictly cash, there is little or no opportunity to capture potentially valuable utilization, quality, or other data.

In health care, affinity benefits have come to include a wide array of health care and wellness services. The growth of this affinity benefit approach gained notice when Oxford Health Plans became one of the first nationally known health maintenance organizations (HMOs) to offer CAM services. CAM providers are identified and organized to one degree or another into credentialed networks. Members of the health plan have access to these credentialed providers, with the added value of some assurance of access to quality providers. This strategy may be seen as beginning the process of integration. Weeks (1998) identifies the basic elements of this approach:

• The product is not a covered benefit but a "value-added" service.
• The network of providers contracts at a 10% to 25% discount.
• Providers are credentialed, giving confidence to consumers or purchasers who may want some guidance as to the disciplines and practitioners among the array of alternatives that have received a certain level of scrutiny.

- The member or individual consumer usually (but not always) pays an annual fee. In some cases, access to discount panels is made available to the public at no charge as a form of marketing for the health plan (for example, Blue Shield of California).
- The fee is discounted if paid by a larger group (such as an employer or a health plan).

Affinity benefits have been a part of many service sector industries for quite some time. Frequent flier plans with most airlines, for example, have accompanying "affinity benefits," ranging from discounts on car rental and lodging to access to specialized credit cards and telecommunications services. Companies view this "value-added" approach as a cost-effective way to build customer loyalty and enhance product offerings without the added overhead of intensive product development.

PREFERRED PROVIDER ORGANIZATIONS AND INDEPENDENT PRACTICE ASSOCIATIONS

Basic Definitions

Independent practice associations (IPAs) have been defined as networks of independent practices, typically within a single therapeutic specialty, such as chiropractic (Vickie Ina, written communication, June 1999). Participants in the network have contractually organized themselves to negotiate contracts with health plans and employers. These practices may also work with programs such as workers' compensation, disease management organizations, or other IPAs. They are generally able to provide their services based on fee-for-service or a capitated risk-based agreement. The IPA normally establishes a fee schedule for contract negotiations with health plans and medical groups. These provider groups are also able to accept risk and negotiate reimbursement rates. Examples of this type of model are:

- Acucare—a statewide network of acupuncturists
- AcuNet—an affiliation of acupuncturists throughout California that contracts with managed care organizations

Organizational Structures: CAM PPOs and IPAs

With the maturation of managed care, two basic types of physician organizations have emerged: the individual (or independent) practice associations and preferred provider organizations (PPOs). These organizations are defined classically in terms of their ownership, governance, structure, functions or services, and the financial relationships among the patients, practitioners, and the payers.

The IPA is characterized by Wagner (2000) as an organization that contracts with a health plan on a capitation basis and, in turn, contracts to pay physicians for services on a fee-for-service or a capitation basis. He contrasts this model with the PPO, which essentially pays physicians directly on a discounted fee-for-service basis. The PPO arrangement also typically involves incentives for patients to seek care from PPO (preferred) practitioners and may or may not bear risk. Although these definitions may be useful conceptual models, in reality, the nature of practitioner organizations that have emerged in the diverse managed care arena defies ready characterization and precise definition.

The fundamental distinctions between IPAs and PPOs, as characterized by Wagner (2000), have become obscure with the development of a wide variety and diversity of practitioner networks. A recent evaluation by the American Association of Preferred Provider Organizations (Greenrose, 2000) documents a wide range of organizational structures and functions that all reputedly fall under the umbrella of the PPO.

ECONOMIC FUNCTIONS OF PPOS

Medical PPOs have arisen in the gap between traditional fee-for-service delivery and financially managed HMOs. Traditional features of PPO arrangements have been agreements among purchasers, payers, and providers to offer services to insureds at a discount or subject to utilization management controls of the PPO. Patients may be free to obtain services outside the network of contracted providers but usually with disincentives for seeing these "nonpreferred" providers.

Characteristics of PPOs

Wagner (2000) has identified several key features of PPOs:

- *Select provider panels.* PPOs seek to manage cost and quality by selecting high-value providers, those delivering high-quality care at low cost.
- *Negotiated payment rates.* PPO participation agreements require providers to accept payment from the PPO as payment in full for services. PPOs seek to negotiate rates with providers that produce a competitive advantage, relative to the rest of the market.
- *Rapid payment terms.* PPOs frequently offer participation incentives to providers in the form of commitments to prompt payment for services. Turnaround time on bills is reduced for the provider, in return for discounts from usual and customary fees.
- *Utilization management.* Many PPOs offer payers assurance of cost control through various utilization management strategies. Preauthorization of services and a variety of diagnosis-based treatment algorithms are used to restrain utilization.
- *Consumer choice.* The health care consumer is usually free to seek services outside the network of preferred providers. Use of these nonpreferred services, however, comes at increased cost to the consumer in the form of deductibles, higher copayments, or reduced benefits. Preferred services may be covered at 80%, with only a small copay. Nonpreferred services, in

contrast, would be covered at a lower percentage, for example, 60%, with a larger copayment at the time of service.

Managed care organizations have frequently been compelled by outside forces to build relationships with CAM providers. Statutorily mandated benefits, such as insurance equality laws, for example, have induced managed care plans to offer certain CAM services—typically, chiropractic. Workers' compensation systems also frequently mandate the availability of some CAM services—again, most often, chiropractic. Organizations in these arenas have come to adopt PPO relationships as an effective way to integrate CAM providers in response to these mandates. PPOs have pursued two basic approaches to offering the services of CAM providers: contracting with individual CAM practitioners or seeking out existing networks of CAM providers for contracting.

Traditionally, PPOs have developed strategies to identify cost-effective, high-quality medical providers to bring into the network of preferred providers. Medical managers in PPO settings have felt confident in their ability to recognize "good care" from orthodox medical providers and to be able to identify those providers who render it. Similarly, utilization and quality management issues are familiar ground for PPO medical directors and others concerned with medical management. Each individual provider is credentialed by the PPO according to well-known medical criteria. Each provider's utilization is managed by the PPO. This same model has been used by many managed care organizations in the assembly of PPO panels of CAM providers.

CAPITATING CAM IN HMO ENVIRONMENTS

Networks of Managed Care Organizations— Basic Definitions

Managed care or integrated networks are administrative organizations that establish, contract, and manage services provided by practitioners in their networks (Vickie Ina, written communication, June 1999). Within complementary medicine, these organizations typically consist of a group of health care administrators who set up panels and networks and provide credentialing. Many are able to accept capitation and risk for their network, but this will vary from state to state, depending on the specific regulatory requirements of state law.

In contrast, IPAs (and, in some cases, PPOs) are managed by the practitioner-members themselves. Managed care organizations (MCOs) within complementary medicine usually provide health care services that include a number of major alternative disciplines. Operations are usually supervised by the network, through a team made up of administrators and clinicians. They contract with health plans and employers and provide utilization and quality management services for their network. Examples of managed care networks include:

- Alignis—a nationwide MCO that provides a network of chiropractors
- Alternare—an MCO that provides services in Washington state. It has a significant breadth of providers available to members through participation in their managed care programs
- OneBody.com—a California-based MCO providing complementary medicine and wellness services on a nationwide basis through both physician and nonphysician providers
- Landmark—a California-based MCO that offers primarily acupuncture and chiropractic services, with expansion into massage and nutrition

Provider Risk Sharing

As the needs of providers, patients, and payers are considered in turn, MCOs have implemented a number of strategies to sensitize physicians and other practitioners to the costs of care. For example, capitation arrangements for primary care physicians are structured, in part, to realign the incentives for a provider's use of health care resources. Rather than seeing the provision of more care as a direct source of increased revenue, capitation compels providers to regard utilization not as revenue, but as expense.

This cost-consciousness, however, also bears the burden of potential underutilization of health care. The withholding of appropriate care to restrain cost risks the consequent sacrifice of quality of care for the patient. The challenge for providers is to strike a balance between constant mindfulness of cost and the assurance of a continuing focus on the highest quality of health care for the patient. It can be suggested that seeking this balance provides the greatest value for the purchaser in the delivery of health care. Success in managed care is the maximization of value for the "customers" of the enterprise—both patients and purchasers. The extent to which practitioners support this ideal and the extent to which the systems in place facilitate it provide an accurate measure of integration.

The ability of providers to accept and manage risk is the hallmark of provider–system integration in the financing of health care. The power of capitation is its ability to sensitize providers to the costs of care. This radical shift of incentives away from the provision of care as representing a revenue stream and toward incentives for the economic use of health care services that come to be seen as health care expense brings providers more into harmony with the desires of the other stakeholders in the managed care enterprise to maximize efficiency—the greatest number of "units" of health care for the available "units" of health care resources.

Capitation and CAM

More fully integrated health care systems rely heavily on risk sharing with individual practitioners and with groups of practitioners. Financial integration of CAM providers in this model has been achieved with some of the CAM disciplines, notably, chiropractic in some settings. The ability of either CAM provider groups or MCOs to accept or share risk has been limited by two essential factors: inadequate provider group organization and lack of practical understanding concerning CAM practices. CAM practitioners traditionally have not been organized to accept risk. As noted previously, they may lack the essential knowledge of the process of communicating with health care plans. Managed care organizations lack experience with CAM services and, consequently, do not have the actuarial data and other technology to share risk confidently with CAM providers.

Health plans are confronted with the dilemma that both patients and purchasers are asking for prepaid CAM services, but the plans themselves are unable to price a capitated benefit. A recent Capitation Management Report (Alternative Medicine, 1998) noted "the problem is that consumer demand for CAM has overtaken the availability of utilization data, and providers are loathe to accept risk for member populations without historical experience." Given these uncertainties, plans have opted for reimbursement strategies other than capitation, such as discount affinity benefits (discussed previously) or restricted access to CAM through referral from risk-bearing primary care physicians.

In the absence of effective risk-sharing arrangements, numerous alternative avenues to financial integration are being pursued. In terms of integration per se, the assortment of financial relationships that have been implemented in a variety of settings represents clearly different measures of integration, but all can be seen as mechanisms to bring CAM into MCOs.

Case Study: Capitated Chiropractic

As individual physicians and physician groups have struggled with risk bearing, so too have CAM providers begun the process of rationalizing the use of health care resources. An early effort to capitate a CAM benefit was the development of a relationship between Kaiser-Permanente Northwest (KPNW) and ChiroNet, a chiropractic IPA based in Portland, Oregon.

KPNW is a respected group model HMO in the Pacific Northwest that has its historical roots in the Kaiser shipyards in the Portland area. For years, KPNW was the sole source of managed care in Oregon and Southwest Washington. It enjoyed a reputation for quality care and affordable prices for decades preceding the market-driven health care reform of the 1980s. The advent of new HMOs in Portland presented KPNW with major competitive challenges. In a concerted attempt to reinforce its position in the Portland market, KPNW proceeded with focus group activities among its clients to identify their needs and desires. Member requests for a chiropractic benefit were the impetus for an alliance between KPNW and ChiroNet.

To date, CAM services are available to purchasers affiliated with KPNW on the basis of an added-to-premium rider benefit, on top of the usual capitated health care service offerings. An array of benefit designs with various levels of copayment requirements, dollar caps, or limits on number of visits permits the health plan to offer its customers several options for CAM coverage. Table 30.1–1 provides a few of these arrangements. As experience with CAM benefits accumulates and confidence in ChiroNet increases, the intention is to incorporate the chiropractic benefit into the core benefit offering for all members.

BARRIERS TO FINANCIAL INTEGRATION

In managed care settings, the integration of CAM providers is sometimes inhibited by the nature of CAM practice. The typical CAM practitioner is in solo practice, in a partnership, or in a small group setting. Achieving effective financial integration out of this context is difficult, at best. The ability to accept and manage risk is nonexistent for solo or small-group practitioners. The development of larger, better-organized provider groups has proved to be a necessary precursor to financial integration beyond the cash discount models of affinity benefits or discounted fee-for-service PPO arrangements. As conventional physicians have responded to this need with the formation of group practice

Table 30.1–1 Network Models

Setting	Access Model	Utilization
Regional HMO, contracted network of CAM practitioners	Primary care provider—referral for specified clinical conditions	Approximately 1 patient per 1 million members
National CAM MCO—Practitioners contracted with various payers	Direct access, preauthorized services	Approximately 4 patients per 1 million members
Regional IPA contracted for prepaid HMO members	Open access (direct access, no preauthorization)	Approximately 6 patients per 1 million members

and associations of individual practices, so, too, have CAM providers begun the process of joining together into larger and larger groups. It is predicted that this trend will gradually set the stage for the potential of more complete and effective integration of CAM providers.

Another barrier to effective financial integration that confronts CAM practitioners is the perceived ethical challenge inherent in prepaid, capitated health care. CAM practitioners pride themselves on their traditional role as advocates for patient care. In their usual cash-based financial relationship with patients, CAM practitioners have cultivated a heightened sensitivity to a patient's willingness to pay for health care services. This has been addressed throughout the history of CAM practice by an intense focus on the patient as a customer. This exhaustive patient-centered approach probably underlies the findings of very high levels of patient satisfaction with CAM care. Patient loyalty has not unexpectedly produced most of the current consumer demand for CAM services in managed care programs.

THE PROVIDER'S PERSPECTIVE

From the CAM provider's perspective in a health system, the basic relationship between the practitioner and his or her patient is fundamentally challenged. This dilemma has not escaped the attention of orthodox medical practitioners, either. Kassirer (1998) describes this double bind, wherein the provider in a managed care arrangement becomes both an advocate for the individual patient's need for care and an agent for the financial success of the health plan. He worries that trying to care for a population of patients within a global budget, represented by capitation payment methodologies, requires providers to become "agents for the plan instead of agents for their patients." Many CAM providers look at the experiences of their orthodox medical colleagues who are caught on the horns of this dilemma and simply choose to remain in the status quo and to accept only fee-for-service cash payment. However, this approach creates a circumstance that frequently limits the pool of potential patients to those who have disposable income. It unavoidably promotes underutilization of CAM services.

Countervailing motives also exist, however, that drive CAM practitioners to creating relationships with managed care. As increasing numbers of Americans have their health care purchased exclusively through managed care plans, access to CAM services becomes increasingly difficult. CAM practitioners who hold to the vision of expanding the availability of their services to the public must necessarily work toward resolving this dilemma.

CONCLUSION

Transformation of health care delivery in the United States has been rapid and thorough, and all aspects of the health system have been affected in the ongoing process. Practitioners, patients, and payers have had to adapt to new relationships and accountabilities. As CAM has assumed a greater role, it is inevitable that the impact of health care reforms and managed care have also affected CAM practitioners.

Complementary medicine networks reflect the diversity and variety of structures and functions seen in these same organizations in mainstream medicine. As with their mainstream counterparts, networks of CAM practitioners seek to meet the needs and requirements of the reformed health care marketplace. As health care markets move to make CAM services more readily available and as CAM practitioners become more fully engaged in health care delivery systems, the imperative will increase for CAM networks to maximize their effectiveness on behalf of all stakeholders—patients, payers, and providers.

REFERENCES

Alternative medicine: A big unknown under capitation. *Capitation Management Report.* 1998;5(6). Marietta, GA: National Health Information, LLC.

Eisenberg DM, Kessler RC, Foster C, et al. Unconventional medicine in the United States. *N Engl J Med.* 1993;328(4):246–252.

Greenrose K. *Rise to Prominence: The PPO Story.* Washington, DC: American Association of Preferred Provider Organizations/URAC; 2000.

Kassirer JP. Managing Care—Should we adopt a new ethic? *N Engl J Med.* 1998;339.

Wagner ER. Types of managed care organizations. In: Kongstvedt PR, ed. *The Managed Health Care Handbook,* Fourth Edition, Gaithersburg, MD: Aspen Publishers; 2000: 28–41.

Weeks J. *Alternative Medicine Integration and Coverage.* 1998;2(12). Reston, VA: St. Anthony's.

30.2 Checklist: Evaluating Specialty Plans, PPOs, and Other Types of Networks

Marla Jane Orth

Specialty networks require industry-specific clinical and administrative expertise that is different from the traditional medical insurance model. Health plans or employers considering the inclusion of CAM services and products in their benefit designs need to scrutinize carefully their options by asking, then evaluating answers to, critical questions. A few of the more important points to consider are summarized below

Marla Jane Orth, MS, MPH, is a consultant who provides health management, organizational development, and capital investment expertise to a broad array of constituents and is the former President/CEO of Landmark Healthcare, Inc.

OPTIONS FOR EVALUATION

Infrastructure

- Does the network demonstrate sufficient administrative infrastructure to discharge all of the legal, financial, medical, marketing, membership servicing, and contractual responsibilities of managing a successful network?
- Is there a financial structure in place that includes checks and balances over financial accounting methods? Are there sufficient operating reserves in place to cover anticipated medical and administrative costs by the network? Are the network principals, officers, and directors bonded? Are there

documented provisions in place to ensure protection in the event of an insolvency, so that your members will be protected? Are there mechanisms in place to ensure continuity of care for your members if there is an action by regulators, an event of insolvency, or a reorganization that causes services to be discontinued?

- Does the network demonstrate sufficient capitalization to achieve and maintain financial break-even and fiscal solvency on a continuous basis?
- Does the network demonstrate the ability to service your members' or employees' needs adequately? Do they offer a toll-free number that is staffed at least 12 hours a day? Is the call center professionally staffed with trained personnel, and supported to handle volume requirements?
- Determine how the network handles inquiries from practitioners regarding patient eligibility and coverage inquiries, including limitations, copayments, and other requirements; authorization of care; and other specifics. Is there a call center that is professionally staffed, to handle inquiries from the *professionals* in the network, given its size?

Regulatory Compliance

- Are the networks appropriately licensed to do business in the states in which they operate? Is the network licensed or is the license rented from another entity? Are there any restrictions placed on the licenses or any limitations on the network's ability to operate within a particular state? Is there any licensure action or investigation in progress or pending?
- Do not be shy. Ask for copies of state filings to ensure compliance or make inquiry of the state licensing authority for verification of compliance with rules and regulations. Also ask to be provided with a summary of complaints, as applicable, from clients, members, practitioners, or the public at large.

In many states, these are a matter of public record.

Governing Boards/Committees

- Does the network have representation (beyond ownership interests) of persons from the business community, practitioner community, patients or members, and other stakeholders that affords a balance between fiscal and patient care interests?

Grievances and Complaints

- Is there a formalized process in place to evaluate objectively and consistently patient or practitioner complaints and grievances for administrative and medically related matters?

References

- Always check references of networks as you would with any other subcontractor. Ask for the names of a half-dozen or more network clients and randomly select the ones you would like to interview, rather than letting the network make the decision for you. Also consider interviewing network practitioners to ask their opinions about the working relationship with network administrators and their perception of the quality of care provided by the network. Do not hesitate to ask open-ended questions and allow sufficient opportunity to have those providing the reference comment on areas and issues they believe are important to consider. You will likely learn a great deal.

PRODUCT CONSIDERATIONS

Despite surface appearances, not all product designs are equal, and, in many instances, there may be more differences in product design than you might believe. For example, some acupuncture networks offer a more restricted category of diagnoses that will be covered under their programs. Some may require the written referral of a medical doctor. When evaluating price, make sure you are assessing comparable product offerings, limitations, and other variables that will be important to you and your membership.

Network Parameters

- Are the network panels owned and operated or are they leased from an unaffiliated third party? If the latter, you need to ascertain who has the authority to enforce reimbursement policies, peer-review actions, and other contract-related issues. Unless the network has privity of contract—a direct contractual relationship with the practitioner—compliance will be virtually impossible to enforce.
- Does the network accept credentialing by another entity? Ask who sets the standards and determines what mechanisms are in place to ensure that all practitioners meet minimum standards of participation.
- Verify that practitioners have executed a binding contract and are in good standing in the network. Confirm that they accept new patients and have the administrative and clinical capacity to serve your members. It has been documented that some networks list practitioners who are in limited academic practices or whose practices have been closed to new patients, or whose availability to treat patients is so sporadic as to cause serious concerns about the availability, continuity, and quality of care.
- Verify that network practitioners are not marketed as available prior to the completion and verification of credentialing.
- Take the time to document the number of unique practitioners in the network and objectively evaluate the size, location, and availability of network providers to service your members' needs. Having practitioners clumped in one geographic area will not address the needs of the work force of today, which is highly mobile and dispersed. Although a network of 10,000 practitioners may sound impressive, if you find that they

are clustered sporadically over 50 states, you may not be so impressed.
- Document that the network carries coverage for medical malpractice for its administrative and clinical rulings. Also document that each and every practitioner has malpractice coverage in force at the coverage levels indicated by the network. Be suspect of networks that allow practitioners to "self-insure" their malpractice coverage—in other words, pay the network directly for coverage in the event of a malpractice suit instead of utilizing traditional risk insurance companies. This practice is highly questionable and places clients at increased risk of malpractice exposure. The standard in the industry is $1 million per occurrence and $3 million in the aggregate from an accredited and admitted insurer.
- Ask your clinical consultants to evaluate the soundness of the clinical protocols and pathways utilized by the network. Are these approaches applied objectively and consistently?
- Evaluate the credentials of the network's clinical management team. How adequately are they trained to coordinate patient care? Ask about clinical training and experience. Ask whether they are full- or part-time employees. Do not be afraid to establish the credentials of the network to ensure that care is being provided at the highest level, with objective and consistent oversight.
- Determine what type and level of quality of care evaluation is conducted. Determine who conducts these evaluations and ask to see copies of their reports. Determine how frequently these audits occur and whether they meet your requirements.

Satisfaction Surveys

- Determine whether satisfaction surveys of members, practitioners, and clients are performed; if so, by whom and how often are they performed? Are these data collected and evaluated independently and free from bias or manipulation by a third party? Determine whether the network will share the surveys of their members or employees with you on a reliable periodic basis.

Reports

• Does the network have the capability and willingness to comply with standardized reporting on utilization, cost, member and practitioner complaints, and regulatory and third-party audits?

CONCLUSION

In summary, developing and managing a specialty network are not as easy as it may appear. It generally is also more expensive to build and manage your own network than to contract for these services through a qualified third-party network. It takes considerable time and money to recruit, credential, and manage networks. Specialty networks are no exception. To maintain your own reputation and mitigate financial and malpractice exposure, careful consideration needs to be given to every aspect of the network. Many health plans do not want to bear the administrative burden or the costs associated with developing and managing a specialty network.

Treat the relationship as you would a marriage. The relationship needs to be built on solid foundations, complete with trust, respect, and commitment, for it to be successful in the long term.

CHAPTER 31

Phasing in CAM through Discount (Affinity) Services

31.1 The CAM Discount (Affinity) Model: Consensus Health
Alan M. Kittner
31.2 Perspective: Discount Networks in Hawaii
Cliff K. Cisco
31.3 Profile: Member Services in a Discount Model—Telephone and Internet Interface
Tony Knox

31.1 The CAM Discount (Affinity) Model: Consensus Health

Alan M. Kittner

In highly competitive markets, health plans need to build brand equity in order to increase market share and membership loyalty. Market differentiation is important to a health plan for growth and member retention. This is particularly true in markets in which there is a greater penetration of managed care products over indemnity products, and major providers compete on the basis of price as opposed to product differentiation.

This trend is also true in markets where there has been extensive consolidation in the health

Alan M. Kittner was founder and Chief Executive Officer of OneBody.com, formerly known as Consensus Health, from 1996 to October 2000. He has been a partner at Montgomery Medical Ventures LP and Montgomery Medical Ventures LP II, a health care venture capital partnership with $135 million under management that specializes in seed and early stage investing. He has also worked with the Senate Health and Welfare Committee in California and as a legislative advocate for a statewide health care membership organization. He is a graduate of University of California at Berkeley and holds a master's degree from Yale School of Management.

plan choices offered to consumers; where managed care has significant market share, this is particularly evident—on the West Coast, in the Northeast, and in other areas such as Minnesota. A desire for brand identity and product differentiation is characteristic of these maturing markets, in which two to five corporate health plans control 40% to 60% of the market share. Any legitimate opportunity that enables a health plan to distinguish itself with purchasers will be particularly compelling.

Health plans must establish their product not only on the basis of cost, but also on some other distinguishing feature, because similar products are typically similarly priced. Plans have begun to focus on product quality to build goodwill. In particular, they have become interested in targeting services to members interested in complementary and alternative medicine (CAM). In the current market, one successful strategy is to offer products and services that meet the consumer's definition of health and wellness. CAM is a service that fulfills these criteria.

MARKET DEMOGRAPHICS OF CAM

It is important to note that although there appears to be greater utilization of CAM among particular segments of the population, there is also very significant interest on a national basis. In this context, Eisenberg (1998) has documented an increased use of CAM services of approximately 25% in 7 years, totaling an estimated 629 million visits to CAM practitioners in 1997. That exceeds the number of visits to primary care physicians in the same year (386 million). Clearly, interest in CAM is not a limited phenomenon.

Demographic findings by Eisenberg (1998) with 1997 data include a number of trends:

- Although the interest in CAM is occurring nationwide, this interest tends to be greater in the West.
- There is also greater interest among more highly educated populations and those in which individual income is more than $50,000 a year. This suggests that urban areas have greater utilization compared with rural areas.
- Interest is greater among certain age groups, particularly those 35 to 49 (the baby boomers), compared to younger or older populations.

Eisenberg conservatively estimated the market in 1997 at $21.2 billion (1998). Since that time, utilization has increased to $27 billion. In the study done at Stanford by Astin (1998), data suggest that the greatest use of these services is by people who have specific health problems that have not been fully addressed by conventional medicine. They have sought solutions that were unconventional, not because of a particular ideological or psychological predisposition, but because their needs were not being fully met and they were looking for ways to resolve a health condition or manage chronic illness.

Yet these services are not just used by people who have chronic illness. Research suggests that although almost 50% of consumers who use these services are addressing specific health conditions, the other 50% use them for prevention and health maintenance (Eisenberg, 1998). There are probably differences between the demographics of individuals in each of these two categories. This information suggests that people are using CAM in a meaningful, purposeful way.

Although health plans may be highly motivated to offer complementary therapies, programs cannot be successful without the necessary demographic requirements. The first and most obvious is the nature of consumer or membership interest in these services.

The Employer's Perspective

A CAM benefit can be a viable marketing tool for employers. In highly competitive job markets, employers may be more attractive to job seekers if they offer health plans that include CAM as part of the benefits package. This seems to be true among employers who are either part of large corporations or early-stage technology companies. These demographics are important to take into consideration when designing health benefits because there is evidence of significant overlap between CAM health care users and technology users. In fact, alternative health care is reported to be the single topic of greatest interest in searches for health information on the Internet.

Employers are interested in attracting technology-savvy employees with higher educational and income levels, who are market innovators or leaders and who think independently. People with this profile also tend to be motivated to use CAM. In a competitive job market, employers can distinguish themselves by offering coverage for CAM.

The Consumer's Perspective

Increasingly, health plans in competitive markets are coming to regard the consumer as a major decision maker. Today, consumers are paying a higher and higher percentage of out-of-pocket costs for health insurance. In fact, the percentage of employees required to pay a portion of their health care premiums has grown from about 50% in 1989 to more than 70% in 1997. As a result, consumers are playing more of a role in decision making. Consumerism is influencing the development of health care as plans realize their customers are not just the health benefits representatives or the employers, but the actual users of the service.

Many employers provide several health plans and periodically offer open enrollment when employees can select among competing benefit packages. It is no longer enough just to be one of the plans that an employer offers. Health plans want to appeal to the consumer, be recognized as consumer-oriented, and be the first choice.

ELEMENTS OF PRODUCT DESIGN

Designing a CAM Product for Wellness and Preventive Care

The affinity discount program for CAM services is a flexible, cash-effective, value-added model for offering CAM services through a health plan. This is the model developed by Consensus Health dba OneBody.com for Blue Shield of California through a strategic relationship that began in 1997. The product "mylifepath" is designed to focus on health and preventive care, while providing value-added, discounted services. The initial vision can be credited to Ken Wood, chief operating officer at Blue Shield of California, who had already taken steps to create an organization responsive to consumer needs. Blue Shield pioneered consumer open-access products by developing a health plan that provided consumers direct access to specialists without a referral. The tremendously positive market response to open access made it clear that there is untapped potential in benefit design that empowers consumers. It became apparent that there was more that could be done to meet consumer expectations. As a next step, Blue Shield looked to CAM.

The Multidisciplinary Network

Consensus Health's approach from the very beginning to the development of a CAM network has been multidisciplinary. Staff knew that the first integrative networks evolved with chiropractic practitioners. In developing a new network, Consensus Health decided that practitioners from a variety of healing traditions should be included in this offering, provided that they met certain standards. The panels that were developed reflect many different skill sets and traditions, including practitioners trained and credentialed as physicians, osteopaths, nurses, licensed acupuncturists, chiropractors, and certified massage therapists. The services offered encompass 8 different modalities and at least 12 different types of credentialed practitioners. Other health professionals are also represented in the network, such as registered dietitians, nutritional counselors, and mental health professionals with specific expertise. The inclusion of such a breadth of services has enabled Consensus Health to provide a product that appeals to a very broad population. For example, in California, Consensus Health now offers:

- chiropractic
- acupuncture
- massage and bodywork (from 40 different subspecialties)
- somatic education (movement awareness such as Feldenkrais and Alexander technique)
- access to spas and retreats
- access to fitness centers and health clubs, including personal trainers
- yoga
- stress management
- nutritional counselors (both certified nutritional counselors and credentialed dietitians)
- healthy dining and cooking classes

In North Carolina, the panels also include naturopathy.

A selection of these and other services such as T'ai chi and Qigong are available. Each health plan chooses their selection based on local market considerations and the availability of providers.

Cost Containment

The affinity discount product has an impressive economic profile. Cost containment is a daily economic reality, and employers are highly sensitive to added costs and premium increases. In addition, the health plan's concern about the medical loss ratio is an ongoing consideration. The affinity program provides a low-cost, low-price option—a very consumer-oriented, market-driven product made available to a broad population.

This benefit can be compared with supplemental riders for chiropractic care that are sold to employers. In order to offer rider coverage, the employer has to be willing to pay an additional $1.50 to $3 per member per month. Although the rider benefit is then available to all employees, perhaps only 3% of their population will actually use those services. In addition, employees in that plan still do not have increased access to other CAM services.

When Consensus Health offers an affinity program that includes multiple specialties, it is able to provide wellness and complementary services that are of interest to at least 15% to 20% of the population. Since these services are not insured covered benefits, they are provided to the consumer at a tenth of the cost. They are still of real economic value to the consumer because the services have been carefully evaluated, rigorously credentialed, and significantly discounted.

Consensus Health has been able to price the payers' cost so low that some health plans, including Blue Shield, became interested in offering the product at no cost, rather than passing the expense on to their employers. This arrangement has proved so favorable to Blue Shield that in 1998 they made it available to all members, and currently, the program is open to all Californians if they sign up through the Internet. Access is available through <http://www.mylifepath.com>.

Quality

Quality assurance is an essential consideration in the development of a CAM product. The role of Consensus Health dba OneBody.com has been to develop new standards and screening criteria for alternative practitioners to ensure that their credentials and practice standards are of the highest caliber. In-depth standards have been developed for the alternative therapies through Consensus Health's work with experts, practitioners, and national professional associations to understand the educational and clinical requirements within each specific discipline. To ensure safety and the highest quality service, the concerns of the health plans regarding malpractice insurance and certification have been addressed. The goal is to develop credentialing criteria that provide everyone the assurance that networks of the highest quality are being created.

These programs have proven to have definite value.

- The credentialing process increases the safety factor and builds consumer confidence.
- The credentialed panel is a source of reliable referrals to competent CAM practitioners.
- The program enhances the legitimacy of CAM because the product has met the standards of credentialers and of respected health plans.
- It enables health plan physicians to become more comfortable with a range of disciplines and provides physicians with experience in referring patients to CAM practitioners.
- It has served as a highly successful educational tool for consumers.
- The credentialing process has provided the basis for development of practice guidelines and a knowledge base for CAM medical management.
- It is laying the groundwork that will eventually facilitate the integration of these therapies and protocols into conventional medicine.

In an environment in which integration is occurring along a continuum, discounted, multispecialty affinity benefits will eventually be covered, once a significant body of evidence is accumulated. In the meantime, this program has allowed Consensus Health to move forward quickly and meet consumer demand with the assurance of a significant level of safety.

Accessibility

The affinity model successfully addresses several aspects of the accessibility issue. The first is the geographic coverage of providers. There must be a sufficient pool of trained practitioners in any given area in order to offer programs of this type. If consumer demand has existed in a particular region, practitioner density typically will have already developed to fill the need. From a managed care perspective, one needs to offer services to a region large enough to cover access standards, whether the region is defined by regulatory guidelines or marketing characteristics. In a managed care environment, it is essential to provide a product that meets the members' needs in both urban and rural areas. To meet the requirement for broad geographic coverage in the development of this product, the most effective approach has been to develop a discount program that includes a broad diverse offering of disciplines and practitioners. As a result, Consensus Health is able to provide practitioners in more than 2,500 locations in California.

Issues of Safety

Safety is the primary consideration in designing a CAM program benefit. A focus on quality is one way to ensure safety. Consumer protection and liability are also important considerations. It is vital that the health plan address these issues, either directly or through a consultant who will conduct efficient credentialing and set essential safety standards.

Physicians also have a primary concern for the health and safety of their patients, as part of their sacred role. Health plans have a brand to protect, as well as their reputation for integrity. When offering new products and services, the design must address all these considerations. It is essential to make sure that sufficient quality standards are built in, so that service delivery does not jeopardize consumer safety, health plan accreditation (National Committee on Quality Assurance), or the physician-patient relationship. This is true even when the product has historically been in existence for some time, but is somewhat new to health plans and physicians.

Liability Issues

Each practitioner carries his or her own malpractice and liability insurance. The intermediary, such as Consensus Health dba OneBody.com, also carries insurance. Since Consensus Health is separate and independent from the health plan, the health plan is protected from any corporate liability. It is noteworthy that in the history of liability within CAM services, malpractice claims are very rare. Not that there have not been abuses, as in any field, but the overall history of CAM has been very positive. Consensus Health's research indicates a notable absence of complications. Problems are rare enough to be considered minor, if not completely insignificant.

There has been concern that liability claims will increase as this industry becomes more recognized within mainstream medicine and associated with companies that are viewed as having deep pockets—resources that a disgruntled consumer might be tempted to take advantage of. On this issue, it is the role of the network to make sure that consumers are seen by quality practitioners, with no history of past problems, either clinically or legally. It is also important to ensure that there is sufficient malpractice insurance coverage at every level to protect the affiliated parties.

The affinity design provides an opportunity to build a track record for these therapies. Information on utilization goes into Census Health's database, enabling staff to document activity by consumers and practitioners and then share that data with the health plans.

ORGANIZATIONAL FACTORS

Market Demographics

In designing any health program benefit, it is essential to determine the environments most conducive to the provision of discount, direct-access health care services.

There are several factors that influence this issue:

- What are the competitive dynamics in the market?
- What are the demographics of that marketplace from the perspective of all the stakeholders? These include the membership and consumer points of view, as well as employers' and practitioners' perspectives.
- What are the characteristics of the organization? What are the issues? Within the health plan, which components will be necessary to develop this program to its full potential? What type of program can be provided that will offer maximum benefit to the consumer?

Program Design and Organizational Support

Another aspect of planning involves an assessment of the level of commitment of the organization.

A number of different indicators are suggestive of a health plan's predilection for success:

- the history of commitment to consumer-oriented products on the part of senior management
- managerial and financial commitment to marketing support in terms of both budget resources and creativity
- physician acceptance and orientation to these services

To be successful as a product innovation, any health product must fit within the overall philosophy and commitment of the company. In order to succeed, it must receive strong support. Unless the new services are viewed as important by the health plan, they will not receive enough support to become an ongoing component of a successful brand equity strategy. Without sufficient marketing support, the product may not reach consumers. Without organizational support, it may not be successfully implemented in terms of quality standards and integration into the health plan's other services. If the services are viewed merely as a fad or a product add-on to generate short-term interest, the chances for success are significantly decreased.

When developing partnerships in this area, Census Health looks for market leaders who are advocates and innovators within health plans, who understand and respond to the needs of their particular markets in creative ways. Census Health looks for those who are willing to use their managerial and financial resources to implement new programs. Census Health seeks providers with a commitment to marketing, public relations, and education, both within the health plan and in the employer-consumer community.

If the program is not well defined by both the vendor and the health plan, it will merely be viewed as a discount program similar to current discount programs available through health clubs. Although these types of programs are utilized, their full value is not realized because they are not part of an overall medical wellness philosophy. Such a program requires the support of the medical staff in order to achieve congruence within the organization. This requires appropriate staff education.

It is also important to achieve some degree of physician buy-in. Organizational solidarity can be furthered by insisting on standards for complementary practitioners that meet physician criteria for accountability. Maintaining high-quality standards will increase respect for CAM by both physicians and consumers.

Marketing

The other issue in terms of organizational commitment is whether the health plan has a marketing orientation. Health plans do not all market, and they do not all necessarily understand the importance and subtleties of marketing. It is important to determine whether the plan has a marketing infrastructure and an orientation that can support a CAM product. This support is essential in achieving recognition at a level that reaches a sufficient audience of consumers and employers. This commitment goes beyond philosophy in terms of how health insurance is sold. It also requires a certain budgetary commitment to reach the target audience, as opposed to simply offering the product through an employer list and relying on brand identity and market position to achieve recognition and market share.

Health plans are increasingly coming to recognize that consumers are active participants in the selection of their own health coverage. When a new product appears on a list of employer benefits, health plans can no longer rely on their brand equity or product differentiation as a sufficient attractant to consumers unless they have actively marketed their product. Marketing and public education provide the basis for product recognition and subsequent popularity.

Limitations to Discounted Services

One of the primary limitations involves the kind of outcomes data that can be captured in an affinity access program, compared to the data available through a covered benefit or supplemental rider. This is because the affinity access program is still a relationship between the consumer and the practitioner. Since no claim is submitted, data capture is limited. There are multiple ways of collecting data, and Consensus Health is doing everything it can to gain as much information as possible, but that will not cover 100% of utilization, and it will not be as detailed as desired.

The other drawback is that the services are not fully integrated into clinical care because the program is self-referred and an out-of-pocket expense. The affinity access program is not a covered benefit, it does not reimburse the consumer for care, and it is not integrated into the referrals from the physician or the health plan. There is no interdisciplinary case management that integrates complementary and conventional medicine, which is why the model is at one end of the continuum, reflecting a limited degree of integration into the system.

CONCLUSION

Discount, open-access CAM benefits are the easiest, the least expensive, most consumer-friendly of all services of this type. These programs offer appreciable benefits; they provide real value from a wellness perspective. They have a good history of safety and a high level of consumer interest. There are other models that are important and make sense along the developmental path in the integration of CAM into conventional medicine. Consensus Health views this program as the beginning, not the end.

REFERENCES

Astin J. Why patients use alternative medicine: results of a national study. *JAMA*. 1998;279(19):1548–1553.

Eisenberg D, Davis R, Ettner S, et al. Trends in alternative medicine use in the United States, 1990–1997: results of a follow-up national survey. *JAMA*. 1998;280(18): 1569–1575.

31.2   Perspective: Discount Networks in Hawaii

Cliff K. Cisco

Hawaii is the only state in the country that has a labor law mandating that every employer provide health care coverage to their employees. As a result, the state has very close to universal health care coverage. Consequently, the state must be very careful about adding benefits to employer-based insurance because the employer has no other option but to pay for them. At this point, given the economy in Hawaii, employers are not particularly eager to add new types of coverage or expenses.

However, there is extensive interest in CAM in Hawaii. With the wide diversity of ethnic backgrounds, both acupuncture and various forms of massage therapy are popular, particularly Hawaiian massage techniques. There is also a vast array of other CAM therapies that have attracted interest. It is hoped that in the next 2 years, discount programs will provide the opportunity to gather data, increase understanding of the interest in the community, and determine how much these programs actually cost. Once this type of information is available, a rider could be developed for employers that would complement the standard health plan benefit. Essentially, this is a phasing-in process—a process of development.

Certain questions need to be answered in order to better define the utilization and benefits of CAM.

- Do people use CAM services in place of conventional medical care?
- Or are these services an add-on, which means an additional expense?
- Do these therapies significantly cut health care costs?

Cliff K. Cisco is the Senior Vice President of the Hawaii Medical Service Association.

- Do they make a difference in health and in health care utilization even when they are only used as adjunctive therapy?

Until this type of data is available, employers and insurers would be hesitant to add coverage for CAM services.

In terms of insurance coverage in the state of Hawaii, there are less than 1 million covered lives. Consequently, researchers watch mainland research and demographics very closely for developing trends. For example, if Washington state were to develop a large data set, Hawaii officials and researchers would be very interested in seeing these data. Although there are regional differences in health, it would be helpful to have data on a larger population to determine the broad patterns of how people use various CAM services. Clearly, the size of the data set lends it greater credibility.

In Washington state, it should be possible to gain additional insight on CAM utilization, because socioeconomic status is minimized as a variable due to universal inclusion. Currently in Hawaii, the funds that pay for CAM are usually discretionary funds, which means that users tend to be more affluent. Given expanded access, it would be worthwhile to know how much people utilize CAM services. Insurers also want more information on the baseline health status of the individuals who are choosing CAM.

Some people believe that these services are used in addition to medical care. The concern is that enrollees would use alternative care and then when they really got sick, they would also use traditional medical care *in addition*. Advocates for CAM suggest that access to these types of programs will reduce the overall need and utilization of health care.

The question becomes, how can the utilization data that insurers want and need be obtained? Since there are large budgets at stake, it is understandable that no one wants to make a mistake. What kind of information will provide the concrete data that insurers need to move forward, to develop other types of CAM benefits, and to integrate them more thoroughly into their coverage?

The hope of the Hawaii Medical Service Association is that it will be able to collect data from its network partners on members who have used complementary services in order to begin cross-tabulating utilization of CAM services compared with medical services covered by the health plan. The goal is to create matched data sets to determine whether there is any replacement of CAM for traditional services, or if the demand for health care in traditional health plans is reduced because of access to complementary programs.

31.3   Profile: Member Services in a Discount Model— Telephone and Internet Interface

Tony Knox

Consensus Health dba OneBody.com has achieved quality member services as a result of a number of ongoing initiatives. These can be summarized in at least three primary categories:

1. staff education
2. technical initiatives
3. quality management

STAFF EDUCATION

The staff has developed an understanding of CAM therapies that is supported through information resources and training. Consensus Health provides an extensive library, which includes alternative health journals, magazines, and textbooks. Consensus Health offers in-service classes presented by the practitioners in the network. For example, when Consensus Health added biofeedback services to the network, it scheduled classes with a provider to review the origin of the practice, the conditions biofeedback treats, the training of practitioners, and other aspects of the practice.

Everyone on staff is welcome to attend these trainings, and those in member services are required to attend. Two different sessions are offered in order to accommodate as many staff as possible. Sessions are also recorded for those who are unable to attend.

TECHNICAL INITIATIVES

Consensus Health provides information to clients both on the telephone and on the Web. On the telephone, the technical interface is designed to provide the most seamless interaction possible. There are easy-to-understand information resources that service representatives can use to effectively convey information to members. Currently, Consensus Health receives approximately 150 to 200 calls a day, requesting referrals. Consumers want to know if they are eligible to participate in the discount program, how it works, and whether they can be referred to practitioners in their area. Through the use of call-processing software, Consensus Health is able to provide members with the names of participating providers in all available specialties, at the nearest possible location. Referrals are organized by ZIP code, county, and other types of geographic information.

Tony Knox is the Supervisor for Member Services at OneBody.com.

For those with Internet access, there are several Web sites, associated with Consensus Health's contracted plans. This information is available to both members and the general public. Anyone can access them online and receive health information. Access to information gives members the opportunity to educate themselves about CAM therapies.

QUALITY MANAGEMENT

Consensus Health ensures top performance on the part of service representatives through periodic real-time phone monitoring with recording capability, and through extensive reporting on overall team performance. Customer service representatives have been averaging less than 15 seconds to respond to a telephone call from the moment the call comes in until a live agent answers the telephone. This involves a streamlined menu of telephone options and an adequate number of well-trained responsive staff. The industry standard for the average speed of answer is 30 seconds or longer.

Abandonment rate is 2%. The average call link lasts up to 5 minutes during the launch of a new program, after a mailing, or following a major press release. At those times, Consensus Health is delivering a tremendous amount of new information regarding the program. At less active times, the average telephone call is approximately 3.5 to 4 minutes. Consensus Health's target is to answer 80% of calls within less than 20 seconds, and, typically, 94% to 96% of the calls are answered within 30 seconds. Initially, Consensus Health staff responded to toll-free calls from the states of California and North Carolina, but its scope of service has since expanded nationwide.

CHAPTER 32

Preferred Provider Organizations

32.1 An Open Access Preferred Provider Organization Model of CAM Delivery:
Complementary Healthcare Plans
Richard D. Brinkley and Charles A. Simpson
32.2 Quality Management in a Practitioner-Managed Network:
Complementary Healthcare Plans
Pamella J. Marchand

32.1 An Open Access Preferred Provider Organization Model of CAM Delivery: Complementary Healthcare Plans

Richard D. Brinkley and Charles A. Simpson

THE INITIAL NETWORK

Complementary Healthcare Plans (CHP) is comprised of networks of CAM providers that were formed to provide professional administration of managed health care services in the state of Oregon. The organization began as a chiropractic specialty network in 1989, contracting with workers' compensation and employer health plans. The initial network formed partnerships with a variety of managed care plans bringing managed chiropractic services to preferred provider organization (PPO) and health maintenance organization (HMO) environments. As the network evolved and expanded, practical experience was accrued in benefit design, clinical management, and administrative integration, working in cooperation with its managed care partners.

Building on models of utilization and quality management from ambulatory care settings, CHP has created systems of provider profiling,

Richard D. Brinkley is President and CEO of Complementary Healthcare Plans. His prior experience includes a variety of increasingly responsible positions at Blue Cross of California in operations, finance, and marketing; president and CEO of Key Health Plan; and principal in TBG Healthcare Consulting. He received his master's degree from Golden Gate University and has taught at the graduate and undergraduate levels. Mr. Brinkley is a member of the board of directors of the American Association of Preferred Provider Organizations (AAPPO).

Charles A. Simpson, DC, is a founder and Chief Medical Officer of Complementary Healthcare Plans of Portland.

Complementary Healthcare Plans, Inc. (CHP) is an Oregon-based preferred provider organization (PPO) with four networks of practitioners. CHP has grown in three years from serving fewer than 50,000 lives to over 330,000 lives in terms of prepaid members. In addition, as a PPO and a managed care organization (MCO), the health plan serves a population of more than 1 million lives. The network provides services through hundreds of practitioners in the fields of chiropractic (ChiroNet); acupuncture (AcuMedNet); naturopathic medicine (NatureNet), and massage (CHP Massage Therapy Network).

Source: Adapted from C.A. Simpson, Integrating Chiropractic in Managed Care, *Managed Care Quarterly*, Vol. 4, No. 1, pp. 50–58, © 1996, Aspen Publishers, Inc.

credentialing, quality assurance, and utilization management that can provide high-quality and cost-effective health care. The chiropractic network of 260 practitioners in Oregon and southwest Washington is a model that illustrates that administrative and structural integration of nontraditional providers can be achieved successfully in organized health care systems. Practitioners of CHP currently have a number of different arrangements with a variety of managed care plans. In each case, the administrative and operational components have been designed to respect the philosophy and accomplish the goals of all the players in the system: members, payers, and practitioners.

An independent study by Performance Marketing of Vancouver, Washington, surveyed chiropractors in southwest Washington to evaluate CHP against all of its competitors in a blinded evaluation (1998). CHP was rated the number one chiropractic organization in every category assessed. The respondents were practitioners from a number of networks. Each organization was rated by its own practitioners and by those in other networks, but there was no indication of which organization sponsored the survey. CHP received 89% of the excellent ratings.

On the member side of the equation, the complaint ratio is less than .06 complaints per 1,000 members. Other organizations have rates of up to 6.5 complaints per 1,000 members—100 times higher. Not only does CHP experience a low member complaint ratio, it rarely receives complaints from employer groups. To sustain quality, the network has refused contracts that we thought were unfair to practitioners because they were based on price, as opposed to quality of care.

NETWORK EXPANSION

The success of ChiroNet in its initial market encouraged health plans to request similar offerings for acupuncture, naturopathic medicine, and massage therapy. Using the administrative models created initially for chiropractic, panels of other complementary providers were developed. AcuMedNet, NatureNet, and CHP Massage Therapy were launched in 1998 and joined with ChiroNet to form the parent organization, Complementary Healthcare Plans (CHP).

The founders of ChiroNet, all chiropractic clinicians, articulated an explicit vision of the effective blending of clinical management with the management of the business. Although clinical policy is determined by clinicians, administration is implemented by professional managers. Achieving a balance between the often competing imperatives of the clinical side of health care with the business side is one of the primary competencies developed in the ChiroNet model. Transposing this same core competence for AcuMedNet, NatureNet, and CHP Massage Therapy was regarded as the key ingredient in the development of these new products under Complementary Healthcare Plans.

Management Processes

Administrative Integration

The first phase of integration was to align the goals of CHP and its managed care partners to achieve quality health care in a cost-effective manner. The networks depend on the plan for membership and benefit information, premium collection, and the marketing of the benefit. The networks provide the plan with utilization and quality management; claims administration; performance monitoring; and data for accounting, actuarial, and planning activities.

Participation of Clinicians in Governance

Clinical policy making and oversight are provided by practitioners. Providers from each discipline are recruited to staff the nucleus of the team of practitioner-managers who formulate essential clinical policies. In the initial organization, issues of credentialing standards, scope of practice, and clinical quality criteria were formulated by these clinical leaders. The involvement of clinicians in policy-making roles has continued to be one of the strengths of the organization. Clinical policies have informed the development of benefit design and premium pricing, along with the administrative details of credentialing, quality, and utilization management.

Protocol Development

Clinical protocols are developed through professional consensus among panel providers and review of the current clinical literature. The protocols provide guidelines for appropriate use of diagnostic and therapeutic procedures. Treatment plans can be reviewed prospectively as necessary in certain plans. Potentially high-risk claims can be identified early and appropriate case-management interventions achieved. Concurrent, real-time case management avoids the frustrations and the ill will inherent in retrospective review and retroactive denial of services. The provider is made aware of potential problem cases early on. The patient benefits by having the most effective and appropriate treatment plan in place. The payer benefits from the most cost-effective use of services.

BENEFIT DESIGN AND ACCESS

Considering benefit design from the perspective of access, there are essentially two different types of models. One is direct access, in which the patient or member can go to a provider of complementary and alternative medicine (CAM) without a referral from a primary care provider. Direct access works best when the risk is shared with the CAM network. When the network is at risk for utilization, the necessary checks and balances can be built into the system's processes and procedures through utilization review. If the network is not at risk and some other entity, such as a medical group, assumes financial risk, tight utilization management, usually involving some form of referral protocol through the network or another gatekeeper, is necessary. It is fundamental to managed care that the provider bear risk. If the provider does not have the opportunity to manage that risk at the provider–patient interface, the system may become unworkable. Threats to patient access arise through rigid referral protocols because there are no longer inherent economic safeguards that respect practitioners' clinical autonomy.

One key ingredient to successful benefit-design implementation is the ability to recognize and deliver reasonable and necessary care. Creating a benefit that includes all of the services and procedures normally used in chiropractic and the other disciplines allows providers the flexibility to deliver the most appropriate treatment to the patient. This improves clinical outcomes, as well as patient and provider satisfaction. It also allows for services to be more compatibly integrated with the medical elements of the plan and keeps the focus on outcomes of care.

CHP promotes direct access to its networks of practitioners in both HMO and PPO settings. One arrangement, a workers' compensation managed care organization (MCO), requires referral from a primary care physician (PCP), but analysis of data collected to date shows no significant difference in utilization between a gatekeeper system and direct access. CHP has negotiated direct-access protocols in all of its HMO plans. Using access to certain medical specialties, such as gynecology and obstetrics, as a model, the plans have assumed that patients can and do self-refer appropriately.

UTILIZATION MANAGEMENT

Utilization management strategies employed by CHP include:

- Benefit design
- Credentialing and practitioner profiling
- Data management and utilization monitoring
- The management information system
- Additional management features:
  –Quality management
  –Medical management
- Risk sharing

Utilization management is overseen by the network medical director and a committee of CHP providers who review related policy and procedures, facilitate consensus among providers on clinical protocols, and act as arbiter in dispute resolution of relevant issues.

Benefit Design

Benefit design is a fundamental aspect of utilization management. Patient copay requirements are an effective brake on the unnecessary use of services. Copayments of $10–$15 are the rule in CHP plans, whether in a PPO or capitated HMO arrangements. Experience with a $5 copay shows this lower level of patient risk to increase utilization by nearly 50%. Benefit caps limit liability of the networks. However, they must be generous enough to provide meaningful coverage for conditions treated by CAM practitioners. Caps average $1,500 annually.

Credentialing and Practitioner Profiling

The credentialing process is used, in part, to identify practitioners whose practice style fits the guidelines of the network. The goal is to recruit providers whose patients neither over- nor underutilize care. Rather, the networks seek practitioners who are not outliers in terms of utilization and whose utilization patterns tend to be under the normal part of the curve. When these providers are identified and credentialed, they are viewed as assets and an integral part of the network. Management also works with them collegially and makes additional training available. The effectiveness of this partnership approach is reflected in the fact that the network has experienced less than 2% turnover since 1989.

In terms of standards, network practitioners adhere to and exceed credentialing criteria set by the National Commission on Quality Assurance (NCQA). In addition to primary source verification and site visits, which are not required by NCQA, CHP also uses three proprietary screens that review a practitioner's economic profile, professional philosophy, and practice techniques.

Data Management and Utilization Monitoring

Once practitioners are members of the network, their practice profiles are regularly re- viewed by the utilization management committee. Profiles that consistently deviate from expected performance help to identify unexplainable variations. Providers so identified are then further reviewed in light of case mix and severity indicators. If performance is found to be outside acceptable norms, the provider has an opportunity to participate in a corrective action process that identifies practice philosophies and procedures not shared by the rest of the panel. Peer intervention in the form of one-to-one contact or recommendations for remedial education is the first level of corrective action. Secondary action consists of focused review of continuing performance. Failure to achieve explicit utilization target goals in a specified time frame may result in termination from the panel.

The Management Information System

The CHP information system is an effective tool for utilization management. The network sees all claims from providers and is able to capture data reported on HCFA-1500 forms submitted for payment. Providers also submit clinical charts with each billing. The combination of claims data with clinical information permits "real-time" case management on a concurrent review basis. Accumulated data provide objective information to create individual physician profiles with each provider's performance. These data are routinely shared with each chiropractor, and individual practice profiles are shown in comparison with panel averages for cost per visit, number of visits per episode, cost per episode, and so on.

Additional Management Functions

Clinical Management

CHP philosophy is that care needs to be managed clinically before it is managed administratively. This essentially means that medical directors within each discipline will work with our network practitioners on issues of health care delivery and behavior before taking any administrative action in terms of disciplinary measures or behavior modification. For example, if the data suggest that a particular provider has patients who are overutilizing services, the only people who contact that provider about those reports are medical directors—not clerks and not CEOs. This is strictly a peer-to-peer intervention, and it's done in a nonconfrontational manner. That has worked out very well, and it contributes to the low turnover among the practitioners in the network. Many other organizations resort to an administrative remedy, which essentially involves cutting reimbursements and denying further health care services. We value continuity of client services and keep health care services as a priority.

Quality Management

The component that enables us to put this philosophy into practice is quality management. Our medical directors and clinical advisors interface and interact with providers on a daily basis, making sure that the quality of health care is maintained and that the health care protocols are consistent. We provide evidence-based health care. Not only are the providers satisfied with this approach, but health plan members are satisfied, as well.

Medical Management

We seek providers who will embrace a philosophy that is essentially one of treating and releasing. We want to restore the health of our patients as quickly as possible and return them to their normal lifestyle. The way we accomplish that is through medical management. Our medical directors serve as mentors to practitioners by maintaining open communication. We are able to use a mentoring approach to utilization management for the majority of the time, and it is an ongoing process that we are developing on a continual basis.

Although some PPOs have focused on deeply discounted fees as a marketing strategy, CHP has committed itself to the philosophy that the delivery of rational care from the hands of reasonable practitioners in a realistic time frame provides the highest quality of health care and

the greatest value. Deep discounts alone as a cost-containment strategy encourage physicians to "game the system" by unbundling procedures, performing more services, extending treatment plans, and seeing patients for shorter visits. There may be discounts on fees, but no real savings are guaranteed, and quality and efficiency may be sacrificed.

Risk Sharing

Another aspect of utilization management is the economic structure through which CHP shares risk with the practitioners. All of the practitioners and physicians are involved in sharing risk with a particular health plan. Consequently, there is a self-correcting feature—a feedback loop that directly involves the practitioner—which has worked very well. Although a practitioner will periodically complain that he or she does not want to subsidize the practice of others, this is rare. There is typically enough business to go around, so that practitioners are able to see and treat patients in a manner in which they feel comfortable, without excessive worry about overutilization.

The fact that the network is managing the risk means that the network will monitor the data, perform utilization review, and provide guidance and feedback to outliers whose patients overutilize. When risk is being managed by the network, all utilization management and quality management activities occur within the network, implemented by peer professionals in the same discipline.

Peer review ensures that the evaluation is made by individuals who have similar clinical experience in making determinations regarding:

- What constitutes reasonable treatment for a given condition
- The appropriate duration of treatment in most cases
- When exceptions are most likely to occur

Medical groups are very reluctant to assume risk for CAM services because they most often do not have baseline data on exposure, utilization, and outcomes. Without an extensive actuarial basis on which to design benefits, there is a tendency to restrict access to services in order to avoid overutilization. As a result, some insurers offer benefits that look generous on the surface but are somewhat restricted, limited in scope, and difficult to access. In a gatekeeper model, which requires the referral of a primary care provider in order to utilize alternative care, the patients must first visit the primary care provider and convince the provider that this is a viable approach to their condition. The provider must develop a reasonable treatment plan that would support the referral. The referral must then go through the system before the patient can access the alternative care.

Complementary Healthcare Plans has increasingly engaged in risk sharing with HMO plans. A variety of arrangements has been developed, with capitation amounts set according to an array of benefit designs. Managed care purchasers are able to select from a number of different access models, copay requirements, and maximum benefit caps. The network currently is moving to share risk directly with the panel providers through zero-based capitation. Each plan (and the corresponding participating providers) shares the capitation pool. Administrative costs are paid to the network, then providers are paid at usual and customary fees or a fee schedule, so long as the capitation pool is larger than total medical costs. The remainder is held in reserve to cover future medical costs. When medical costs exceed the capitation pool, each provider is paid an apportioned percentage of allowed charges, thus distributing the risk throughout the panel.

A DIRECT-ACCESS MODEL

In brief, CHP has found that it is possible to provide open access to patients without having to worry about runaway utilization, if credentialing is used to identify and recruit providers who will maintain a rational attitude and balanced practice with regard to utilization.

- Rather than simply refusing to pay for services, we first work with the practitioner to bring service provision into line with appropriate utilization.
- Our medical directors will intervene or meet with a physician in a nonthreatening manner.
- Peer pressure is in place, because the economic cost of overutilization is spread among all the practitioners in a region.

The risk-sharing model enables us to offer health plan members open access to services without the necessity of first seeing a primary care provider or someone else in a gatekeeper role. This eliminates the need for pretreatment authorizations and essentially removes the hassle factor from health care. It allows our physicians to treat their patients without the additional burden of paperwork because an open access model eliminates the need for rigid referral protocols.

THE CHALLENGES OF INTEGRATION

Successful integration of complementary and alternative disciplines depends on the alignment of goals and incentives among all players in the system, including providers, their network, patients, and the health plan. As managed care markets mature, both individual buyers and corporate purchasing alliances have become more sophisticated in their appraisal of competing plans.

Competition

In a marketplace with expanded choices in plan selection, price-point differential has become only one of a number of considerations available to consumers. Important product differentiators now include provider selection, access to specialty care, and a wide array of health care services. Consequently, there is a growing awareness on the part of insurers that alternatives to standard medical care can create a competitive advantage, particularly the addition of services such as chiropractic therapy or acupuncture.

Program and Benefit Design

The challenge of integrating seemingly incompatible combinations of alternative and traditional services can appear to be a daunting task. Traditionally, allied services such as physical therapy, mental health, or drug and alcohol rehabilitation are seen to fit well into most managed care plans. However, nontraditional health services, such as chiropractic care, may be viewed as problematic. In some environments, administrators and medical managers have had little experience in identifying appropriate utilization of chiropractic services. They may also be unfamiliar with standards for measuring medical quality in the chiropractic setting. A further unknown for plan managers is whether making chiropractic services available increases medical costs.

Practitioners' Issues

In addition, many alternative practitioners are skeptical of integration into mainstream medicine. They fear loss of clinical autonomy, compromise of their clinical values, and immersion in environments focused increasingly on cost containment, to the detriment of quality health care. Maintaining the core values and quality of patient-focused alternative health care in the face of initiatives by HMOs for increasing efficiency is a continuing challenge.

CONCLUSION

Alternative health care services have become increasingly attractive to managed care plans. The marketing advantage created by a mix of traditional and complementary care appeals to increasingly sophisticated health care purchasers. The experience of CHP demonstrates that chiropractic and other alternative medicine services can be offered in a plan at a competitive price. As experience accumulates, the effect of medical cost offset may allow the addition of this service as a basic benefit with no additional premium. In fact, one of CHP's health plan partners has integrated CHP's CAM program into its core benefit.

CHP has developed a management philosophy and administrative capability that meet the needs of the managed care market for accountability, quality, cost-effectiveness, and performance documentation. Although CAM professions have been largely on the fringes of the medical care system, the future of these professions lies in their ability to become an effective part of integrated medical systems. Creating benefit designs and models of access that are appropriate for chiropractic and other complementary disciplines is a continuing challenge. CHP and its partners represent a useful model of the successful integration of CAM therapies into the managed care environment. As managed care markets continue to mature, this inclusion can create comprehensive and fully integrated health care services. Limited health care resources can be more efficiently used, and the health care needs of the community can be most effectively served.

REFERENCE

Performance Marketing Group. Chiropractic Network Survey. Vancouver, WA; 1998.

32.2   Quality Management in a Practitioner-Managed Network: Complementary Healthcare Plans

Pamella J. Marchand

Continuous quality improvement (CQI) is the foundation of a quality management program. The level of quality service provided by an organization and its practitioners establishes the value for the health plan and its members. The CQI process also improves the services being delivered. Complementary Healthcare Plans (CHP) strives to bridge the gap between biomedicine and complementary and alternative medicine (CAM) disciplines by using the same standards and processes for quality management as health care providers use in the mainstream.

PRACTITIONER PARTICIPATION IN QUALITY MANAGEMENT

Organizational Structure

Oversight

The three networks of CHP (ChiroNet, AcuMedNet, and NatureNet) are supervised by a multidisciplinary team composed of practitioners from each of the networks. This joint quality committee performs the majority of the work for the quality program. The committee meets on a monthly or quarterly basis, based on the status of current projects. At the joint committee level, members establish CAM-specific guide-

lines and correlate them with National Committee on Quality Assurance (NCQA) guidelines. Meetings generally focus on a single topic and provide a forum in which to establish and review standards for the network. These standards are then communicated to network practitioners and disseminated through practitioner manuals. This formulation is of value because, in some areas of CAM, the field lacks formal standards.

The Quality Committee

Practitioners are represented at every level of the quality program. Within the three networks, discipline-specific advisory committees establish peer standards as benchmarks in each major area of management. These committees are responsible for setting policies and guidelines and for monitoring quality through various professional and clinical reviews. For example, the acupuncture committee has developed record-keeping standards and a system of chart notes that provides diagnostic categories and clinical documentation for both Western and Chinese medicine.

Practitioner Autonomy within the Network

CAM practitioners are typically accustomed to a great deal of autonomy. This is true of chiropractors, acupuncturists, and, to some extent, naturopathic physicians. Only massage therapists are accustomed to working within larger systems, such as hospitals or clinics. CAM practitioners may have a greater need to maintain an independent style of practice than do those who work in the mainstream. Consequently, although monitoring and quality assurance are provided, the goal is to maximize autonomy and avoid intrusion in the practitioners' delivery of care.

Pamella J. Marchand, MBA, Vice President, Complementary Healthcare Plans, has over eight years of experience in health care on both the provider and corporate sides of the industry. She has successfully managed credentialing, quality management, utilization management, and member services programs for three networks. In addition, she is responsible for provider and health plan contracting, management personnel, communications, and provider relations.

THE QUALITY MANAGEMENT PROCESS

Monitoring the Quality of Service Delivery

Credentialing

Credentialing is an important aspect of quality management. Within CAM credentialing, content varies significantly from that of conventional medicine. Consequently, in some cases, it is necessary to develop new standards within a discipline. Currently, CHP utilizes existing standards of NCQA for chiropractors. However, specific NCQA standards are not in place for acupuncturists, naturopathic physicians, or massage therapists. Therefore, the committee has established its own guidelines for credentialing and recredentialing. Staff continue to monitor and reevaluate guidelines on an ongoing basis.

Site Visits

The quality of client services is verified through site visits, as well as through formal and informal surveys of practitioner offices. CHP's standards align with other benchmarks and guidelines in the industry. Is the office wheelchair accessible? Do office staff members respond promptly to questions or requests for information? Because lifestyle interventions are central to many patient treatment plans, it is important that clinical staff be available to provide patients with training and assistance.

The committee also provides periodic, ongoing oversight, in which it evaluates each major aspect of the program and confirms that standards are being met, based on current regulations and new developments in the industry. For example, the committee recently reviewed all chiropractic offices to evaluate the handling of radiology equipment. Compliance with requirements was assessed with regard to appropriate shielding, quality of films, and record keeping on licensure of equipment and personnel. The committee provides this type of evaluation on an annual basis, across all areas of safety and compliance, to determine what needs to be done to maintain provider services and facilities at a very high standard.

Recredentialing

Biannually, the performance of each practitioner is reevaluated. Program outcomes and surveys are reviewed. Medical record keeping and participation in network quality initiatives are assessed. In addition to recredentialing, the goal is to identify any other major aspects of practice that are characteristic of good providers. This is done primarily through the clinical quality committee, which focuses on three primary components of practice:

1. the quality of the facility
2. the process of clinical care
3. the treatment outcome

Risk management is also an important element in these evaluations.

Linking Quality and Utilization Management

The quality management program is also directly linked to utilization management and credentialing. Information gathered from the utilization management program is used to create profiles of practitioner performance. The economic profiles of practitioners are evaluated to ensure that they are not providing too many or too few services. These profiles also include reports of patient satisfaction and medical record keeping. The information is aggregated with evaluations on patient risk minimization, appropriateness of service, access to care, and other major quality parameters.

Review of Clinical Documentation

Chart Notes

Chinese medicine is one of the disciplines in which chart notes differ most significantly from Western practice. If the practitioners use Chinese notation, they must also include an English translation of their notes. They may have a Chinese medicine diagnosis, but there must also be a Western diagnosis. The majority of our acupuncturists also provide enough information so that practitioners from other disciplines can gain a good understanding of the patient's condition and treatment. CHP works with practitioners who need a little training to enable them to achieve good chart notes.

Medical Records Review

Evaluations are performed on medical records at the time of credentialing. Sample files are scored with a basic quality assessment instrument developed within the organization. Once practitioners are in the system, they are recredentialed every two years. The medical records are collected for recredentialing and reviewed by a committee through the quality program. That review enables us to revise the review tool and to make sure that records are appropriate and understandable.

Training on Documentation

A packet of information on writing good chart notes is available to practitioners. A mentoring program is also in place. Peers on the provider panels work with other providers who need assistance with medical records to help them meet the standards. This form of peer coaching has worked well.

Clinical Content

The second level of medical records assessment is also a form of peer review. Here, the quality committee evaluates the actual clinical content and process. The quality committee reviews the medical records to gain a sense of the clinical thinking and to track treatment plans, which have been selected at random to determine whether the treatment adheres to standard protocol. Where adjustments in the protocol have been made, the committee checks to determine whether the changes are reflected in the notes.

ASSESSING PATIENT SAFETY AND SATISFACTION

Ensuring Patient Safety

Risk Management

This is another aspect of quality that is standard throughout health care. This element in-volves a focus on safety, that is, making sure that patients are not at risk for injury in CHP's providers' offices. It includes basics such as ensuring that steps are marked well with reflective tape, that exits are clearly identified, and that smoke detectors are in place. For acupuncturists, for example, it also means making sure that the needles go in appropriate disposal units. The quality committee also monitors many of the same risk factors found in mainstream clinical environments.

Evaluating Patient Satisfaction

Brief Surveys

The foremost component of the quality program is patient satisfaction, which is monitored primarily through two means. The first is a brief postcard-style survey distributed through providers' offices that asks three or four basic questions of patients. The survey provides the data necessary to meet NCQA standards for the element of patient satisfaction. These brief surveys focus on patient comfort, convenience, and safety. CHP patient satisfaction rates, as reflected on those surveys, have been extremely high for all aspects measured and are typically in the 90th percentile.

In-Depth Surveys

Another way in which patient satisfaction is evaluated is through longer surveys mailed to them at home. These evaluations address issues that are more substantive than are those in the brief surveys. The longer surveys generally consist of 15–20 questions that focus on quality of care, patient outcomes, and patient satisfaction. They are asked about satisfaction in interactions with the practitioners and their staff. Most important, they are asked about the outcome of treatment. At the end of the treatment plan, were the patients happy with their health and sense of well-being? CHP has had good response rates from patients and has found that the longer surveys (again in the 90th percentile) provide useful insight into what is being done right and what needs to be modified.

Providing Patient Education

The providers typically include a preventive component in their approach to treatment. Consequently, they tend to place a greater emphasis on evaluating the patient's overall health. Practitioners are more likely to use patient lifestyle as a means of leveraging health. Consequently, treatment tends to involve a great deal of patient education (for example, responding to questions about diet or providing therapeutic exercises). As in any form of medicine, subsequent follow-up with patients is important to confirm that they are actually applying the regimen.

Evaluating Patient Compliance

Quality management looks at basic compliance in a number of different ways. Medical records usually reflect whether the practitioner has documented all of the specifics and is continuing to follow up with patients regarding their compliance with the intervention—whether it involves exercises, a change in diet, or specific home therapies. The quality committee may also send surveys to patients to determine whether they felt the treatment plans were appropriate and whether they have continued to follow the therapeutic programs.

Applying What Is Learned about Patient Compliance

Practitioners are also surveyed for the methods they find most effective in achieving and enhancing patient compliance, and that information is shared with other providers. These strategies are valued, because patient compliance is one of the more challenging areas of medicine.

Monitoring Care

Timely Care

It is important to ensure that care being delivered is timely and medically necessary. Timely care is relevant to any health system. If a patient needs an urgent appointment, the system must be designed so that the patient can get the needed and appropriate care. The expectation is that a provider will be able to see a patient on the same or the next business day, or that the provider will refer that patient to another credentialed provider within the network who can see him or her in a timely manner.

Assessing Treatment

When the quality committee reviews clinical care, it also reviews the appropriateness of treatment. The goals are to confirm that the physical examination and any medical testing are relevant, timely, and suitable for the condition being treated; that the diagnostic workup is appropriate; and that there is clinical correlation for the treatment and diagnosis. The committee is also interested in identifying the aspects of service provision indicating that this practitioner is a step above other providers.

Establishing Clinical Pathways

Peer-review committees are invaluable in the development of clinical pathways. This is extremely important in the CAM disciplines, which lack well-defined care pathways in many areas. In any discipline, there may be several approaches to achieve the same goal. In addition, CAM care pathways may vary significantly from a biomedical approach. For example, Chinese medicine tends to take a systems perspective to illness, evaluating the vitality of the entire body and the immune response, rather than focusing on only the specific diagnosis or the affected area of the body.

Reviewing Clinical Care

CAM protocols are verified by reviewing chart notes according to the International Classification of Diseases (ICD-9) diagnostic codes. Chart notes are compared with clinical pathways that are in place within our network guidelines to determine whether the practitioner is using a reasonable approach to treatment. Operating as a feedback loop, information from practitioners is used to shape care pathways and to determine whether current guidelines still provide the best procedures for treating a given condition. The notes are also reviewed to verify that the practitioner followed the pathways and whether the notation process or the pathway needs to be upgraded.

The medical directors work collegially with practitioners whose practice style or utilization patterns are significantly different from those of their peers. Through informal discussions, the medical director and the practitioner seek to identify the source of any problems, modify the approach to treatment, where appropriate, or find different ways to work with patients.

Tracking Outcomes

The final phase of our own review focuses on outcomes. We strive to achieve the best outcome for the patient, whether that means providing service or referring them back to their primary care physician. We want the outcomes of our providers to be as good as or better than those of the general community. For this reason, outcomes are evaluated in relation to clinical processes and protocols. This provides feedback that can be used to increase the effectiveness of treatment.

COMPUTERIZED CAM QUALITY ASSESSMENT

CHP is a licensed user of the AmbuQual ambulatory quality assessment system from Ambulatory Innovations, Inc. (1993) and Methodist Hospital of Indianapolis, Indiana (part of Clarian Health Partners). This highly structured program is unique, in that it enables an organization to quantify the ongoing level of quality, using customized indicators (measures) selected by the organization. The assessment tabulation can be performed manually or through the AmbuQual software.

Standards and performance goals of the organization that relate to health care are identified prior to the beginning of the quality assessment activity. The software enables the organization to focus quality assurance efforts on issues that have an impact on the health of patients. Ten ambulatory care parameters are defined, providing both a foundation for indicator selection

and a comprehensive framework ensuring that the program is evaluated from all relevant perspectives. Using the information generated by AmbuQual, the quality committee is then able to evaluate total performance of the program against specific standards and goals.

Quantitative feedback is provided by this system. The software generates both a summary number reflecting the level of quality generated by the organization, as well as specific measurements of all the relevant indicators. This information makes it possible to gain a sense of the quality of both care and service delivered throughout the network. Tracking these numbers over time allows the organization to determine whether quality is really improving and, if not, why not. A quality improvement plan process then ensures that, once identified, quality improvements are actually carried out successfully. The program provides a structured mechanism to survey the quality continually and comprehensively, in conjunction with total quality management (TQM) and CQI programs.

Through the use of the software, there is no doubt when an opportunity for improvement exists and what should be done to be certain that improvement occurs. The roles of management and of the quality management committees are clearly delineated. The structure of the program, implemented by the committee, makes it possible to optimize the limited quality assessment hours that are available to an organization.

The quality-related information requirements for a complementary medicine program are similar in many ways to those of other health care organizations. In other ways, they are quite different. For example, in credentialing practitioners in developing risk-management programs and evaluating patient compliance, the content is specific to the discipline involved. At CHP, we have adapted the AmbuQual program to the specific needs of a complementary medicine network by developing instruments and tools for gathering preliminary data, which can then be fed into the existing parameters in the software. Table 32.2–1 summarizes the differences in the use of software in a complementary medicine

Table 32.2–1 Use of a Quality Evaluation Instrument—AmbuQual—by a CAM Network

Elements Measured	How the Measurement Process Resembles or Differs from the Use of AmbuQual in Biomedicine

1. ***Practitioner performance***	Two checklists have been developed in-house and are used at a preliminary phase to provide data for AmbuQual:
	  1. Credentialing (content is specific to each CAM discipline)
	  2. Clinical performance (again, content-specific)

2. ***Support staff performance***	Site visits are conducted for all new practitioners to determine compliance and identify additional areas for improvement for existing practitioners. The survey instrument developed in-house is provided to evaluate:
	  • Credentials and performance of the practitioner's staff
	  • Systems within the practitioner's office

3. ***Continuity of care***	Same as biomedicine.

4. ***Medical records system***	Two tools for each discipline were developed by the organization:
	  1. The basic tool—utilized at the time of initial credentialing to evaluate essential elements of the medical record. The tool focuses on format and primary content of the medical record.
	  2. An intermediate tool—used at the time of recredentialing (two years later), focused on clinical content. This tool evaluates correlation between the patient examination and treatment, as well as the diagnosis and treatment.

5. ***Patient risk minimization***	The site evaluation tool was developed in-house. Site visits are performed for all new practitioners. Standards are the same for CAM as for biomedicine, but the content is specific to each discipline.

6. ***Patient satisfaction***	Two instruments are used:
	  1. Basic satisfaction cards developed in-house
	  2. Written mail survey developed in-house
	The organization surveys the following elements:
	  • Interaction with practitioners
	  • Length and frequency of treatment vis-à-vis patient satisfaction
	  • Appointment process and waiting time
	  • Patient outcomes
	  • Patient satisfaction with support staff interaction
	Content differs, due to the nature of CAM therapies—in CAM, treatment often involves actual hands-on therapeutics and more extensive patient education.

continues

Table 32.2–1 Continued

Elements Measured	How the Measurement Process Resembles or Differs from the Use of AmbuQual in Biomedicine
7. *Patient compliance*	Seven survey tools have been developed in-house. Surveys are conducted annually; a different tool is used each year. • Data for this element are collected through review of medical records (reviewed for the type of information provided to the patient) and utilization management data (practitioner report cards, number of patient visits, etc.). • CAM practitioners meet different expectations in providing patient education and resources, because treatment frequently involves lifestyle interventions (such as exercise, diet, or stress reduction). • CAM patients are expected to participate actively in treatment; other expectations are similar to mainstream medicine.
8. *Access to care*	Seven tools have been developed in-house to date to measure aspects of this element. One tool is used each year. The tools measure dimensions comparable to those of primary care practices; content may differ. • Time spent with new and returning patients (more extensive in CAM) • Range of accessible hours (for example, practitioner may offer some early evenings, early morning, Saturday hours, etc.) • Patients with emergent needs must be seen with 24 hours or referred to another participating practitioner
9. *Appropriateness of service*	Data for AmbuQual on appropriate use of hospital care are omitted because the vast majority of CAM providers do not have admitting privileges. • Information on prescriptions is typically replaced with specifics on recommendations for botanical or nutritional supplements. Naturopathic doctors can prescribe certain medications but do so to a limited extent.
10. *Organizational performance*	Six tools have been developed in-house to evaluate and measure organizational performance, based on the indicators in this element, including: • Strategic planning • Leadership and management • Quality goals • Practitioner satisfaction • Fee schedules • Training and retraining of personnel

Courtesy of Ambulatory Innovations, Inc., Indianapolis, Indiana.

program, as well as the tools that we have developed in-house to make those accommodations.

CONCLUSION

The quality management program allows our organization to continually review and make improvements in the care being delivered by the contracted practitioners of the network. We make every effort to ensure that efficient and effective health care services are being delivered to patients. The focus on CQI allows any organization to routinely improve the level of quality and service being delivered to patients.

REFERENCE

Ambulatory Innovations, Inc. *AmbuQual II; An Ambulatory Quality Assessment and Quality Management System.* 2nd ed. Indianapolis, IN: Methodist Hospital of Indiana; 1993.

CHAPTER 33

Managed Care Networks

33.1 Case Managed Coverage in a Managed Care Environment
Laura Patton with Nancy Faass
33.2 A Quality Management Program in Complementary Medicine
Lynn McDowell

33.1   Case Managed Coverage in a Managed Care Environment

Laura Patton with Nancy Faass

OVERVIEW

Group Health Cooperative (Group Health) is a large health maintenance organization (HMO) in Washington state, providing complementary and alternative services in chiropractic, naturopathy, acupuncture, and massage therapy. Our program has been in place since 1996. Totally, we insure approximately 600,000 people in the state of Washington, with approximately 450,000 customers in the Puget Sound area of western Washington and 150,000 people in eastern Washington.

The organization is a nonprofit, now affiliated with Kaiser Permanente, but we have maintained a separate organizational structure. In terms of our delivery of care, Group Health is a mixed-model managed care organization. We are a group model in the sense that many practitioners are salaried employees of Group Health Permanente. Most of the physicians work at sites that are identified as Group Health sites, and we see only Group Health members. We also have network arrangements: Farther away from Puget Sound, in counties to the north, the plan is affiliated with primary care doctors under contract in a standard independent practice association (IPA) arrangement. The fundamental structure is the group model HMO.

We developed the program in complementary medicine in response to a state mandate, which went into effect in 1996 after being passed by the legislature in 1995. In the development of the program, we wanted the complementary and alternative medicine (CAM) practitioners to be familiar with and agree to abide by managed care principles. Given that understanding, our goal was to build a system in which managing alternative care would not be substantially different from the management of other health care services. That meant that most of the services offered by CAM practitioners were to be provided based on referrals from a primary care provider. Our task was to develop parameters that would provide the basis for referral.

The analysis of referral parameters was initiated by a task force created in 1994 to explore

---

Laura Patton, MD, has been Clinical Director of the Alternative Services Program at Group Health Cooperative since 1996. She holds a medical degree from the University of Washington and attended Duke University as an undergraduate. She has worked in utilization management and health care administration in the Seattle area for 15 years and is an associate clinical professor at the University of Washington School of Medicine.

alternative medicine. The group looked at the conditions for which CAM coverage might be offered by Group Health. We applied a rigorous process to establish an evidence basis through practitioner interviews and the medical literature. The committee also evaluated educational requirements and common conditions treated by each type of provider.

DEVELOPING THE NETWORK

The Initial Process

Credentialing

The decision was made early on to contract with a network management company for credentialing services. Ultimately, we contracted the entire development of the network with a vendor, which turned out to be a very good decision on our part. The network management company was able to develop a sizable network of acupuncturists, naturopaths, and massage therapists in a relatively short period of time.

Working with CAM Practitioners

In working with a network management company, one of the major challenges we have come to appreciate is that most CAM providers have not had any experience working under an insured model. The vast majority of them are independent practitioners who are accustomed to providing services on a cash-and-carry basis. Some have never seen a claims form before, nor do they know how to go about coding a diagnosis. Consequently, our development of complementary services involved a major educational effort to bring the practitioners into the network initially.

Educating Practitioners about Managed Care

Provider orientations to billing and network procedures required a major investment of time and effort in the beginning, but that was preferable to attempting to catch up after the fact. The management company shared the responsibility for practitioner education. Much of the coaching was literally done one-on-one. In some cases, the process required site visits and walking people through the procedure of filling out the claims forms. We also scheduled orientation sessions to review the processes and the documentation we required from the providers.

Administrative Structure

The program of alternative services at Group Health consists of four staff members. As clinical director of this program, I have been involved since the early stages of program development, although I actually work part-time in that capacity. The program has a full-time coordinator who is a registered nurse with a background of experience in utilization management. She often works closely with the CAM providers. An additional reviewer has been added. There is also a program assistant who maintains the database and who responds to telephone calls from consumers who want information about how their benefits work.

Time Invested

Our coordinator spent a great deal of time working individually with providers to answer basic questions about what was and was not appropriate. We did everything we could initially to provide sufficient information but have come to the conclusion that there will always be new providers who need coaching to make the transition into network participation. We were unprepared for the degree to which practitioners were inexperienced regarding insurance. There is no easy way to avoid this aspect of network development. This must all be considered in the context of the tremendous shifts that are occurring within health care, throughout the profession and for all of the individuals involved.

The Management Process

We found that some of the complementary medicine practitioners were quite comfortable with and supportive of the goals of managed care. As a result, we have been able to develop a stable network that includes more than 500 practitioners—approximately 70 naturopaths, 115 acupuncturists, and 350 massage therapists.

The Chiropractic Network

Chiropractic services became part of the basic covered benefit in 1996, after having been a popular rider prior to that time. Currently, Group Health has approximately 180 chiropractic providers in the network. We have had a chiropractic network in place for a decade. The network has been so stable and has worked so well that practitioners are reimbursed on a capitated basis, which is somewhat unusual.

Contracted Management

The network management company with whom we currently contract is the American WholeHealth Networks, Inc. (AWHN). It managed our original chiropractic network, and it has also developed a network of other CAM providers for us. We now contract with AWHN to provide credentialing and network management for CAM, and it also performs utilization management and quality assurance for our chiropractic network.

Utilization

Our utilization has been somewhat lower than we expected. Our overall referral rate increased approximately 28% last year. Acupuncture in any given month accounts for at least 50% of referrals. Massage represents approximately 30% and naturopathy about 20%. The vast majority of patients have had their conditions for more than a year, which implies a chronic nature to many of them. A recent survey indicated that these patients also found conventional medical care to be quite helpful—51% referred to it as "moderately helpful." In the same survey, approximately 80% found CAM therapists to be at best "moderately helpful."

COVERAGE FOR COMPLEMENTARY MEDICINE

Benefits for complementary therapies are core benefits, rather than riders. The provision of CAM services as a core benefit is required by state law, which addresses every category of provider. Our coverage requires a referral from the primary care provider for specific conditions. The referral specifies a certain number of visits. Table 33.1 1 provides examples of the guidelines in use at the time of this writing, which are updated annually.

When a physician writes a referral, for example, to an acupuncturist, that referral is good for eight visits. For massage therapy, the initial referral is good for six visits. For a naturopath, it is good for three visits. At the end of that treatment period, if the CAM provider wants additional visits, he or she must provide us with a treatment summary that details the progress that the patient has made to date and the treatment plan for future visits. All of this information is reviewed by one of our two review nurses. Most of the time, they are able to make a determination based on the information present in the treatment summary, but in some cases, the request requires further review. In other situations, we may ask that the patient return to the primary care physician who wrote the referral for a follow-up assessment. Based on that assessment, we will either refer the patient again or not. Referrals are based on medical necessity, as opposed to any kind of artificial limits on visits.

We do not stipulate or define how treatment should be provided. Practitioners treat based on their own judgment as to what is appropriate. The referral is good for three months. One of our current goals is to institute greater standardization in the medical documentation. The coordinator reads every one of the treatment summaries. That provides us with a wealth of information about what kind of care is being provided, which practitioners are doing well, and which are not.

AUTHORIZATION USING AN EXPERT SYSTEM

Chiropractic coverage is structured differently and may eventually serve as a model for other

Table 33.1–1 Alternative Medicine Referral Guidelines—Group Health Permanente

Therapy	Acupuncture	Massage Therapy	Naturopathy
Needs a referral?	Yes. With hard copy preauthorization.	Yes. With hard copy preauthorization. Primary care provider may consult with physical therapist before making referral.	Yes. With hard copy preauthorization.
Diagnoses and clinical conditions that are covered:	Chronic* myofascial pain Fibromyalgia as defined by 1990 ACR Criteria† Chronic neck and back pain Dysmenorrhea Chronic headaches including migraine and stress Pain secondary to metastatic disease Chronic neuropathic pain Chronic arthritis Hyperemesis with pregnancy Nausea and vomiting associated with chemotherapy, not responding to usual medical management *Chronic refers to symptoms that are present on a daily basis for greater than a 3-month duration.	Subacute** myofascial pain not responding to usual management (excludes acute and chronic pain conditions). Examples include plantar fasciitis, thoracic outlet syndrome, epicondylitis, neck/back strain. Part of rehabilitation benefit where expected to produce sustainable functional improvement in 60 days. Not covered for relaxation, palliative, maintenance therapy, or other indications. **Subacute refers to duration of symptoms generally between 2 and 6 months.	Premenstrual syndrome Menopausal symptoms Chronic*** fatigue syndrome Chronic arthritis Chronic irritable bowel syndrome Fibromyalgia as defined by the 1990 ACR Criteria† Headaches (persistent sinus, muscle tension, migraine) Chronic sinusitis Chronic serous otitis media (duration of 3 months) Eczema/atopic dermatitis Asthma (nonoral steroid dependent) ***Chronic refers to symptoms that are present on a daily basis for greater than a 3-month duration.
Visit limit:	8 visits and then review by primary care physician and alternative care medical reviewer. Treatment summary within 10 days of eighth visit to health plan's administrative office.	Co-managed with physical therapist/ occupational therapist. 6 visits within 60 days (no extensions) and should occur simultaneously with a physical therapy program. Treatment summary to health plan's administrative office.	3 visits and then reviewed by primary care physician and alternative care medical reviewer. Treatment summary within 10 days of third visit to health plan's administrative office.

continues

Table 33.1–1 continued

Therapy	Acupuncture	Massage Therapy	Naturopathy
Refer to where?	See network provider list.	See network provider list.	See network provider list.
Ancillary services (labs, pharmacy, x-rays):	Labs, x-rays, pharmacy must be ordered via primary care provider and provided through the health plan.	Labs, x-rays, pharmacy must be ordered via primary care provider and provided through the health plan.	Lab services must be obtained through specific providers, among from a range of labs, depending on location.* Health plan encourages naturopaths to phone health plan's lab customer service to obtain results. Pharmacy prescriptions must be filled at the health plan's medical centers. No coverage for botanical herbs, vitamins, food supplements. NTX lab testing is excluded from coverage. All x-rays, EKGs, ultrasounds, procedures (ie, scoping), allergy (scratch) testing, injections to be done by health plan. *Contracted alternative providers must check with the health plan's provider manual for more detailed information. There are specific details for specific geographic areas for laboratory services.

Note: ACR, American College of Rheumatology
Courtesy of Group Health Cooperative of Puget Sound.

forms of CAM coverage. We have a network of chiropractors who work under capitation, as opposed to fee-for-service. Our network management company handles the requests for extended treatment through an interactive voice technology system that can be accessed by telephone. Chiropractors call a toll-free number and respond to a series of questions regarding the type of symptoms and their duration. Most of the time, they will receive an immediate response to their request for the authorization of continued visits. If the system cannot provide a decision, the case goes to a review board for consideration. The system has certain advantages because the guidelines and authorization are based on peer standards, which are just beginning to be developed in the other CAM professions. This is relatively new technology, and only time will determine its effectiveness.

The point in the cycle at which the chiropractor must obtain authorization from the expert system depends on the insurance plan. The guidelines are based on the chiropractic benefits elected by the employers who purchase the plan. The authorizations are based on both the diagnosis and the severity of the condition. The expert system is designed to evaluate the severity of symptoms by asking questions about the nature of the pain that the patient is experiencing (for example, whether the pain is radiating and how far it is radiating).

For chiropractic, these responses are relatively straightforward, because our network chiropractors focus on the treatment of back and neck pain. However, it would not be as easy to tailor this type of system to the practice of a naturopath, in which there is much greater variability in the conditions treated and the therapies used. This reflects both the opportunity for systemization in areas of service and the need to tailor procedures uniquely within other programs in complementary medicine.

33.2   A Quality Management Program in Complementary Medicine

Lynn McDowell

INTRODUCTION

American WholeHealth Networks, Inc. (AWHN), a wholly owned subsidiary of American WholeHealth (AWH), is a corporation that organizes integrative medicine practitioners into networks or programs to make health care services available to policy holders, employees, and

Lynn McDowell is Vice President of Medical Services for American WholeHealth Networks, Inc. and is responsible for quality management services for its nationwide complementary medicine network. Ms. McDowell supervised quality and utilization management for Aetna Health Insurance for 12 years.

members of groups. Approximately 20 million people nationwide have access to AWHN's networks. AWHN has adopted a continuous quality improvement (CQI) process as a means of conducting business. Quality improvement is achieved through a multidisciplinary approach and effective teamwork.

The quality management program focuses on the assessment and improvement of both the service and the quality of the care delivered to patients by contracted practitioners and the services provided to practitioners by AWHN. It provides a framework for the development and measurement of activities representing all functional processes of the organization, as can be seen in its Quality Management Workplan (Exhibit 33.2–1). Although the program is broad in scope, including 32 practitioner types and all 50 states, it attempts to identify those issues relevant to the customer.

As a leading national integrative medicine network company, it is the goal and responsibility of the organization to define the industry standard. AWHN is committed to accomplish this goal by maintaining a comprehensive quality management program, effective practitioner selection and recruitment, consistent high-standard credentialing, and compliance with regulatory and certification requirements.

PROGRAM COMPONENTS

A comprehensive quality management program strives to identify, monitor, and improve the services and care delivered to customers. The program components discussed below are especially important in a CAM program.

Review and Evaluation of Integrative Medicine Services

Identifying the demographics of the population serviced by the network and determining which services are most commonly provided are key to building an effective quality management program. The program should focus on improving the health care and services that are delivered to a wide base of customers, in addition to some of those high-cost and possibly high-risk services. By understanding the types of services provided and the practice patterns of the contracted practitioners, a baseline of data can be built, from which opportunities for improvements can be identified and results can be compared.

AWHN began capitating chiropractic covered benefits in 1988 and complementary and alternative benefits in 1997. Today, AWHN administers both covered benefit and discount plans for millions of patients nationwide. Data on discount services can be difficult to obtain. AWHN has partnered with several health plans and is currently collecting this type of data, in addition to the covered benefit utilization data. When evaluating data, it is important to look at the type of benefit plan available, the limitations of that plan, the availability of the network practitioners, the scope of their practice, and state regulations.

Credentialing and Recredentialing

The National Committee on Quality Assurance (NCQA) has set standards for credentialing that are frequently adopted by network credentialing programs. Although NCQA has developed credentialing criteria for medical doctors, osteopaths, and chiropractors, standard criteria have not been developed for the majority of the CAM specialists. The challenge is to develop criteria that measure quality in a manner consistent with the NCQA standards and allows an adequate number of practitioners to participate.

AWHN has been awarded Credentialing Verification Organization (CVO) certification by NCQA. This means that AWHN's credentialing program has met or exceeded the NCQA standards and that the organization has been recognized for a management structure that monitors and promotes quality improvement. AWHN credentials the following practitioner types: chiropractor, naturopathic physician, physician/osteopath acupuncturist, chiropractor/naturopathic physician acupuncturist, holistic physician (MD/DO), acupuncturist, behavioral health practitioner, dietitian, holistic nurse practitioner, Chinese herbal medicine practitioner, Oriental bodywork therapist, massage therapist, rolfer, myotherapist, reflexologist, naprapathy practitioner, Alexander Technique teacher, Feldenkrais teacher, exercise specialist/personal trainer, Hellerwork therapist, Qi Gong instructor, Reiki practitioner, T'ai chi instructor, Trager therapist, yoga instructor, biofeedback practitioner, guided imagery/hypnotherapy practitioner, meditation instructor, homeopathic practitioner, Ayurvedic practitioner, nutritionist, and herbal consultant.

Exhibit 33.2–1 Quality Management Workplan

Activity	Committee	JAN	FEB	MAR	APR	MAY	JUN	JUL	AUG	SEP	OCT	NOV	DEC
Quality Management (QM) Report to the Board of Directors				X			X			X			X
QM Program Description Review	OQC, Q/UM	X		X									
QM Work Plan	OQC, Q/UM	X											
Annual QM Program Evaluation	OQC, Q/UM	X											
QM Policy Review	OQC, Q/UM	X				X							
Utilization Management (UM) Program Description Review	OQC, Q/UM	X	X										
UM Policy Review	OQC, Q/UM		X	X									
UM Criteria Review	OQC, Q/UM					X							
Interrater Reliability Assessment Review	OQC, Q/UM								X				
Network Analysis	OQC											X	
Utilization Data Review	OQC, Q/UM			X			X			X			X
Access Data/Survey Review	OQC										X		
Availability Data/Survey Review	OQC										X		
Practitioner Change Data Review	OQC			X			X			X			X
Practitioner Data Audit	OQC				X			X					
Complaint/Appeal Data Analysis	OQC, Q/UM		X			X			X			X	
Delegation Oversight Review	OQC	X								X			
Medical Record Documentation Review	OQC, Q/UM						X						X
Member Satisfaction Survey	OQC								X				
Practitioner Satisfaction Survey	OQC									X			
CVO Credentialing Turnaround Time	OQC, CC			X			X			X			X
CVO % of Network Credentialed	OQC, CC						X						X
CVO Committee Satisfaction	OQC, CC						X						X
CVO Audit Results	OQC, CC			X			X			X			X
Customer Reports	OQC, CC			X			X			X			X
Annual File Count	OQC								X				

OQC, oversight committee; Q/UM, quality, utilization management committee; CC, credentialing committee; CVO, credentialing verification organization

Courtesy of American WholeHealth Networks, Inc., Hartland, Wisconsin.

The credentialing program focuses on data collection, analysis, reporting of findings, and evaluation of customer satisfaction with the program. The program activities include:

1. Application review and comparison with business criteria
2. System data entry and file development of professional documentation
3. Primary verification of professional credentials
4. Data comparison with credentialing criteria
5. Telephone interview for identified specialties
6. On-site office visit, as requested by customer
7. File/system audit, data analysis, and report preparation
8. Review of performance indicators
9. Evaluation of both practitioner and network satisfaction with the credentialing process

AWHN credentials an average of 200 practitioners monthly. From the date that the credentialing file is received until the date that the file is marked "ready for committee," there is an average turnaround time of 20 days. From the "attestation date" on the file until the file is approved by the credentialing committee, there is an average turnaround time of 48 days.

On-Site Visits and Medical Record Audits

Site visits have most commonly encompassed the primary care physician and high-volume or high-risk practitioners. Performing site visits to CAM practitioners' offices offers credibility and a sense of security to some customers. It also allows the network an opportunity to identify educational needs. Although safety and patient confidentiality are requirements that must be met, AWHN views site visits as an opportunity to partner with practitioners in improving the service site. It is not uncommon for some networks to request photographs of a practitioner's practice site, and an on-site visit offers the most protection. The professionalism and safety of the site are a common concern of the customer.

Because site visits are a topic of interest to customers, AWHN works with each customer individually to recommend a plan specific to his or her needs. Two examples have been found to be quite effective.

Plan 1:
• Initial site visits to all practitioners participating in a customer-specific network
• Site visits every two years to the high-volume practitioners, as determined by number of patients seen and number of visits per patient
• Site visits every two years for practitioners in remote locations

Plan 2
• Initial site visits performed for those specialties that the customer has identified as being of high risk. This would be a random selection of practitioner sites, based on the customer's patient demographics, for example, 50% of one specialty type and 25% of two others
• Site visits every two years to an additional 20% of network practitioners, based on volume of services rendered
• Site visits to practice sites that have received complaints

Clinical Practice Guidelines

Development, implementation, and monitoring of clinical practice guidelines comprise another activity in the evolution of CAM quality assurance. AWH, in conjunction with integrative medicine clinics and practitioners, has developed clinical practice guidelines for more than 100 diagnoses typically treated by CAM practitioners. The clinical practice guidelines have been tested in the clinics and are being integrated into the network organization. Use of consistent clinical practice guidelines provides the groundwork for effectively measuring outcomes.

Guidelines need to be shared with practitioners and performance measured against the guidelines. Networks that have developed or adopted certain clinical practice guidelines are often reluctant to share them at this early stage in the development of integrative medicine services. Measuring performance against guidelines can be accomplished through on-site medical record reviews or at desktop audits.

Complaints and Appeals

Basic to any quality program is the review, resolution, and tracking of patient and practitioner complaints and appeals. Patients and practitioners can complain about any service provided by the network or a contracted practitioner or any decision made by the network or a network customer. Appeal and complaint data provide information on practitioner performance, compliance with network policy, quality of care, and customer satisfaction. Networks need to have written policies on the handling of complaints, appeals, and grievances. Policies need to address the various types of complaints and appeals. These include: how complaints and appeals are tracked, how peer-review committees are involved, who is involved in the investigation and resolution, what actions are possible, the time frames in which they need to be resolved, and what types of issues are reported.

In addition to resolving complaints and appeals, networks need to analyze the data and look for opportunities for improvement. Trends that are typically monitored may include practitioners with multiple complaints, similar or repetitive administrative issues, and noncompliance with network policy. Networks need to be extremely sensitive to quality of care issues.

AWHN categorizes complaints and appeals as: credentialing appeals, utilization management appeals, quality of care appeals, and general appeals. There were a total of 56 complaints in 1999. Fifty were administrative, and six were quality of care complaints. The most common administrative complaints were balance billing and incomplete treatment plans. There were no

reportable actions in 1999. The analysis showed no complaint patterns and no practitioners with more than one complaint.

Complaint and appeal information for each practitioner should be included in the recredentialing process. The number and type of complaints may be an indicator of future behavior and future risk. This information is also effectively used in individual practitioner profiling.

Regulatory and Certification/Accreditation Compliance

Current and proposed regulations in the field of integrative medicine are complex. Regulations vary from state to state and by practitioner specialty type. Some states are highly regulated, and others have no regulations at all. States commonly regulate a practitioner's scope of practice; more and more states are licensing, and some cities now also provide licensure.

AWHN contracts with practitioners in all 50 states and, therefore, must be informed of regulations in all states. The following is a sampling of the data collected by AWHN.

Patient and Practitioner Satisfaction

Surveys. Organizations use surveys as a means of assessing both compliance with quality management programs and satisfaction of its customers with the network and network services. Among the variety of surveys utilized, satisfaction surveys and access and availability surveys are the most common. It is important to survey the practitioners' satisfaction with the network organization, including its credentialing process and its utilization management programs. Surveys are also an effective way of assessing patient satisfaction with the network, network programs, and practitioner services.

Survey results provide excellent feedback to organizations on the stability of the network, the likelihood that customers will continue to contract, and the strengths and weaknesses of both network and contracted practitioners. The major weaknesses of a network should be incorporated in the quality management work plan as opportunities for improvements. The quality committee, along with contracted practitioners, should determine which interventions would be most appropriate to achieve the desired results.

Practitioner Access. Networks should have access and availability policies as a condition of practitioner participation. AWHN has standards that address the time frame in which practitioners are able to accommodate urgent, emergent, and routine services. Standards vary for practitioners in covered benefit networks versus the discounted networks, and standards vary among practitioner types.

AWHN uses on-site visits, telephone surveys, and patient satisfaction surveys to ensure that practitioners are complying with these standards. Practitioners who do not meet this requirement will be notified of the need to correct this deficit. Follow-up is conducted within three months of initial survey, if needed.

AWHN requires that practitioners have provisions for 24-hour availability. Patients need to know how to access care in emergency situations and during hours when the practitioner's office may be closed. *The provision for 24-hour availability may be accomplished in one of several ways:*

1. A prerecorded answering machine message that includes the telephone number of the practitioner on call or instructions on what to do in case of an emergency
2. Call Forwarding to the residence of the practitioner on call when the office is closed or the primary practitioner is unavailable
3. Call Forwarding to an answering service to take messages for the practitioner on call, with assurance to the patient that his or her call will be returned within one hour

AWHN conducts telephone surveys and uses on-site visits and patient satisfaction surveys to evaluate compliance with this standard. Failure to provide 24-hour availability is identified as a quality issue, and the practitioner will be notified of the need to correct this deficit. Corrective measures will include education of the practitioner. Recurrent failure to meet this policy could result in sanctions.

Program Resources

AWH and AWHN executives locally and nationally are dedicated to the continuous quality improvement process. Medical and professional staff, system support, and financial resources are sufficient to meet the program objectives. The local Medical Services Department administers the quality management program. Program resources include a medical director, two associate medical directors, a medical director consultant, a vice president, medical services, two network managers, seven network representatives, and two receptionists/administrative assistants.

Credentialing, member and practitioner satisfaction, access and availability, and complaints and appeals are handled by the local network representatives. Customer service is handled by staff at locations closest to the customer. The Operations Department provides additional customer service support. System support, including data retrieval and analysis, is provided by Information Services.

CONCLUSION

Although complementary medicine clearly reflects unique aspects, fundamentally, quality management for CAM resembles quality management for any medical service. It is important that CAM practitioners and CAM services be held to the same standards and the same high level of quality as other disciplines. Consistent focus on quality is one of the endeavors that will ultimately facilitate integrative medicine.

PART IX

Integrative Medicine Centers

CHAPTER 34

Designing the Integrative Medicine Center

34.1   Planning and Development in the Integrative Medicine Center

Linda L. Bedell-Logan with Nancy Faass

STRATEGIC PLANNING

As a consulting firm, Solutions in Integrative Medicine (SIM) provides on-site evaluation for the development of integrative medicine centers. At each evaluation, a thorough assessment is performed to provide the basis for a complete set of recommendations. The consultant works with the management of the center to develop a business plan. If the center is new, the planning process will also involve the development of clinical operations. Currently, there are three primary types of integrative medicine centers: academic centers, hospital-based facilities, and freestanding centers. SIM has participated in the development of all three types of centers, including programs at Harvard, Stanford, and Yale, as well as numerous other universities and health systems—more than 65 integrative programs to date.

On-Site Evaluation

In the on-site assessment process, the consultant meets with everyone in the organization, from the receptionist and the billing staff to the CEO. The consultation includes a tour of the facility by a member of the staff, rather than by management, which provides an opportunity to see the organization from a different perspective. As a focal point of the visit, the consultant also confers with the director and the managers. The organizational chart is reviewed, and the entire operation of the center is evaluated in the context of the center's mission and the long-term goals. At that point, all of the information is analyzed, and an executive summary with recommendations is submitted.

It is important to determine the mission of the organization. Why is there interest in creating a program in integrative medicine? Are patients the source of the motivation? Has the initiative arisen out of a desire to change the health delivery system? Is the impetus primarily economic? These issues are important because, ultimately, the development of a viable integrative program requires a great deal of expertise and patience. If an organization is not genuinely committed to this process, management may not have the

---

Linda L. Bedell-Logan, President and CEO of Solutions in Integrative Medicine, has worked in health care administration for Medicare and the private sector and has been a consultant in the development of complementary medicine for a decade.

patience to follow through, and it is not likely to commit the financial resources required to sustain the effort over the long term.

The Relationship between the Center and the Stakeholders

Every new center entails an entirely new set of challenges. The needs of each environment are unique, and, although there are developmental models, the models must be adapted to the specific circumstances and requirements of the individual center.

Relationships must be built with the community. Those relationships involve not only potential clients, but also physicians, practitioners, the hospitals, and insurance companies—all of the major stakeholders, from patients to payers. The model focuses on how those relationships work—how they are initiated and how they are sustained. In some states, there is a very friendly regulatory climate that provides the requisite structure for professional licensure and for insurance reimbursement. In those regions, insurance companies are willing and able to participate in pilot projects. In other states, the legislative climate is unfriendly to complementary and alternative medicine (CAM); as a result, project development is more difficult and must be approached very differently. It is important to anticipate a wide range of responses to any integrative medicine initiative as the program relates to each different constituency.

The Relationship between the Center and Other Providers

Most of the integrative medicine centers that SIM has assisted in developing are designed specifically as disease management centers. The community-based healing philosophy addresses the medical needs of the community as a whole and focuses on the diseases that create overutilization in our health care system. This approach involves identifying and targeting the most prevalent clinical conditions in any given region and designing programs around these identified needs. Programs are then developed to provide state-of-the art integrative treatment and care for patients suffering with pain syndromes, heart disease, cancer, and other major chronic disorders.

It is assumed that patients of the integrative medicine center will retain their primary care physician or health care provider to treat them outside the integrative setting. SIM does not recommend that centers set themselves up as primary care facilities, because one primary care physician cannot keep five complementary practitioners occupied. CAM practitioners must rely on outside referrals. Primary care providers are hesitant to refer patients to other providers who also offer primary care services. Typically, they would be concerned that they might lose patients. Rather, the integrative centers are developed as specialty centers only. This provides the basis for ongoing relationships and referrals from primary care providers in the community and eliminates the concern that patients will be co-opted.

An Integrative Model

The integrative medicine model involves holistic nurse practitioners in a central role, providing coordination at the hub of the organization. There are typically two medical directors: a director of natural medicine, who is a naturopathic doctor, and the director of biomedicine, a medical doctor. The nurse practitioner serves as the coordinator of complementary practitioners from a range of disciplines.

Physicians most often see patients initially for screening, to rule out more serious conditions or to provide an alternative perspective on the patient's condition. For example, it is possible that a massage therapist with only 100 hours of training might not detect a cancerous tumor and may treat it as though it were simply a knotted muscle. To bring safety and choice to medical care and to the process of disease management, integration is essential. This means that medical oversight and a holistic perspective are merged in the treatment process. The naturopathic physician works in partnership with the medical doctor to coordinate a team of providers, including massage therapists, acupuncturists, mind-body practitioners, chiropractors or osteopaths, and others. Working as a multidisciplinary team, they make decisions collaboratively to develop care plans through the forum of team meetings.

MAXIMIZING PATIENT SERVICES

A Developmental Model

It is important that the center be designed to create a different experience in total for the patient, rather than one that merely adds new clinical options. The goal is to stimulate improvement by reaching the patient on a human level and eliciting a healing response. Every interaction can provide an opportunity for healing.

Staff Training. Informal education by the consultant begins at the time of the initial evaluation. Staff are trained in the special qualities that are essential to client services in a successful integrative medicine center. The staff must develop a keen sense of what it means to be chronically ill and how important the response of the staff is to patients.

Quality of Communication. Mechanisms are built into the program to maximize the quality of the patient's experience in both initial and ongoing contacts. A therapeutic response can be encouraged in the initial interaction with the receptionist, the first person with whom the patient has contact. Every effort is made to relate to the patient in a manner that is not rushed or harried.

Initial Contact. In-depth new patient contact is not initiated with the telephone receptionist but through a patient educator. New patients are either connected with this liaison immediately or given a timely telephone appointment to speak with an educator in a day or two.

Patient Education. Before the initial consultation, the patient is typically seen by a holistic nurse and receives an intake, screening, and re-

ferral. That first appointment includes explanations of how the center works; the services provided; the philosophy, approach, and responsibilities of the clinical staff; and the patient's responsibilities. When the patient is given a protocol, there is much homework to be done—the patient is expected to be an active partner in the treatment process. Patient education may be provided by a nurse, a practitioner, or a patient educator. In any case, patient education and participation are fundamental to integrative medicine. Complementary care and lifestyle interventions involve an approach that is more proactive and demands more of the patient. The patient is asked to participate in problem solving, prioritizing options, and setting treatment goals.

The Mind-Body Connection. The psychological aspects of illness are also important. Counseling may be recommended to identify areas of high stress, negative attitudes, or habits of self-care that sabotage the healing process. In one case, we learned of a patient diagnosed with advanced prostate cancer who recovered through psychotherapy and without chemotherapy. It is sometimes vital to make the mind-body connection.

The Therapeutic Encounter. The pressure to serve many clients may create a rushed process, and the perception of haste tends to compromise the potential of the therapeutic encounter. Conversely, the patient encounter can be one of the most healing aspects of the service provided. It is essential to take a compassionate approach. The patient must be touched in a caring manner, with healing intention.

The importance of the therapeutic encounter has been further validated in the *Current Procedural Terminology* (CPT) manual of the American Medical Association (2000). Now the element of time may be considered "the key or controlling factor" to qualify a patient encounter as a particular level of "evaluation and management service." Never before has time alone been considered a controlling factor in defining the level of service and, therefore, of reimbursement. Physicians can now bill for time spent counseling patients and not be penalized for allegedly overbilling.

Maximizing the Multidisciplinary Team. Developing a cohesive team can be a challenge. Therefore, it is important to seek out practitioners who are interested in working collaboratively. The hiring process involves the identification of flexible team players in preference to those who are less willing to participate, whether due to their training or to the need for a high degree of autonomy.

Developing Patient Protocol

Once the integrative team has been established, there is the opportunity to develop protocol for the treatment of chronic conditions such as diabetes, migraines, cancer, and asthma. Initially, the care pathways of an immature center are relatively speculative. However, as more clinical experience is accumulated, the protocols become more mature, and the evidence base is informed by the additional clinical experience. Working with feedback from physicians, patients, and clinical outcomes, there is the opportunity to refine the multidisciplinary treatment approach. Data and clinical experience inform both general protocol development and the evolution of more subtle individualized treatment approaches.

Maximizing the Synergy of Treatment. Integrative medicine provides the possibility of developing new approaches to treatment—new therapeutic protocols and care pathways. The goal is to maximize the synergistic effect. For example, when chiropractic treatment and massage are provided in combination, clinical experience suggests that the adjustments tend to hold longer. Healing may occur more rapidly as a result of this dual treatment, and there is a cost benefit, as well. This demonstrates the type of protocol refinement that will occur as outcomes data are accumulated and aggregated regarding the clinical applications of complementary therapies.

Individualized Protocol. In protocol development for specific patients, the predominant therapy is refocused periodically, based on the response of the patient. When the client indicates that one therapy is working better than another, the protocol is adjusted accordingly. The deciding factor in the development of the protocol is the patient's response to treatment.

Reimbursement for Disease Management. SIM is interested in the development of a flexible capitated insurance product that would provide a flat rate for patients with expensive chronic conditions. The payment would be predicated on the idea of applying the flat rate reimbursement flexibly, based on the individualized requirements of each particular patient and his or her diagnosis, unique circumstances, and treatment needs. The money could be spent on appropriate evidence-based therapies deemed appropriate for that particular disease, as prescribed by the primary care provider or the multidisciplinary team. Disease management centers would be empowered to apply that money in flexible patient-oriented, individualized multidisciplinary protocols that enable the center to treat a range of degenerative diseases using highly flexible approaches, with the goals of reducing human cost and maximizing cost benefit. Medical savings accounts could be applied in a similar fashion.

THE FUTURE

Visionary leaders in health care are creating new delivery systems that integrate conventional technological advances with alternative and complementary therapies and reemerging traditional approaches to clinical intervention. Our challenge is to create a system that—through individual choices, belief systems, and informed consent—will increase the quality of care rendered in the United States. It is vital to lower expenditures in this area in an effort to enhance our federal and private health care delivery systems and improve the overall quality of life for our citizens.

REFERENCES

American Medical Association. *Current Procedural Termi-nology CPT™ 2000*. Chicago: American Medical Association; 2000, 8.

34.2 Case Study: Planning and Reimbursement in an Integrative Medicine Center

Lon Hatfield

Integrative medicine is in a state of intense evolution. What it looks like today is not what it will look like in a year. The evolutionary process is occurring very rapidly and is assuming different forms in various environments. There is no model that is right for everyone. Consequently, there is no nice, neat prescription for success. Most centers continue to be very much in a learning mode.

BUILDING ON AN EXISTING RELATIONSHIP WITH THE COMMUNITY

It is important to strive for a high degree of excellence. The Healing Arts Center in Colville, Washington, developed out of another medical practice that had been established in the community for more than 20 years. That practice began with five physicians and grew to about 25 doctors in a multispecialty group, affiliated

with a hospital that was voted one of the most stable rural hospitals in the United States by the American Hospital Association. That original medical group has been recognized as one of the 18 best rural clinics in the United States and the best in the state of Washington. The integrative medicine center has built on that history.

The second center has also forged a new path. In the decision to create an integrative program, it became important to decide whether the second center should be part of the original or be developed in a new setting. It was decided that the new center should have its own distinct identity to bring the concept more fully to fruition.

Providing Value-Driven Services

Many complementary care programs lack clarity and intent. In some cases, they reflect an economic decision spurred by the market that has been identified with alternative medicine. In other situations, major shortcuts are being taken in order to offer CAM services in a timely manner. To create the right environment, the first step is to make sure your goals and motivations are clear. Get your integrity clear. Define what you are trying to achieve. Study everything you can and immerse yourself in the work.

Lon Hatfield, MD, PhD, is a family practice physician and biochemist now specializing in integrative medicine. He is founding medical director of the Healing Arts Center in Colville, Washington, an alternative medicine center with 10 practitioners, and cofounder in 1979 of the nationally recognized Northeast Washington Medical Group, an allopathic medical center that now has 25 physicians.

BUSINESS PROFILE

Colville Healing Arts Center, which was founded in May 1998, is unusual among large clinics. The 10,000-square-foot clinic successfully hit operational break-even in just 12 months of operation (Weeks, 1999). The following profile in Table 34.2–1 reflects data averaged over a four-month period.

The monthly charges are billings, rather than collections, in cases in which third-party payment applies. The goal is an 80% collection rate, which puts the center just above the $92,000 monthly operating expenses. Collections average approximately 80–90% at the previous conventional medicine clinic. In the development of the integrative medicine center, the importance of management is often overlooked. The role of the administrator is vital in monitoring financial management and promoting staff development.

Working with Insurers

One strength of the Colville facility is the extent of reimbursed services. Nearly two-thirds of services (65%) are paid through traditional indemnity insurers, and another 5% are reimbursed through managed care contracting. One factor in this high level of coverage is the clinic's location in the state of Washington, where a 1995 state law requires all plans to include "every category of provider." Consequently, services of naturopathic physicians, acupuncturists, and massage practitioners are more likely to be reimbursed than in many jurisdictions.

In addition, the clinic's ability to obtain coverage can also be attributed to positive communication and relationships built with insurers. In billing, the administrators work cooperatively with the insurance companies as a resource to help them determine how to relate to an alterna-

Table 34.2–1 Colville Healing Arts Center: Business Profile

Provider/Service Type	No. of Staff	Types of Services	Monthly Charges
Osteopathic physician	1	Physical medicine, adjustments	$24,000
Naturopathic physician	1	Natural medicine—primary care	$11,000
Medical doctor	1/2	Part-time; also provides management, outreach; 50% conventional medicine	$13,000
Education, counseling	1	Psychological orientation	$12,000
Acupuncturist/physical therapist	2	Dual license, provides mixed services	$21,000
Natural pharmacy		Separate corporation	$12,000
Laboratory			$3,000
Other clinical services	6	Nurse practitioners, massage therapists, yoga, biofeedback	$43,000
Total Receipts	14		Approximately $136,000
Adjusted Receipts			
Total Operating Expenses			$92,000

*All figures adjusted down slightly at second yearly evaluation, except acupuncture, which was increased from $12,000 to $21,000.

Source: Reprinted with permission from J. Weeks, Monthly Review Spread from 10,000 Square Foot Center, *The INTEGRATOR for the Business of Alternative Medicine*, Vol. 4, No. 2,3, p. 7, © 1999.

tive medicine clinic. Another important factor is the way in which claims are worded: They must make sense to an insurer.

The insurance firms cover standard procedures, but in some cases, they also provide coverage for new types of treatment. For example, the author, as medical director of the center, worked closely with insurers to assist in the conversion of traditional Chinese medicine diagnoses into ICD-9 (International Classification of Diseases) codes.

In billing for new techniques that have not yet been assigned ICD-9 codes, the approach is to describe the treatment method to the insurer, as well as other treatment options. For example, in the treatment of allergies, one option would be to write an ongoing prescription for medication or desensitization shots. However, when patients are treated with the Nambudripad Allergy Elimination Technique (NAET), it is sometimes possible to eliminate the allergy completely. The center cannot charge for the treatment because, at the time of this writing, there is no ICD-9 code for NAET therapy. Rather, there is simply a charge for the office visit, which the insurance company has agreed to cover. Thus, the approach to insurance coverage has been

to communicate with insurers, explain the treatment for a particular diagnosis, and ask the insurer how it wants staff to word the claim so that it is intelligible to the underwriters.

It is important that CAM disciplines develop a means of coding not only specific treatments, but also the services of providers. For example, one of the traditional Chinese medicine practitioners at the center is an acupuncturist-physical therapist. Under her physical therapy license, she cannot make a medical diagnosis. Under her acupuncture license, she can make only an Eastern diagnosis, and there are no ICD-9 codes for Eastern diagnoses, so there has been no way to bill an insurance company directly. She is not allowed to provide Western diagnoses through her acupuncture license. However, as a medical doctor working in conjunction with her, the author can provide the Western diagnoses for some of her patients. Essentially, this is a matter of reconceptualizing treatment within a Western framework and communicating the protocol to an insurance company in terms that make sense. In this phase of integrative medicine, there is a great need to translate and reword basic concepts, definitions, and descriptions.

REFERENCE

Weeks J. Monthly revenue spread from 10,000 square foot center. *Integrator.* 1999;4(2,3):7.

CHAPTER 35

Three Free-Standing Integrative Medicine Centers

35.1 Perspective: Community Health Centers of King County

Thomas Trompeter with Nancy Faass

ADMINISTRATIVE STRUCTURE

Organizational Model. Community Health Centers of King County is a nonprofit community health care organization, which means that it is a primary medical corporation with a mission to provide care to people who are underserved. There are six health centers in the corporation. The Kent Community Health Center is an integrative primary care clinic.

Clinical Focus. Its clinical focus is primary care.

Management Model. The management of the clinic resembles that of a nonprofit center with an administrative team, rather than that of a pri-

vate practice. Clinical supervision is provided by a medical director, who oversees both integrative and complementary services. The natural medicine program was developed in collaboration with Bastyr University. The initial medical director was quite knowledgeable regarding natural medicine—an important criterion for that role. Administrative operations are overseen by a chief financial officer, a deputy director, and a number of other managers. The author serves as executive director. Governance is also provided by a board of directors that functions appropriately for a nonprofit, community-based service organization.

CLINICAL SERVICES

Triage Protocol. Patient utilization of CAM is a matter of patient choice. The clinic has a list of conditions for which patients must first see a physician. These are primarily the kinds of conditions that could result in hospitalization or that are extremely acute. This approach also respects the scope-of-practice laws for acupuncturists, naturopathic physicians, and medical doctors.

Thomas Trompeter, MPA, is the Executive Director of Community Health Centers of King County, a private non-profit corporation providing primary health care services for underserved residents of King County outside the city of Seattle and home of the King County Natural Medicine Clinic. Prior to joining CHCKC, Mr. Trompeter was the Executive Director of the Northwest Regional Primary Care Association. He has worked with nonprofit providers of care to underserved people for over 20 years.

Interdisciplinary Communication. The clinic care at Kent is a collaborative operation. Practitioners interact on a daily basis. The clinic also has regular sessions in which the providers meet once a month. Clinical issues are discussed rather broadly for all of the providers present. Conferences focus on the needs of specific patients, as well as on a policy level. In addition, time is set aside to discuss specific approaches to treatment from the perspective of natural medicine. There are six medical clinics in the system, and the integrative clinic is located in the Kent clinic.

Categories of Licensed Providers. The categories of licensed providers include medical doctors, osteopaths, naturopathic physicians, acupuncturists, physician assistants, and nurse practitioners.

Patient Referral. Practitioners in the clinic refer patients out as necessary to a range of psychiatrists and other specialists who are all medical doctors. The clinic also has referral relationships with chiropractic practitioners and with massage therapists, although therapeutic massage is also provided in-house.

Handling of Emergent Situations. The clinic is a primary care facility with primary care physicians working within the scope of family practice. The physicians have referral relationships with four different hospitals, depending on the location of the clinic where they practice. Physicians are all on staff at local hospitals, admit and attend their patients in the hospital, and provide services such as the delivery of babies. They do not, however, perform surgeries; surgical care patients are referred out to specialists.

Primary Conditions Treated. The clinic treats diagnoses appropriately treated within the scope of family practice.

Cases Appropriate for Integrative Care. If a patient comes to the clinic with unspecified chest pain, he or she will be seen by a medical doctor because that could be a symptom of a potential heart attack. If a patient comes in with a broken bone, he or she will certainly be seen

by a medical doctor first because these physicians have the training to provide the appropriate treatment. The clinic prefers to see those conditions that are within the scope of practices of its providers.

In terms of an integrative approach, there is a great deal of communication and referral among the providers. To use a somewhat simplistic analogy, the practitioners basically use the tools in the tool box that seem to make sense at the time. Many of the medical doctors have developed a sophisticated understanding of the use of vitamins and supplements, and will prescribe them out of the natural medicine dispensary at the clinic.

Chronic Conditions. The patient population seen at the clinic has a disproportionately high incidence of diabetes, cardiovascular disease, hypertension, and asthma.

EVALUATION AND REIMBURSEMENT

Assessment of Patient Satisfaction. These assessments are performed through periodic surveys. The clinic also has post cards available in all waiting rooms that ask, "How are we doing?" In addition, as a provider of services under Medicaid, the state agency also conducts periodic client surveys. The clinic also works with a managed care program that conducts client surveys. As a result, there is a variety of ways to assess patient satisfaction.

The clinic receives patient feedback on the integrative services from time to time, which is positive. Another reflection of the success of the program is the fact that it is being expanded to other centers—a corporate decision as to the direction in which the program should move.

Assessment of Provider Satisfaction. The clinic performs annual staff surveys, so the focus is not just on the providers. It is on all staff members and practitioners who work with the clinic.

Utilization Management. The clinic has a consolidated utilization management and quality improvement program, whereby quality and utilization measures are monitored very carefully.

Reimbursement. About half of the clinic clients have low incomes and no insurance at all. The remaining patients are either covered by Medicaid or have coverage under a low-income health care insurance program sponsored by the state of Washington. Care for those who have low incomes and no source of coverage is funded by grants.

ADDITIONAL ASPECTS OF THE PROGRAM

Patients of Community Health Centers of King County have wanted an integrative medicine program for some time, as evidenced by the result of a 1995 survey. Sixty percent of patients responding indicated that if the clinic were to provide services considered to be complementary or alternative medicine, these patients would use those services. Because the clinic constantly strives to determine its patients' needs and to provide for them, these survey results were a fairly significant force behind the clinic's decision making.

Clinic management and staff believe that the combination of the two spheres—mainstream and complementary medicine—really is the best of both worlds. Both areas have strengths and weaknesses, but providing them in combination and encouraging honest and collegial relationships among the various providers enable the clinic to provide a system that maximizes benefits for its patients.

35.2   Perspective: The Center for Comprehensive Care

James Blair with Nancy Faass

ADMINISTRATIVE STRUCTURE

Organizational Model. The Center for Comprehensive Care, Inc. (CCC) is comprised of three independent, self standing business entities that work in a coordinated fashion under an incorporated umbrella. The centralized center management acts as a point of service contact

---

James Blair, LAc, Dipl Ac, is a licensed acupuncturist with the Seattle Acupuncture Associates, Center for Comprehensive Care in Seattle, Washington. The Center for Comprehensive Care began as a clinical affiliation in 1989, and incorporated as an independent practice association (IPA) in 1992. The objective of the Center is to provide comprehensive rehabilitation services to the community, based on the philosophy that cost-effective quality patient care, delivered in a timely fashion, will produce the best patient outcome.

for third party payers, physician groups, hospitals, and direct patient populations. The individual businesses beneath the corporate umbrella function to provide each service in an integrated manner. This program of care is facilitated by a nurse care coordinator for more complex cases and between individual practitioners at other times. Each of the business entities has different clinical focuses ranging from physical and occupational therapy to vocational rehabilitation, mental health services, and natural and preventive medicine interventions. A list of services provided can be found in Exhibit 35.2–1.

Clinical Focus. The CCC's individual business patient load ranges the full spectrum of standard metropolitan outpatient clinics. Due to the nature of the services provided and the triaging capacity of the nurse care coordinator, the Center receives a large number of physician and other health practitioner referrals for integrated individualized and programmatic care. These referrals tend to have a high degree of complexity and require innovative care and reimbursement models. The most complex cases are triaged into Chronic Care Programs, which are treatment/education groups, 4 to 16 weeks in length. Each group consists of 6 individuals who meet weekly for 4 hours. A comprehensive program is designed from the list of services offered within the CCC for the needs of each group based on a standard model developed by the CCC. Each individual and group are assessed by standard outcomes measures to provide ongoing assessment and guidance for educational and treatment evolution.

Management Model. There is a part-time administrator for the Center who is also a business manager for one of the businesses comprising the CCC. The administrator is responsible as the point of contact for assessing individual third-party reimbursement for individual and group treatment care. All facility and service contracts are administered and tracked by the person in this position. The administrator is the staff person for the nurse care coordinator and his or her schedule. Overflow help and support for this position are available from the other business administrators on an as-needed basis.

CLINICAL SERVICES

Triage Protocol. Patients are referred by their primary care physician (PCP), other health care provider, or self-referred. Each clinical service triages its own patient load to a level of complexity comfortable within its scope of practice. Clinical care pathways, which describe levels of disease and prognosis and are developed by the CCC, are used to evaluate and trigger need for consultation with another service, the physician, or the nurse coordinator.

Provider Communication. In any integrated care offering, communication and case planning

Exhibit 35.2–1 Services Provided by the CCC.

Occupational Intervention Services

- Occupational Therapy
- Vocational Counseling
- Return to Work Interventions
- Environmental Assessment and Planning
- Home Access and Safety Assessment
- Cognitive and Functional Therapies
- Job Site Assessment/Modification
- Daily Living Skills Intervention
- Adaptive Therapies/Conditioning
- Work Hardening/Conditioning

Physical Intervention Services

- Physical Therapy
- Postural Alignment
- Spinal Assessment and Treatment
- Sports Rehabilitation
- Massage
- Physical Capacity Evaluations
- Muscular Conditioning and Strengthening
- Injury Prevention and Education
- Acute Injury Care
- Personal Fitness Programs

Natural Health Services

- Acupuncture
- Biofeedback
- Massage Therapy
- Nutritional Counseling
- Herbal Intervention
- Acupressure
- Tai Ch'i/Ch'i Kung Instruction
- Traditional Chinese Medicine
- Traditional Chinese Nutritional Counseling

Courtesy of the Center for Comprehensive Care, Seattle, Washington.

are necessary and the most time-consuming. In the best of all worlds, daily case planning detailing interventions and desired outcomes would be done. In the real world of clinical medicine, weekly staffings are a luxury and bi-weekly meetings are more likely. The most common form of a case staffing are "hallway consults." These meetings are frequent, short, pithy, and can cover most if not all of the less complex case load. The more complex cases are considered and planned in the standard group case staffing.

Categories of Licensed Providers. The Center provides physical therapy, occupational therapy, physical trainers, vocational rehabilitation counselors, mental health counselors, psychotherapists, biofeedback nurses, nurse practitioners, acupuncturists, massage therapists, and traditional Chinese herbal medicine practitioners. Nutrition is provided through the traditional Chinese medicine practice.

Patient Referral. When services at the Center are insufficient as might be the case when the need of a specialty consult is required, the patient is triaged into the surrounding community to the appropriate service or institution for support. The CCC is functionally affiliated and enjoys a healthy referral relationship with the Minor and James physician group that houses most standard care services and has one of the largest rheumatology practices in the western United States. Due to the nature and specialty of the CCC and surrounding physician practices, the Center receives a large number of consults from around the Northwest. These patients are triaged, examined, and, in some cases, treated before being sent back to their communities for continued intervention. This referral into their community is usually done with referral recommendations to the local provider.

Handling of Emergent Situations. Few emergent conditions are seen at the Center. Most cases have been well screened; however, occasionally there is an emergent condition that is then appropriately treated in-house or urgently referred to an outside practitioner or service.

Primary Conditions Treated. The hallmark of care at the CCC are the chronic cases that comprise 20% of patients who consume 80% of the health care dollars. Due to the comprehensive manner in which patients are cared for and the timely triaging from one specialty service to another, we believe the number of treatments and overall costs are reduced. These are practices common to the CCC and its programs of care. Common case loads include rheumatoid arthritis, lupus erythematosus, chronic fatigue and fibromyalgia, undifferentiated connective tissue disorder, polymyalgia rheumatic, and osteoarthritis. More traditional case loads seen in a less integrative manner include traditional musculoskeletal disorders, mental health, migraine and chronic headache patterns, digestive, and menopausal symptoms.

EVALUATION AND REIMBURSEMENT

Assessment. Assessment at the Center has historically been by way of group treatment programs described in previous sections. The standard forms of measurement are the Functional Status questionnaires, both the SF-12 and SF-36, to assess functional improvement in individual and patient populations. The Quality of Life Assessment Tool is also employed. Individual practices have a wide range of assessment tools that are used from the MMPI to visual analogue scales in the rating of pain. The CCC has compiled and presented statistical outcomes for the chronic fatigue/fibromyalgia group treatment programs to the American College of Rheumatology at many of their annual conventions.

Utilization Management. Utilization is monitored through the nurse care coordinator, who assesses the limits of care based on what various insurance plans will cover.

Reimbursement Received for Complementary Medicine. Each part of the country is different. Indeed, each practice within a given region is varied due to the sophistication of CAM providers and complexity of reimbursement systems. Comprehensive Care, the natural medicine service, sees approximately 200 visits per week.

Of these, 65% are third-party reimbursement. Outside billing agencies are utilized to expedite reimbursement that averages 3 to 6 weeks.

Use of CAM Services. In the state of Washington and generally in the Northwest, what are referred to as CAM services have a high degree of utility and viability. Unfortunately, they are often referred to *en masse* although frequently have little in common with one another. They must be triaged individually as should all specialties. As health care reimbursement changes the face of medicine, it is not uncommon to find "alternative" services filling in where more traditional therapies have been limited by reimbursement reform. When this is done well, not only do patients recover more quickly, we often feel that a more complete, cost-effective,

and timely recovery is achieved. In the worst case scenario, CAM services become an add-on expense creating frustration in all avenues of care.

Quality Improvement. Quality assurance is surveyed in-house, but the data calculations and statistical analyses are performed by outside contractors. The Center engages in periodic self-assessments of how patients are doing, how well various programs are running, and whether there are ways that services and processes can be performed better. There is also quality assurance, in the sense that the practitioners and managers all sit down to talk about how the Center is actually doing. The process is comparable to that of a hospital that has a quality assurance committee into which each department has input.

35.3   Perspective: Seattle Cancer Clinic

Kim M. Carlson with Nancy Faass

ADMINISTRATIVE STRUCTURE

Organizational Model. The Seattle Cancer Clinic is owned by a larger company based out of Chicago, but is managed as an individual private practice in Seattle.

Clinical Focus. The focus of the Clinic is the provision of services to patients with cancer. This particular practice brings together medical

---

Kim M. Carlson is Administrator of the Seattle Cancer Treatment and Wellness Center. She also served as administrator for 10 years for a medical oncology practice in Dayton, Ohio, and for 5 years with a hospice in Omaha, Nebraska.

The Seattle Cancer Treatment and Wellness Center integrates medical oncology with natural, scientifically based nutritional medicine that includes naturopathic medicine, nutrition, and Oriental medicine.

oncologists, naturopathic physicians, oncology nurses, Chinese medicine practitioners, and a dietitian. The entire team sees the patients.

Management Model. The Seattle Cancer Treatment and Wellness Center integrates medical oncology with natural, scientifically based nutritional therapies that include naturopathic medicine, nutrition, and Oriental medicine. The focus of the Center is care for the whole person. While treatment occurs in the context of medical oncology, the clinicians of the Center are experienced in using Eastern and Western medicine in combination to address severe chronic conditions. Consultations and interventions are also provided through a range of complementary therapies that, for some patients, may promote comfort and healing.

The two medical oncologists of the Center have trained and participated in treatment and research at a number of facilities, including University of California, San Francisco; Fred Hutchinson Cancer Research Center; the University of Washington Cancer Center; Harbor UCLA; and City of Hope National Medical Center in Los Angeles. The clinical staff also include two acupuncturists trained as physicians in China who teach Oriental medicine at Bastyr University. One supervises clinical acupuncture at Bastyr, and the other has participated on research teams evaluating the use of Chinese herbal medicines in the treatment of chronic conditions. The two naturopathic physicians on staff trained at Bastyr; both also hold master's degrees and have participated in botanical and pharmaceutical research.

Triage Protocol. Typically, patients call for information, and the physicians call them back to discuss the case. The clinic frequently sees patients who are not newly diagnosed. They may have already been through one or two protocols, and they want to know what services the Clinic has to offer. The retention rate of the Seattle Cancer Clinic is about 96% (Seattle Cancer Treatment and Wellness Center, 2000). Patients seem to appreciate the high level of support in the program. The nurses invest a great deal of time providing patient education and thorough explanations. The Clinic has its own support groups. The professional staff members are available on call and go out of their way to be responsive.

Provider Communication. The medical oncologists lead each case. They typically see the patient together with a naturopathic physician, and both follow the patient. The medical oncologists determine whether there are any symptoms best treated by the naturopathic physician and/or the Chinese medicine practitioner. In-house tumor boards are held with all six of the physicians and the dietitian every Thursday for an hour, and the patients are discussed. This time is used to focus the care and determine what is working the most successfully. For example, sometimes the Chinese medicine is working

better for a particular patient than is the naturopathy, or vice versa.

Categories of Licensed Providers. There are two medical oncologists, two naturopathic physicians, two Chinese medicine practitioners (both licensed medical doctors from China), an acupuncturist, and a dietitian.

Patient Referral. The physicians refer patients to a broad range of services, as needed, including surgeons, radiologists, urologists, and so forth. The approach is truly integrative.

Handling of Emergent Situations. There are seldom emergencies in this field. Obviously, if a patient has had a pleural effusion or if a tumor suddenly obstructed breathing, an immediate referral is provided and the patient is admitted to a local hospital.

Primary Conditions Treated. The Clinic treats all types of cancers and hematology conditions.

Conditions Not Treated. Children are not treated at the Clinic. The preference is to treat adults.

Conditions Seen. The Clinic sees all cancer patients, regardless of the type of cancer involved. With the complementary care of naturopathy and the Chinese medicine, it is the observation of the Clinic that patients do much better when they go through chemotherapy.

Most Difficult Cases. In some cases, patients come to the Clinic with cancer at a very advanced stage. Although the disease process may not be controllable, the Clinic still gives these patients as much quality of life as possible because it is able to provide them extensive care. Supplements may be used to support them during chemotherapy. Acupuncture may be provided to decrease the pain. The latest antiemetic medications are used so that patients do not experience excessive nausea and vomiting. These drugs may also be used in combination with acupuncture, if necessary.

Additional Interventions. Massage therapy has just been added and has been well received. Initially, the service is provided two days a week.

EVALUATION AND REIMBURSEMENT

Assessing Patient Satisfaction. Patient surveys are provided to clients. The surveys are mailed off-site so that they cannot be altered by anyone in-house. There is also a suggestion box on-site to track immediate problems that should be brought to our attention. Patients can make suggestions anonymously. We also find it gratifying that we serve an unusually large population of blind and deaf people who have cancer. The data on patient satisfaction are analyzed off-site by an outside contractor, which provides the clinic with indications of what is working and what needs adjustment.

Assessing Provider Satisfaction. In terms of the satisfaction of providers who refer patients to the clinic, there has been a tremendous increase in recent referrals. Two years ago, the clinic patient population was 100% patient referral, with no referrals from physicians as evidenced by the marketing team report on referral patterns. At the present time, 30% of Clinic patients are referred by physicians. Usually, patients are sent by surgeons, urologists, family practice doctors, and internists. They have seen the results in their patients, and that has brought additional referrals.

Patient Satisfaction. The clinic surveys patient satisfaction quarterly. A separate company evaluates the clinic by surveying the patients.

The satisfaction ratings have been approximately 96% (Press Ganey Survey 5, 2000).

Utilization Management. Patients are provided with the services that they need. Services are essentially bundled. For example, the Clinic does not bill for visits to two physicians on the same day of service.

Reimbursement. Approximately 40% of patients have Medicare, which does not currently cover any kind of alternative medicine services provided by the Clinic. In certain cases, patients will pay cash for those additional services. Patients who pay out of pocket represent about 10% of the client population. Approximately 50% of patients have secondary insurance. Indemnity coverage is nearly 10%. Approximately 30 to 40% of reimbursement represents a combination of physician practice organization and HMO payments. However, in some cases, the Clinic absorbs the difference, because full coverage is not yet available.

Effect of CAM on Medical Costs. The observation at the Clinic is that complementary medicine tends to decrease health care costs. It tends to keep people out of the hospital; patients are not hospitalized with malnutrition and other ailments that accompany radiation and/or chemotherapy treatment. Often, they do not need pain medication when they have acupuncture as an adjunct to traditional medical oncology. The experience of the Clinic patients suggests that costs are decreased significantly by using an integrative approach.

Most patients have had prior treatment at a more traditional oncology clinic. Their reports suggest that they feel the cost is substantially less than their prior experiences.

REFERENCES

Press Ganey Survey 5. Seattle, WA; 2000.

Seattle Cancer Treatment and Wellness Center, *Internal Review of Patient Charts*; 2000.

CHAPTER 36

A Multispecialty Group Practice: East-West Health Centers

H. Phil Herre with Nancy Faass

East-West Health Center is a group practice that integrates traditional health care services with complementary and alternative medicine (CAM) therapies. The practitioners come together in a multispecialty group to deliver care selected from the best of all the worlds of medicine. The center is staffed by practitioners who collaborate on patient care, drawing on expertise in biomedicine, Oriental medicine, and CAM therapies. A strong emphasis is placed on education and patient personal responsibility. A range of services is provided at one location, in a comfortable, professional, and aesthetically pleasing environment.

PROGRAM DESIGN

Therapies

The choice of therapies is based on an in-depth review of the medical literature. Initially, East-West hired a physician to investigate the scientific efficacy of all of the CAM therapies currently in use. More than 60 forms of CAM were evaluated, and those with the best record of safety were closely scrutinized. As a result, the therapies offered in the Center are basically those for which there is the strongest evidence of safety and efficacy.

Practitioners

The types of practitioners in the Center include two family practice physicians; a nurse practitioner; two chiropractors (one of them provides acupuncture as well); two acupuncturists who also practice herbology (one of them is a doctor of Oriental medicine with 6 years of training in Oriental medicine); a naturopathic doctor who also practices homeopathy; two psychotherapists; a physical therapist; a nutritionist; six massage therapists; two Rolfers; and trainers in yoga, meditation, and T'ai chi.

THE SITE

East-West Health Center is a freestanding, two-story building with about 7,500 square feet of office space and ample parking. The company began in 1996 and opened its first center early in 1997. The site is located in the central metro area of Denver, which is very accessible to both downtown and the freeway.

Aesthetics

The lobby is a very aesthetically pleasing environment; it is painted in soothing tones—shades of light colors and pastels. There are Chinese paintings and other types of art work on the walls. A waterfall is the centerpiece of the lobby, which was designed especially for the Center by a sculptor. The background sound of trickling water has a pleasant effect. The sculpture depicts a globe with the Eastern and Western worlds coming together—a theme that reflects what the Center is trying to accomplish.

The Use of Space To Minimize Overhead

There are approximately 20 rooms or treatment areas. The exam and massage rooms are

---

H. Phil Herre is the Chief Executive Officer of East-West Health Centers in Denver and one of the organization's owners and founders.

about 8 or 9 feet by 10 feet. Some of the rooms serve more than one purpose and can be used by more than one practitioner, based on scheduling. Patients are seen individually and privately, but for administrative tasks, space is shared by the practitioners. This flexibility enables the Center to keep overhead down. No one has a private office, including the owners. For office space, employees double up with two desks in each room. In some cases, there is a desk and an exam table in the same room. There is a provider area where a number of practitioners gather to work on medical records, check their schedules, or eat lunch.

STAFFING

Most of the practitioners are full-time; a few are part-time. When the Center first opened, practitioners were not sure how successful the business would be, so many of them continued to work part-time in their previous jobs. When it became apparent that the Center would succeed, they dropped their employment at other locations to make East-West the only location where they practice. Some found it difficult to practice in two different locations. At present, the psychotherapists and Rolfing® practitioners provide scheduled hours by appointment.

Recruiting and Credentialing

East-West developed the Center by recruiting the very best practitioners available. The Center conducts its own credentialing process and requires a very high level of credentials for providers. For example, naturopathic doctors are not licensed in Colorado, but they are licensed in 11 other states. The Center requires that its naturopathic doctor be licensed in one of those 11 states.

Training

As an example of the Center's high standards, the naturopathic doctors must have a postgraduate degree in naturopathic medicine from one of the three recognized and accredited naturopathic

colleges in the United States. There is one in Portland, Oregon; one in Seattle, Washington; and one in Scottsdale, Arizona. There are also relatively new naturopathic colleges in Connecticut and in Canada.

Malpractice Coverage

All practitioners are required to carry malpractice insurance. Some of them did not consider carrying this insurance when they were in solo practice. For example, the naturopath originally noted that naturopathic doctors never get sued, and, therefore, he did not require malpractice insurance. However, when he investigated the insurance he found that his national association provided malpractice insurance and concluded that it was a professional asset.

Staff Meetings

Weekly staff meetings are held. All practitioners have an equal voice in decision making. In that way, everyone will feel that he or she is part of the group practice.

CLINICAL MANAGEMENT

The Global Medical Record

There is one centralized chronological medical record in the facility used by all the practitioners. Through that global record, each practitioner has access to information on the care provided by all the other practitioners. The record fosters integration. For example, the physician sees what the massage therapist has done, and the naturopathic doctor sees what the acupuncturist has done. Each practitioner has an equal role in the creation of these records.

Case Conferences

There are case conferences (called grand rounds) in which the charts are reviewed, and the patient's needs are evaluated by the integrative team. On occasion, patients are included in those conferences so they can gain additional input from each practitioner. Then it is the patients' choice as to the treatment they elect. The Center wants to give patients as much control over their own health care as they would like to have.

Triage

Patients decide which providers they want to see. Most clients already know who they would like to see when they make their initial appointment. However, Center staff can also provide patients with guidance by triaging them into the system.

The Herbal Pharmacy

Most of the patients who require some kind of botanical product obtain it in conjunction with their visit. The Center has an herbal pharmacy that stocks between 200 and 300 herbs, either in liquid or in dry form. The naturopathic doctor tends to use more of the liquid herbal extracts. The traditional Chinese medicine doctor uses more of the dry herbs in formulations prepared by prescription for the client. Having the pharmacy on-site enables the Center to provide any of the herbs recommended by the practitioners and provides some sense of control over the quality of those herbs. The Center also sells a very limited number of herbs in the lobby.

Providing Services by Gender

In order to accommodate patient preference, the Center has a male and a female practitioner in each major discipline (acupuncture, chiropractic, and massage). When patients call to make an appointment, the receptionist asks which gender they would prefer to see. Touch is a very personal experience. The Center gives its clients a choice as to whom they want to see. Physician referral is not required before seeing alternative practitioners.

INSURANCE BILLING

Insurance Coverage

East-West accepts all insurance plans, and the Western doctors participate in all of the major insurance plans. Some of those plans are health maintenance organizations, some of which are capitated. As a result, patients who have insurance coverage will be covered when they see East-West's conventional physicians. In addition, physical therapy services are covered if they are provided by prescription.

Alternative Coverage

Insurance plans vary as to whether they will pay for alternative medicine services. In this area of the country, the insurance companies have not yet decided to pay for CAM services. Insurers will pay for chiropractic in most cases, particularly under coverage for automobile accidents. Workers' compensation will also frequently pay for chiropractic and sometimes massage therapy. Insurance companies have also paid for acupuncture and massage therapy following automobile accidents. In addition, more insurers are beginning to cover acupuncture. Typically, they evaluate these services on a case-by-case basis. Increased coverage is also becoming available for therapeutic massage. When there is confirmation that a service will be paid for by the insurance company, the Center will perform the billing.

Noncovered Services

Currently, there are few plans that provide coverage for naturopathic medicine. Consequently, all naturopathic doctor visits are on a cash basis, as are most of the visits for therapeutic massage. Rolfing® treatments are paid for out of pocket by patients, as are nutritional counseling, yoga, T'ai chi, and meditation. These out-of-pocket payments do not seem to be deterring clients since the largest group of potential clients are typically those with disposable income.

PATIENT SERVICES

The data from the *New England Journal of Medicine* (Eisenberg et al, 1993) suggest that a third of Americans use alternative care. In 1990, patients spent more than $13 million out of pocket for alternative medicine. In that study, the demographics of those most likely to use CAM were women ages 25 to 49 with college educations, incomes of more than $35,000, and disposable income.

A third of the patients are seen at the Center to receive their regular health care; they see the physicians for the types of problems seen by any primary care provider. They may have little interest in integrative medicine and want to see the doctor without seeing any of the other practitioners. Obviously, the Center's physicians are very open-minded toward complementary medicine; they would not be working at the Center otherwise.

The physicians reflect two of the many practice styles within medicine today. One of the physicians is board-certified in preventive medicine. His practice focuses on lifestyle, wellness, fitness, prevention, and nutrition. He may recommend herbs on occasion, but he is a Western doctor. The other physician tends to be more mainstream with an open mind toward alternative approaches, but he does not prescribe herbs. Rather than prescribing them himself, he would be more likely refer that patient to the naturopathic doctor, who has 6 years of training and education in the use of herbs.

Another third of the patient population is attracted to preventive medicine. The remaining third use the Center's services to address chronic problems, including back pain, headaches, chronic pain, depression, and anxiety. As the population ages, chronic conditions are projected to increase significantly. It seems that chronic disorders are those that are the most difficult to treat. Complementary medicine is useful in addressing chronic conditions, and that is where the future integration of medicine ought to occur.

Fees and Services

Client fees are right at the median of charges in the Denver metropolitan area (or a little lower). Fees are neither high nor low, but are very competitive. The Center's philosophy regarding cus-

tomer service involves all the constituents of the Center: the providers and the staff. The goal is to always put the patients first. In order to treat the patients well, it is essential to also treat the providers well.

PROVIDER RELATIONS

Contracts and Salaries

Each practitioner is incorporated as a professional corporation. It is not uncommon for doctors to have their own professional corporations (PCs), but it has generally been common for alternative practitioners to have PCs. The Center provides the facility, all of the equipment and supplies, and administrative support services, including staffing and marketing—everything a health care professional needs to practice. Providers practice at the Center knowing that all they have to do is what they have been trained to do. All of the administrative hassles of running a practice are the Center's responsibility—scheduling the patients, performing the billing and collections, and paying the bills.

Practitioner Contracting for Administrative Services

The charges to practitioners for administrative services are a little lower than market rate. The practitioners like not having to worry about the administrative component of running a practice. Most of the CAM providers have been on their own in solo practices or in small offices in their homes, in malls, or in health clubs. Consequently, they have not had access to the professional stimulation that is available in a multidisciplinary environment. They find they learn from the other providers in the Center while still having a great deal of autonomy.

Salaries

Practitioner salaries are based on a percentage of collections. That percentage varies by specialty. It is a competitive rate for all of the providers. The Center's goal is to provide services that are very economically viable for both patients and practitioners.

Overhead

The administrative services are provided at a price that is as good as, or better than, anywhere else in the area. In fact, even if the practitioners provided their own services, they would not be able to do better. Consequently, practitioners come out a little ahead. In addition, they receive stock options.

For example, the Center hired a chiropractor who had a successful solo practice a few miles away for 10 years. However, when he came to East-West, he received an immediate increase in salary (about 10%) because our percentage of overhead was less than he had been paying as a solo provider. The reason he joined East-West was that he was tired of doing all the administrative work himself and wanted the professional stimulation of working in an environment with other providers—the salary boost was an added bonus.

Provider Incentives

The Center's goal is to build a team of practitioners who want to be here for the long term. One of the ways the Center retains practitioners is by offering an executive stock plan—a form of profit-sharing arrangement under which it distributes shares of stock in the company at the end of the year, based on how well the company has done. Consequently, all the providers become partial owners in the firm.

Fiscal Issues

The cash flow of the company must be managed on a daily basis. It has been challenging, and there are certain things that will be done differently when the second center is set up, but the project has ultimately been satisfying.

Stability

The Center experiences low turnover in its provider population. Many of the practitioners

have been with the Center since the day it opened, including the two acupuncturists, one of the chiropractors, and one of the physicians. Other practitioners are added as East-West continues to expand. The second chiropractor was recruited about 1 year ago, and he has been a very positive addition.

A Site for Interns

The Center is currently a training site for student interns. There is a medical student doing part of his rotation here, and a marketing student who is fulfilling some of her degree course requirements. The Center is attractive to some of the universities because there are so many aspects to the practice, in one location.

MARKETING

Informal Marketing and Referrals

A good deal of the Center's marketing takes place informally in the waiting area where there is a bookcase with educational materials on less familiar therapies, such as naturopathic medicine. Patients can pick up brochures about any of the therapies and learn what they are and which conditions they treat. Making information available to patients empowers them. The Center provides them with a safe, professional environment in which they can try therapies that may be new to them.

There have been patients who comment on their first visit that they do not anticipate using any services but those of the physician. Over time, these same clients may gradually expand their use of services. Not everyone uses all of the services. Some people use just one service, but others use many of the services that are here.

For example, a patient may have always wanted to try acupuncture. However, he or she may not want to just go to the place down the street with the acupuncture sign or to choose a practitioner at random from the Yellow Pages. The patient wants to go to a place that he or she feels is safe. In addition, as patients get to know the staff, they become aware of the exceptional caliber of the practitioners and that builds trust.

For example, a patient who comes in with chronic tennis elbow can be seen by either of our physicians; both have backgrounds in sports medicine. (In fact, one of them is the physician for one of the local university basketball teams, and one was one of the Olympic doctors in Atlanta, Georgia.) The doctor can give the patient a shot of cortisone, which will work for a while, but the patient may have to return for periodic injections to relieve the pain. In an integrative practice, the physician also has the option of bringing in the acupuncturist, who can explain viable alternative treatment options for the condition.

The physician will not want to simply make a general referral for acupuncture, unless he can refer to a specific practitioner, based on the practitioner's training and credentials. The capacity to make these referrals to other practitioners on site tends to have a different effect than simply making a referral to a practitioner across town. If the physician brings in the acupuncturist for an informal consult at the time of the office visit, the patient tends to be more interested in actually trying acupuncture. This an important aspect of integration, which goes beyond case conferences. In addition, by the practitioners working collegially, the patients are less likely to be lost to follow-up, and the Center's physicians are more likely to get feedback from the CAM practitioner.

Other Forms of Marketing

- Since some of the Center's providers had existing practices when they joined and they brought clients with them, the Center had a base of patients when it opened its doors.
- The Center is in an excellent location with very visible signage on Interstate 25, which runs north and south through the center of Denver.
- Many patients learn of the Center through word of mouth. From my work as a hospital chief executive officer, I knew many physicians and people in the insurance industry.
- The Center provides corporate wellness and health promotion programming and serves as the corporate wellness department for companies such as Johns Manville in the Denver area. Coors is also a client, and the Center provides practitioners and massage therapists to Coors' corporate wellness site.
- East-West actively participates in community service events such as screenings and health fairs, which also serve as a form of marketing.
- Prospective patients can read about providers on East-West's Web site <www.East-West-Health.com> before making an appointment.

CONCLUSION

Complementary medicine is here to stay. The consumer is embracing it more and more as time goes on. Integrative medicine is the way in which medicine will be practiced in the future, combining the best of both worlds and involving patients to a greater extent in the health care decision-making process.

REFERENCE

Eisenberg DM, Kessler RC, Foster C, et al. Unconventional medicine in the United States. *N Eng J Med.* 1993:328(4):246–252.

CHAPTER 37

An Integrative Medicine Clinic in a Teaching Hospital

Debra Canfield

The program in alternative medicine at Hennepin County Medical Center (HCMC) has been in place since 1993. The program is a division of the department of medicine, located within HCMC, which is one of the teaching hospitals affiliated with the University of Minnesota. The program director, Patricia Culliton, was involved with the development of acupuncture programs in public health before she initiated the Alternative Medicine Division. Her early work was in research and focused on the treatment of addictions.

PROFILE OF THE PROGRAM

There are three components within the division: (1) the clinic itself, (2) a research component, and (3) two education components. The educational aspect of the program has included seminars, conferences, and community education.

At this point, approximately 20% to 22% of the clinic's referrals are made by physicians in other parts of the department or the hospital. It has taken years to reach this stage, but there has been an increasingly positive trend. Additionally, since the National Institutes of Health (NIH) Consensus Statement on Acupuncture, the clinic has received very specific referrals

from physicians. Before the consensus statement was issued, the clinic never received referrals from oncologists.

At this point, the clinic receives referrals with increasing frequency. When patients are scheduled to receive chemotherapy, they are referred to acupuncture by the physician before the chemotherapy begins to minimize nausea and vomiting. There are also many referrals for musculoskeletal pain from general practitioners and internists, and in some cases from orthopedists and rheumatologists. The clinic receives numerous referrals for chronic conditions such as fibromyalgia and chronic fatigue. Patients with these chronic conditions often first seek help within the system and eventually exhaust the available resources.

Management

The program has a medical director who is an internist and serves as medical supervisor of the clinic. The program director, Patricia Culliton, has a master's degree and is a licensed acupuncturist. There is a clinic supervisor who oversees day-to-day clinical activities and administration who is a licensed acupuncturist and a certified Chinese herbalist, with experience as both a practitioner and an administrator. The operations coordinator has responsibility for the supervision of the front desk and two medical receptionists. Administrative activities include management, quality improvement, documentation, report writing, and coordination.

Medical Oversight

When a patient is seen here for the first time, the medical director reviews the patient's entire

Debra Canfield has been Operations Coordinator since 1996 for the Alternative Medicine Division at Hennepin County Medical Center in Minneapolis. She has also served as public information specialist for the NIH-funded Center for Addictions and Alternative Medicine Research and as a supervisor in the home care division of Caremark of Minnesota. She has presented in national forums on the topics of operations and quality improvement in integrative medicine.

medical history. He monitors the first progress notes and all the medical forms for red flags that might suggest a patient needs to be seen by a primary care physician for a diagnostic workup. However, the practitioners are so experienced, the medical director rarely finds that they have missed any aspect of the case. This type of review and oversight is provided on an ongoing basis by the medical director for all patients. The practitioners do not function as primary care providers.

Services Provided

The clinic offers acupuncture, acupressure, Shiatsu, bodywork, herbs, and chiropractic. In addition to six acupuncturists, there is a practitioner who sees patients exclusively for Shiatsu massage. There are also two bodyworkers who provide primarily neuromuscular reeducation, myofascial release, and deep tissue work (rather than Eslan-style massage, which is primarily just for relaxation). The clinic does not provide mind-body medicine. However, when a patient comes in for acupuncture, the treatment involves the whole person. Questions are asked about all aspects of the patient's life, not just the localized symptoms. The practitioner uses tongue diagnosis and reads the multiple pulse points monitored in Chinese medicine. Although the actual treatment is very specific, it is based on an assessment that takes the patient's entire situation into consideration. The clinic also provides chiropractic services.

Policies

The clinic has been precedent-setting in many of their initiatives over the years so they have had to develop new systems. There was essentially no information available to help develop a credentialing and privileging program, job descriptions, and competencies and to establish necessary policy guidelines. They were developed for the Hennepin system and now Hennepin consults with other programs on these topics.

Research Component

The medical director, Milton Bullock, MD, and program director, Patricia Culliton, MA, Lac, started research in 1981 on the use of acupuncture for the treatment of addictions. They were pioneers in the use of randomized controlled clinical trials in acupuncture research. Their work became the foundation for the clinical services that were eventually developed. The first clinical services were offered to study participants after the studies were completed. When the clinic was established in 1992, data collection was of primary importance. Alternative medicine at Hennepin has now had several grants funded by the National Institutes of Health (NIH). The Center for Addiction and Alternative Medicine Research is the longest-standing center funded through the National Centers for Complementary and Alternative Medicine (NCCAM). There have also been several publications based on the outcomes data gathered on the patients at the clinic.

SERVICE PROVISION

Caseload and Clinical Staffing

Practitioners provide approximately 1,000 patient visits a month that cover a wide range of symptoms and complaints. Two acupuncturists work full-time in the clinic and several other providers work part-time. As a result, the mix of practitioners varies from day to day, with an average of five practitioners in the clinic on any given day. One of the practitioners is a registered nurse in the oncology clinic at the hospital; she is also an acupuncturist and herbalist, and in our clinic, specializes in treating oncology patients with traditional Chinese medicine. Another member of the staff is a registered nurse in the cardiac intensive care unit and is also a chiropractor and acupuncturist. The clinic receives referrals through their work at the oncology and cardiology centers. In the alternative medicine clinic, they are able to work independently and integrate their skills and knowledge. It has been easier to integrate treatment for this type of care since the NIH Consensus Statement regarding acupuncture.

Programs in the Treatment of Addictions

The clinic initially developed out of a research project that was studying acupuncture as a treatment for addiction. When the data were published, the community requested acupuncture services in the treatment facilities. The acupuncture practitioners currently see more than 2,000 patients per month in such facilities. Minnesota is well known for its excellent addictions treatment facilities. Alternative medicine services are available in treatment facilities that are targeted to specific populations such as women, men, African Americans, Native Americans, pregnant women, mothers, or geriatric or incarcerated individuals. In addition, the Twin Cities recently initiated an inner-city drug court providing young people with alternative treatment as an option to incarceration. This range of programs is funded by the county, the state, and private grants.

MEDICAL OVERSIGHT AND ACCESS

One of the primary goals of the clinic's integrative approach is safety. The initial intake assessment and database were developed out of concerns for safety. Unlike in some integrative clinics, there is no gatekeeper—a concept whereby a physician is the initial contact for all patients coming into the clinic. The physician then refers the patient to the most appropriate complementary therapy. In the HCMC Alternative Medicine Clinic, prior authorization or referral is not a requirement. Instead, the clinic provides medical monitoring and oversight through the medical director. There is one exception to access without a referral, and that is managed care. Some insurance policies require a referral from a physician before a patient can be seen by any specialist, including complementary medicine.

Conditions treated at the Alternative Medicine Clinic are primarily chronic or subacute conditions and patients with any potentially serious complaints would be referred immediately to their primary physician or another physician. The provider assesses the patient's condition through an interview and review of the intake forms completed by the patient. The provider then uses this assessment as a basis for the treatment plan. If the patient's condition warrants a referral to another medical provider or alternative medicine practitioner, the referral will be made. The patient will also be informed if the practitioner feels the condition is not appropriate for alternative therapies available at this particular clinic.

Focus on the Provision of Complementary Care

The philosophy of the Alternative Medicine Clinic is to provide patients with another health care option beyond conventional medicine. All practitioners are licensed or certified in their area of expertise. An evaluation is completed for each patient at the initial visit. Medical oversight occurs under the thorough supervision of the medical director. The medical director reviews all new patient charts to determine if the patient needs a work-up through conventional methods prior to their treatment, as well as for appropriateness of the treatment plans. The medical director is available on a regular basis for consultations with the practitioners regarding ongoing care.

DEFINING THE LEVEL OF INTEGRATION IN AN INTEGRATIVE MEDICINE CENTER

John Weeks, noted author, has described essentially three levels of integration in physician practice that can be used to define the type of physician services to be provided. A clinic must determine the level of knowledge it will expect from the physicians.

The type of medical oversight provided in the Hennepin County clinic is considered the first level. A physician providing integrative care knows the vocabulary of complementary and alternative medicine (CAM), reviews the charts, looks for red flags, and checks to ensure the patient is seeing a primary care physician. However, the physician does not provide clinical treatment in any area of CAM. Some insurance companies (and some states) require a prescription from a physician before the patient can have access to a particular therapy or treatment such as massage. The clinic works primarily by referral. However, when additional documentation or a more detailed treatment plan is required, the supervising physician has a working knowledge of the various therapies and may prescribe a particular therapy and the appropriate number of treatments.

CLINICAL PATHWAYS

Clinical pathways are currently at an early stage of development in most institutions. The Hennepin Center guidelines are in development and are not yet ready to be published. However, it is clear clinical pathways for CAM will be a necessary and beneficial tool in the future. These guidelines will be useful to physicians because they will establish expectations for treatment. They will be useful to the insurance companies to guide reimbursement and assist them in judging the appropriateness of the treatment plans. Clinical pathways will assist in the development of an accessible knowledge base that will indicate the most cost-effective approaches to treatment. For example, it may be determined that the most cost-effective treatment for low-back pain may be anti-inflammatories, acupuncture, and massage, and this combination may help reduce the need for back surgery for some types of conditions. As the program and the staff expand, the availability of clinical pathways will help new clinicians master the learning curve more quickly and effectively.

Integrated Medical Records

The clinic's medical histories are quite extensive; they include the notes from the patient's physical and the records from any and all treatments the patient may have received in any of the other ambulatory clinics. The progress notes for the Alternative Medicine Clinic are completely integrated with those of the other clinics. There are 13 distinct clinics, including primary care, pediatrics, ophthalmology, and multispecialty clinics, and all share a centralized medical record. For instance, if a patient comes to the alternative medicine clinic and then sees a nurse practitioner in the internal medicine clinic, and 2 weeks later sees a physician in gastroenterology, all of the providers the patient sees will have access to the chart notes for all the other practitioners and have information about what the patient is being treated for, which medications and/or herbs he or she has been given, and any other relevant information. This communication could be further enhanced by the use of clinical pathways for alternative medicine, which would explain the patient's alternative treatment protocol to physicians in other specialties and departments.

Using Clinical Pathways To Integrate Care

The long-term goal is to develop not only clinical pathways for alternative medicine, but also to have alternative medicine included in conventional clinic pathways for treatment and referral. For example, in the case of a woman receiving chemotherapy for breast cancer, once the condition has been diagnosed and the treatment has been scheduled, she could be referred immediately for acupuncture to set up complementary treatment that would address nausea or vomiting following the chemotherapy. Over time, the protocols would become part of the clinical pathway, and eventually part of the standard care. Although some physicians currently make these types of referrals, it is not yet a formal written protocol, but rather a palliative option they elect for patients. Ongoing outcomes research may facilitate the development of these protocols.

RISK MANAGEMENT

By actively networking with colleagues, administrators can be kept abreast of critical issues in risk management. Through such contacts, administrators may learn of problems that have occurred at other hospitals and clinics and how these situations were resolved. Armed with such valuable information, administrators can then write policies and procedures that anticipate risk and address its management even before problems develop. Obviously, no policy will cover all possible scenarios, but a well-informed manager can develop a useful policy based on case histories and medical precedents.

Steps To Minimize Risk

Administrators should ensure that all practitioners have malpractice insurance. This can be done through the organization hiring the practitioner, or through a policy that the practitioners will carry their own malpractice insurance. Health care organizations will have minimum requirements for coverage amounts and these will vary by organization.

At the Alternative Medicine Clinic, a physician reviews all cases; doing so provides an additional level of supervision and oversight. In the management of complex cases, a weekly staff meeting provides additional clinical review. Practitioners present cases that have raised questions, such as those that may require referrals, as well as patients who are not responding to treatment. These meetings resemble those of any multidisciplinary team. Practitioners describe the details of complex cases, voice their concerns about patient progress, exchange recommendations, and decide when the patient should be referred back to the primary care physician.

The Alternative Medicine Clinic has also developed an extensive database that not only assists with outcomes research, but is also a tool for risk management. Patient visits, herb sales, and incident reports are recorded in the database and reports are run on a regular basis to monitor these issues and address them as needed. Reports tracking trends can also be run.

The Details of Safety in Acupuncture Treatment

When a patient is receiving acupuncture, how does the practitioner make sure that the needles are not left in for too long once they have turned on the soft music, dimmed the lights, and left the room? When six or seven treatment rooms are being used at once, and each practitioner is seeing two or three patients, it is possible to forget the order of treatment. How does the practitioner make sure he or she goes back to the room to check on the patient in a timely fashion? At the clinic, there are timers outside each room that go off in 20 minutes. The practitioner must return to the room to turn off the beeper, and then checks on the patient. The timers are useful because they remind practitioners of the status of each patient.

THE HERBAL PHARMACY AND RISK MANAGEMENT

The herbal apothecary can be an area of risk unless it is managed well. Many hospitals do not yet have an herbal pharmacy. The clinic initiated this service many years ago in order to control the quality of the herbs its patients were taking. The clinic's large herbal pharmacy carries both Chinese and Western herbs. The focus is not retail sales, however. The patients must see an herbalist before they are allowed to purchase herbs from the pharmacy. This procedure is a means of regulating and monitoring the use of the herbs that are dispensed. This has become a very important issue in integrative centers.

The clinic requires that manufacturers send documentation about their use of good manufacturing standards. Good Manufacturing Practice (GMP) standards are an international standard for production. The clinic also buys herbs only if there are lot numbers and expiration dates on the herbs. Every herb dispensed is documented in the clinic database, consequently, giving the clinic a record of every herb bought by any patient in the clinic. If the clinic were to ever receive information suggesting a contaminated lot, or some other type of adverse event, it would be possible to contact every one of those patients and notify him or her of the possible problem. In addition, the clinic also tracks expiration dates. Although it is not likely that the herbs will lose their potency, there is much still to be learned about herbs. The clinic believes it is better to have more documentation, rather than less.

The clinic maintains flowsheets in the charts that document the use of botanicals and medications. This information is part of the patients' medical records, and any physician, nurse, or staff member in any of the clinics can determine which herbs the patients are taking, particularly in conjunction with any medications. The herbal flowsheet also serves as a reminder to nurses and physicians to ask their patients about use of over-the-counter herbs and other supplements. Many people are now buying herbs such as gingko, garlic, and St. John's wort in drugstores. These safeguards have been instituted on behalf of the patients in order to maintain a high level of safety.

The occurrence of side effects is low, and they are typically quite minor when they do occur. There can be interactions when herbs are taken concurrently with certain medications, however. In some cases, the herb may stop or slow the effect of the medication. In other cases, the herb may enhance it, which could produce an increased response. Documentation is even more important when there is a lack of data regarding drug-herb interactions. Dietary and herbal supplement studies are being performed, but the information will not be available for some time to come.

CHART NOTES

Traditional Chinese Medicine Chart Notes

Two types of information are maintained within each patient's medical record. If a Western diagnosis has been given to the patient by the physician, this will be included in the chart note, as well as a treatment plan written in Western terms. The acupuncturists record other information in their chart notes, including Chinese medicine diagnosis. Both the Western and Chinese diagnoses will be included in the chart for the physician or other staff. A physician may ignore the description written in terms of Chinese medicine; most physicians will not be interested in the specific points treated. However, the treatment plan will include when and how often the patient should return for treatment.

The format for the TCM chart notes has been developed specifically for use in this clinic. Initially, the practitioners were interviewed to determine the information they felt was essential to include in the charts, and the scope of service developed under the Minnesota Board of Medical Practices was reviewed; then a specific format was developed.

The final documentation requirements were ultimately based on the state scope of practice. The regulations require that a consent form be obtained from all patients who receive acupuncture and that practitioners must record the traditional Chinese medicine diagnosis in their charts. In order to keep the chart relevant to all practitioners, the acupuncturist includes progress notes that are clear to physicians and administrators. The physicians must be able to understand the treatment plan and follow the progress of the treatment. The notes are written in parallel form, with notations that are meaningful to both types of practitioners. When a practitioner or another acupuncturist picks up the chart before seeing that patient, he or she will know what the patient was being treated for.

Other CAM Chart Notes

Other alternative medicine practitioners also work in the clinic, and chart notes have been designed for those practices as well. All practitioners are expected to write SOAP (Subjective Objective Assessment Plan) notes and documentation audits are done on a regular basis. Chart notes also include information about the patients' ability to learn and their religious and cultural beliefs, and any patient education that is provided must also be documented.

Staff in other clinics are more likely to read the information contained in the charts if it is described in terms of Western biomedicine. This holds major implications for Chinese medicine. The integration process may occur more rapidly when the core concepts of Chinese medicine are also provided in the terminology of Western medicine.

DISCUSSION: THE ROLE OF MANAGEMENT

A program in integrative medicine requires administrative services that go beyond writing budgets. This type of program development involves writing policies, researching credentialing standards, and performing background checks to credentialing providers. The administrator must also be able to communicate well with physicians. A background in management, medicine, or legal administration is helpful. In addition, the administrator serves as a liaison to the program, sitting in on committee meetings throughout the system. The clinic's division plays a central role, and staff make an effort to be aware of activities throughout the organization that relate to alternative medicine. This networking is important to the clinical programs because more than one-fifth of the clinic's referrals come from within the hospital.

CHAPTER 38

The Integrative Multidisciplinary Spine Center: The Texas Back Institute

John J. Triano, Ralph F. Rashbaum, Daniel T. Hansen, and Barbara Raley

INTEGRATING CHIROPRACTIC INTO SPINE CARE

The Integrative Spine Care Center

The concept of focused facilities in health care is relatively new (Coile, 1995). They have evolved in part from the attempts to price health care under capitation as "carve-outs" for certain procedures or specific diseases (Pristave et al, 1995). In some types of services, this approach has resulted in reasonable value in care for these patients, for example, in the management of diabetes and of end-stage renal diseases. Focused facilities and provider networks for specific disorders offer a comprehensive set of health services that maximize economies of scale and depth in expertise for treating a narrow range of problems. The focused facility is a single-site "one-stop shop," where all services likely to be needed are available.

As a result, the integrated delivery system focusing on specific disease entities has become an emerging practice style that offers many attractive features to payers and patients. There is growing sentiment that the fragmented system in which a primary care provider at one site attempts to manage care of specialists scattered in other sites is inefficient and as costly as health care before reform. Not only does this disrupt continuity of care, introducing expensive delays in appropriate treatment, but it also requires the new case management industry to make multiple contacts and office visits at higher administrative expense to the benefits plan.

Advantages

A multidisciplinary facility for spine care, for example, affords several advantages. First, treatment administered under one roof and managed by a single primary contact provider centralizes communications and medical records. It minimizes the number of case manager contacts and travel costs. Early detection of patients failing to respond to therapy can be made, with rapid transition to alternate approaches. These advantages can have an impact on outcomes achieved.

For the practitioner, there are equally compelling advantages. Each provider sees a significant increase in value of practice support by participating in economies of scale. That is, providers get more support for the money. Teams of staff can be afforded that focus on modern health administrative services ranging from credential-

John J. Triano, DC, PhD, is the Director of the Chiropractic Division and Co-Director of Conservative Medicine at the Texas Back Institute, and Adjunct Faculty, University of Texas, Southwestern and Arlington Joint Biomedical Engineering Program.

Ralph F. Rashbaum, MD, is the Medical Director and an orthopedic spine surgeon at the Texas Back Institute.

Daniel T. Hansen, DC is Assistant Medical Director for Quality and Outcomes Management, Texas Back Institute.

Barbara Raley, LVN, OMA, is a clinical orthopedic/chiropractic nurse at the Texas Back Institute.

The Texas Back Institute (TBI) is a multispecialty integrative spine center in Plano, Texas. The center provides sophisticated spine care, drawing on the expertise of physicians, physiatrists, surgeons, and chiropractic practitioners.

Source: Adapted from J.J. Triano and B. Raley, Chiropractic in the Interdisciplinary Team Practice, *Topics in Clinical Chiropractic*, Vol. 1, No. 4, pp. 58–66, © 1994, Aspen Publishers, Inc. and J.J. Triano, R.F. Rashbaum and D.T. Hansen, Opening Access to Spine Care in the Evolving Market, *Topics in Clinical Chiropractic*, Vol. 5, No. 4, pp. 44–52, © 1998, Aspen Publishers, Inc.

ing providers, billing and collections agencies, and patient precertification services to practice marketing. Administrators can administrate, and doctors can focus their attention on the delivery of care. Payer groups are increasingly inclined to credential entire groups of providers as a unit because they tend to result in greater subscriber satisfaction with continuity of care and availability of specialists.

Consensus

The provider network consists of a multidisciplinary group that works closely with common consensus on appropriate care. In doing so, they can meet the clinical needs of the patient with increased efficiency. For instance, by nature of having a common medical record, redundancy of diagnostic procedures can be avoided. It is not uncommon for diagnostic imaging obtained by one provider or at an emergency department to be unavailable to the doctor who ultimately becomes the manager of the case. With a common medical record, those results are immediately available, and management decisions can address the need for advanced imaging or a modification in the treatment plan without delay or added cost.

Patient Population: Injury Care

Injured workers and motor vehicle accident victims are good examples of a focused population. Injury care represents a significant portion of neuromusculoskeletal practice. Disorders range from the uncomplicated strain or sprain to more complicated fractures, total joint failure, or central or peripheral nerve syndromes. The commonality of mechanisms of injury and the knowledge of typical course and outcome permit predictions that generally apply. Evidence-based protocols can be applied that give guidance from triage to rehabilitation. Progress can be monitored with valid outcome measures to anticipate the need for changing the treatment plan early when progress begins to lag. The effect is to address the expectations of the patients and payers with focus to reduce work-time loss and enhance

functional status upon return to work. It is hoped that all of this can be accomplished at a minimum for both direct and indirect health costs. Although there is ample evidence of significant regional variations in practice (Jarvis et al, 1991; Carey et al, 1995), it is clear that chiropractic practice can be cost- and time-effective (Jarvis et al, 1991; Mosley et al, 1996; Triano et al, 1992). Appropriately coupled as a part of the health care team, there is every reason to believe that such efficiency can be leveraged, even for chronic, severe, and complex cases.

Patient Population: Complicated Cases

Clinical outcomes depend on a balance between the constellation of factors that affects patient status and the effectiveness of treatment administered (Exhibit 38–1) (Triano et al, 1998). Depending on the individual case complexity, that effectiveness may rely on the dexterity with which the managing physician coordinates multiple providers and services. The effects of age, pathology, comorbid disease, postsurgical anatomy, and psychosocial factors most often define complexity. The greater the complexity, the more resources may be necessary to bring the patient's problem under control.

For example, segmental instability, failed back syndrome, pseudoarthrosis, degenerative scoliosis, and even severe osteopenia are all physical features of pathology or postsurgical anatomy. Each requires modification and adaptation of manipulation techniques to accommodate the more fragile issues. Similarly, patients with diabetes, peripheral vascular disease, or neuropathy may not be able to tolerate adjunctive thermal therapies. Those with gastric sensitivity may not be able to have a referral for anti-inflammatory medications.

CASE STUDIES

As all practicing physicians know, academic discussion of patient care never adequately conveys the experience (Triano and Raley, 1994). The two case studies that follow have been se-

Exhibit 38–1 Factors Affecting Clinical Outcomes

Patient Clinical Status

- Age and sex
- Comorbid illness
- Primary diagnosis
- Condition severity
- Clinical stability
- Financial status
- Work or life habits
- Cultural, ethnic attributes
- Psychosocial functioning

Treatment Methods

- Manipulation
- Mobilization
- Modalities
- Muscle energy technique
- Exercise

Complementary Services

- Advanced diagnostics
- Medication
- Psychologic counseling
- Physical therapy
- Occupational therapy
- Injection techniques for muscle, joint, and disc

Source: Reprinted with permission from *Risk Adjustment for Measuring Health Care Outcomes, Second Edition*, by Lisa Iezzoni (Chicago: Health Administration Press, 1997).

lected to show how a vertically integrated system can operate with the chiropractic component serving multiple provider roles, from case manager to consulting physician.

Case Study 1: Back Injury, Construction Worker

SR, a 44-year-old Hispanic male, is a construction worker. On April 16, 1992, SR was employed at a work site, erecting the super-

structure of a multistory office building. While working on the ground, he was bent over at the waist when a four-by-four piece of lumber fell from the sixth story of the construction site. The wooden projectile struck the patient in the lumbopelvic region. SR was driven to the ground and lost consciousness. He was taken by ambulance to the local hospital, where he was found to be paraplegic with severe low-back and leg pain. Anteroposterior and lateral radiographic views were taken at the emergency department, demonstrating traumatic ileus and patent renal function by intravenous pyelogram. In addition, inspection of the hemipelvis on the right demonstrated a clear fracture line through the body of the ilium. On the lateral view, a traumatic spondylolisthesis, resulting from dislocation of the articular processes, was seen at L-5/S-1.

Early intervention consisted of internal fixation by bone screws and plates through the pedicles and into the vertebral bodies, performed by surgeons at another site. Following the operation, SR's pain was managed medically with acetaminophen with codeine, and spinal support was provided by a claim-shell rigid external brace.

On May 11, 1992, hydrotherapy was initiated, along with upper extremity strengthening exercise and cardiovascular endurance training with bicycling and stretching. Passive treatment to increase flexibility was initiated through use of myofascial release techniques by physical therapists. On June 15, 1992, SR graduated from his brace to ambulation with a walker and lower extremity exercises, using the Total Gym exercise equipment.

A functional performance capacity assessment (FPCA) was performed on September 14, 1992, and was contrasted to SR's expected job task demands to identify therapeutic goals and create an individualized program to return the patient to work. As an index of his capability at the start of the program, he was able to lift 18 pounds, using a combined leg and back lift posture, compared with expected job requirements of 100 pounds. Return to work, full time, on duty limitations of 50 pounds was achieved after a second FPCA on November 13, 1992. Although a number of chiropractors specializing in rehabilitation would have been able to facilitate this patient's recovery, no chiropractic services were a part of the initial health care recovery.

Regardless, this outcome would be the happy ending of an unfortunate injury in a well-motivated patient. However, on March 2, 1993, SR was shopping for groceries when a metal display shelf fell on top of him, striking his left upper quadrant. He fell to the floor, and the shelf and its contents landed on top of him. Severe renewed pain was experienced from the thoracolumbar region to the buttock and groin areas. He consulted medical physicians at the Texas Back Institute (TBI), and a diagnosis of strain was made. Anti-inflammatory, antispasmodic, and analgesic medications were prescribed. Flexion/extension radiographs were obtained on April 16, 1993, due to severe pain and persistent limitation of motion. Subsequent bone scan, searching for evidence of undisclosed fracture, was obtained on May 28, 1993. The intervening time was used to administer physical therapy in the form of exercise and soft tissue work by physical therapists.

On August 4, 1993, a chiropractic physician was added to the multidisciplinary team and asked to consult on the case. Examination revealed a patient who presented in obvious distress and wearing a heavy elastic lumbar support with reinforcing elastic belts. The gait was markedly abnormal, with stride length nearly one-third of normal and an antalgic forward tilt to the trunk. All neurologic testing was normal. Further assessment revealed a severe Maigne's syndrome (thoracolumbar FSL with radiation to the iliac crest), quadratus lumborum myofascial pain, sacroiliac fixation, and status post surgical fusion with instrumentation. Therapy was changed to continuous passive motion in flexion and flexion coupled with lateral bending. High-velocity procedures were utilized to restore function to the thoracolumbar junction, and a pelvic drop technique was applied. Treatment was initiated on a daily regimen for 2

weeks, followed by a progressive reduction in frequency.

On August 20, 1993, Williams' flexion and torsional exercises were added. Pool therapy and progressive resistance exercises were initiated with the aid of a lumbosacral support belt on September 15, 1993, under orders of the chiropractic physician.

One month of functional restoration was initiated by FPCA on October 11, 1993, and the patient returned to full duty on November 15, 1993. One episode of recurrence was experienced beginning April 15, 1994, from work-related lifting. The patient was taken off work for 10 days, and a new regimen of three treatments was resolved within a 2-week interval, at which time, full-duty work status was restored.

Case Study 2: Torn Ligament, Salesman

WB, a 30-year-old male car salesman, was injured on the job on February 8, 1993. He was struck from behind by a slowly moving vehicle when a co-worker was "playing" and intended to "nudge" WB from behind with the bumper of a showroom car. When the bumper contacted the back of his leg, WB spun to the left, pivoting on his left foot. Because he was wearing crepe sole shoes with a high friction coefficient, the left knee sustained torsional injury and disruption of the anterior cruciate ligament. Surgical reconstruction was conducted by an orthopedic surgeon, and the patient was entered into a rehabilitation program postoperatively. During isokinetic exercise of the leg, the left lumbosacral, sacroiliac joint regions were injured. Therapy was discontinued, and WB consulted a local chiropractor for relief of pain. Spinal manipulation, transcutaneous electrical nerve stimulation, and biofeedback therapy were administered. The surgeon who had performed the knee operation had also attempted a cortisone injection to the sacroiliac area without obtaining relief.

After several months of continued therapy and short-term relief, WB was transferred to the multidisciplinary spine care center at TBI, which had a chiropractic physician on staff. During the intervening time, WB's financial resources dwindled. At the time of evaluation, he had undergone bankruptcy and loss of his home. He presented on October 26, 1993, for evaluation as an angry, bitter, and frustrated man who was highly skeptical of any possible favorable outcome from more treatment. His examination revealed a 73-inch, 200-pound male who was in pain on walking and rising from a chair. A noticeable limp was observed involving the left side. Orthopedic testing showed full range of motion, positive Kemp's and Gaenslen's signs, positive drawer test, positive patellar scrape test, vastus medialis atrophy, and snapping left hip. He was diagnosed with status post anterior cruciate ligament (ACL) reconstruction; secondary chondromalacia patellae; quadriceps deconditioning; and facet, sacroiliac, and snapping iliopsoas syndromes. With the multiple problems and possible psychologic overlay, a series of interventions was coordinated under chiropractic supervision. The patient was referred to a general orthopedist to obtain clearance for an appropriate rehabilitation program. Restrictions were placed on activities of daily living to limit bending and lifting activities. Pool therapy was ordered to permit full range-of-motion exercise while unloading of the back, hip, and knee, due to the buoyancy of the water. Simultaneously, a consultation was obtained from the pain management group for lumbar facet joint (Marcaine and methylprednisolone) and sacroiliac (lidocaine) injections to get the inflammation of these structures under control. Early results were excellent, with reduction of symptoms and the beginning of functional gains with exercise.

On November 29, 1993, WB reported on follow-up evaluation with renewed sharp lumbosacral pain, initiated by twisting while clearing the Thanksgiving Day dinner table. Manipulation of the spine and pelvis was initiated on an "as-needed" basis in the form of continuous passive motion, followed by mobilization and high-velocity, short-amplitude thrusting, if warranted by findings. Two treatment sessions resolved the episode, and he was returned to a follow-up routine for evaluating rehabilitation program progress. All totaled, WB experienced eight similar short-term episodes of exacerbation lasting up to 2–3 days each over the interval until January 24, 1994.

Despite the recurrences, his functional gains continued in spin and extremity performance; muscle mass of the left thigh expanded in response. However, the patient again began to exhibit anger and signs of depression over the repetitive episodes of pain. A behavioral medicine consultation was obtained to offer counseling for his frustration and coping strategies to contend with his chronic pain and damage to his sense of self-worth.

On February 9, 1994, the patient was sent for disability evaluation and discharged as having reached maximum therapeutic benefit. Limitations were expected for the patient with a 5% permanent disability rating. At discharge, he was pain free, provided that he not overexert in lifting from the floor. His upper leg dimensions were symmetrical, and the chondromalacia patellae and snapping iliotibial band were resolved. WB's emotional resources were rebuilding, with evidence of becoming more self-reliant. His discharge was timed with transfer to a work training program for a new job in another city and to continued home care exercise to maintain his functional gains.

Case Conclusions

Both of the cases selected for illustration involve complex musculoskeletal health problems that had failed to respond under earlier care—one medical and one chiropractic. The chiropractic roles required integration of the appropriate treatment, in conjunction with the coordination and management of care by several professionals. The common feature is the central focus on patient need and the acquisition of resources to meet those needs.

For both of the cases shown here, a strong communication line was maintained with the precertification staff for workers' compensation in order to have authorization for the services rendered. In the foreseeable future, triage of patients will not always be controlled internally. Some managed care purchasers will require an external gatekeeper, whereas others will permit patient self-selection of providers from credentialed panels. Clinic success should be defined by the uniqueness of each case. At times, it is appropriate to expect and reach for complete symptom relief. At other times, where this objective is unlikely to be reached, rapid recruitment of supportive resources—once it is evident that therapy is lagging—will usually return the patient to a functional and more satisfying life of self-reliance. Finally, the judicious use of skills from other disciplines can augment the benefits of chiropractic care to salvage otherwise failed therapy cases.

SUCCESSFUL INTERDISCIPLINARY COLLABORATION

Team Composition

The specific composition of an interdisciplinary team will vary from one system of delivery to another. Whether the collaborative practice of the future is conducted in solo practice, under the umbrella of a loosely coordinated confederation of providers, or under the umbrella of a defined multidisciplinary structure, the requirements for more frequent and intense collaboration in case management can be expected. Members of various professional disciplines representing diverse, even averse, viewpoints are being brought together to work out new systems of practice that take advantage of the training and expertise of each group.

Due to the overlap of subspecialty topics (ie, radiology, rehabilitation, pain management) between disciplines, the professional credentials of team members may vary. The grounds for membership should be dictated primarily by the anticipated service needs of the population of patients likely to be encountered and the professionals whose personal training and experience are best suited to meet them. Logical sets of

subcategories that may survive under health care reform are primary care, obstetrics and gynecology, pediatrics, and treatment of musculoskeletal disorders.

The structures of interdisciplinary teams can vary in scope, constituency, and method of operation. Influencing factors include regional variation in health industry regulation, the growth of managed care, more vocal health consumerism, and the advent of volume purchasing of services. Individual and group provider decisions on how to organize themselves will develop out of the focus on the needs of the patient population to be served, the health care environments they select for utilization, and the local resources available. Increasing trends in consumer and purchaser expectations for convenient access to multiple disciplines and patient willingness to make an effort to obtain "one-stop" provider services are becoming driving forces for restructuring (Main, 1993). A higher degree of formal structure, using elements of total quality management and economic credentialing, embody an emerging trend.

There are several ingredients likely to be needed for a successful interdisciplinary practice. First, appropriate service utilization must reasonably be assured. In practical terms for chiropractic, this factor means that a comparable degree of risk sharing exists across all provider classifications. The incentive for a health care purchaser or gatekeeper to dissuade utilization is minimized or canceled in this way. Thus, patients who need chiropractic care will not be discouraged from its use for economic reasons. Members must be individually compatible in order to foster attitudes that permit an open and receptive dialogue on the plethora of unresolved scientific and clinical issues.

The final objective is for the organization—horizontal or vertical—to be able to ensure that patients being seen by any entry-level, first-contact provider will receive similar effective treatment, to the extent that the preponderance of scientific evidence will support. Again, using musculoskeletal disorders as the example, any symptoms suggesting the need for urgent or emergent care or clinical evidence of infection, cancer, metabolic bone disease, and so forth will lead to appropriate biomedical diagnostic workup and referral. Once these possible explanations of the patient's pain are addressed, the initial treatment intervention can follow the provider's preferred method to case resolution or until signs indicate that the patient is not responding. The time frame considered appropriate is usually based on the natural history of the disorder, combined with the risk of chronicity and other mitigating factors from the specific patient's circumstances. Then the resources of an interdisciplinary collaboration become particularly valuable assets to both the provider and the patient.

Considerations in Triage

As more cooperative care opportunities develop, natural questions emerge that serve to illustrate the practice issues:

- How is the patient triaged to different provider types?
- Who is to act as the principal manager of patient care during the treatment encounter?
- What criteria should be used to judge the need for specialty testing and services?
- What are the acceptable limits for the change afforded to any given method of treatment to achieve a clinical success?
- Is clinical success defined the same way for all patient categories and disorders?

Coordinated Integration of Chiropractic Services in the Multidisciplinary Setting

The services offered by providers in neuromusculoskeletal practice often overlap with other groups having a related primary area of expertise, such as chiropractors, physical therapists, occupational therapists, pain management and rehabilitation, and, in some cases, orthopedists. Many of these disciplines use similar

evaluations and the same array of diagnostic technologies for differential diagnoses.

There is logic in bringing all of these resources together into one complementary group with a common mission—the prevention and treatment of neuromusculoskeletal disorders:

1. *Initial assessment.* The provider identifies the need for urgent or emergency care (progressive neurologic deficit, fracture, infection, cancer, or systemic disease).
2. *Optimum approach.* If need for urgent or emergent care is absent, the treatment plan is focused on evidence that there is an optimum approach that should be followed initially.
3. *Contraindications.* If evidence for a preferred treatment method is absent, identify any contraindication to the approach primarily used by the provider performing the assessment. If there is none, initiate a trial of therapy.
4. *Review of results.* Review the results of the initial therapy plan within a short interval (2 weeks). If there is progress toward resolution, proceed. If the patient is not responding as expected, modify the treatment plan or refer to an alternative methodology.

DISCUSSION

Development and Applications of Clinical Guidelines

Historically, case management has been conducted by independent practitioners acting alone or in a loose confederation of providers who are structured more or less informally. Mechanisms for facing a complex set of patient needs in the traditional setting can be represented by a horizontally integrated system. Complaints are triaged by the preferred provider whose advice has been sought by the patient. Occasionally, multiple providers with competing or overlapping approaches to treatment may be consulted simultaneously. This conclusion contributes to increased costs of care, misunderstandings between provider groups, and patient confusion. Without distinct contraindications, early treatment alternatives offered to the patient are likely to represent the provider's preferences. These clinical decisions may or may not reflect the best or most appropriate care available and are the foundation for wide variations in practice.

There is little evidence of benefit and strong suggestion of significant cost associated with these discrepancies in treatment approaches. The current trends in health care policymaking, represented by the activities of the Agency for Health Care Policy and Research, are an attempt to minimize the number of treatment options and resulting variations used in practice that have little foundation (Bigos et al, 1994). Guideline recommendations direct the initial treatment efforts according to the available scientific information on effectiveness. Where compelling data are unavailable, as is often the case, opinion derived from formal consensus proceedings will suffice as a basis for guideline development. This approach has the added advantage of focusing debate and sharpening the search for answers to critical health-related questions.

In the context of the multidisciplinary team, administrative services (credentialing, precertification, billing, collections, and marketing), financial risks, and benefits are available among all participants. Perhaps the simplest way to achieve this is through the development of consensus-based treatment protocols and pathways. Consensus requires time invested in regular, substantive, and focused interactions between all of the providers who are a part of the team. The exercise of developing the protocols reveals the evidence supporting referral, the ambiguities remaining, and the clinical logic that permeates the group. As patient comanagement progresses, cross-referrals can speed patient recovery and strengthen the cohesion of the group.

REFERENCES

Bigos S, Bowyer O, Braen G, et al. *Acute Low Back Problems in Adults.* Clinical Practice Guidelines No. 14. Rockville, MD: AHCPR; 1994. AHCPR Publication No. 95–0642.

Carey TS, Garrett J, Jackman A, McLaughlin C. The outcomes and costs for acute low back pain, seen by primary care practitioners, chiropractors, and orthopedic surgeons. *N Engl J Med.* 1995;333:913–917.

Coile RC. Chiropractic treatment: an "alternative medicine" becomes mainstream health care. *Health Trends.* 1995;7(9):1–8.

Jarvis JB, Phillips RB, Morris EK. Cost per case comparison of back injury claims of chiropractic versus medical management with identical diagnostic codes. *J Occup Med.* 1991;33:847–852.

Main DC. *Forming Physician Networks.* Chicago: American Medical Association; 1993.

Mosley CD, Cohen IG, Arnold RM. Cost-effectiveness of chiropractic in a managed care setting. *Am J Manage Care.* 1996;2(3):280–284.

Pristave RJ, Becker S, McCarthy LI. Development of provider networks for specific diseases. *Health Care Innovations.* 1995;Sept/Oct:9–37.

Triano JJ, Hondras M, McGregor M. Differences in treatment history with manipulation for acute, subacute, chronic and recurrent spine pain. *J Manipulative Physiol Ther.* 1992;15(1):24–30.

Triano JJ, Raley B. Chiropractic in the interdisciplinary team practice. *Top Clin Chiropract.* 1994;1(4):58–66.

Triano JJ, Rashbaum RF, Hansen DT. Opening access to spine care in the evolving market: integration and communication. *Top Clin Chiropract.* 1998;5(4):44–52.

CHAPTER 39

Hospital-Based Integrative Medicine: The Institute for Health and Healing

William B. Stewart with Nancy Faass

THE PROCESS OF DEVELOPMENT

The Institute for Health and Healing (IHH) at California Pacific Medical Center (CPMC) was created in 1994 by the coming together of several longstanding efforts: an education forum in integrative medicine, the Planetree library, and the hospital chaplaincy.

Initially, educational programs of exceptional quality were provided to the community sponsored by the program in medicine and philosophy. The forums included monthly lectures by noted experts and authors, periodic grand rounds, workshops, and courses. These endeavors were never seen as a separate theme outside the mainstream institution—rather, they have always been viewed as another aspect of the broader evolution of medicine. The programs offered the public and medical communities the opportunity to meet clinicians, writers, indigenous healers, theorists, and other experts from all over the United States and the world. It is possible that the interest generated by these forums eventually coalesced in the creation of the Health and Healing Clinic. When the op-portunity became available to develop the clinic, a broad base of support had been in place for some time among both the public and some sectors of the medical community.

The work of the Institute has contributed to the development of the Clinic by furthering an institutional culture that is tolerant of our position and our ideals. The integrative approach of the Institute has led to the development of a comprehensive array of programming including clinical care, public and professional education, and research. The goal has been to increase awareness of other perspectives in healing in a way that is respectful and honors the accomplishments and the realities of contemporary biomedicine.

The Initial Development Phase of the Clinic

The initial impetus and funding for the Clinic came from a patient who wanted to receive care in a setting in which conventional and alternative treatment could be integrated. She wanted a facility where practitioners from multiple disciplines could communicate and collaborate in assessment and treatment. Her timing was right—there was receptivity at the medical center and in the public's mind and mood. Furthermore, she had the financial resources to energize such an ambitious project. She accomplished this with a start-up gift that was matched by a foundation grant.

The idea of creating a clinic was further developed by a steering committee that included Institute staff, working in partnership with leaders of the medical center administration, medical staff,

William B. Stewart, MD, is the Medical Director of the Institute for Health and Healing of the California Pacific Medical Center, San Francisco, and Marin General Hospital, Greenbrae, California.

Source: Adapted from *Healthcare Forum Journal*, Vol. 41, No. 6 by permission, November/December 1998, Copyright 1998, by Health Forum, Inc. and Reprinted from *San Francisco Medicine*, the official publication of the San Francisco Medical Society.

and the CPMC Foundation. The community-based volunteer executive committee of the Institute considered and endorsed the concept.

A comprehensive business plan for the first three years of operation was devised through the office of the vice president of business development at CPMC. At that point, a task force was formed, which included administrators, physicians, nurses, designers, alternative practitioners, Institute staff, Foundation personnel, and executive committee members. The task force included supporters, as well as skeptics. They worked together to define the program and its appropriate environment; plan facilities; design and create a calm, supportive healing environment; recruit personnel; establish policies and procedures; devise budgets; and organize internal and external communications (marketing and public relations).

Guided by information from several focus groups (made up of users and nonusers of complementary medicine) and multiple discussions with members of our medical staff, the Clinic was developed based on the specialty, referral model, rather than the provision of primary care. All patients, even those who are self-referred, must have a primary care physician. The Clinic does not want to compete with either medical staff who have primary care practices or with complementary practitioners in the area. Rather, our goal is to support their work. This is a model that is consistent with the institutional culture; this is not necessarily the case for other integrative medicine centers. The Clinic is designed to be part of the established, conventional medical system.

CLINICAL SERVICES

Providers

The Clinic is directed by Western-trained physicians who have additional training in complementary medicine. The Clinic's objective is to provide a comprehensive assessment by a physician, practicing integrative medicine from a broad perspective. Currently, there are four board-certified physicians—two internists, a pediatrician, and a psychiatrist. One is a fully trained homeopath who is also a board-certified internist; another is highly trained in infectious diseases and herbals and is a Reiki master; a third has special expertise in the influence of psychosocial factors and prayer on illness and health; and the fourth is an expert in nutrition and eating disorders, as well as a board-certified internist. To complement these services, we chose a core staff of several practitioners.

A traditional Chinese medicine practitioner/licensed acupuncturist, several certified bodyworkers, a meditation teacher, a chaplain, the medical director, a manager, and a receptionist complete the clinical staff. Additional practitioners are used as consultants and will be added as required, in response to patient needs and in alignment with the Clinic's financial profile.

The physical environment of the Clinic, although a standard physician's office in shape, is designed and remodeled to enhance healing. Patients are greeted by a receptionist who sits at a small desk with a fountain on it, rather than behind a high counter. Massage tables replace the standard exam tables. Practitioners meet with patients seated in comfortable chairs instead of behind a desk. Live plants and open windows provide atmosphere and fresh air.

Patient Services

Every patient who comes to the Health and Healing Clinic at CPMC in San Francisco undergoes a process of assessment and collaborative care management. At the same time, every patient's experience is different, not just because patients come with different diagnoses, but because they come with different beliefs, temperaments, and lifestyles. There are no formulas—no cookie-cutter approaches. The Clinic seeks to respond to the patients' needs and requests. It brings together knowledge and practices from many cultures and systems of health and medical practice within an established medical center.

Since the Clinic opened early in 1998, approximately 30 to 40 new patients have been seen per month, with patients typically averaging 3 to 6 visits. The patients, family, and involved practitioners collaborate to develop an individualized health management plan. Each patient fills out an extensive intake questionnaire prior to his or her visit with one of the Clinic physicians. A multidisciplinary conference meets weekly to review new and challenging cases. The center's physicians participate in these reviews, as do the Clinic's manager, medical director, hospital chaplains, certified bodyworkers, and other involved practitioners, from both conventional and complementary disciplines.

Through this type of comprehensive assessment, a management plan emerges. Follow-up is shared among the involved practitioners and the patients' primary care providers. The full resources of the medical center and the community are available for consultation, diagnosis, and treatment. The patient may be referred outside the medical center as necessary to complete the collaborative treatment plan that has been established between the team, the consulting physician, and the patient. We seek to complement and potentiate ongoing medical care—not to replace it.

Viewing the data from an initial survey, it is apparent that patients are coming to the Clinic with significant illnesses, rather than just for preventive or wellness maintenance services. The profile of the Clinic's patients differs somewhat from that of the findings of Eisenberg et al (1993, 1998), which indicated that the majority of patients surveyed were using complementary and alternative therapies for wellness or prevention. An analysis of patient profiles, conducted in 1999, showed that patients were being seen most often with the following conditions: cancer (particularly breast cancer); stress, anxiety, and depression; gastrointestinal disturbances (from irritable bowel syndrome to ulcerative colitis); chronic pain (particularly low-back pain); immune-mediated diseases; chronic allergic responses; and pediatric problems such as attention deficit disorder. Approximately 7 percent of our patients receive financial aid through our patient assistance fund.

WORKING WITHIN THE INSTITUTION

Communication

Effective communication—outgoing and incoming—is essential in all work but particularly in this emerging field of integrative medicine. Communication venues range from one-on-one discussions to publications that are distributed throughout the Sutter Health Network of affiliated medical institutions, of which CPMC is a member, and beyond. We describe, explain, review, respond, seek comment, and invite questions from our constituencies, including patients, collaborators, and competitors.

Among traditionalists at the medical center, the response to the Clinic has run the full gamut, from zealous support to zealous resistance. At every step of the way, some have shown support, some healthy skepticism, and others disapproval. Resistance is part of the process as it is with any new frontier, and it is handled by listening respectfully, modifying plans when appropriate, and continuing to educate and be educated. The Clinic's intent is to receive feedback graciously, with openness and interest. Our supporters and skeptics work extremely well together, and, on any given issue, we usually reach consensus. Clinic personnel also work to ensure that we practice evidence-based medicine by staying current with the literature and emerging information and practices.

Quality Improvement

The Health and Healing Clinic is operated under the same rigorous standards for credentialing and quality/performance improvement as those of any clinic of Western medicine and is surveyed and licensed by the state. The Clinic was reviewed by the Joint Commission on Accreditation of Healthcare Organizations (Joint Commission) in 1999 and found to be compliant in all ways; the evaluation occurred in conjunction with Joint Commission review of CPMC. We hold high standards for both the program and the providers.

Components of the Quality Assurance Program

Physician Quality. Clinic physicians are credentialed through their respective medical staff departments and held to the same benchmarks of performance and ethics as other hospital physicians and specialists. The Clinic's organization is consistent with the medical center model, so all the physicians are members of the medical staff and of a hospital department.

Licensed Practitioners. Selection for other types of practitioners is also based on well-accepted rigorous Western scientific criteria that are broadly in place, which include graduation from accredited institutions and appropriate licensure. State-licensed practitioners, such as registered nurses, acupuncturists, and chiropractors, must meet state-mandated standards. The practitioners are subject to competency and quality reviews, as are all employees of the medical center. Rather than pursuing their own specific disciplines in isolation, they are part of the Clinic's team, which reinforces the multidisciplinary approach to patient care and helps ensure quality practice through peer review.

Nonlicensed Practitioners. Certified massage therapists and nutritionists are held to the standards of national certifying organizations. Each practitioner's credentials and job description are set out in the policy and procedure manual of the Clinic. These policies and procedures are consistent with those of other hospital-based clinics licensed under the institution's acute care license. In sum, assurances are provided through practitioner credentialing by the medical staff, through bylaws, institutional guidelines, and laws of the city of San Francisco and the state of California.

Quality Improvement. Internal and external quality and performance improvement protocols are also applied to the Clinic with the same rigor as other program units within the hospital. Peer review, chart review, and case presentations are performed weekly at regularly scheduled meetings within the multidisciplinary conference. Planning and implementation of problem-solving measures are included in the ongoing process of quality assurance. The Clinic is overseen in this arena by the hospital's Committee on Ambulatory Care Quality and Performance Improvement. This willingness to be subject to biomedical and institutional standards is one of the strengths of the program, and, to some extent, that ensures a higher standard of quality. It is the policy of the Clinic to "play by the same rules."

Quality Process. Ultimately, providing a quality product is the result of working with high-quality people. The quality of service provision also comes from the internal process of each individual practitioner. In addition, it grows out of constant dialogue among the staff about how, as practitioners, they can continue to improve and grow professionally and personally.

A Research Orientation

To remain responsive to new information and practice, clinical activities are linked to research instruments that assess parameters that include treatment efficacy, cost-effectiveness, and patient satisfaction. The Clinic also participates in basic research through the Complementary Medicine Research Institute, which contributes to the development of integrative medicine through basic and clinical research.

While it is challenging to design research in the field of integrative medicine, it is mandatory that we do so. Complementary therapies and practice must be subject to the same scientific rigor as the practice of conventional medicine if they are to be incorporated into contemporary medicine in an enduring way.

The clinical work is closely linked with research and the commitment to study efficacy, safety, outcomes, and mechanisms of action—both theoretically and in the clinical setting. Studies related to acupuncture, guided imagery, and distant healing intentionality are ongoing for patients with conditions such as stroke, cancer, and HIV/AIDS. A multiyear grant was received from the NIH in association with Bastyr University in Seattle for projects related to patients with HIV/AIDS. Other research conducted in the past has included a study of massage in the neonatal ICU and an in vitro study of the efficacy of Chinese herbal medicine in combination with standard chemotherapy for breast cancer.

Economic Considerations

On the institutional organization chart, the Health and Healing Clinic is in the reporting line of the vice president for medical affairs. Both CPMC and the CPMC Foundation and the medical center oversee the Clinic's finances. All of its budgets and financial plans are subject to the same scrutiny as any other medical center project. Although the Clinic is responsible for raising a significant proportion of its budget, even proposals that are not linked to a specific monetary request are reviewed by a standing institutional committee of medical staff and administrators at CPMC. One component of the ongoing discussion is how the Institute for Health and Healing can best be managed from a business perspective.

Talk of sustainability raises the abiding question: How will these services be funded over the long term? By and large, at the present time, the responsibility for payment for complementary medicine lies with the patient. However, this is changing. For example, the Clinic is currently in discussion with several organizations that are considering potential coverage.

As business entities move into the relationship between healer and patient, the Clinic makes conscious efforts to retain the bond with each patient. The concern is that the time-intensive interaction between complementary practitioner and patient could be diluted to increase volume and profit margin while reimbursements are ratcheted down. Then the attributes often ascribed to complementary practitioners—unhurried, caring, hands-on service—will vanish under the pressures of economic reality.

COMMUNITY EDUCATION

The IHH provides a range of community educational programs promoting integrative medicine and spirituality including an annual Mini Medical School that expands the community's access to information and research about complementary and alternative medicine practices, special guest lectures by leaders in the field, and wellness classes in which patients learn specific health-enhancing practices such as mindfulness meditation, yoga, Qigong, and guided imagery.

Professional Education

For health professionals, the Institute provides integrative medicine education programs through departmental grand rounds and training programs at CPMC and Marin General Hospital. We bring together physicians, nurses, massage therapists, guided imagery therapists, expressive arts therapists, and spiritual care givers (chaplains) to learn integrative medicine and spirituality through year-long programs. These programs involve clinical care in a hospital setting, group and individual clinical supervision, didactic presentations, interdisciplinary case conferences, and workshops. The inclusion of these diverse healing practices in hospital inpatient and outpatient settings is also an indicator of the expansion in integrative services.

In the sense of a system, one of the frontiers of the Clinic's current work is to bring more complementary medicine knowledge and practices to other hospitals in the Sutter Health System in Northern California. Throughout, the goal is not to be a model focused on modalities as much as a model focused on approaches and perspectives in medicine. The community education programs of the two institutions, Marin General Hospital and California Pacific Medical Center, working in collaboration, have served approximately 60,000 people in the past year through inpatient and outpatient programs.

Wellness Programming

When the Institute was developed in 1994, only two community wellness programs were available for our public and professional constituencies. In partnership with Marin General Hospital, more than three dozen programs are currently provided, including cancer support groups, guided imagery and expressive art therapy for hospitalized patients, meditation, T'ai chi, Qigong, and yoga.

Design for Healing

The patient resource library and the Clinic are examples of sites that have been redesigned and remodeled with the recognition of the effect of the environment on healing. The chapel has also been redone with an ecumenical motif, including careful consideration of color, lighting, privacy, function, and feeling.

Two San Francisco designers, Agnes Bourne and Victoria Stone, have played leadership roles in the creation of these and other healing environments on the CPMC campuses. This is most dramatically represented in the full sized labyrinth installation in the entry courtyard of the largest of CPMC's acute care hospitals. The image has drawn interest in the media, nationally and internationally. It is used regularly by patients, their families, employees, and staff, and for special events sponsored by the department of pastoral care.

Resources

The community has access to the extensive resources of the Institute for Health and Healing Resource Center/Planetree library, recognized by *The Consumer Health Source Book* as "the best of the medical search services." The resource center was one of the first Planetree libraries in the nation. Last year, the library served more than 20,000 clients through telephone, Internet, and on-site services. Patients, their families, caregivers, and health care professionals can access books and journals, search the Internet, and obtain individualized customized information packets on conventional and complementary medicine.

A goal at the Institute for Health and Healing is to provide opportunities for dialogue, for questioning, and for exchange. Education has become an area of great emphasis for the Institute within the health professional community and the general community. Our educational activities relate to the delivery of information, to the development of skills, to learning about the practices of other cultures, other ways of knowing, and other systems of medicine. Another educational objective is self-knowledge and our own journeys of self-awareness, and consciousness. Here "our" includes practitioners, patients, and the public.

CONCLUSION

This is the evolution of medicine, rather than a revolution of medicine. Over time, some of the glow on complementary, integrative, and alternative medicine will diminish as the good parts, the efficacious parts, the safe parts, and the cost-effective parts are incorporated in the healing practices of the dominant form. We are having an impact and will continue to have an impact. In so doing, we will gradually influence medicine.

At California Pacific Medical Center and Marin General Hospital, complementary practices have already been integrated into radiation oncology, women's health, occupational health, physical and occupational therapy, rehabilitation, and cardiology. Ultimately, the success of the Clinic and of the Institute will be known when we disappear—when complementary medicine is so much a part of the mainstream that a separate clinic is not needed. Then there will no longer be a separate program for integrative medicine—rather, the principles that are valuable will be incorporated throughout medicine, in the protocols and pathways where they are found to be appropriate and effective.

REFERENCES

Eisenberg D, Davis R, Ettner S, et al. Trends in alternative medicine use in the United States, 1990–1997: results of a follow-up national survey. *JAMA*. 1998;280(18): 1569–1575.

Eisenberg DM, Kessler RC, Foster C, et al. Unconventional medicine in the United States. *N Engl J Med*. 1993;328(4): 246–252.

PART X

Hospital-Based Programs

CHAPTER 40

Disease Management: The Ornish Program

40.1 The Potential of Integrative Medicine in Disease Management

Richard Sheff

HOSPITALS AS INTEGRATIVE MEDICINE CENTERS

One of the greatest opportunities for hospitals in the integrative environment is to become centers of excellence in integrative disease management. Hospital-based medical centers of this type will be uniquely equipped to assist patients in the integration of their care in cases of complex or chronic illness, such as cancer, coronary artery disease, and spine care. The development of hospitals as integrative centers will attract patients who want to use complementary and alternative services but who also require the conventional services that are the basic "bread and butter" of the hospital. The need for services of this type appears to be quite extensive. According to a study by Hoffman et al (1996), more than 44% of the ambulatory U.S. population has some form of chronic illness. It has been suggested that a significant percentage of complementary and alternative medicine (CAM) use reflects patient attempts to address unresolved chronic illness (Astin, 1998; Druss and Rosenheck, 1999).

These factors may be more relevant to hospitals than they are to health plans. It is clear that this strategy could significantly expand the present scope of hospital-based treatment of chronic illness. A good example of this integrative approach is the successful inclusion of the Ornish programs for heart disease offered at hospitals throughout the United States.

Hospitals currently range across the spectrum in their current levels of interest in complementary medicine. There are a large number of hospitals that have been seriously evaluating CAM. This exploration is frequently driven by individuals in leadership within the organization who have had personal experience with the effectiveness of complementary and alternative therapies. These leaders are looking for meaningful ways to integrate CAM disciplines into hospital programs.

In addition, the hospitals are exploring new markets to compensate for their loss of revenue as they increasingly become outpatient-based environments. They are also experiencing decreased utilization, due to shorter lengths of stay

---

Richard Sheff, MD, is the Chairman of the Board of CommonWell, a company that provides consultation to health care organizations to determine how best to integrate complementary therapies. His background includes 12 years of clinical practice in family medicine; founder and manager of an independent practice association; medical director of a physician hospital organization; vice president of medical affairs for a hospital; president of incorporated physician practice groups; and vice president of a medical insurers' group.

as the trend toward outpatient surgery increases, often provided at separate surgery centers. Consequently, hospitals are considering new lines of business, seeking opportunities that improve their relationships with the community and approaches that will bring in additional patients.

HOSPITAL CAM PROGRAMS

Numerous hospitals have launched CAM programs. George Washington University in Washington, DC, has a CAM clinic, and UCLA has had an affiliated physician-acupuncture education program for almost a decade. The integrative hospital programs at Columbia-New York Presbyterian utilize mind-body medicine in conjunction with acute surgical care and aftercare follow-up services. Memorial Sloan-Kettering Cancer Center in New York has developed an integrative medicine service. Other academic medical centers that offer integrative clinics include the University of Arizona, Dartmouth, Duke, Harvard, the University of Maryland, the University of Minnesota, Stanford, and Tufts.

Griffin Hospital in Connecticut has become the home of Planetree, an organizational leader in the movement for patient-centered care. Hugh Chatham Hospital, a small rural facility in Elkin, North Carolina, has integrated a CAM approach to overall hospital care in a significant way, with a grant from Duke University. This is an example of a hospital that developed a CAM program by building on grassroots support from the staff, rather than by creating a "bricks and mortar" clinic.

Consultants who work with hospitals across the country also observe a conservative perspective on the part of some physicians and a tendency toward strong skepticism regarding complementary therapies. Consequently, hospitals are trying a number of different approaches to integration. I am impressed by the sense that there is a great deal of ferment occurring in hospital environments. Despite the conservatism, some elements are pushing for change, and it is taking place. For example, many hospitals now have task forces that are evaluating opportunities to move the integrative process forward.

It is important that complementary medicine be viewed as more than a marketing tool by the health care industry. Many hospitals have launched CAM clinics in an effort to capture new revenue, especially self-pay revenue. Unfortunately, most CAM clinics either lose money or do not make enough money to justify the capital investment. The business models that have been developed for integrative medicine are at risk of simply adding costs or skimming profits unless this field can truly improve effectiveness and outcomes. The best approach to this goal is through programs in disease management, bringing together the best of conventional, complementary, and alternative medicine in well-thought-out programs with measurable outcomes. Over time, the integration of conventional and complementary medicine has the potential to provide greater cost-effectiveness, increased patient satisfaction, and better clinical outcomes. That will realize the positive potential for health care, patients, and practitioners.

REFERENCES

Astin J. Why patients use alternative medicine: Results of a national study. *JAMA*. 1998;279(19):1548–1553.

Druss BG, Rosenheck RA. Association between use of unconventional therapies and conventional medical services. *JAMA*. 1999;282(7):651–656.

Hoffman C, Rice D, Sung HY. Persons with chronic conditions: Their prevalence and costs. *JAMA*. 1996;276(18):1473–1479.

40.2   Disease Management: Avoiding Revascularization with Lifestyle Changes

Dean Ornish

BACKGROUND

Approximately 500,000 coronary artery bypass graft operations and approximately 600,000 coronary angioplasties were performed in the United States in 1994, at a combined cost of approximately $15.6 billion, more than for any other surgical procedure. The total cost of treatment of coronary artery disease in the United States was estimated to be $56.3 billion in 1994 (American Heart Association, 1994). Thus, there is a potential for significant cost savings if safe and comparably effective, but less expensive, alternative interventions can be implemented.

The idea that the progression of coronary artery disease is often reversible was once a radical concept but is now becoming mainstream. Numerous interventions have been shown to arrest or reverse the progression of coronary atherosclerosis. These include comprehensive changes in diet and lifestyle (Esselstyn et al, 1995; Ornish et al, 1990; Schuler et al, 1992), lipid-lowering drug therapy (Brown et al, 1995; Kane et al, 1990; Blankenhorn et al, 1987), partial ileal bypass surgery (Buchwald et al, 1990), and parenteral nutrition (Gould et al, 1994).

The Ornish program—the Multicenter Lifestyle Demonstration Project—was designed to determine

1. Whether other teams of health professionals in diverse regions of the country could be trained to motivate their patients to follow a program of comprehensive lifestyle changes.
2. Whether this lifestyle program may be an equivalently safe and medically effective but more cost-effective alternative to revascularization in selected patients with severe but stable coronary artery disease.
3. What the resulting cost savings might be.

In other words, can patients avoid revascularization by making comprehensive lifestyle changes at lower cost without increasing cardiac morbidity and mortality?

Dean Ornish, MD, is the founder, President, and Director of the nonprofit Preventive Medicine Research Institute in Sausalito, California; Clinical Professor of Medicine at the University of California, San Francisco (UCSF); and a founder of UCSF's Osher Center for Integrative Medicine. He received his medical degree from Baylor College of Medicine in Houston and was a clinical fellow in medicine at Harvard Medical School. For the past 22 years, Dr. Ornish has directed clinical research on the efficacy of lifestyle interventions in the treatment of coronary artery disease. His research and writings have been published in major medical journals, and he is the author of five best-selling books. Dr. Ornish has served as a physician consultant to President Clinton and has received several prestigious awards.

Source: Adapted from *American Journal of Cardiology*, Vol. 82, No. 108, Dean Ornish et al., Avoiding Revascularization with Lifestyle Changes: The Multicenter Lifestyle Demonstration Project, pp. 72T–76T, Copyright 1998, with permission from Excerpta Medica Inc.

SUMMARY OF FINDINGS

Can Patients Safely Avoid Revascularization?

This study found that 150 of the 194 experimental-group patients were able to avoid revascularization, and the frequency of adverse cardiac events was not increased. The number of cardiac events per patient-year of follow-up, comparing the experimental group with the control group, was as follows: 0.012 versus 0.012 for myocardial infarction; 0.014 versus 0.006 for stroke; 0.006 versus 0.012 for noncardiac deaths; and 0.014 versus 0.012 for cardiac deaths.

Cost-Benefit Analysis

The average cost of the 1-year intensive lifestyle intervention was $7,000. The average cost for angioplasty (with catheterization) was $31,000, and the average cost for bypass surgery was $46,000. All of the experimental group patients were eligible for revascularization in terms of both medical criteria and reimbursement criteria from Mutual of Omaha. However, only 31 angioplasties were performed on the 194 experimental group patients (0.064 events per patient-year of follow-up), and 26 bypass procedures were performed on the 194 experimental group patients (0.053 events per patient-year of follow-up) after entry. The costs in the experimental group included the costs of angioplasties (31 × $31,000); bypass procedures (26 × $46,000); and program costs (194 × $7,000). Thus, the total for the experimental group was $3,515,000—approximately $18,119 per patient.

All of the 139 control group patients were selected for having had a recent angioplasty or bypass before entry: 66 underwent angio-plasty, and 73 underwent bypass. In addition, there were 23 angioplasties and 11 additional bypass surgeries in the control group after entry. Thus, the costs of the control group were: (66 × $31,000) + (23 × $31,000) + (73 × $46,000) + (11 × $46,000). Consequently, total health care expenditures in the control group equaled $6,623,000—approximately $47,647 per patient (see Table 40.2–1).

The average savings per patient in the lifestyle program was $47,647, less $18,119—approximately $29,528 per patient.

OVERVIEW OF APPROACHES TO TREATMENT

A Multifactorial Program of Lifestyle Change

Earlier studies demonstrated that the progression of even severe coronary artery disease often can begin to reverse in many patients by an intensive, multifactorial program of comprehensive lifestyle changes. These lifestyle changes include:

- a very low-fat, low-cholesterol diet (approximately 10% fat, not greater than 10 mg/day dietary cholesterol)

Table 40.2–1 The Multicenter Lifestyle Demonstration Project

Intervention	Experimental Group	Control Group
Angioplasties	31 x $31,000	66 x $31,000 (initial surgeries) 73 x $46,000 (after program began)
Bypass procedures	26 x $46,000	23 x $31,000 (initial) 11 x $46,000 (after program began)
Ornish Program	194 x $7,000	
Totals	$3,515,000—approx. total $18,119 per patient	$6,623,000—approx. total $47,647 per patient
Cost Savings	$29,528 per patient	

Source: Adapted from *American Journal of Cardiology*, Vol. 82, No. 108, Dean Ornish et al., Avoiding Revascularization with Lifestyle Changes: The Multicenter Lifestyle Demonstration Project, pp. 72T–76T, Copyright 1998, with permission from Excerpta Medica Inc.

- a whole-foods vegetarian diet that is high in complex carbohydrates and low in simple sugars
- stress management techniques
- moderate exercise
- psychosocial support.

Endpoint measures included quantitative coronary arteriography to assess coronary artery stenosis and cardiac positron emission tomography (PET) scans to assess myocardial perfusion (Ornish et al, 1990; Gould et al, 1995).

In the past, insurance companies, managed care organizations, and Medicare have been reluctant to pay for lifestyle interventions, in part because these have been viewed as prevention—increase costs in the short run for possible savings years later. Also, because approximately 20–30% of patients change their insurance plans each year, even if cost savings result from lifestyle interventions, they may accrue to another insurance company.

However, a program of comprehensive lifestyle changes may be offered as a much less costly alternative treatment to revascularization for selected patients who are eligible for bypass or angioplasty (under the supervision of the referring physician), thereby resulting in immediate and substantial cost savings. Also, providing lifestyle changes as a direct alternative for patients who otherwise would receive bypass or angioplasty may result in significant long-term costs savings. Despite the expense of bypass surgery and angioplasty, 30–50% of bypass grafts reocclude after only 5–7 years, and 30–50% of angioplastied arteries restenose after only 4–6 months (Bourassa, 1994; Hirshfeld et al, 1991). When this occurs, bypass surgery or angioplasty is often repeated, thereby incurring additional costs.

Coronary Artery Bypass and Angioplasty

Coronary artery bypass is effective in decreasing angina and improving cardiac function. However, when compared with medical therapy at 16 years of follow-up, bypass improved survival in only a very small subgroup of patients—those with decreased left ventricular function and stenotic lesions of the left main coronary artery of greater than 59%. Median survival was not prolonged in patients with left main coronary artery stenosis less than 60% and normal left ventricular function, even if a significant right coronary stenosis greater than 70% was also present (Alderman et al, 1990; Varnauskas, 1998; Chaitman et al, 1981; Coronary Artery Bypass Surgery Cooperative Study Group, 1984).

Angioplasty was originally developed with the hope of providing a less-invasive, lower-risk approach to the management of coronary artery disease and its symptoms. Although widely used, it has never been compared with medical therapy in a randomized trial in stable patients with coronary artery disease; therefore, the mortality, morbidity, and benefits of angioplasty are unknown.

The use of various types of stents (the insertion of a mesh brace into the lumen of the coronary artery during angioplasty) may slow the rate of restenosis, but there are no randomized controlled trial data supporting the efficacy of these approaches. The use of the left internal mammary artery in bypass surgery may reduce reocclusion, but vein grafts also must be used when patients have multivessel disease. Thus, in addition to the costs of the original bypass or angioplasty, there are costs of further procedures when restenosis and reocclusion occur.

The majority of adverse events related to coronary artery disease—myocardial infarction, sudden death, and unstable angina—are due to the rupture of an atherosclerotic plaque of less than 40–50% stenosis. This often occurs in the setting of vessel spasm and results in thrombosis and occlusion of the vessel (Fuster et al, 1992). Bypass surgery and angioplasty usually are not performed on lesions less than 50% stenosed and do not affect nonbypassed or nondilated lesions, whereas comprehensive lifestyle changes (or lipid-lowering drugs) may help to stabilize all lesions, including mild lesions. Also, mild lesions that undergo catastrophic progression usually have a less well developed network of collateral circulation to protect the myocardium than do more severe stenoses.

Bypass surgery and angioplasty have associated risks of morbidity and mortality, whereas there are no significant risks from eating a well-balanced, low-fat, low-cholesterol diet, stopping smoking, or engaging in moderate walking, stress management techniques, and psychosocial support.

LIFESTYLE INTERVENTIONS

Thousands of dollars are saved immediately for every bypass candidate who can avoid the procedure by making intensive changes in diet and lifestyle. However, cost savings in avoided revascularization will occur only if patients who are trained in this lifestyle program adhere to it over time. If patients do not adhere, costs would increase, rather than decrease, because insurers would ultimately pay for both lifestyle training and subsequent revascularization. The missing link, therefore, are the data to demonstrate whether patients will adhere to this intensive lifestyle program. One goal of this study was to determine whether patients who are motivated to make comprehensive lifestyle changes can maintain these changes in an ambulatory setting, if given the proper support.

The Multicenter Lifestyle Demonstration Project

To address this question, the Multicenter Lifestyle Demonstration Project was established in 1993 at eight sites. Also, trained practitioners were put in place at eight additional sites, whose data are not included here. These sites are geographically, socioeconomically, racially, and culturally diverse. Approximately 40 insurance companies are now reimbursing at least part of the cost of this program at these sites for selected patients.

Staffing

Teams of health professionals were trained at each of these clinical sites, including cardiolo-

gists, registered dietitians, exercise physiologists, psychologists, chefs, stress management specialists, registered nurses, and administrative support personnel. These teams, in turn, worked with their patients to motivate them to make and maintain comprehensive lifestyle changes.

Criteria for Patient Inclusion and Exclusion

Patients were selected who had angiographically documented coronary artery disease severe enough to warrant revascularization and who were approved for insurance indemnity to undergo a procedural intervention. Patients were excluded for any of the following:

1. greater than 50% stenosis in the left main coronary artery
2. bypass surgery within 6 weeks or angioplasty within 6 months
3. chronic unresponsive congestive heart failure
4. malignant uncontrolled arrhythmias
5. myocardial infarction within 1 month
6. homozygous hypercholesterolemia
7. psychosis
8. hypotensive response to exercise
9. alcohol or drug abuse
10. life-threatening comorbidity

Program Design

Patients and staff met three times per week for 12 weeks, plus once per week for the remaining 9 months. Most sessions were 4 hours long: 1 hour of exercise, 1 hour of stress management techniques, 1 hour of group support, and a 1-hour meal. The cost of the 1-year program averaged $7,000 per person (shorter and less-expensive versions of the program are now available for people with less severe coronary artery disease).

Data Collection

All hospitals sent data directly to the independently funded data coordinating center at the Massachusetts General Hospital. Matched control-group patients were provided by Mutual of

Omaha. Patients were matched for age, gender, left ventricular ejection fraction (less than 25%, 20–40%, or greater than 40%), and cardiac score defined as the sum of the severity score for each of the three main coronary arteries rated as 0 (less than 50% percent stenosis), 0.5 (50–70% stenosis), or 1.0 (greater than 75% stenosis). All control group patients were within 1 month of having undergone revascularization.

Self-Selection Factors

Although a randomized controlled trial intervention comparing comprehensive lifestyle changes with revascularization may seem ideal, it is not feasible in practice. The attitude of someone willing to make comprehensive lifestyle changes is often quite different from that of someone who wants to undergo revascularization. The decision to make comprehensive lifestyle changes requires commitment, discipline, and a willingness to assume personal responsibility for one's health. The decision to undergo revascularization is often made by patients who tend to be less involved in directly affecting their condition—the other end of the personal responsibility spectrum. This is not a value judgment, but a reflection of different approaches, both of which may be valid. To be randomized, a patient has to be willing to undergo either treatment (revascularization or comprehensive lifestyle changes). Because the mindset is so different, it would be very difficult to find patients who were willing to accept either choice as determined by someone else; most patients want to choose one or the other for themselves.

Baseline Demographics

A total of 333 patients completed this demonstration project. Of these, 194 were in the experimental group, and 139 were in the control group.

At baseline, there were no significant differences between the experimental group and control group in age, gender, marital status, employment status, or history of hypertension, hypercholesterolemia, diabetes, smoking, or family

history of heart disease. In the experimental group, the average age was 58 years; 79% were male, and 77% were married. Of particular note is that 63.5% of these patients were currently working but were able to find time to adhere to the intervention of comprehensive lifestyle changes. Furthermore, 50% were hypertensive, 62% had hyperlipidemia, 19.6% had diabetes, 66% had smoked cigarettes, and 58% had a family history of heart disease. As a final note, 54% of the experimental group patients and 32% of control group patients were taking lipid-lowering drugs.

Severity of Condition

Angiographic severity of coronary artery disease was comparable in both groups. However, 55% of experimental group patients had a prior myocardial infarction, compared with only 28% in the control group; also, experimental group patients had a longer history of coronary artery disease than did those in the control group. Taken together, these factors may bias toward higher morbidity for the experimental group than the control group during the demonstration project.

RESULTS

Incidence of Angina

As described above, a primary benefit of revascularization is reduction of angina. The Multicenter Lifestyle Demonstration Project used a very conservative measure of angina: no angina at all during the prior 30 days. For example, if a patient who had frequent angina at baseline—as many as 10 episodes per day—had even a single episode in the prior 30 days, the patient was still considered to have angina.

After 3 months, 49% of participants had no chest pain during the prior 30 days; after 1 year, 65% had no chest pain during the prior 30 days; after 2 years, 61% had no chest pain during the prior 30 days; and after 3 years, 61% had no chest pain after 30 days (see Table 40.2–2). These reductions in angina are comparable with

Table 40.2–2 Reports of Incidence of Angina

Variable	Baseline	3 Months	1 Year	2 Years	3 Years
Percent of participants having no chest pain during prior 30 days*	Unknown	49	65	61	61

*These reductions in angina are comparable with those that can be achieved through revascularization, but without the morbidity and costs.
Source: Adapted from *American Journal of Cardiology*, Vol. 82, No. 108, Dean Ornish et al., Avoiding Revascularization with Lifestyle Changes: The Multicenter Lifestyle Demonstration Project, pp. 72T–76T, Copyright 1998, with permission from Excerpta Medica Inc.

what can be achieved with revascularization but without the morbidity and costs.

Patient Response to Program Indicators

Patients usually show rapid decreases in the occurrence of angina and other symptoms within weeks. These rapid improvements in well-being help to sustain motivation and to explain the high levels of adherence in these patients. Patients also experience significant changes in their capacity for exercise and their ability to manage stress (Table 40.2–3). They gain a greater sense of control over their diets (Table 40.2–4) and can observe the reflection of these changes in lowered cholesterol levels (Table 40.2–5) and decreased weight (Table 40.2–6).

DISCUSSION

There is no way to know for certain how many of the patients who were eligible for revascular-

Table 40.2–3 Patient Participation in Exercise and Stress Management

Variable	Baseline	1 Year	2 Years	3 Years
Exercise (hours per week)	1.6	3.5	2.9	2.7
Exercise Capacity	9.59	11.66	10.88	11.03
Stress Management Activity (hours per week)	.19	4.5	2.6	2.0

Source: Adapted from *American Journal of Cardiology*, Vol. 82, No. 108, Dean Ornish et al., Avoiding Revascularization with Lifestyle Changes: The Multicenter Lifestyle Demonstration Project, pp. 72T–76T, Copyright 1998, with permission from Excerpta Medica Inc.

Table 40.2–4 Intake of Fat Calories and Cholesterol*

Dietary Compliance	Baseline	1 Year	2 Years	3 Years
Total Calories from Fat (expressed in percent)	6.5%	6.8%	7.4%	8.3%
Total Cholesterol Intake (mg per day)	14.1 mg	19.0 mg	22.7 mg	25.7 mg

*Based on Food Diaries
Source: Adapted from *American Journal of Cardiology*, Vol. 82, No. 108, Dean Ornish et al., Avoiding Revascularization with Lifestyle Changes: The Multicenter Lifestyle Demonstration Project, pp. 72T–76T, Copyright 1998, with permission from Excerpta Medica Inc.

Table 40.2–5 LDL and Total Cholesterol Measured over a Three-Year Period in Conjunction with a One-Year Intervention

Laboratory Values of Cholesterol and Fractions	Baseline	3 Months	1 Year	2 Years	3 Years
LDL (Low-density Lipoprotein)	122.9	106.1	104.2	107.7	101.7
Total Cholesterol	202.0	183.7	182.6	187.3	183.4
HDL (High-density Lipoprotein)	36.7	32.8	36.1	40.1	42.2
Triglycerides	229.8	235.7	228.9	213.0	200.8

*Measured in mg/dL

Source: Adapted from *American Journal of Cardiology*, Vol. 82, No. 108, Dean Ornish et al., Avoiding Revascularization with Lifestyle Changes: The Multicenter Lifestyle Demonstration Project, pp. 72T–76T, Copyright 1998, with permission from Excerpta Medica Inc.

Table 40.2–6 Weight Decreased

Variable	Baseline	3 Months	1 Year	2 Years	3 Years
Mean Weight*	187.3	178.0	177.0	176.6	179.9
Percent Body Fat Decrease	25.7	22.9	21.3	22.4	23.4

*(p value 0.0001 to 0.0007)

Source: Adapted from *American Journal of Cardiology*, Vol. 82, No. 108, Dean Ornish et al., Avoiding Revascularization with Lifestyle Changes: The Multicenter Lifestyle Demonstration Project, pp. 72T–76T, Copyright 1998, with permission from Excerpta Medica Inc.

ization actually would have undergone revascularization in the absence of the lifestyle program. Whether a patient undergoes revascularization is a function of many factors, including disease severity, patterns of practice in the local community, individual preferences among cardiologists and cardiac surgeons, and methods of reimbursement. Revascularization rates tend to be much higher when reimbursed on a fee-for-service basis than on a capitated basis. One of the sites in our demonstration project, for example, performed more angioplasties (17) than did the other seven hospital sites combined (14).

Given the large differential between the cost of revascularization and the cost of the year-long lifestyle intervention program, it would have been cost-effective to offer comprehensive lifestyle changes even if only 18% of patients who were eligible for revascularization actually would have had it, in the absence of this program.

In practice, this research suggests that there is value in offering patients with coronary artery disease a range of therapeutic options, including comprehensive lifestyle changes, medications (including lipid-lowering drugs), angioplasty, and bypass surgery (Leaf, 1993).

Comprehensive lifestyle changes are not for everyone. It is not known how many patients with coronary artery disease in the United States would be interested in choosing to make comprehensive lifestyle changes, rather than to undergo revascularization. To date, the primary limiting factor has been the lack of widespread insurance coverage, rather than a shortage of motivated patients. However, approximately 40 insurance companies are covering this lifestyle program at the sites that have been established, and the program is now being offered at 16 sites nationwide.

This is a particularly rewarding and emotionally fulfilling way to practice medicine—for patients, the physicians, and for other health care professionals who work with them. Much more time is available to spend with patients, addressing the underlying lifestyle factors that influence the progression of coronary artery disease, but costs are substantially lower. Since the major reason that most stable patients undergo bypass surgery or angioplasty is to decrease the frequency of angina, it is encouraging to observe that comparable results can be obtained by making comprehensive lifestyle changes alone. This is a different approach that is caring and compassionate, as well as cost-effective and competent.

In summary, the Multicenter Lifestyle Demonstration Project found that experimental group patients were able to avoid revascularization for at least three years by making comprehensive lifestyle changes at substantially lower cost without increasing cardiac morbidity and mortality.

REFERENCES

Alderman EL, Bourassa MG, Cohen LS, et al. Ten year follow up of survival and myocardial infarction in the randomized Coronary Artery Surgical Study. *Circulation.* 1990;82:1629–1646.

American Heart Association. *Heart and Stroke Facts.* 1995 Statistical Supplement. Dallas, TX: American Heart Association; 1994.

Blankenhorn DH, Nessim SA, Johnson RL, et al. Beneficial effects of combined colestipol-niacin therapy on coronary atherosclerosis and coronary venous bypass grafts. *JAMA.* 1987;257:3233–3240.

Bourassa MG. Long-term vein graft patency. *Curr Opin Cardiol.* 1994;9:685–691.

Brown G, Stewart BF, Zhao XQ, Hillger LA, Poulin D, Albers JJ. What benefit can be derived from treating normocholesterolemic patients with coronary artery disease? *Am J Cardiol.* 1995;76(suppl):93C–97C.

Buchwald H, Varco RL, Matts JP, et al. Effect of partial ileal bypass surgery on mortality and morbidity from coronary heart disease in patients with hypercholesterolemia. *N Engl J Med.* 1990;323(14):946–955.

Chaitman BR, Fisher LD, Bourassa MG, et al. Effect of coronary bypass surgery on survival patterns in subsets of patients with left main coronary artery disease. *Am J Cardiol.* 1981;48:765–777.

Coronary Artery Bypass Surgery Cooperative Study Group. Eleven-year survival in the Veterans Administration randomized trial of coronary bypass surgery for stable angina. *N Engl J Med.* 1984;311:1333–1339.

Esselstyn CB Jr, Ellis SG, Medendorp SV, Crowe TD. A strategy to arrest and reverse coronary artery disease: A 5-year longitudinal study of a single physician's practice. *J Fam Pract.* 1995;41:560–568.

Fuster V, Badimon L, Badimon JJ, Chesebro JH. The pathogenesis of coronary artery disease and the acute coronary syndromes. *N Engl J Med.* 1992;326:242–318.

Gould KL, Martucci JP, Goldberg DL, et al. Short-term cholesterol lowering decreases size and severity of perfusion abnormalities by positron emission tomography after dipyridamole in patients with coronary artery disease: A potential noninvasive marker of healing coronary endothelium. *Circulation.* 1994;89:1530–1538.

Gould KL, Ornish D, Scherwitz L, et al. Changes in myocardial perfusion abnormalities by positron emission tomography after long-term intense risk factor modification. *JAMA.* 1995;274:894–901.

Hirshfeld JW Jr, Schwartz JS, Jugo R, et al. Restenosis after coronary angioplasty: A multivariate statistical model to relate lesion and procedure variables to restenosis. *J Am Coll Cardiol.* 1991;18:647–656.

Kane JP, Malloy MJ, Ports TA, et al. Regression of coronary atherosclerosis during treatment of familial hypercholesterolemia with combined drug regimens. *JAMA.* 1990;264:3007–3012.

Leaf A. Preventive medicine for our ailing health care system. *JAMA.* 1993;269:616–618.

Ornish D, Brown SE, Scherwitz LW, et al. Can lifestyle changes reverse coronary atherosclerosis? The Lifestyle Heart Trial. *Lancet.* 1990;336:129–133.

Schuler G, Hambrecht R, Schlierf G, et al. Myocardial perfusion and regression of coronary artery disease in patients on a regimen of intensive physical exercise and low fat diet. *J Am Coll Cardiol.* 1992;19:34–42.

Varnauskas E, for the European Coronary Surgery Study Group. Twelve-year follow-up of survival in the randomized European Coronary Surgery Study. *N Engl J Med.* 1998;319:332–337.

CHAPTER 41

Designing a Healing Center: North Hawaii Community Hospital

Patrick E. Linton and Karl J. Toubman with Nancy Faass

DESIGNING A HEALING ENVIRONMENT

North Hawaii Community Hospital (NHCH) was built with funding from the State of Hawaii and philanthropic support, in a rural community on the northern end of the Big Island. The hospital grew out of the grassroots support of the community and the vision of Earl Bakken, inventor of the first transistorized, wearable pacemaker. The hospital offers the latest in modern Western medical technology in an environment that honors the Hawaiian culture and integrates complementary medicine. As a hospital, it is designed with special emphasis on the healing aesthetic aspects of the environment. The architectural design highlights the natural beauty of the region by providing direct access from patient rooms to peaceful gardens and fountains, with views of the nearby mountains. It is also a full-service, state-of-the-art, acute care medical center.

Patrick E. Linton, MHA, served as founding CEO of North Hawaii Community Hospital in Waimea, Kamuela, Hawaii. He has also been CEO of hospitals in Wisconsin and Arizona and has held other senior positions in hospital administration. He completed his graduate work at the University of Minnesota and is currently a consultant with the Five Mountain Medical Community in Kamuela.

Karl J. Toubman, LAc, LMT, has been on the medical staff of North Hawaii Community Hospital since the hospital opened in 1996 and has been a founding member of the hospital's integrative healing committee since 1994. He is a graduate of the Oregon College of Oriental Medicine and received advanced training in acupuncture from the Red Cross Hospital in Hangzhou, China. He has been in private practice since 1989 and is active in community projects relating to health and Oriental medicine.

The hospital, which opened in 1996, is centrally located in the town of Waimea and currently serves the 30,000 residents and visitors to the area. In its first two years in operation, NHCH provided more than 50,000 total patient services, including 2,000 surgeries, 80% of which were same-day procedures. More than 10,000 emergency conditions were treated, and nearly 500 births were facilitated.

NHCH is a community-owned nonprofit hospital and is governed by a local board of directors. The hospital offers a full spectrum of acute care services with a commitment to patient-centered care—mind, body, and spirit—in the context of family, culture, and community. The design of the building was developed through an extensive and thoughtful process that involved people in the community, practitioners, and all the major stakeholders. This process has resulted in a soothing and yet efficient environment in which every detail is intended to further healing.

The physical setting includes amply sized single-patient rooms, natural lighting, and garden views with sliding glass doors in every patient room. Common areas are enhanced by skylights, spacious windows, landscaped gardens, and courtyards with water features. The interior design incorporates warm colors, textures, and original art to reflect a homelike ambiance. The sense of a place of spirit and healing is created through music, art, aromatherapy, landscaping, and painstaking architectural design.

Healing services provided to patients include a selection of art, music, entertainment, humor, relaxation, and guided imagery, as well as information resources. Healing touch is available through trained staff at no cost and is a noninvasive therapy used to promote health and well-being through the restoration of harmony and balance. All the staff members make an effort to reflect healing intention in their work and the care that they provide. This perspective extends to housekeepers, food service staff, patient care professionals, volunteers, and admitting, billing, and accounting personnel.

Complementary Therapies

NHCH has also become a prototype for the careful integration of select complementary and holistic healing practices. As part of the process in developing the hospital, a consensus process was also developed for credentialing complementary practitioners. NHCH includes, as members of the consulting or affiliate medical staff, licensed complementary practitioners in the following disciplines: acupuncture, chiropractic, clinical psychology, massage therapy, and naturopathic medicine.

Complementary healers on staff are licensed in the state of Hawaii and meet similar credentialing requirements to those of the physicians and osteopaths on the hospital staff. Complementary practitioners work in collaboration with patients and admitting physicians. Patients can receive consultation or treatment from these licensed complementary providers through a request to their attending physician, who must order the consult. The integration of complementary therapies has been carefully developed, focusing on evidence-based modalities with a history of safety and effectiveness. The integration of these therapies is a gradual process that is occurring over time.

LEADING-EDGE MEDICAL TECHNOLOGIES

The hospital is also expanding its programs in areas that include rehabilitation therapies, sports medicine, and spine care.

- In 1997, the hospital won a national award, having received the highest patient satisfac-

tion ratings in three categories of any hospital in the 50 states.
- In 1998, NHCH passed its first Joint Commission on Accreditation of Healthcare Organizations (Joint Commission) accreditation with excellent scores in the mid-1990s.
- In 1999, a highly specialized form of eye surgery was performed by an ophthalmologic surgeon with the assistance of telemedicine. This was one of the first cases in the world in which telemedicine was used to guide eye surgery.
- NHCH provides patients with leading-edge technology, including a spiral computed tomography (CT) scanner and an exceptionally powerful magnetic resonance imaging (MRI) unit that will soon be installed.

The goal at North Hawaii Community Hospital is to provide patients with integrated healing services that include premiere quality clinical care and the latest technology, combined with complementary healing options. It is important to note that the use of these healing techniques is highly individualized and integrated with medical care according to the preferences of the patients and their attending physicians. The program also places a strong emphasis on community education through outreach services. One of the objectives of the hospital is to provide patients with the information they need to participate with their physicians in making sound decisions about the type of care that is best for them.

INTEGRATING ACUPUNCTURE INTO HOSPITAL SERVICES

At its inception, Northern Hawaii Community Hospital was designed to provide a holistic approach and to include complementary, adjunctive therapies. To implement these programs, the hospital formed the integrative healing committee early on to determine how to integrate complementary medicine within the hospital setting. As an acupuncturist credentialed to provide services in the hospital since it opened, Karl Toubman has periodically participated in a number of procedures.

Applications of Medical Acupuncture

Acupuncture Anesthesia. Recently, Toubman had the privilege of providing acupuncture anesthesia in the surgical unit for an older patient who was allergic to conventional anesthesia. Working in conjunction with the gynecologist, acupuncture anesthesia was administered during a dilatation and curettage procedure. The anesthesiologist was present in the background in case his services were needed, but the patient did well throughout the procedure, and no anesthesia was required. This type of service is potentially a major application of acupuncture within the hospital (Han, 1997; Tsibuliak et al, 1995).

Research performed in China indicates that, for highly invasive surgical procedures, small amounts of anesthesia are used in conjunction with acupuncture (Lao et al, 1995; Lewinth and Vincent, 1996). The finding is that less pharmaceutical anesthesia is required, which provides quicker recovery time. Because patients tend to spend less time recovering in the operating room, the recovery room, and the hospital, there is a cost savings.

Pre- and Postoperative Pain Control. The prospect of surgery tends to be stressful for patients; consequently, benign interventions that calm or relax them in preparation for surgery have value. Acupuncture can increase endorphin levels, promoting relaxation. Following the operation, the application of acupuncture can reduce the need for pharmaceuticals to manage pain so that the patient does not require as much medication. As with anesthesia, decreased use of pharmaceuticals for pain can make it possible to release the patient sooner, cutting down on the hospital stay and costs (Dundee et al, 1989; NIH Health Consensus Panel, 1997).

Obviously, patients also benefit when their pain can be managed effectively. For example,

abdominal surgery tends to be fairly painful after the medication wears off. If an acupuncturist can see patients soon after they are out of the operating room, the level of discomfort can be significantly reduced.

Obstetrics and Gynecology. Acupuncture can be a useful adjunct to the birthing process, first to assist with the induction of labor, and then, as labor proceeds, for pain control. The author's experience in this area has been highly positive. This approach also offers the potential to decrease the need for medication and to reduce the number of Caesarean sections, and expands the options for pain control in a more natural approach to childbirth (Cardini and Weixin, 1998; Li and Wang, 1996; Summers, 1997; Ternov et al, 1998).

Detoxification Treatment Programs. Periodically patients who are addicted to pain killers or recreational drugs are seen in the hospital. There is a need for additional options for both inpatient and outpatient treatment. One of the goals of NHCH is to develop a detoxification program within the hospital that will address this need in the community. There is an extensive background of research and clinical experience in acupuncture detoxification (He et al, 1997; Konefal et al, 1995). In particular, the application of auricular (ear) acupuncture, promoted through the work of Michael Smith, MD (Lipton et al, 1994), is now applied in more than 1,000 comprehensive addiction treatment programs worldwide.

Physical Therapy Programs. A supervised intern has provided acupuncture within the physical therapy department at no cost to patients, and that has worked well. Acupuncture is used in other medical programs, such as the Kaiser system in both Portland, Oregon (Weih, 1999) and Vallejo, California (Kaiser Permanente, 1999), where acupuncture services are integrated within the outpatient physiatry and orthopedic departments. These services are used for pain management and integrated with traditional physical therapy services, frequently in conjunction with massage therapy and hypnosis. This is another clinical arena in which acupuncture is relevant to the work of a hospital (Berman et al, 1995; Bullock et al, 1997).

THE INTEGRATIVE PROCESS

Challenges and Strategies: Practical Initiatives in Integrative Medicine

The process of integration will require time. The greatest challenges encountered at NHCH include the lack of familiarity with acupuncture, limited American research, and minimal insurance coverage. NHCH has evaluated each of these issues and explored a variety of strategies to overcome them, with mixed success.

Credentialing. One of the first major steps of the hospital's integrative medicine committee in 1994 was to establish standards for credentialing practitioners of complementary medicine. At that time, there were very few benchmarks for the provision of complementary therapies within a hospital setting. To establish a baseline, the committee interviewed complementary and alternative medicine (CAM) practitioners who had provided outpatient services in health systems. It also sought models for credentialing, malpractice, and insurance coverage but found only a limited number of programs available. However, the research did result in the development of a good set of bylaws that have provided a sound basis for credentialing acupuncturists and other complementary medicine practitioners as adjunctive providers.

Clinical Information Resources. One of the problems in obtaining the buy-in of physicians has been the limitations in the research, particularly in 1996, when the committee began developing the program. What the physicians have most wanted are the abstracts and the clinical studies to substantiate the claims for CAM therapies, rather than general statements about their benefits. Since that time, the National Institutes of Health has produced the Consensus

Statement on Acupuncture (1997), and the National Center for Complementary and Alternative Medicine (NCCAM, 2000) has funded studies and centers focused on the discipline. In addition, the MEDLINE database was opened to CAM research in 1996 and now contains more than 7,000 studies on acupuncture (MEDLINE, 2000).

In-Service Training. NHCH provides training and in-service workshops for the staff that describe and demonstrate the many applications of these therapies.

Patient Information. Hospital and nursing staff do not always have the time to explain all the care options to patients. To keep patients well informed, NHCH has developed a video that patients can view when they first enter the hospital. The video describes the various complementary modalities that are offered.

Grant Funding To Cover Complementary Therapies. The hospital has recently considered creating a grant for patients for the use of complementary medicine that will function as a pilot grant. Patients are often hesitant to use alternative therapies when they learn that they will have to pay out of pocket. They are already uneasy about potential copayments and deductibles they may owe for their care. The thought of additional outlays on top of these charges makes the therapies far less desirable. The availability of grant funding will make these services available to patients and will provide feedback on the level of patient interest in CAM when the issue of reimbursement is removed.

Potential Programs

In the future, medical acupuncture subspecialties may be developed to provide focused training, certification, and clinical protocols for applications in anesthesiology, obstetrics, and pain management. In particular, pain management has broad potential applications in hospital environments ranging from surgical units to the emergency room. These subspecialties could be established through pilot projects in research, education, and clinical practice. As the benefits and safety of these options are more clearly defined, the use of acupuncture in hospital environments is anticipated to increase.

REFERENCES

Berman B, Lao L, Bergman S, et al. Efficacy of traditional Chinese acupuncture in the treatment of osteoarthritis: A pilot study. *Osteoarthritis Cartilage.* 1995;3(2):139–142.

Bullock ML, Pheley AM, Kiresuk TJ, Lenz SK, Culliton PD. Characteristics and complaints of patients seeking therapy at a hospital-based alternative medicine clinic. *J Alternative Complementary Med.* 1997;3(1):31–37.

Cardini F, Weixin H. Moxibustion for correction of breech presentation: A randomized controlled trial. *JAMA.* 1998;280:1580–1584.

Dundee JW, Ghaly RG, Bill KM, Chestnutt WN, Fitzpatrick KTJ, Lynas AGA. Acupuncture prophylaxis of cancer chemotherapy-induced sickness. *Br J Anaesth.* 1989;63(5):612–618.

Han JS. Acupuncture activates endogenous systems of analgesia. *National Institutes of Health (NIH) Consensus Conference on Acupuncture, Program and Abstracts.* Bethesda, MD: Office of Alternative Medicine and Office of Medical Applications of Research, NIH; 1997.

He D, Berg JE, Hestmark AT. Effects of acupuncture on smoking cessation or reduction for motivated smokers. *Prev Med.* 1997;26(2):208–214.

Kaiser Permanente. Program brochure. Vallejo, CA: Kaiser Permanente; 1999.

Konefal J, Duncan R, Clemence C. Comparison of three levels of auricular acupuncture in an outpatient substance abuse treatment program. *Alternative Med J.* 1995;2(5):8–17.

Lao L, Bergman S, Langenberg P, Wong R, Berman B. Efficacy of Chinese acupuncture on postoperative oral surgery pain. *Oral Surg Oral Med Oral Pathol.* 1995;79(4):423–428.

Lewinth GT, Vincent C. On the evaluation of the clinical effects of acupuncture: A problem reassessed and a framework for future research. *J Alternative Complementary Med.* 1996;2(1):79–90.

Li Q, Wang L. Clinical observation on correcting malposition of fetus by electro-acupuncture. *J Tradit Chin Med.* 1996;16(4):260–262.

Lipton DS, Brewington V, Smith M. Acupuncture for crack-cocaine detoxification: Experimental evaluation of efficacy. *J Substance Abuse Treat.* 1994;11(3):205–215.

MEDLINE. National Library of Medicine. <www.ncbi.nlm. nih.gov> Accessed 6/00.

National Center for Complementary and Alternative Medicine (NCCAM). <http://nccam.nih.gov> Accessed 5/00.

National Institutes of Health Consensus Panel. *Acupuncture.* National Institutes of Health Consensus Development Statement. Bethesda, MD: Office of Alternative Medicine and Office of Medical Applications of Research, NIH; November 3–5, 1997.

Summers L. Methods of cervical ripening and labor induction. *J Nurse Midwifery.* 1997;42(2):71–89.

Ternov K, Nilsson M, Lofberg L, Algotsson L, Akeson J. Acupuncture for pain relief during childbirth. *Acupuncture Electrother Res.* 1998;23(1):19–26.

Tsibuliak VN, Alisov AP, Shatrova VP. Acupuncture analgesia and analgesic transcutaneous electroneurostimulation in the early postoperative period. *Anesthesiol Reanimatol.* 1995;2:93–98.

Weih J. Oral communication, 9/99.

CHAPTER 42

Integrative Medicine at Memorial Sloan-Kettering Cancer Center

Simone B. Zappa

OVERVIEW

Memorial Sloan-Kettering Cancer Center (MSKCC) is the oldest and largest private institution in the world devoted to cancer treatment, prevention, patient care, research, and education. The institution has consistently set the standard of care for people with this condition by providing the most effective treatment and the best possible quality of life for patients.

The Integrative Medicine Service builds on this philosophy. The program is designed to emphasize three primary components: clinical services, research, and education. In the clinical program, complementary therapies, selected on the basis of sound research, are now being integrated into mainstream cancer care. The peer-reviewed literature has been carefully evaluated to identify a core program of complementary services, under the supervision of program chief Barrie Cassileth, PhD, a well-known researcher in this field. Note that the service does not offer alternative medicine remedies, unproven therapies promoted in place of conventional care.

Simone B. Zappa, MBA, RN, is the Program Director/Administrator of the Integrative Medicine Service at Memorial Sloan-Kettering Cancer Center. She holds a bachelor's degree in nursing from Hunter College/Bellevue School of Nursing and an MBA in health care administration from Baruch College/Mount Sinai School of Medicine. Her background in health care management includes experience in both the administrative and clinical arenas, with expertise in programmatics. Ms. Zappa has also worked at Mount Sinai Medical Center and Bellevue Hospital Center in New York, as well as Fairview Riverside Medical Center in Minneapolis, and has developed several innovative, patient-focused programs at major academic medical centers.

Rather, complementary, adjunctive therapies are provided in conjunction with mainstream treatment.

The Integrative Medicine Service at MSKCC was designed to support the mission of the hospital by providing therapies found to improve patient quality of life and enhance the healing process. Therapies were selected on the basis of their ability to decrease pain, depression, or fatigue and to improve patients' sense of well-being. There are also indications of cost-effectiveness, although research is not yet available to confirm the economics of these therapies. For example, the use of massage or acupuncture in pain management can be less expensive than long-term pain medication. Patients with decreased pain and stress levels can go home from the hospital sooner, suggesting a potential cost savings.

A THREE-TIERED APPROACH

Clinical Services

Inpatient Programs

The complementary medicine program consists of three clinical units. The inpatient program provides complementary therapies to patients as adjuncts to their primary treatment program. At present, several therapies are available to hospitalized patients: massage, acupuncture, mind/body therapies, and music therapy. There is no charge for those interventions. Referrals to integrative medicine can be made by a member of the health care team or at the request of the patient or a family member. Music therapy, for example, receives a highly positive response from patients in the hospital and is a well-regarded service in the inpatient arena. Staff of the integrative medicine service function as part of the hospital team. They review charts to determine appropriate therapies for patients, confer with the nurses and physicians, and document the therapies provided and then the outcomes in the medical record.

The Program at Rockefeller Outpatient Pavilion

The integrative medicine program at the hospital's Rockefeller Outpatient Pavilion is one of two outpatient programs. At the Pavilion, select supplemental therapies are available to patients coming to be seen by their physician or undergoing tests or treatment. For example, patients can receive a massage for 30 minutes before their chemotherapy treatment, or massage can be provided in the chemotherapy areas during the initial part of the treatment. Massage helps patients to relax, which seems to minimize the nausea and side effects associated with chemotherapy treatment. Meditation and relaxation techniques also appear to improve the patient's experience when provided either just before or during the initiation of chemotherapy.

The Integrative Medicine Center

The third clinical site, the Integrative Medicine Center, is considered the crown jewel of the program. The facility looks more like a spa than a medical facility. It is a beautiful environment of approximately 3,700 square feet, decorated in muted tones—very serene and elegant. A full array of services is provided, including acupuncture, Swedish massage, Shiatsu, reflexology, Reiki, nutritional counseling, and various mind-body therapies (Table 42–1). Classes are available in yoga, T'ai chi, Pilates, and Alexander Technique, as well as dance and movement. Art therapy also has become a popular and successful program. Counseling and nutrition guidance are available to patients in response to their questions and interests.

Although the program is focused in the field of cancer treatment, the services of the Integrative Medicine Center are also open to people in

Table 42–1 Memorial Sloan-Kettering Cancer Center—Integrative Medicine Services

Individual Therapies	Classes
Swedish Massage	T'ai chi
Shiatsu Massage	Hatha Yoga
Reflexology	Alexander Technique
Reiki	Pilates Mat Class
Meditation	Chair Aerobics
Hypnotherapy	Dance and Movement
Acupuncture	Therapy Series
Nutrition Counseling	Creative Journey
Music Therapy	Healing through Ancient
Sound Therapy	Tibetan Sound Therapy
Art Therapy	

Courtesy of Memorial Sloan-Kettering Cancer Center— Integrative Medicine Services, New York.

the community with other diagnoses, including the need for stress management. All therapies are also available to staff at reduced cost to help them deal with the day-to-day stresses associated with their work as health care providers. In addition, classes in yoga and T'ai chi are provided specifically for staff.

Research

In addition to clinical services, the program is designed to conduct research and provide education. Research protocols currently are under development. Research emphasizes quality of life improvement with complementary therapies and botanical remedies that may work to destroy cancer.

Education

Another aspect of the program's mission is to provide educational programs to the community and to professionals. Integrative cancer treatment is a new discipline, unfamiliar to many clients, and there tend to be a great many misconceptions regarding this field. The program offers presentations to the public to provide background and research on the services provided. Professional education includes ongoing in-service training for physician and nursing colleagues. Supervision is available to graduate students in nursing and in music therapy who are performing their internships in the program. The Integrative Medicine Service is also initiating training seminars for health care professionals. Currently, a series on medical massage for the cancer patient is scheduled in a series of four seminars over the next year (two and one-half days each), and all have full enrollment at this time.

PROGRAM DEVELOPMENT

Support of Leadership

The Service at MSKCC was initiated by hospital leadership. In many organizations, a constituency within the program must make a major effort to sell the idea to senior administration. At Memorial Sloan-Kettering, the concept has been backed by institutional leadership since its inception, which has made it possible to develop programs more rapidly.

Evidenced-Based Approach

The program is based on a strong foundation of research data, and continues to monitor clinical research on an ongoing basis. This approach provides the evidence basis for the clinical programs and is integral to the program's mission. If a therapy offered in the program proves not to be beneficial (contrary to the existing literature), it is eliminated. As new research becomes available and data are accumulated about complementary therapies, they are reevaluated and considered for inclusion in the program. However, it is necessary to be exceptionally careful about the therapies that are selected for inclusion. Although there is research on many of the alternative therapies, the quality of the studies varies.

Consider, for example, the questions associated with the use of acupuncture, a therapy that can be very useful for posttreatment nausea and for pain management. Individual responses to acupuncture vary widely and are unpredictable. It works well for some people but for others

has no effect. Acupuncture has indications of effectiveness historically and in both clinical and animal research. Program leadership is interested in conducting additional acupuncture research because there is a limited amount of information and data available on the applications of acupuncture in the field of cancer treatment.

Credentialing

To establish and maintain the credibility of a new program in a new area of medicine, it is extremely important to staff the program with high-caliber, highly experienced staff and practitioners. Many of the practitioners in the program are health care professionals who have a background in clinical medicine and have also become very skilled in the use of complementary modalities. Everyone who works in the center holds a New York state license: There are no unlicensed personnel. In addition to licensure, staff typically have more than five years of experience in a related field and in-depth expertise. Hiring selection is highly individualized. In selecting massage practitioners, the program hires clinicians who have worked in therapeutic programs, rather than spas. Overall, we seek the finest practitioners—those who will genuinely enrich the program.

Flexible Programming

From the standpoint of programmatics, the development of the center has been atypical. Under most circumstances, an entire program is fully developed before it opens. As with other programs, MSKCC's Integrative Medicine Service was developed with a business plan clearly stating its organizational structure, mission, and goals. However, unlike other new programs, the operational policies and procedures were kept loose. In a new complementary medicine program, there are few prototypes or benchmarks available. In addition, we have kept the program development process flexible in order to accommodate the patient population. For example, do patients want late hours or morning hours? Working in an area in which there is little real history, one cannot simply call colleagues to ask what has been done, because currently there are so few programs.

Starting Small

Based on the author's experience in program planning, the center was initiated on a moderate scale and has been developed in response to patient demand. At present, the Integrative Medicine Service sees more than 800 patients a month. As the program gains additional clients and requests for services, it will continue to expand. New programs are initiated based on client interest and response. In this approach, the first step is to identify the availability of well-qualified practitioners and to advertise the program. Based on the response, the program administration then decides whether to offer the program. Only when the skilled practitioners are in place does the program attempt to attract the audience or the market.

Phasing in New Services

The program has a number of per diem employees who are available on an on-call basis. They are practitioners who have already been interviewed, identified as skilled, and credentialed. This approach allows us to draw from a pool of highly competent practitioners. Initially, practitioners work in the program as needed. Frequently, new practitioners—particularly massage therapists—attract their own following, which builds patient volume. As the demand for their services grows, the program is able to offer them permanent part-time or full-time positions. Consequently, it is possible to expand programs incrementally, with less financial risk to the institution.

BUILDING A CLIENT BASE: EMPHASIZING A SERVICE ETHIC

Focus on Quality

The quality of service and the quality of the practitioners provide the foundation for this program. It is very important to strive toward optimal patient satisfaction. If service excellence is not provided to clients, patient volume cannot be maintained. This type of program involves a different approach than that of inpatient services. In complementary medicine, the competition is intense. There are a great many good practitioners, particularly in New York. The quality of practitioners and of service provision must be exceptional to remain competitive and to maintain a program consistent with the high-quality norms of our parent institution.

Ensuring Patient Safety

Patients often report that experiencing a life-threatening illness creates a great sense of insecurity and that coming to this program restores a sense of safety. Patients know that any therapy offered at MSKCC has been thoroughly researched, evaluated, and reevaluated. In fact, an initial rationale for this program was to establish a baseline of safety in the provision of cancer services. If patients want these approaches, it is better to provide them in an environment in which the therapies are evaluated and monitored. Patient safety is the focus of the rigorous quality standards of this program.

Benefits of Complementary and Alternative Medicine

Complementary modalities enhance patients' sense of security. The biomedical treatment for almost any life-threatening condition can have an invasive aspect. Patients often report feeling that they have lost control. When they come to Memorial Sloan-Kettering Integrative Medicine Service, they are able to exert an element of control. All services provided are elective therapies. Patients decide whether and how they wish to participate in this program. As they begin to heal, they come to like their bodies again and regain a sense of well-being. They can experience pleasure through massage or movement therapies and peace of mind through meditation or yoga. They find a way to feel good again about the body that has so betrayed them.

Service

Ultimately, clients are attracted by the quality of service provided by staff. The goal of the program is to provide clients with the sense of being taken care of exceptionally well. Staff do as much as possible to accommodate clients within the reasonable limits of good customer service and good business practice. The goal is to set limits yet make people feel special and enhance their healing.

Staff Development

From the management side, it is important to promote the morale of staff and to let them know that they are appreciated. The other task of management specific to integrative medicine is to help practitioners learn to work within the structure of a larger institution. Many practitioners come to the program from private practice, rather than from a hospital or corporate background. Consequently, it is important to explain budget, policies, and procedures, and to keep them generally apprised of developments that occur within the hospital. For example, staff may not realize the nature of regulatory constraints placed on a hospital and the impact of those constraints on the services they provide.

Communication is key and occurs through venues such as hospital orientation programs, regular staff meetings, team-building workshops, and in-service training. Mentoring and coaching are provided through both group and individual supervision. For example, the manager of massage therapy uses one-on-one supervision to monitor correct technique and to teach new methods. Individual mentoring is also provided for the development of clinical and interpersonal skills. To the degree that management can cultivate a positive environment, staff members convey that positive outlook to patients.

Staff development takes a different form for practitioners who already have a professional background. In the acupuncture program, all of the providers are physicians. Our mind-body practitioners are psychologists with doctoral degrees. At this level, professionals take personal responsibility for staying current in their fields, and the institution supports their attendance at clinical conferences, workshops, and trainings.

Integration within a Hospital Environment

When complementary services are provided in a mainstream medical institution, certain aspects of program development take on particular importance:

1. *Working within the medical model.* The clinical programs of any hospital are ultimately defined by the administration and by the physicians. The role of the program needs to be aligned with the work of the physicians. Physician support and referrals make an enormous difference to a program. Integrative medicine must be able to integrate its services into the MSKCC structure, within the guidelines of the conventional protocol and practice.

2. *Development of a strong administrative component.* In any new program, there is constant demand for a committed administrative presence to provide monitoring, decision-making, and staff support. This requires leadership on several levels: a spokesperson who can network extensively on behalf of the program; an on-site administrator who makes policy, supervises staff development, and shapes the program into the larger organization; and a front-line supervisor who will deal with day-to-day operations and staffing.

3. *Adapting and remaining fluid.* In the development of a new program, policy is being made on-site in real time. Situations constantly occur for which there is no existing policy or established precedent.

4. *Establishing a visible presence.* Like most other CAM programs, we must ultimately become self-supporting. Because word of mouth is still one of the ways in which a program grows, a new program must attract patients in order to build a following and create volume. Communication is vital to growth in this field. Everything done to make the program well known keeps it strong and viable, including participation in edu-

cational activities such as lectures and conferences, the use of marketing, and the provision of consultations and tours for visiting physicians.

CONCLUSION

Memorial Sloan-Kettering continues to be at the forefront of cancer treatment and research. The institution's Integrative Medicine Center expands the options available to patients by providing complementary medicine to support the healing process. Applying the tools of integrative medicine such as stress reduction, movement therapies, and good nutrition offers additional resources to patients to nurture and strengthen themselves during and after treatment. The Integrative Medicine Center reflects Memorial Sloan-Kettering's ongoing commitment to the most comprehensive approaches to treatment and to patient quality of life.

CHAPTER 43

Architectural Design

43.1   An Investigation To Determine Whether the Built Environment Affects Patients' Medical Outcomes

*Haya R. Rubin, Amanda J. Owens, Greta Golden,
and David O. Weber*

OVERVIEW

Surprisingly little modern scientific research has been conducted to test the premise that aspects of the health care environment (other than cleanliness) have effects on therapeutic outcomes. Given the need for additional data in this field, a major review of the medical literature was performed in 1995 and updated in 1997 and 1998 at Quality of Care Research, The

---

Haya R. Rubin, MD, PhD, Associate Professor of Medicine and Director of Quality of Care Research at The Johns Hopkins Medical Institutions is a general internist and health services researcher specializing in the assessment and improvement of health care quality. Dr. Rubin was awarded an MD and PhD in Pathology from Case Western Reserve University, completed an internal medicine residency at The Mount Sinai Medical Center, and a research fellowship in the Robert Wood Johnson Clinical Scholars Program at UCLA, where she also received an MSPH studying patient satisfaction and end-of-life care. As a faculty member at University of California, San Francisco, RAND, and Johns Hopkins, she has worked with health care provider organizations, monitoring accreditation agencies and health care payers to develop methods to measure and improve the quality and outcomes of health care.

Quality of Care Research is an interdisciplinary unit of the Johns Hopkins School of Medicine and the School of Hygiene and Public Health and Johns Hopkins Medicine, an integrated health system. The mission of the unit is to advance knowledge regarding health care quality assessment and improvement and to assist organizations that provide or monitor care to improve quality and performance. The affiliated faculty represent a range of disciplines, including medicine, health services research, epidemiology, the behavioral sciences, statistics, psychometrics, and survey research.

The Center for Health Design (www.healthdesign.org) is a nonprofit, nonmembership organization headquartered in Martinez, CA, whose mission is to promote life-enhancing health care environments by demonstrating the value of evidence-based design in improving health and the quality of life. Since 1988, when the CHD founders established the Symposium on Healthcare Design, the Center has been providing education, research, and resources to a community of more than 25,000 health care and design professionals worldwide.

Courtesy of the Center for Health Design, Lafayette, California. The full report is available in print or CD-ROM from The Center for Health Design at <www.healthdesign.org>.

Johns Hopkins University, under the auspices of The Center for Health Design.

After culling more than 78,761 potentially relevant titles from medical databases, the research team identified only 1,219 articles that appeared to describe investigations into the impact of environmental elements on health outcomes. Nevertheless, only a few dozen reports in the medical literature since 1966 contained data that relate a particular design feature to a specific clinical outcome for a particular population. Of the more than 78,000, a total of 84 studies were judged relevant.

For example, one study (Giradin, 1992) tested the impact of artificial light on babies in hospital nurseries by randomly assigning a sample of 50 newborns to cribs under blue light (the highest-intensity visible wave length), while another matched sample of 50 babies was placed in cribs under red light (the lowest-intensity visible wave length). The researchers observed and reported that the babies subjected to blue light were more wakeful, slept more often but more briefly, and had more irregular patterns of sleep. Yet for all its strength of research design, a single study of 100 babies—all healthy and sharing a single ethnic background—leaves open the question of whether the same results would pertain among babies of other ethnicities or among sick or premature babies, for whom regular, sound sleep may be an important factor if they are to thrive.

Another small subset of the studies were experimental trials with paired data or observational studies with paired data, both of which are also considered by scientists to be reasonable constructs for drawing relatively reliable research conclusions, when well crafted.

An instance of the former involved a 1975 study (Belgaumaker and Scott, 1975) of 19 premature infants whose incubators were set first at high humidity, then at low humidity. Eight of the infants experienced severe breathing problems, and episodes of apnea occurred in significantly greater proportion when the humidity was kept low. Here again, however, a single study of a very small group of subjects is not sufficient to support broad generalizations, even when the

method is sound. Similarly, a 1992 observational study (Harris et al, 1992) of nearly 14,000 patients in a state mental hospital indicated that when rock or rap music was played in a common area, the patients exhibited more incidents of "inappropriate behavior" than when country or "easy listening" music was played. The unusually large cohort of subjects involved lends weight to the finding, but the study did not control for the various rhythms or lyrics of the music that could possibly be provocative factors.

Few, if any, scientific studies produce incontrovertible evidence. Unshakable judgments based on one or two trials, no matter how large or tightly controlled to eliminate chance, confounding factors, and experimenter bias, are rarely, if ever, drawn by circumspect scientists. However, analysis of this body of research is at least suggestive that a cause–effect relationship exists between some health care environmental factors and therapeutic outcomes for some types of patients.

One conclusion from the evaluation team's initial assessment is that research in this field holds promise but that more and better studies are vitally needed. The effort would appear to be justified on the evidence of the best of the studies surveyed, a high proportion of which did find significant associations between the environmental variable investigated and a health outcome.

Rationale: Improving Patient Outcomes through Design of the Health Care Environment

Wise use of health care resources to improve patient health and well-being, promote efficiency, reduce employee turnover, and avoid wasteful spending dictates a careful examination of the ways in which such an encompassing factor as the built environment can affect patients' health outcomes. If it is, in fact, an important contributor to health care effectiveness, it can be easily manipulated. Without knowing which, if any, aspects of the physical setting make a difference, however, health facility design decisions will continue to be made on the basis of untested propositions. Money could be saved and a greater payback realized if design decisions were grounded in scientifically valid information.

These were the premises upon which The Center for Health Design contracted in 1995 with Quality of Care Research at The Johns Hopkins University to develop a concept paper for a research master plan that would address whether and in what ways patients' clinical outcomes might be improved through designed elements of the health care environment. Three tasks were included in the contract:

1. To review the literature to determine what is known about the effect of health care environmental design on patient health outcomes
2. To suggest design applications based on selected findings in the literature
3. Based on the literature review, to make initial recommendations for developing a research agenda in this area for the next 20 or more years

In an era of intense concern over the rising costs of medical care, improving therapeutic results through the most efficient allocation of finite resources has become the touchstone of health care practice and processes. If, in fact, the very environment in which patients receive treatment has a significant influence on physical responsiveness and prognosis, it is important to determine which elements can promote more satisfactory outcomes under what circumstances. Health care facilities can then be designed to take advantage of such knowledge. This concept was stated well by Florence Nightingale in *Notes on Nursing*, republished in 1960:

> Eventually scientific findings will go beyond subjective responses . . . . The doctor will then know how to write a prescription for environment even as he now does for drugs, and technology will modify and maintain it to his pre-

scription, applying all beneficial variables, including . . . temperature; air content of solids, liquids, and gases; air pressure and movement; light in all its aspects, including movement and color; other forms of radiation; ionization; size and shape of enclosure; physical movement of the enclosure; pattern and texture of materials; sound, both generated and absorbed; and the physical form.

REVIEW OF THE LITERATURE

Defining the Key Environmental Factors

The first step was to review the literature to determine what is already known. The health care environment was defined to include anything that can affect a patient through the senses. In a brainstorming session with staff from The Center for Health Design, a list of environmental design features was compiled. The Center's Healthcare Design Research Committee then reviewed, amplified, and refined the list, resulting in the selection of elements included in the search keywords in Exhibit 43.1–1. More formal

---

Exhibit 43.1–1 Patient Outcomes Included in Literature Search

- Physical, anatomical, or physiological health
- Diagnosis or diseases
- Adverse events or complications
- Patients' reports or evaluations of aspects of their health
- Symptoms
- Functional status
- Well-being
- Patient evaluations of health care
- Health care environment

Courtesy of The Center for Health Design, Evanston, Illinois.

studies toward the definition of the health care environment would be helpful in tailoring future research agendas.

Defining Health Outcomes

In 1995, the computerized literature search used the National Library of Medicine Health Planning and Administration and MEDLINE electronic databases to find any articles containing data about how one or more of the variables related to the health care environment. Variables were selected to include any terminology that reflected clinical patient outcomes (Exhibit 43–1). In 1997, the Health Star and MEDLINE databases were used to expand the original search.

Results

As of September 1998, the Johns Hopkins reviewers had examined 78,761 articles for possible inclusion, on themes listed in Exhibit 43.1–2. Thus far, the search revealed only 84 articles published in the medical and design literature in the last 30 years that contain relevant data. These studies have been abstracted and critiqued, and are available in a report from the Center for Health Design.

Seventy-four of the studies (88%) demonstrated that some health care environmental feature was related to at least one patient outcome parameter. Those features that were found by at least one study to influence at least one health outcome are:

- intensity of artificial lighting
- placement of ultraviolet lights
- temperature (this and the previous feature were studied in premature infants)
- humidity (effects on premature infants, geriatric patients, and mechanically ventilated patients)
- ventilation system contaminants (affecting intensive care units, ambulatory surgery units, and leukemia and bone marrow transplant patients)
- temperature of respired air (with mechanically ventilated patients)

Exhibit 43.1–2 Selected Features for the Health Care Environment Included for Literature Review

- Room scale
- Room size
- Room privacy
- Room organization
- Environmental control by patient
- Room flow or interactivity (How much it permits interactions with staff and others)
- Lighting
- Color of walls, furnishings
- Texture or finish of walls or furnishings
- Pattern of walls, furnishings, artwork
- Air and ventilation
- Aroma
- Noise
- Music
- Temperature
- Type of furnishings
- Relationship with nature
- Equipment design
- Windows
- Type of window view

Courtesy of The Center for Health Design, Evanston, Illinois.

- tapes of music, therapeutic suggestion, and sound simulation (effects on patients undergoing coronary artery bypass surgery, gynecologic surgery, emergency laceration repair, and arthroscopic surgery; on children undergoing dental cavity preparation; and on newborns)
- type of ambient music (effects on psychiatric patients)
- noise levels (effects on intensive care and postoperative patients)
- natural window view (effects on patients in intensive care after major surgery; after cholecystectomy; and on neonates)
- room exposure to sunlight (effects on depressed patients)
- exposure to outdoor sunlight (elderly patients in geriatric facility)

- amount of available space, effects of its layout and decor on social interaction, staff use for patients with disabilities or wheelchairs, and outdoor areas (in psychiatric and substance abuse treatment facility patients)
- furniture placement (effects on psychiatric and rehabilitation patients)
- carpeting (in units for elderly patients)
- bedside computers (for geriatric medical and surgical patients)
- newly built versus refurbished wards (for geriatric patients)
- bed enclosures (for burn patients)
- privacy or openness of room or of ward (effects on acute medical patients and on patients undergoing cataract surgery).

CRITIQUE OF METHODS

Many of the research studies had significant methodologic flaws that weakened the validity of their conclusions. First, some study designs are better than others for deciding whether an environmental feature matters. There were 23 randomized controlled trials. This is the best way of organizing a scientific investigation. There were also experimental studies with paired data, another strong study design. Most of these involved premature infants who were evaluated under different incubator conditions.

The majority of articles described observational studies; that is, research that compared groups of patients who had been located in different environments in the course of their routine care. In several studies, the groups of patients were observed in different units or hospitals. This raises the concern that unspecified and unmeasured differences between the two study sites were, in fact, responsible for the differences reported. In these studies, most of the researchers also neglected to measure important patient characteristics that could have caused different outcomes in different environments.

A few observational studies (Davis-Rollans and Cunningham, 1987; Sauer et al, 1984; Shi-

roiwa et al, 1986) used paired data, where patients serve as their own controls. This is a stronger study design because it eliminates the concern that differences among the patients in different groups are responsible for the variance, rather than the environmental factor or factors under investigation.

Are investigators finding what they're looking for? Methodologic flaws may influence the likelihood that a study would find a relationship between an environmental feature and a patient outcome. This phenomenon permeates the history of medical research, in which loosely constructed experiments tend to give the answer sought by the investigators. Of the studies with weaker study designs, 37 of 39, or 95%, concluded that the environmental feature under investigation affected at least one health outcome measure.

Of the 45 studies with relatively stronger research methods—that is, randomized trials, experimental trials with paired data, or observational studies with paired data—37, or 82%, also found positive correlations. Both studies with strong and weak methodology found measurable associations between the environment and clinical outcomes. Therefore, methodologic flaws probably are not responsible for the preponderance of published research studies that have found associations between environmental features and clinical outcomes.

Conclusion

The analysis of the body of existing research leads to three important conclusions. First, the large majority of published studies characterized by better research designs has found that an environmental feature is related to health outcome. At least in the short term, improvements in outcomes may, indeed, be available through design interventions guided by sound scientific inquiry.

Second, studies that contain data about the effect of the environment on health outcomes are surprisingly scarce. The need for a broadened research effort in this area is striking. Many aspects of the health care setting and many patient populations have never been investigated.

Third, many published studies have significant methodological flaws that render their conclusions suspect or cast doubt on their ability to generalize their findings. Future research into the effects of the health care environment on patient outcomes should be more carefully designed and performed with greater methodological rigor. In particular, researchers should make strong efforts to ensure that groups of patients being compared under varied environmental conditions do not differ in other ways that may skew the results.

EXAMPLES FROM THE RESEARCH: EFFECTS OF THE AUDITORY ENVIRONMENT IN HEALTH CARE SETTINGS

To illustrate how the design of the physical environment might be based on scientific evidence of what promotes better patient outcomes, the Johns Hopkins team focused on studies of the auditory environment that were characterized by relatively strong research methods. Translated into design principles, the study conclusions can be applied pragmatically to representative health care settings.

The expanded status report (1998) includes a new application on air quality. This application was selected because there were several high-quality studies indicating that contaminated air causes hospital-acquired infections. Therefore, better design of ventilation systems in health care facilities may improve patient outcomes by preventing such infections.

Example 1: Quiet in the Coronary Care Unit

Research Question: Does cardiac care unit (CCU) noise affect random eye movement (REM) sleep? (Topf and Davis, 1993)

Methods. Seventy healthy women were randomly assigned to sleep in a sleep lab under quiet conditions or listening to an audio tape recording of CCU sounds. Ten measures of REM sleep were assessed, including REM activity and duration during the first and second halves of the night and throughout the night, and the interval between first and second REM cycles.

Findings. Women exposed to CCU noise had less REM activity, shorter REM durations, and longer intervals between REM cycles.

Limitations. Use of volunteers in a lab means that we cannot be sure that the results apply to patients in the CCU, although less REM sleep for critically ill patients could reasonably be assumed to be more problematic than for healthy volunteers. The relationship of REM sleep in the CCU to longer-term outcomes is unknown, although more sleep is a desirable short-term outcome for patients with myocardial infarction.

Conclusion. CCU noise may suppress REM sleep.

The Design Principle. Dampen ambient sound in critical care units to the extent possible.

Sample Design Application. A critical care room incorporating design strategies to promote quiet, including:

1. ceiling utilizing specialty acoustic tile with a noise reduction coefficient (NRC) in the range of 0.85 to 1.0
2. all chairs upholstered with sound-absorbent fabric
3. flooring in all areas consisting of acoustical-resilient sheet vinyl with sound-deadening properties
4. sound absorbent wall panels
5. noise-cancellation headphones.

Example 2: Effects of Music on Adults during Minor Surgery

Research Question: Does music chosen by patients and played through a headset change their vital signs or reduce their pain or anxiety during laceration repair in the emergency department? (Menegazzi et al, 1991)

Methods. Thirty-eight emergency patients who underwent laceration repair with local anesthesia at the University of Pittsburgh teaching hospital were randomized to receive headset music or not to receive music during the repair. Patients in the music group chose from 50 available styles and artists, and controlled the volume themselves. Investigators monitored heart rate, blood pressure, and respirations before and after the repair, and obtained pain ratings and a state of anxiety scale after the procedure. The group that heard music was asked to rate how beneficial the music was, as well.

Findings. Patients who listened to headset music that they chose experienced anxiety levels similar to those in the control group, but reported less pain. Of those who heard music, 89% thought it was very beneficial, and 100% said they would use it again if it were offered.

Limitations. A small study at one hospital can give spurious results, so it should be repeated at other hospitals to confirm the findings.

Conclusion. Patient-selected headset music during laceration repair in the emergency department helps to reduce pain.

Example 3: Effects of Music on Children during Dental Procedures

Research Question: Does ambient music during dental cavity preparation affect children's anxiety levels during the procedure? (Parkin, 1981)

Methods. Twenty-five children scheduled for two different visits to the children's department of a dental hospital for cavity preparation were assigned to be exposed to ambient music on one visit and not to receive music on one visit. Children ranged in age from 7 to 14 years old. Children were recorded on silent videotape for a period of 60 seconds at each visit. Four inde-pendent observers, blinded to the presence or absence of music, graded the child's anxiety using a visual analogue scale.

Results. Patients were graded as less anxious during the visit at which they heard music.

Limitations. Investigators themselves raised, but could not answer, the question of whether it was the music or the novelty of the music that created the effect.

Conclusion. Ambient music may reduce children's anxiety during cavity preparation.

The Design Principle. Provide a way for patients undergoing minor surgery to listen to music, preferably of their choice, during the procedure.

Sample Design Application. An operating room was designed to provide music during minor surgery, including the following features:

1. speakers installed in the ceiling
2. headphones for playback of personally selected music available for use at the discretion of the patient and/or surgical personnel
3. speakers attached to the underside of the operating table
4. TheraSound® Body Mat on the operating table to provide the patient a full-body experience of sound and vibrational resonance before, after, or throughout the procedure, at the patient and surgeon's discretion.

CONCLUSION

Data and conclusions from the research suggest significant effects that can result from the environment:

- *The designed environment can support or hinder caregiver actions and medical interventions, making it harder or easier for clinicians to do their jobs and facilitating helpful actions or preventing harmful ones*. For example, the call bell enables patients to summon nurses or doctors to the bedside when emergency assistance is needed, and carpeting reduces the hubbub of clinical personnel going about business.

- *The designed environment may impair or strengthen patients' health status and personal characteristics by alleviating or exacerbating already existing conditions and by opposing patients' natural strengths.* For example, loss of sleep due to noise may prolong recovery time after a procedure. The impact may be greater on those who are in a worsened state, with more severe preexisting health problems, than for those who are comparatively well to begin with. Conversely, equipment designed to make activities of daily living possible and easy—a bedside commode or speakerphone, as ex-

amples—may prevent dysfunction for some patients with physical impairments who might otherwise be unable to reach and use them.

- *The designed environment can protect patients from or expose them to causes of illness.* For example, excessive noise may alter sleeping patterns, reduce REM sleep, and thereby cause irritability and dysfunction (Topf and Davis, 1993). Several high-quality studies indicated that contaminated air causes hospital-acquired infections. Therefore, better design of ventilation systems in health care facilities may improve patient outcomes by preventing such infections (Cotterill et al, 1996; deSilva and Rissing, 1984; Fridkin et al, 1996; Humphreys et al, 1991).

REFERENCES

Belgaumaker TK, Scott KE. Effects of low humidity on small premature infants in servocontrol incubators. *Biol Neonate*. 1975;26:348–352.

Cotterill S, Evans R, Fraise AP. An unusual source for an outbreak of methicillin-resistant *Staphylococcus aureus* on an intensive therapy unit. *J Hosp Infect*. 1996;32:207–216.

Davis-Rollans C, Cunningham SG. Physiologic responses of coronary care patients to selected music. *Heart and Lung*. 1987;16(4):370–378.

deSilva MI, Rissing JP. Postoperative wound infections following cardiac surgery: Significance of contaminated cases performed in the preceding 48 hours. *Infect Control*. 1984;5(8):371–377.

Fridkin SK, Kremer FB, et al. *Acremonium kiliense endophthalmitis* that occurred after cataract extraction in an ambulatory surgical center and was traced to an environmental reservoir. *Clin Inf Dis*. 1996;22:222–227.

Giradin BW. Lightwave frequency and sleep-wake frequency in well, full-term neonates. *Holistic Nurs Prac*. 1992;6(4):57–66.

Harris CS, Bradley RJ, Titus SK. A comparison of the effects of hard rock and easy listening on the frequency of observed inappropriate behaviors: Control of environmental antecedents in a large public area. *J Music Therapy*. 1992;29:6–17.

Humphreys H, Johnson EM, Warnock DW, et al. An outbreak of aspergillosis in a general ITU. *J Hosp Infect*. 1991;18(3):167–177.

Menegazzi JJ, Paris P, Kersteen C, et al. A randomized controlled trial of the use of music during laceration repair. *Ann Emerg Med*. 1991; 20:348–350.

Nightingale F. *Notes on Nursing: What It Is and What It Is Not*. London: Harrison; 1960.

Parkin SF. The effect of ambient music upon the reactions of children undergoing dental treatments. *ASDC J Dent Child*. 1981;48(6):430–432.

Sauer PJ, Huib DJ, Visser HK. Influence of variations in the ambient humidity on insensible water loss and thermoneutral environment of low birth weight infants. *Acta Paediatr Scand*. 1984;73:615–619.

Shiroiwa Y, Kamiya Y, Uchibori S, et al. Activity, cardiac and respiratory responses of blindfolded preterm infants in a neonatal intensive care unit. *Early Hum Dev*. 1986;14:259–265.

Topf M, Davis V. Critical care noise and rapid eye movement (REM) sleep. *Heart and Lung*. 1993;22(3):252–258.

43.2   Perspective: A Patient Focus Group on Design

The Picker Institute

Working with The Center for Health Design, The Picker Institute facilitated a series of focus groups with consumers to learn which factors are most important to patients in a health care environment.

The findings from those focus groups can be summarized in seven areas:

1. *Connection to staff.* In ambulatory settings, patients expressed concerns that, while waiting for an appointment, they would not be able to see or hear the clinic staff who would call them, because of the shape of the lobby, the location of the reception desk, or the seating arrangements. In acute care settings, it is important to patients and families to know that staff can see them or reach them in an emergency.

2. *An environment conducive to well-being.* In ambulatory settings, patients want an environment that is "conducive to well-being"—one that facilitates relaxation and makes people who are anxious or bored feel more comfortable. In acute care settings, an environment that promotes well-being is one that is comfortable in terms of noise and control over the environment (lights, temperature, and the ability to move around), and it offers comfort and positive distractions, through aspects such as color schemes, comfortable beds, music, and art.

3. *Convenience and accessibility.* In ambulatory settings, features that help the patient get in and out of the facility more quickly and easily are described as "convenient." This includes proximity of services and visual cues to help patients know what to do when they arrive or to help them find their way. In acute care settings, focus group participants spoke more about the need to have easy access to the hospital, including parking and drop-off areas, and easy access once they were inside the building, including clear signage.

4. *Confidentiality and privacy.* In ambulatory settings, patients were concerned about confidentiality and privacy while in waiting rooms during intake interviews and during clinical encounters. In acute care settings, patients and families emphasized the needs for privacy—especially in patients' rooms—and for places where they could get away from the noise and bustle of the nursing unit.

5. *Caring for the family.* In ambulatory settings, patients look for areas designed with the needs of children in mind. They want extra seating for family and more space to make room for family members. In acute care settings, patients look for quiet areas, including visitors' rooms and chapels for family members, convenient restrooms, phones, food and coffee, the ability of rooms to accommodate family members, or the availability of sleeping chairs or couches for overnight stays.

6. *Consideration of impairments.* In ambulatory settings, patients who do not feel well place additional importance on restful, quiet waiting areas; appropriate, well-placed signage; and adequate comfortable

The Picker Institute of Boston is a nonprofit affiliate of CareGroup, Inc, founded with support from Harvard's Beth Israel Hospital and The Commonwealth Fund. The Institute's products and services include surveys to assess patient experience and satisfaction with care; to develop educational programs, publications, and media; and to provide consulting services.

Courtesy of the Picker Institute, Boston, Massachusetts

seating. In acute care settings, patients want to be able to maneuver through space with equipment. They want comfortable beds and short distances between services.

7. *Close to nature.* In ambulatory settings, patients would like windows to the outside, indoor plants or fish tanks, and fresh air. In acute care settings, they especially appreciate access to outside areas via balconies; outside sitting areas or walking paths, indoor plants or gardens, or pictures of natural scenes; and windows in patients' rooms with outside views.

CHAPTER 44

Service Delivery

44.1   Redesigning the Hospital Environment

David H. Freedman

METAMORPHOSIS

At Griffin Hospital, which serves a mix of the modest-income clients in south central Connecticut, patient satisfaction has soared to 96%—an astounding level in any type of business. Not coincidentally, Griffin has boosted admissions an average of 2% per year over the past four years, with healthy revenues and cash flow, despite proximity to no fewer than seven competing hospitals.

The secret of Griffin's success has been a clear three-step process. First, Griffin's management has cultivated a decade-long obsession with re-conceptualizing every element of the business around customers' desires. Second, they have implemented the resulting insights with thoroughness and attention to detail usually reserved for manned space flight. In addition, Griffin is known for its excellence in providing patient-centered care.

Although Griffin's journey has demonstrated how basic the formula for business transformation can be, it also indicates why most organizations attempting metamorphosis are challenged. Qualities that most managers consider to be the building blocks of a successful business—stability, reasonable compromise, moderation, and careful prioritization—can also be the very qualities that forestall major, lasting change. Griffin's in-house, do-it-yourself makeover suggests that thorough uncompromising revision may be what makes real change possible—in Griffin's case, paired with common sense.

For almost 80 years, nonprofit Griffin Hospital had been able to count on the steady patronage of the citizens of Derby, Connecticut, and the surrounding townships. It had served a population bound by tradition and by its dependence on the rubber and metal mills, the core of the community's economy. However, in 1985, a new highway joining two of the state's main commuter routes passed right through town, and Derby suddenly became just a convenient commute away from New York City, Hartford, and other faster-paced,

David H. Freedman is a contributing writer at Inc. magazine.

Source: Reprinted with permission, *Inc.* magazine, October 2000. Copyright 1999 by Gruner + Jahr USA Publishing, 38 Commercial Wharf, Boston, MA 02110. Inc. is a registered trademark of Gruner + Jahr Printing and Publishing.

affluent cities. Factories closed, and upscale companies moved in. Over a period of four years, housing prices tripled as many long-time residents sold to young couples.

Griffin began losing patients at an alarming rate. The newcomers all seemed willing to travel 10 or even 30 miles to be cared for by Griffin's competitors. In response, the hospital commissioned a survey of local residents. More than a quarter of the respondents labeled Griffin as a hospital they would avoid. The reasons given included outdated facilities and lack of parking. Many of the people who leveled the harshest criticisms also noted that they had never so much as driven by the hospital. Board members realized the effect that word-of-mouth was having.

During that period of reevaluation, a vice-president at Griffin was in a serious car accident and was hospitalized for nearly three months in another city. The wife of the chief executive officer (CEO) went into a diabetic coma and died in the hospital; another Griffin vice-president lost a breast to cancer; and the father of one of the administrators suffered a heart attack and was hospitalized on Long Island.

When the executive staff members reconvened to evaluate Griffin's image problem, they happened to compare notes on their personal experiences with hospital environments. They reached an immediate consensus: Hospital experiences could be improved upon. To determine how Griffin could do better and win new patients, they decided to return to their potential customers for more detailed research.

The question arose, Which customers? Griffin's board wanted to focus on geriatrics, noting that the population was aging. Others proposed a focus on obstetrics and maternity services, with the idea of attracting young families and establishing lifelong loyalty.

Griffin distributed detailed questionnaires to its obstetrics patients and ran focus groups in the community. The board soon assembled an impressive wish list for maternity services. For example, not only did mothers want their husbands present during delivery, but many also wanted their children and their own parents in the birthing rooms. They wanted rooms that did not look like hospital rooms. They wanted double beds, so that their husbands could sleep next to them. They wanted Jacuzzis. They wanted big windows and skylights. They wanted fresh flowers. They wanted big, comfortable lounges where the family could gather. They wanted nurses who paid close attention to them and very thorough follow-up on problems.

Posing as expectant parents who wanted to tour the facilities, two managers visited every obstetrics and maternity ward within an hour's drive. Other managers searched the industry literature to identify the few hospitals in the country with the best reputation in delivery and maternity services, and then flew out to visit them. Team members gathered again to compare notes and to select the hospital that would serve as their template for customer satisfaction. What they had discovered was that the model did not exist, so they decided to build it themselves.

It seemed obvious to everyone involved that the first step should be to prioritize the wish list and narrow it down. Some of the ideas, such as skylights, seemed frivolous. Others, such as Jacuzzis, seemed downright dangerous—bathing during labor carries a risk of infection. Double-size hospital beds did not seem to exist. How was the hospital to change the behavior of doctors and nurses, who tend to be fiercely protective of their routines? After vigorous debate, it was decided that they would do it all.

The new obstetrics and maternity unit opened in 1987. It had rooms where families could gather. It had fresh flowers. It had skylights. It had a Jacuzzi and custom-built double beds. It had birthing-helper classes for children and grandparents. It also had primary-care nursing—each patient was the responsibility of a single nurse who would make sure that all the patient's needs were met and that the doctors were kept informed of any and all developments.

Obstetrics admissions doubled over the next few years, reflecting enthusiastic patient response. Not only did most of the nurses get used to the extra demands of the new unit, but they also began to like them. Turnover among the nursing staff, always a problem, dropped. Nurses began taking it upon themselves to find more ways to cater to the patients. For example, they developed a program that provides a free examination of mother and baby three days after discharge—either at the hospital or at the mother's own home, should a hospital return be inconvenient. Ninety-six percent of mothers were soon availing themselves of that exam, and in one-third of the cases, a nurse identified a problem that might have otherwise gone untreated, such as jaundice or lactation difficulties. Most amazing of all, only a small percentage of the patients asked to have a nurse come to their home to conduct the exam; they all seemed perfectly happy to return to the hospital.

Now the hospital found that top-notch obstetricians, including female doctors often favored by expectant mothers, were actively seeking out Griffin, which was encouraging because, historically, the hospital had experienced difficulty in attracting good physicians. What is more, because the new unit's philosophy was clearly established, the doctors who signed on tended to be physicians who preferred working in this patient-driven model. The board found that the new environment was becoming a recruiting tool.

In 1990, the executive team was asked whether it could build an entire hospital on the same model.

REALITY

No matter how much you have been warned that Griffin does not look like an ordinary hospital or how carefully you have followed the signs that clearly indicate, "Hospital," you cannot help wondering whether you have made a mistake when you enter Griffin's lobby. Think of the lobby of a high-powered law firm: expensive-looking wood; curving, sophisticated structures; and an energetic, pleasant, and efficient-looking young receptionist sitting alone behind a massive desk, smiling at you as though you were the firm's most important client. A finely tuned player piano provides light jazz in the background.

Throughout the hospital, corridors are generously trimmed in maple and nicely carpeted (special wheel bearings were purchased to keep gurneys from bogging down in the thick pile carpet), and they feature warm, indirect lighting. There are no gurneys, wheelchairs, crash carts, or food-tray dollies lining the corridors. There are no public-address-system pages, announcements, or gongs.

The rooms are furnished at a level of taste and comfort roughly equal to that of a typical upper-middle-class hotel. Some rooms are oversized, with couches that fold into double beds. Those are the care partner rooms, in which family members who help provide care are allowed to stay with the patient. None of the rooms is more than a dozen feet or so from a nurses' station. Nor are they more than 100 feet or so from a well-stocked, home-style kitchen that is open to all patients and visitors 24 hours a day. Sometimes, patients cook as a kind of therapy. At other times, families gather in the kitchen to make life-and-death decisions. Everywhere you turn, you see similar touches, inspired by ideas solicited from clients.

When Griffin initially focused on maternity, it had selected hospital services most amenable to change and most likely to meet with success. Expectant mothers tend to be young and healthy. They are generally not actually ill, are in the hospital for only a few days, and do not require extensive treatment. Maternity services tend to provide good revenues, relative to what this type of care costs the hospital.

In contrast, providing an emotionally satisfying, minimally inconvenient experience to a broad population in a hospital environment is a different story. The care of clients who are suffering from heart attacks, having parts of their bodies removed, or fighting for breath through failing lungs is typically more challenging. Nevertheless, the Griffin team again prepared community surveys and focus groups to determine what it would take to make people more comfortable in a hospital environment. This time, the groups focused on the needs and desires of an older population.

Again, the resulting wish list was staggering. They wanted nice furniture. They wanted kitchens. They wanted carpeting. They wanted nurses by their beds essentially all the time. They wanted their pets to visit. They wanted spouses or family members to have beds there in the room with them and to be allowed to help take care of them. Additionally, they wanted a better understanding of what was happening to them, medically speaking.

Again, the decision was to proceed. The hospital was operating in a 60-year-old building, which had not been renovated since 1969; it was due for a new building. Why not design it to meet all of these newly identified needs?

Extensive community-hospital building projects need approval from a state commission. The commission finally agreed to let Griffin do what it wanted, as long as it did it for no more than the average cost of adding on a similar-sized conventional hospital building—about $145 per square foot. That meant doing a first-class job on everything but providing first class inexpensively.

Developing a basic layout for the new rooms—normally a "boilerplate" sort of process—turned out to be a painstaking experience. The design not only had to meet patient demands for a homey environment, but it also had to accommodate medical equipment and extensive gas and plumbing fixtures, and to provide convenient access and movement to nurses, technicians, and the housekeeping staff. The management team and the project architects sketched ideas and employed a computer-aided design system, then worked with cardboard models, and finally built a full-scale mock-up of a hospital room in a warehouse across the street from the hospital. Hundreds of patients, staff members, technicians, builders, and board members explored the room, each one submitting ideas for modifications.

The chief administrator personally selected the furniture, favoring warm, semi-contemporary wooden designs. No detail seemed too unimportant. Handrails were tried out in a bewildering variety of materials, shapes, and heights. Hospitals almost always go with stainless steel, but wood was chosen for its added warmth—not to mention the fact that it costs less. Fluorescent lighting was eliminated.

Another request was for double rooms that would provide the companionship of a roommate but not a lack of privacy. No one could think of a way to design a double room that met all of those criteria. However, one of the managers discovered an unusual double room in a trade journal, went to check it out while vacationing in Florida, and, upon his return, excitedly described the room he had seen: an L-shaped room with the two beds arranged at right angles to each other, each along one of the two limbs of the L. Because the room entrance and bathroom were located at the bend of the L—the entrance on the outer bend and the bathroom on the inner—caregivers could enter and walk directly to either bed, and neither patient would have to walk by the other to get to the bathroom. The patients' views of one another were partially blocked by the outside walls of the bathroom that jut into the room. Working with the layout, the team hit on the idea of placing cabinetry at the bend, which would further block the patients' views of each other and would offer privacy, as long as one or both beds were in the flat position. If both patients felt like a little companionship, they could raise the heads of their beds, angling themselves forward enough to clear the obstructions visually and see each other. Unfortunately, putting a window at both ends of the room was out of the question. However, the team was able to devise a compromise. If they placed the window directly alongside one of the beds, the patient in that bed would be close to the window but would have to turn to the side to see it, whereas the patient in the other bed would be farther from the window but would have a full view. When the full-scale mock-up was tested, it was clearly a success.

Designing better access to the nurses' station was another priority. In almost all hospitals, every wing has a central nurses' station, and typically some patients are located the equivalent of a block away, which raises their anxiety levels. The solution: replacing the central station with individual nurse workstations, each with four patient rooms arranged fanlike around it. In that arrangement, every patient can actually see the primary-care nurse from bed, only 15 feet away. Some of the nurses objected, insisting that they needed to be near other nurses to share information and to socialize to ease the pressure of the job. However, the new design was implemented and has been a tremendous success with both nurses and patients.

That focus on patient needs is evident throughout the hospital today. A large health resource center, open to the public, includes medical information for lay readers and computers linked to health-related Web sites. The medical library in which the doctors do their research is adjacent to the resource center and is open to the public, so it is possible to find patients and visitors sitting next to doctors, reviewing medical journals.

Although state regulations require too many procedures to make it feasible for patients to receive visits from their pets, Griffin has half a dozen dogs who keep patients company. These personal touches are everywhere. Patients point out that they are constantly receiving unexpected acts of kindness. All employees of the hospital are considered caregivers, whether they are processing bills in accounting or cleaning labs. Griffin also has an open chart policy. Some physicians worried that letting patients see their charts would lead to lawsuits, but the medical director reports that not a single negative experience has resulted.

Although its reputation for pleasantness is attracting a growing number of patients from outside the immediate community, Griffin is aiming for a national market by establishing niche services within the hospital. One of those is a comprehensive pain- and headache-treatment center. Another is a hyperbaric wound-treatment center, where patients are placed in high-pressure, high-oxygen tanks that speed the healing of difficult wounds. Perhaps most remarkably, Griffin has even managed to construct an intensive-care unit that provides virtually all the same patient amenities, including private rooms that are only slightly less hotel-like than the other inpatient rooms. To make patients accessible to visitors without restricting physicians' ability to rush in for emergencies, each room provides a door at opposite ends: one that opens into a nurses' station and the other opening into a lounge area from which family and friends can enter whenever they wish, day or night.

This continued commitment to change is reflected in every aspect of Griffin. It is a fundamental requirement. From Griffin's perspective, there is no middle ground in transformation.

44.2   Vantage Point: The Planetree Model

Susan B. Frampton

Planetree, Inc., is an alliance of progressive health care facilities and individuals committed

Susan B. Frampton, PhD, Executive Director of Planetree, Inc., has master's and doctoral degrees in medical anthropology from the University of Connecticut. She has worked with hospitals in New England over the past 20 years in the areas of community health, wellness, and integrative and holistic medicine.

Courtesy of Planetree, Inc., Derby, Connecticut.

to the creation of patient-centered health care environments. The Planetree model has been in existence for more than 20 years, and includes innovative programming, unique approaches to patient services, the provision of resources and information for patients, and a focus on the design of the healing health care environments. The Planetree Organization is now a subsidiary of Griffin Health Services Corporation and can be accessed at <http://www.planetree.org>.

BASIC CONCEPTS OF THE MODEL: EXPANDING PATIENT-CENTERED HEALTH CARE

Planetree recognizes that the experience of illness has potential to transform the patient. It can be a time of great personal growth as life goals and values are reexamined, priorities are clarified, and inner resources are discovered.

Programs and Resources

Educational Materials. A variety of information resources is made available to the patient, the family, and the community through consumer-friendly health resource centers and satellite centers. Planetree resource centers aid those in search of information as they review broad collections of books, medical texts, and journals. Video and audio tapes, computerized resources, databases, research services, and a wealth of other resources are provided to support patients' increasing hunger for information about their health and medical care.

Human Interactions. Planetree encourages healing partnerships between patients, family members, and caregivers. All employees in Planetree hospitals are considered to be caregivers, and they will impact the experience of the patient. Staff training is provided to enhance sensitivity to the patient's experience while hospitalized.

Enhancing Social Support Networks. Social support has been shown to be vital to good health. Medical and social science research indicates that healing is promoted when love, intimacy, connection, and community are fostered. Planetree supports and encourages the involvement of family and significant others wherever possible. The Care Partner Program offers education and training to empower family participation in the care of patients while they are hospitalized and at home after discharge. Significant others can make a valuable contribution in the quality of the patient's hospital experience. Care conferences are held within 24 hours of admission with the patient, family, nurse, and physician to discuss treatment plans together. Patients are encouraged to read and make entries in their own medical records.

Spirituality in Healing. Planetree recognizes the vital role of spirituality in healing the whole person. Patients, families, and staff are encouraged to connect with their own inner spiritual resources. The model promotes the creation of sanctuaries that provide opportunity for reflection and prayer, such as chapels, gardens, and meditation rooms. Chaplains are considered vital members of the health care team.

The Importance of Human Touch. Touch is an essential way of communicating caring and may be omitted from the clinical setting. Therapeutic full-body massage or chair massage are made available for patients, families, and staff. Internship programs for massage therapists and training for volunteers to give hand and foot rubs are also available and help keep program costs minimal. Families, as part of the Care Partner Program, can also be taught to give massages to loved ones. Health care staff and professionals also benefit from the use of chair massage as a useful way to relieve stress and reenergize themselves.

Healing Arts. Music, storytellers, clowns, and other forms of humor are used to create an atmosphere of serenity and playfulness in the Planetree model. Aesthetic touches are included to enhance the ambiance of the hospital environment through artwork in patient rooms, in treatment areas, and on art carts. Volunteers work with patients who would like to create their own art. The involvement of artists, musicians, poets, and storytellers from the local community expands the resources available in the health care facility.

Complementary Therapies. Use of complementary and alternative therapies has increased substantially in the last decade. The data suggest that a growing number of patients desire treatment options that are more natural and holistic to complement biomedical approaches. To meet the growing consumer demand for complementary therapies, Planetree affiliates have instituted a range of options including heart disease reversal programs; acupuncture; mind-body medicine interventions such as meditation and guided imagery; meditative exercise such as T'ai chi and yoga; therapeutic massage, therapeutic touch, and Reiki.

The Importance of Nutrition. Sound nutrition is recognized as an integral part of health and healing. It is essential not only for health, but as a source of pleasure, comfort, and familiarity. The scientific data also demonstrate the role of nutrition in health and disease. In a hospital environment, nutrition can be emphasized in the entree selections of the cafeteria and by providing healthy choices in the vending machines. Some Planetree hospitals offer room service in patient areas of the hospital; the availability of kitchenettes makes it possible for the family to prepare favorite foods or meals for their loved ones. The kitchens also serve as gathering places for patients and families, much as they do at home, thus enhancing the sense of a more personalized environment. Cooking demonstrations and classes are provided by nutritionists and volunteers. Nutrition education focuses not only on the patient's current illness but on healthy living for the entire family, as well.

Architectural Design. The Planetree model encourages the development of physical environments that are conducive to the healing process of the patient. Facility design includes efficient layouts that support patient dignity and autonomy. Domestic aesthetics, art, and warm, homelike settings are emphasized. Architectural barriers are minimized. Designing and maintaining an uncluttered environment encourages patient mobility and a sense of "safe shelter." The design of a Planetree facility provides patients and families with spaces for both solitude and social activities, and includes libraries, kitchens, lounges, activity rooms, chapels, and gardens. Comfortable accommodations are available so families can stay overnight. Healing gardens, fountains, fish tanks, and waterfalls are provided to connect patients, families, and staff with the relaxing, invigorating, healing, and meditative aspects of nature.

Supporting the Care Providers. It is as essential to create healing environments for the staff as for patients. Physicians, nurses, and ancillary staff are very much affected by their working environment. Consequently, lounges and areas for meditative retreat designed especially for staff are another important component of the Planetree model. All of these elements in concert enhance the sense of healing that can be created in a hospital environment.

44.3 Perspective: How You Can Become Involved

Nancy S. Moore

PERSPECTIVES FOR ADMINISTRATORS

These are challenging times for hospital administrators and health systems. Everyone recognizes the need for change. However, the questions of what, how, and when change should occur are not easy to answer. Hospitals are in uncharted territory. The options for change and the course to be taken are individual decisions for each program, based on the developmental stage of the organization and the needs of the community and customers. One thing is certain: Change will occur, whether we choose it or not.

Approaches

If you like some of the ideas in this section, the following are suggestions for getting involved:

1. *Check in with yourself.* Do the ideas and approaches presented make sense to you? Are they stimulating? If so, consider the words of Lathrop: "Few will challenge the goals of the patient-focused hospital. Many will question the means—telling us 'you can't get there from here.' The simple imperative is: we must get there, and here is the only place we can start. As long as we keep patients and common sense foremost in our minds, we will succeed" (1991).

2. *Gather information.* Consider the reading materials listed in the resources section of Chapter 65. A wealth of information is now widely available on innovative approaches to programming and service delivery.

3. *Get others involved and obtain their buy-in.* This involvement should start with top management, but it must also include middle management. A well-aligned management team is a key to the success of patient-focused healing. It pays to take the time to develop a fully informed and committed management team. To involve staff without management's support is a setup for organizational conflict and stress.

4. *Perform an internal assessment.* Where are you in relation to where you want to be? Some questions to consider include:
   - *Is there a quality improvement process already in place?* Patient-centered concepts can be integrated as options in these processes.
   - *How do you compare on the elements of the patient-centered model?* You may want to evaluate your organization using objective quantitative measures, such as the Planetree values described in this chapter.
   - *Where can you begin right now to gain immediate benefits?* What type of

Nancy S. Moore, RN, PhD, is one of the founders and Vice President of Healing Health Services at St. Charles Medical Center in Bend, Oregon. Her educational background includes degrees in nursing and in counseling, and a doctorate from Greenwich University, having studied under Leland Kaiser. She is also a member of Kaiser Consulting Network. With more than three decades of experience as a practicing hospital nurse and administrator, she has both experiential and theoretical knowledge of health care in this country. Ms. Moore is listed in the *National Distinguished Registry in Nursing* (1988) and *Who's Who in American Nursing* (1990–1993), and she is coauthor of *Patient-Focused Healing* (Jossey-Bass, 1993).

programmatic efforts will help people see the value of your program? We began by redesigning the pain management program using a more patient-centered healing approach.

- *What is the financial status of the hospital, and what is its projected status?* Programs described in this book have found that patient-centered models enhanced the bottom line. These programs tend to attract new patients. As health systems implement them, many find that they have become preferred providers in their community and attract new patients.
- *How can these same models be applied to employee growth and development?* We have found this approach to improve morale, customer service attitude, and, ultimately, cost savings.
- *Are grants or foundation money available to fund these projects?* The return on investment is long range, so the financial issue is a big one for hospitals.
- *Are you ready to embark on remodeling or renovation?* If so, this can provide an opportunity to integrate new approaches into the design of your facility.

5. *Use site visits to gain a sense of the available options.* Include leadership in on-site evaluations of the best models. Site visits are powerful, tangible ways to change people's minds. Not only do they see what is possible, but they can see the process in action. Site visits provide a good opportunity for networking. The collegial relationships that evolve as a natural consequence are invaluable when it comes time to implement a new program and questions arise.

6. *Attend relevant workshops and conferences.*

7. *Initiate a study group.* For example, consider beginning an advisory group for alternative therapies that includes physicians, complementary practitioners, pastoral care, administrators, physical therapists, and others that meets and reviews the literature to develop white papers and recommendations.

8. *Develop a vision for what you want to create.* Use the tension between the reality and the vision to create the energy for change.

9. *Appoint a person to spearhead the project.* Although CEOs must generate the excitement and energy with their vision, it is unlikely that they will have the time to keep the project moving forward. Ideally, project leaders are selected on the basis of their knowledge and skill for project management, as well as for their enthusiasm for the project itself. This enthusiasm is an important element to overcome the natural inertia inherent in any change process and to sustain the momentum over time.

10. *Consider involving outside consultants.* Use them strategically. Focus their services so that their contribution is feasible, strategic, and economically practical. Most hospitals look to consultants when undertaking projects that affect major systems. When shifting an organization's paradigm, it can be useful to involve outside perspectives at regular intervals, such as a consultant who is sympathetic to what you are trying to achieve but who is not a part of the day-to-day politics of the organization. This person can hold the organization accountable, yet avoid polarization and organizational politics. The outside consultant can monitor the process and minimize blame, particularly blame directed at those who are initiating the change. It helps to have an outsider come in to uncover the inevitable problems and facilitate their resolution.

11. *Develop champions.* Many CEOs who have been through this process recommend identifying a few people representing key constituencies and gaining their support for your ideas. It helps to

focus your energy on a few key individuals at first. They can then aid in getting the word out and gaining the support of others.

12. ***Initiate the project in pilot units.*** Once you have identified what you want to do, Kaiser (1991) recommends trying the idea in one area at first. People who do not want to participate can choose to work elsewhere in the organization. The effects of the new design can be studied and refined before moving on to other areas. Of course, the administrator will need to weigh the economic benefits of expanding the project to a larger scale. As models for patient-focused healing are refined, they will become easier to implement.

PHYSICIAN INVOLVEMENT

How can physicians get involved? They, too, have been caught by the speed of change demanded by consumers. Physicians have a tremendous influence on patient care. New models of care will not succeed unless physicians are involved.

A number of relevant approaches to current issues bring physicians into the process:

- Identify and develop champions, preferably opinion leaders. Begin by recruiting a few supporters who can enlist the support of their colleagues.
- Have physicians teach physicians. Doctors learn best from doctors.
- In expanding patient-focused healing services, provide physicians with specific data from patient focus groups or surveys. In addition, provide doctors with aggregated data about their patients.
- Make research available that documents the efficacy of these approaches to care. Physicians want hard data and research before considering fundamental shifts in their style of practice. Also provide annotated bibliographies, clinical reviews, and venues for continuing education.
- Involve the physicians in your hospital in a collaborative team effort with other doctors.
- Link new programs to systemwide quality initiatives. Physicians, on the whole, strive for excellence and are likely to support aspects of the program that set rigorous standards and promote top-quality clinical care.

NURSING AND OTHER PROFESSIONS

New models of care delivery have evolved during this transitional period that emphasize collaborative approaches. Consequently, nurses now have the opportunity to expand their leadership role in health care. Many of the new models are based on the foundational perspectives and values of nursing: caring for the whole person, advocacy for patients, integration of care, and coordination of resources based on patient needs. In fact, the basic concept of holistic health draws on the traditional values of nursing as a caring and healing science. In addition, nursing continues to be key to quality of care in the hospital environment. Research has shown that community members and physicians often select hospitals based on the quality of nursing staff (Advisory Board, St. Charles Medical Center, 1999).

At the same time, no one profession can do it all, and we must leverage the best in the practice of each of the health care professions. The current collaborative model of care—which has been highly successful—is based on teams formed around patient needs. This multidisciplinary approach involves the coordination of social services and physical, occupational, and respiratory therapies, as well as other professionals, as needed. Even in physician practices, the use of physician extenders is considered good practice, particularly in the context of disease management for patients with complex medical needs.

However, the current speed of the change has caught most health care professionals by surprise, and there is the need to move to a more proactive mode.

Now is the time to expand collaborative planning, using the tenets of innovative models of care and healing:

- Make the patient the center of care. Services should be designed around the patient's needs.
- Encourage active patient and family involvement and education.
- Maximize the healing aspects of the environment.
- Expand the continuum of care.
- Incorporate mind/body/spirit therapies.
- Decentralize services to the patient-care unit whenever practical, based on utilization. For example, if a group of patients requires 8 hours of social services a day, make a social services person a permanent member of the team.
- Become as flexible as possible through cross-training. Multiskilled practitioners are an absolute must. The days of widespread specialization are over. Specialization is not affordable in today's health care environment.
- Leverage skills so that professionals are freed up to do what they are educated to do and identify lesser-skilled people to assist them with tasks.
- Monitor and improve quality on an ongoing basis. Eliminate waste and redundancy.

LEARNINGS: ORGANIZATIONAL DEVELOPMENT

Challenge as Opportunity

Crisis Presents Two Polarities: Danger and Opportunity. Time and time again in the process of our development, what has seemed to be a crisis became an opportunity for our next step in growth. Each crisis along the way has required that we become clearer and reexamine our values or change.

One excellent example of this occurred in the last quarter of 1998, when we found that, for the first time in our history, our expenses exceeded revenue. This realization sent a shock wave through the organization. We began an in-depth exploration to determine how we had lost control. Our leadership council came together and set targets for cost reductions. Each manager reviewed his or her operations for opportunities to reduce cost. Managers went back to their departments to involve staff and physicians in brainstorming to find solutions. We feared that we would not be able to afford some of our newest, most innovative programs. This spurred a deep look inward and an exploration of our values and mission. We found the cost savings by modifying certain programs. We affirmed that our core service is our patient care, and our relationships with our patients and each other— each employee and every physician—are our most valuable assets. Our investment in relationship-centered care, rather than being a luxury, was what got us through the crisis. This approach pulled the entire hospital together to find the internal resourcefulness that made it possible for us to manage our way through the crisis. We are now fully back on track and are exceeding our financial targets.

Conflict Can Be Used Constructively. It is to be engaged and openly explored. A good example of this was seen during the development of our Center for Health and Learning. One potential initiative was the development of an integrative primary care clinic as an exemplar for providing relationship-centered care and alternative care in tandem. Some members of the medical staff had grave concerns about both the primary care clinic and alternative therapies. The medical director for the center invited debate. Our medical staff meetings had record attendance as the director and opponents put on a point-counterpoint style of debate. It energized the medical staff (Moore, 2000). We applied what we had learned from this debate and adapted our model, eliminating the primary care clinic and some of the specific alternative services from our initial program. The hospital developed an advisory group of physicians, hospital representatives, and alternative therapists to review the research on alternative therapies and to develop white paper recommendations for the hospital and medical staff. As a result, our medical symptom reduction program and other ventures are enjoying excellent physician referrals.

The Dynamic of Change

The Process of Change. There is a statistical bell-shaped curve for human behavior in implementing major change processes. It is wise to empower the strong proponents on the leading edge of the project as its champions. Identify them for each discipline. Then focus on disseminating the information to those in the middle of the population through education and dialogue to bring them along in the change.

Responding to Dissent. Although it is important to listen to and learn from those at the dissenting edge of the curve, human values are not usually changed through words alone. A judgment call is involved in evaluating the magnitude of the dissent. If the forces for change significantly outweigh the dissent, we have learned that it can be worthwhile to move forward. As the implementation occurs and health care professionals can see the benefits for their practice and their patients, they begin to come along. Generally, people have to experience the new program. It is difficult for most people to become enthusiastic about abstractions. Remember that change takes time; it usually takes years.

Planning. We have learned that planning is important, but you should not spend too long in the planning phase. The entire project cannot usually be fully envisioned in the planning phase. We have learned to define our vision, create a good plan, then set out to achieve it. As the project is implemented, it becomes apparent what is working and what is not. Course corrections can then be made on this information.

Leadership

Leadership is everything. By empowering people at all levels of the project, you can maximize buy-in—people want to support what they help to create. We view leadership as embodied in Gandhi's statement, "You must be the change you wish to see in the world." In health care, where health and healing are our mission, we ourselves must be healthy and healed.

One example of the importance of commitment has occurred through the leadership of our vice president, who has instituted monthly administrative rounds on each shift for four hours. Initially, staff did not fully understand the approach. They wondered why she was making rounds, asking them how they were doing, and what was working (and not working) in their jobs. Then they began to notice that the concerns they identified were actually being addressed. Now, when it is time for her visit to their shift, they are waiting to see her with ideas and stories. Administrative rounds provide a tremendous opportunity for leadership to learn how the plans and policies of the hospital actually translate into patient care. This is also a dynamic example of the value of relationship building between leadership and staff. It has tremendously enriched the work of the administrator by increasing staff support and maximizing program effectiveness.

CONCLUSION

Transforming health care is everyone's business. No one group or individual can do it alone. It will require a collaborative effort. To renew health care, we must be bold. We must be willing to consider new initiatives, while maintaining our focus on the highest quality. It is not an easy task to change the form of structures already in place. However, we have no place to begin but where we are.

REFERENCES

Advisory Board Company. *Nurse Executive Center: The Journey Begins, Chicago 2000.* Washington, DC, 1999.

Kaiser L. *Healing Health Care.* Presented at the St. Charles Medical Center, Bend, OR, 1991.

Lathrop JP. The patient-focused hospital. *Healthcare Forum J.* 1991(July/Aug):17–20.

Moore N. *Norman Cousins Award Application, Fetzer Institute.* St. Charles Medical Center, Bend, OR, 2000.

SUGGESTED READING

Moore N, Komras H. *Patient-Focused Healing: Integrating Caring and Curing in Health Care.* San Francisco, CA: Jossey-Bass; 1993.

Part XI

Wellness Programs for Hospital Systems and Employers

CHAPTER 45

Health Promotion and Complementary Medicine: Expanding the Continuum of Care

Roger Jahnke

The continuous transformation of health care is requiring great flexibility in an environment of constant change. All organizations are affected, including managed care, provider networks, indemnity insurers, hospital groups, and medical centers. For many health systems, the fiscal mandate of the current market has required a focus on core business. This implies that the key objectives are to build market share, ensure that staff members continue to improve clinical outcomes, and sustain profitability. Organizations have responded with a variety of strategies, including the development of new products and service lines.

This transition includes a shift in focus from a delivery system based on disease intervention to one that includes a major focus on health promotion. New programs with a health-improvement focus are appearing throughout every level of health care. Many of these initiatives involve complementary and alternative medicine (CAM)

and ultimately are targeted at an integrated model of delivery.

Health promotion programming integrates quite logically with CAM concepts and therapies. This same congruence is evident for a multitude of program derivatives, including wellness, health enhancement, disease management, behaviorally based health improvement, and mind-body healing.

Currently, there is a common presumption that CAM is founded primarily in therapeutic modalities such as acupuncture treatment, chiropractic adjustments, massage, and herbal medicines. In fact, all of the utilization studies of CAM have demonstrated that the largest percentage of consumer activity in the area of alternative or unconventional medicine has not been in treatment, but rather in health promotion activities, including exercise, nutrition, visualization, and other approaches (Eisenberg et al, 1993; Eisenberg et al, 1998; Astin, 1998).

THE BUSINESS CASE FOR HEALTH PROMOTION

The business rationale includes the opportunity to decrease medical costs and to create new revenue streams. Even in the most utilization-intensive populations—those already receiving treatment for disease—there is the capacity for major medical cost reduction. The well-documented Ornish program for the reversal of heart disease has demonstrated average savings of $30,000 per patient per year (Ornish, 1998). Savings in well populations are also impressive. A Procter and Gamble study in which 4,000

Roger Jahnke, consultant, futurist, and CEO of the Health Action Consulting Group in Santa Barbara, California, has assisted numerous health systems in the design of comprehensive health care delivery strategies. See http://HealthAction.net.

The Health Action Group is a consulting and training organization in Santa Barbara, California, that collaborates with large health care organizations to improve health outcomes, build market share, and create new or expanded revenue streams. Health Action also trains trainers and facilitators in the use of innovative programs in medical symptom reduction, support group process, wellness, and health enhancement.

Courtesy of Roger Jahnke, Ph.D., Santa Barbara, California.

employees participated in health enhancement programs accrued a savings of more than $1.6 million in just one year (Goetzel et al, 1998) (see Chapter 49).

Health promotion is now being viewed as the source of a viable revenue stream. The market for nutritional and herbal supplements, natural foods, and products is now $28.2 billion a year (Traynor, 2000). This sector has experienced increases from 4% to 45% annually in various market channels, one of the most rapidly growing segments of the health care industry. Spas, health clubs, and fitness centers reflect this trend. In hospitals and health maintenance organizations (HMOs), fitness centers, health education programs, and mind-body programs are often the first initiatives, particularly for building market share and enhancing clinical outcomes. Revenue-generating programs in wellness and personal effectiveness enhancement for business are now being provided by innovative hospital systems and HMOs, as well as by entrepreneurial training companies.

EXPANDING THE CONTINUUM OF CARE

For decades, health care has focused on treatment targeted at the major causes of death (see Table 45–1). A conceptual breakthrough published in the *Journal of the American Medical Association* suggests that the leading causes of death are secondary to the actual causes of death (McGinnis and Foege, 1993).

Although the ten leading causes imply that we are the victims of diseases, the nine actual causes reflect the more accurate idea that we frequently choose behaviors that cause disease. Depending on one's perspective, perhaps six and as many as all nine of these causes are preventable, many of which are directly related to personal behavior and choice.

In the context of industrial societies, the major diseases occur from preventable behavioral causes. The data can be viewed as a mandate to reengineer health care delivery to include a major focus on health promotion and prevention. It is then appropriate to ask, What are the underlying causes of high-risk behaviors? What causes a person to choose to smoke, overuse alcohol, use recreational drugs, agree to high-risk sex, carry firearms, neglect seat belt use, or indulge in high-risk diet and activity patterns? The answer to this question includes factors such as lack of access to information, internal and external stressors, low self-esteem, poor communication skills, and social or peer pressure.

Although heart disease and cancer can be treated with medical procedures in clinical facilities, personal choices are not the domain of

---

Table 45–1 Leading Causes of Morbidity in the United States

10 Leading Causes of Death	9 Actual Causes of Death
Heart disease	Tobacco
Cancer	Diet and activity patterns
Cerebrovascular disease	Alcohol
Accidents	Microbial agents
COPD	Toxic agents
Pneumonia and influenza	Firearms
Diabetes	Sexual behavior
Suicide	Motor vehicles
Liver disease	Illicit drug use
HIV/AIDS	

Courtesy of Roger Jahnke, Ph.D., Santa Barbara, California.

treatment. This raises the question of the most appropriate approach to high-risk behaviors. When there is a focus on upstream, preventive interventions, the options are expanded. In that context, these are not only medical issues; they are behavioral issues with solutions that are more likely to be associated with education and empowerment.

From this perspective alone, it is obvious that health promotion and disease prevention through behaviorally based health improvement programming is likely to be the foundation of the health care delivery system of the future. The potential financial benefits are also significant (see Chapters 46 through 49).

The Potential for Prevention

Consider these findings:

- Of current health care expenses, 70% result from preventable illnesses, according to the U.S. Department of Health and Human Services, Healthy People 2000 (1991) and Healthy People 2010 (2000).
- Eight of every nine diseases have preventable causes, reported by former U.S. Surgeon General C. Everett Koop, MD, and James Fries, MD, of Stanford University (1993).
- Herbert Benson, MD, has suggested that 75% of illness is the result of stress (Benson and Friedman, 1996; Friedman et al, 1997).

These impressive facts, applied in conjunction with an expanded vision of service delivery, have the potential to transform and reshape the world of health care. They point to a profound breakthrough for the health care industry: Caring for, sustaining, and even improving health is a fundamental health care objective, but it is not inherently a clinical activity, nor one based in medical diagnostics and medical treatment. As consumers, employee groups, and self-funded pools continue to refine their health strategies aggressively, it will become more and

more important for hospitals, clinics, payers, and provider organizations to understand the importance of integrating health promotion as a complement to treatment.

For almost a decade The Health Project, a consortium of agencies and corporations originating from a White House Round Table initiative, has been presenting the C. Everett Koop Award to businesses and communities that demonstrate this capacity to save or reallocate health care dollars through health promotion. In a ground-breaking 1993 article from the *New England Journal of Medicine* (Fries and Koop, 1993), it was predicted that awardees from The Health Project and similar programs could generate billions of dollars in medical cost savings. The prediction was correct, and the momentum of this program is increasing (see the Web site http://www.healthproject.stanford.edu for more information).

Examples of the cost benefits of health promotion include Husky Injection Molding Systems (Ontario, Canada), which saves an estimated $1.4 million each year through reduced absenteeism with a highly successful worksite wellness clinic that includes naturopathic medicine (Baron, 1997); Steelcase achieved a 50% reduction in medical claims with its health promotion programming (Health Promotion Update, 1992), and Johnson and Johnson has generated savings of nearly $2 for each $1 spent on prevention. Blue Shield of California decreased medical visits by 15%, achieving a savings of $6 for every program dollar spent. Equally innovative are the community programs that have received the Koop Award (The Health Project, 1999).

THE EMERGING DESIGN OF HEALTH PROMOTION

Although health promotion has been a foundation of public health programming and an evolving component of employee group health cost reduction since the 1980s, the nature of health improvement and its role in health care are currently being redefined. This expanded vision of health promotion can be integrated within health systems, as well as in employee groups, to create a continuum of services from those that enhance health and prevent illness to those that address acute needs.

As a meaningful complement to these foundational approaches to health improvement, initiatives from mind-body medicine and CAM provide a new generation of health promotion services (Table 45–2).

Mind-body methods are expressions of the biopsychosocial model of health care. These kinds of programs use self-care, behavioral methodologies, and health education to link conventional medicine, health promotion, and alternative medicine into a seamless, comprehensive, and far-reaching system of services with a focus on health improvement. We have the profound opportunity to redesign the delivery of health care to integrate the best of these methods into a comprehensive system that is therapeutic when it must be and preventive whenever it can be. With direct and integral linking of the best of modern medicine to the best of health promotion and alternative therapies, we are on the threshold of perhaps the most remarkable era yet in the history of health care and medicine.

Complementary Medicine: Peripheral or Central Issue

Health care organizations are focused on improving economic viability and sustaining the "core" business of health care delivery while retaining customers and expanding market share. Complementary medicine currently has the powerful advantage of public approval and increasing momentum from very positive media. CAM has, as has been noted, an inherent connection with health promotion.

Is complementary medicine a distraction from the business of delivering good medicine? Is CAM a peripheral issue in the evolution of health care delivery? Or is CAM a central component of the solution to the health cost and quality challenge? Is it possible that CAM is not so much an end in itself but more of a tool in the redesign of health care? To achieve the goal of a more comprehensive system of health creation, could complementary medicine be of greatest value in leveraging the expansion of the health care system to include lifestyle interventions, mind-body approaches, and preventive service delivery?

Time will tell, of course. However, it is guaranteed that the evolution of the design of delivery will include a major focus on health improvement. In its many permutations, CAM will rarely emerge in isolation from health promotion. As health enhancement is integrated into the system, it will provide a foundation for the inclusion of the best of the complementary therapies. As CAM is integrated into delivery, it will typically include an expansion of lifestyle interventions that take the form of health promotion

Table 45–2 Complementary Systems of Health Promotion

Mainstream Health Promotion	Mind-Body and CAM in Health Promotion
Preventive health screenings	Stress reduction
Health Risk Appraisals (HRA)	Biofeedback
Risk reduction programs	Yoga, T'ai chi, and Qigong
Smoking cessation programs	Health coaching
Drug and alcohol management	Support groups
Preventive and therapeutic nutrition	Meditation
Fitness and exercise	Visualization and imagery
	Spiritual and religious practices

Courtesy of Roger Jahnke, Ph.D., Santa Barbara, California.

in both prevention and patient care. For example, acupuncture is just a clinical tool without a wide array of naturally complementary behavioral components (such as diet, Qigong, and T'ai chi, etc.). Acupuncture in complement to these behavioral components becomes a complete system—traditional Chinese medicine.

Consumers Want a Health Focus More Than Alternative Therapies

A careful reading of the seminal survey of Eisenberg and colleagues (1993) reveals a finding that is frequently overlooked. Less than one-third of the respondents were using alternative therapies provided by practitioners. Most importantly, more than two-thirds of the responses reflected the use of self-care activities such as exercise and nutrition, products such as vitamins and herbs, and behavioral activities such as meditation and stress reduction.

Similar findings were reported by Astin in the *Journal of the American Medical Association* (1998). In that study, more than two-thirds of respondents reported using self-care alternatives to complement mainstream medicine. The data from this study indicate that the use of alternative or unconventional health care resources was not so much a reflection of consumers' dissatisfaction with conventional medicine. Rather they were indicative of consumers' active interest in a wide variety of health care options that were more aligned with their personal preferences and philosophical biases. A follow-up study by Eisenberg and colleagues (1998) confirmed this, as well as the necessity for a more evidence-based approach of both alternative therapies and alternative behavior practices. These three studies suggest a high level of consumer interest in health, fitness, and prevention. The obvious conclusion is that despite the consumer and media interest in alternative therapies, there is a far greater demand for self-care activities and products focused on health improvement than the demand for alternative clinical treatments.

For hospitals, health systems, and managed care organizations, this is an encouraging trend

that must be acknowledged and carefully explored. CAM programming that accurately reflects consumer interest and utilization trends ideally includes a strong focus on self-care, health promotion, and lifestyle change—perhaps even more than on the inclusion of CAM therapies.

For organizations that are interested in integrating CAM concepts and programming but are simultaneously experiencing some internal resistance, this information suggests an initial focus on health promotion, rather than on alternative medical modalities. Health systems nationwide are finding that this staged or phased transition to the eventual integration of complementary therapies is economically sound and addresses the internal pressures present in many health care organizations (see Chapter 6).

THE RELEVANCE OF HEALTH ENHANCEMENT ACROSS ALL POPULATIONS

Health care decision makers have been accustomed to the perspective that wellness and health promotion are luxuries, rather than medically necessary. However, in employer-based systems, the health of all employees—well and sick—is the ultimate focus of programming. Similarly, in managing populations—at-risk groups, "baby boomers," Medicare, low income, uninsured—health maintenance and demand management are of interest at every point in the continuum. Consequently, the business of health care is evolving to include the improvement and maintenance of health not only in populations that are at risk, but also those that are well. New-era wellness initiatives are dynamically reframed in this perspective.

Health improvement is then seen as applicable and relevant across the entire continuum of care in the provision of services for:

- well populations
- those at risk
- early intervention
- chronic illness and rehabilitation
- disease treatment.

Currently, a number of frugal, low-tech health enhancements, such as nutritional counseling, stress reduction, support groups, and therapeutic exercise, are proliferating in hospitals, managed care organizations, medical centers, and community education programs throughout the United States. In fact, the most impressive medical and economic results in health promotion have been in populations with life-threatening conditions and intensive medical needs, such as the heart disease patients served by the Ornish model. Where this approach is relevant, cases in need of the highest concentration of expensive medical services generate the most profound savings (see Chapter 40.2 on the Ornish program). Preliminary clinical reports suggest that lifestyle interventions may be relevant to other populations with acute or chronic conditions as well, such as the management of cancer, diabetes, and arthritis (see also Chapter 9). As health care delivery continues to develop programming that focuses on this expanded continuum, mature applications specific to each of these levels of the continuum of health care will emerge.

The expansion from a focus on disease to include a focus on health makes eminent sense in the context of changing epidemiological patterns. It makes sound financial sense, particularly in the context of capitated populations, corporate self-funded programs, and medical savings accounts. Health promotion also meets increasing consumer expectations for wellness, empowerment, life extension, and health longevity.

NEW MEDICINE REQUIRES A NEW PARADIGM

The emerging models for the delivery of health care—comprehensive delivery, complementary medicine, holistic health care, integrated medicine, and others—have one thing in common: They all involve expanding the continuum of care. The new paradigm includes health promotion as a foundational element.

Complementary approaches have a significant place in the spirit and developing practice of prevention and health promotion across the continuum of care. Although specific CAM therapies may or may not become enduring components of the new standard of health care delivery, health promotion is required to maximize outcomes and manage costs. Preventive and self-care programs that address health and illness are critical to demand management, risk management, new forms of disease management, wellness, and performance enhancement. Although alternative medicine is the current focus of much attention in the evolution of health care, health promotion may actually be the more powerful tool for achieving the most critical health care goals: decrease risk, enhance access, minimize costs, expand revenue, and improve clinical outcomes.

REFERENCES

Astin J. Why patients use alternative medicine: Results of a national study. *JAMA.* 1998;279(19):1548–1553.

Baron RA. Benefits of integrating naturopathic medicine in the work place: An introductory report. *J Naturopathic Med.* 1997;7(2):56–60.

Benson H, Friedman R. Harnessing the power of the placebo effect and renaming it "remembered wellness." *Annu Rev Med.* 1996;47:193–199.

Eisenberg D, Davis R, Ettner S, et al. Trends in alternative medicine use in the United States, 1990–1997: Results of a follow-up national survey. *JAMA.* 1998;280(18): 1569–1575.

Eisenberg DM, Kessler RC, Foster C, et al. Unconventional medicine in the United States. *N Engl J Med.* 1993; 328(4):246–252.

Friedman R, Sedler M, Myers P, Benson H. Behavioral medicine, complementary medicine and integrated care. Economic implications. *Prim Care.* 1997 Dec;24(4): 949–962.

Fries J, Koop CE. Reducing health care costs by reducing the need and demand for medical services. *N Engl J Med*. 1993;329:321–325.

Goetzel RZ, Jacobson BH, Aldana SG, Vardell K, Yee L. Cost savings through worksite health promotion. *J Occup Environ Med*.1998;40(4):341–346.

Health on the Net Foundation. Utilization survey.

<http://www.hon.ch> Geneva, Switzerland, 1999. Accessed 10/99.

Health Promotion Update, Body Bulletin Fact Sheet. 1992.

The Health Project, Koop Award Listing

<http://www.healthproject.stanford.edu>, 1999. Accessed 3/00.

Healthy People 2000 National Health Promotion and Disease Prevention Objectives. Washington, DC: Department of Health and Human Services, 1991, #91-50213.

Healthy People 2010: Understanding and Improving Health. Washington, DC: Department of Health and Human Services, 2000, #017-001-00543-6.

McGinnis JM, Foege WH. Actual causes of death in the United States. *JAMA*. 1993;270(18):2207–2212.

Ornish DM. Avoiding revascularization with lifestyle changes: The Multicenter Lifestyle Demonstration Project. *Am J Cardiol*. 1998;82(10B):72T–76T.

Traynor M. Natural products market tops $28 billion. *Nat Foods Merchandiser*. 2000;21(6):1, 21.

CHAPTER 46

Maximizing Benefits to the Patient and the Bottom Line:
Akron General Health and Wellness Center

Douglas Ribley

PROGRAM DEVELOPMENT

Akron General Health System includes three hospitals, several physician office practices owned by the system, and community health centers throughout the county. The recently opened Akron General Health and Wellness Center is located 12 miles from the main campus of the hospital in a suburban area that is one of the health system's important markets. The project was completed in 1996 and is currently one of the most financially successful components of the entire system (Akron General LifeStyles, Responsibility Summaries, 1996–2000). In terms of membership, the health facility has full enrollment. In 1997, LifeStyles won a distinguished achievement award from the Medical Fitness Association as the number one hospital-based center in the country and received several NOVA 7 awards from *Fitness Management Magazine*, including facility design, pro-

Douglas Ribley, MS, is Development Team member and Director of LifeStyles, the award-winning fitness component of the Akron General Health and Wellness Center. He has been active in a variety of leadership roles in the fitness industry for the past 20 years, having served as executive director of the Houstonian Institute (a successful health and fitness country club in Houston) and vice president of the Steuben Athletic Club (a fitness facility to more than 100 corporations in the Albany area). He has also served on advisory boards to state government, the national fitness industry, and nationwide community service organizations and is an original board member of the Medical Fitness Association.

motion, operations and finance, and exercise programming. As a result of these successes, the hospital is convinced that this is an efficacious approach, and management is exploring the possibility of replicating this type of center throughout the system.

The Health and Wellness Center is a facility of approximately 197,000 square feet with a wide range of clinical and retail components, including diagnostic, outpatient, surgery, rehabilitation, physical medicine practices, and wellness services. Within the Center, the LifeStyles facility is strictly a membership component. The entire project has been extremely successful financially. The clinical focus of these various services has meshed very successfully with the mission and purpose of the hospital. Cross-referrals are now generated in both directions. Understandably, the people who use this center build a relationship with the health system, so that when they need hospital services, our facility is their preference. Membership surveys bear this out (Akron General LifeStyles, Membership Demographic Statistics, 1996–2000; International Health, Racquet, and Sports Association, 2000).

The project began about 8 years ago, through planning efforts by the health administration to determine the future trends affecting the health care market. In health care organizations traditionally focused on disease, illness, and injury, there has been an evolution toward systems that include prevention, early detection, and outpatient treatment. In the past decade, many hospitals have considered expanding the continuum of care. The difference at Akron General is that the health system believed in the concept so strongly that it reached into its metaphorical pocket, pulled out $35 million, and built a center that embodies this new paradigm. The Health and Wellness Center reflects this expansion in the offerings of a full-service hospital system.

ECONOMIC PROFILE OF THE FITNESS COMPONENT

The fitness unit of the new center, LifeStyles, opened in November 1996, following a 6-month presale in which memberships to the facility were marketed before the building was actually available for use. As a result, the center opened with an enrollment of 2,600 members. That presale was very important to the success of the project.

Once the fitness unit became operational, it led the project for the first 2 years of the program. Now that the program has been in operation for 4 years, all of the other departments are experiencing success and in some cases have surpassed the fitness membership component (Akron General LifeStyles, Responsibility Summaries, 1996–2000). This is understandable, because it requires time for the clinical programs to become established. Physicians develop preferences in their referral patterns; these habits and preferences do not change immediately.

In contrast, the LifeStyles unit has been successful since its opening, despite the fact that it was initially considered the greatest area of risk because it required so much square footage in the facility. Since that time, the revenue stream has been steady and building. The LifeStyles program has experienced significant growth every year and, in 1999, membership generated a net profit of approximately 22% of LifeStyles' total revenue (Akron General LifeStyles, Responsibility Summaries, 1996–2000). The success of the program has exceeded expectations.

The fitness component offers another advantage to the health system—cash retail business. In the context of a large multifaceted institution with all the inherent reimbursement issues, the LifeStyles program is a viable retail business. On the first of every month, the business manager pushes a button on the computer, and a significant amount of cash is automatically deposited into the hospital's account through electronic fund transfer and credit card debit.

This has been a new experience for the administration, which has been accustomed to struggling with insurance companies to obtain 50 or 60 cents on a dollar. This money has helped to support the entire health system. At this point, Akron's administration and board of trustees are confident in this concept and are considering replicating this model elsewhere in our service area. Hospital administrators from all over the country come to visit us regularly. This appears to be a reflection of interest in programs on prevention by health systems as they become interested in expanding their continuum of services. The Health and Wellness Center, which is now 4 years old, is one of the most financially successful centers of this kind in the nation.

THE OUTPATIENT CENTER: A CONTINUUM OF SERVICES

Outpatient Services

The Health and Wellness Center is a 197,000-square-foot outpatient facility that provides the complete continuum of medical services.

Diagnostic Unit. The Center offers a full range of diagnostic capabilities: cardiopulmonary function, magnetic resonance imaging (MRI), X-ray, computed tomography (CT), ultrasound, and other state-of-the-art technology. There is also a women's breast health center that provides mammography and bone densitometry.

Outpatient Surgery. To respond to the needs of patients using these diagnostic services, the outpatient center is designed to provide all of the outpatient services necessary for treatment. The outpatient surgery center includes four state-of-the-art outpatient surgical suites and two endoscopy suites. Consequently, there is extensive capacity to diagnose disease and treat illness within the Center. Outpatient treatment is available on site: The building also includes 37,000 square feet of physician office space, which is fully occupied.

Wellness Programs and Facilities

Rehabilitation Programs. Following treatment, services are available for rehabilitation, including sports medicine, physical therapy, neurotherapy, occupational therapy, and cardiopulmonary rehabilitation. In sum, the Center offers diagnostics, treatment, rehabilitation, and prevention.

Lifestyle Modification and Fitness. Patients frequently require services for secondary prevention following rehabilitation. To complete the continuum of care, they can enroll in the LifeStyles unit, a membership facility focused on the prevention and treatment of lifestyle-related disease and illness through physical activity and lifestyle modification. The LifeStyles unit constitutes the largest portion of the facility, occupying a site of 56,000 square feet. Overall, the basic premise is to provide all components under one roof, offering the complete continuum of care.

Conference Center and Amenities. The Center also includes conference facilities with five rooms of various sizes. The largest can accommodate up to 300 people in a classroom style setting and is used for a range of activities from medical conferences to receptions. The conference area is basically available to the general public for any type of public event. Frequently, it is the site of wedding receptions. There is also a restaurant, the Crystal Cafe, that serves healthy entrees. The cafe also offers the option of hamburgers and french fries, but people who want to eat in a healthy way can do so in this cafe.

Day Spa. The most recent addition to the building is the spa. In the development of the wellness center, one of the goals was to provide spa services to address an aspect of health and wellness that involves relaxation and personal rejuvenation. The original intention was to provide these services in-house. However, a joint venture was arranged with Mario's International Spa, an organization in Northeast Ohio that has provided spa services successfully for more than 20 years, ranked as one of the top 10 spas in the country. The spa is housed in a 2,300-square-foot area adjoining the exercise facility. Spa services include manicures, pedicures, facials, massage therapy, paraffin treatments, seaweed wraps, mud treatments, hydrotherapy, and complete hair and beauty services, for example. Those services have been extremely successful for the Center.

The Fitness Component

LifeStyles offers all services that one would expect to find in a state-of-the-art health fitness or wellness center for both cardiovascular training and muscular strength and endurance. The facility includes more than 200 pieces of computerized cardiovascular exercise equipment, six full circuits of strength-training equipment, and a six-lane, 25-yard competition swimming pool.

The Pool. A complete schedule of water exercise classes is offered in the pool area, including kayaking and canoeing programs, so it is in constant use. The pool is used for swimming lessons to youth and master swim teams. The Center has also donated pool use to the local school system for its high school swim team; the pool serves as the team's home pool. The facility includes a therapy pool, a 20-yard pool with 2.5 lanes that is kept at 93 or 94 degrees. It is used primarily for physical therapy patients, but LifeStyles members also have access to it at designated times.

Weight Training and Fitness. There is a 2,000-square-foot free-weight area, and there are two group exercise studios. Seventy exercise classes are offered each week. Classes range from T'ai chi to aerobics, including high-impact and low-impact classes, step-and-slide aerobics, and boxing. There are also classes in group cycling, yoga, Pilates, karate, and many other programs. There is a full high-school-size gymnasium used for adult volleyball and basketball leagues and tournaments, as well as for open gym time. A running track is located above the gym, on the perimeter of the building. The gymnasium is also used extensively by the cardiopulmonary rehab program for its patients and by physical therapy for gait analysis and other activities that require more space.

Facilities for Children. The LifeStyles unit offers a program called KidStyles, which is a fitness center for children 6 through 12 years old. That program is conducted in an area of the center that provides reduced-size strength-training equipment designed for circuit training with lighter weights. The goal is to instill exercise habits in young people, rather than to emphasize heavy weight training. The scaled-down equipment and weights allow the children to become accustomed to the equipment and to expand their range of motion using proper technique. LifeStyles also hosts summer and winter camps for children. During the school year, there are weekend sports-enhancement programs.

AN INTEGRATED REHABILITATION UNIT

The LifeStyles Center has been recognized as one of the most successful hospital-based centers in the country, receiving several national awards. The program has been described as the first to successfully integrate rehabilitative clinical services into a membership component focused on preventive services. The general concept has received a great deal of attention as a rational approach to the continuum of care. This approach suggests that costs savings can be achieved with the variety of economies that result when duplication is avoided through pro-

gram integration. This cost-effective programming allows the provision of better services and programs at a reduced price. Historically, very few health systems have been able to integrate services successfully.

Achieving Economies by Avoiding Duplication

Nationwide, there are many facilities across the country that describe themselves as integrated. We have visited a number of these facilities. Many of them have a beautiful fitness facility, but their physical therapy departments completely duplicate all the same exercise equipment provided in the fitness center. When a cardiopulmonary rehab unit is included, it is housed in a separate environment with another set of staff and more of the same equipment found in the fitness and the physical therapy areas. These centers have been described as integrated because they are under the same roof, but they do not enjoy the true economies that come with total integration.

In the Health and Wellness Center, there is no duplication of services. The rehab and the fitness components share staff, exercise equipment, and space in the 56,000-square-foot LifeStyles fitness unit. In sharing, we have access to more of everything, but our costs are lower. Consequently, integration has been an important factor in our success.

There is no wall separating these two programs. The patients and members are totally intermingled throughout the exercise area. This enables the Center to provide exceptionally well-trained staff to both patients and members, including exercise physiologists, cardiopulmonary rehab nurses, physical therapists, and personal and athletic trainers. Consequently, a tremendous amount of expertise is present in the facility and available to clients and members at any given time. All patients and clients have access to a wide variety of equipment in a roomy, expansive environment. Because these different programs share space, they also share building costs and other operating costs. As a result, Life-

Styles is able to deliver very high-quality services at a very reasonable price, creating a major breakthrough in programming within health and wellness facilities.

Benefits of the Integrated Approach

Benefits to Patients

Over the years, many of the professionals in this field have expressed the belief that it is not possible to program for rehabilitation patients and healthy club members together in the same environment. The Health and Wellness Center has accomplished that, and the result has been tremendously positive. Patients pulling oxygen tanks behind them exercise side-by-side with apparently healthy people. We have many clients in wheelchairs and many with orthopedic and mobility issues. Patients report that they find it normalizing to be exercising along with club members who have no apparent health problem. As they exercise, mixed in with the healthy people in the center, it is a reminder that they have something to strive for.

Benefits to Members

The inclusion of the rehabilitation program in the fitness center broadens the range of ability among participants and, if anything, increases the comfort level of older club members who are able-bodied. Healthy members come to appreciate their own health and the level of fitness they have achieved through their efforts. Members also experience a certain sense of freedom. Life-Styles is not the type of environment in which members have to be wearing the right clothes or makeup. This is a medical fitness facility. The average age of our primary member is 48 years old (the center now has 7,900 members). That can be compared to the commercial club industry norm, in which the average age is 32 years old. The program has attracted a somewhat older population.

An Expanded Clientele

More than 50% of our members have never been a member of a health club before (Akron General LifeStyles, Member Survey Results, 1996–2000). These are typically people who know they should be involved in fitness and who want to do something to better their health, who want to reduce their incidence of morbidity and live longer through involvement in a physical activity program. Our members would likely feel uncomfortable in a commercial health club, where everyone may seem younger and healthier. This can be an intimidation factor and can affect the motivation for fitness. However, our members are comfortable in the LifeStyles program. The facility is glamorous, but we serve such a broad range of clients of different ages, abilities, and fitness levels that the intimidation factor has been removed. As a result, the program takes on some of the sense of a big family of people who have mutual respect as they all work together to better their health and wellness on all levels.

Relationships with the Community

Participation in the Center also grows out of long-standing relationships that the hospital has built throughout the community over many years. Participants came to us when they were sick or when they had their babies, so there is a level of confidence in this particular health system. Consequently, when it is time to make the decision about choosing a fitness program, they feel comfortable coming into this setting.

Advantages of a Hospital-Sponsored Facility

Our members are also here because they believe, correctly, that we provide a very high level of expertise. They are in an environment that is safe, with people who are qualified to answer their questions about improving their health. Another issue for many of our members is cleanliness. Our focus groups have indicated that a significant number of potential members were motivated to join because they were concerned about cleanliness and believed that a hospital-based facility would adhere to hospital standards of cleanliness. That was an important consideration expressed in the focus groups and later in the member surveys of those who had elected membership (Akron General Life-Styles, Member Survey Results, 1996–2000; Focus Group Summary, 1995).

REPLICATING THE PROJECT

Over the long term, the health system plans to make this type of service and programming available to the entire community that we serve in the Akron and Summit County area, which is our greater community and our target market. We are currently located in the northwest portion of Summit County, so our services are not yet available to everyone in our locale. Eventually, we would like to provide these services to all of the potential clients within our market.

When we initiated this project, there was concern that it might draw business away from the hospital. This is also a question that is frequently raised when we are hosting site visits for other hospitals considering this type of project. Our experience has been that, after four years of operation, we have not reduced utilization of the hospital in any way. Other centers around the country are reporting similar findings. Rather, the Health and Wellness Center has added a new revenue stream to the economic basis of our health system. When the Center conducted a member survey, we found that 30% of our respondents indicated that they are using Akron General clinical services or seeing physicians in the health system for the first time (Akron General LifeStyles, Member Survey Results, 1996–2000). That phenomenon has been consistent since opening.

A unit for complementary medicine is anticipated. The center has had some challenges in obtaining physician support as it relates to the complementary medicine component. The first step in the inclusion of complementary approaches was the spa, which encompasses massage therapy and related services. Over time, the addition of acupuncture, chiropractic services, and nutriceutical products may be considered. The Health and Wellness Center is the logical place to integrate these services and products into the health system.

Convenience is another important factor in our success. The Center would not be as successful as it has been without the inclusion of the clinical components. The program provides services that expand the continuum of care. In the Center, the LifeStyles program is part of that continuum, and we coexist with the diagnostic, surgery, and rehabilitative services that are located here. It reflects a logical progression in the range of services, all focused in one location that is convenient for our patients and members.

REFERENCES

Akron General LifeStyles. Focus Group Summary. Akron, OH; 1995.

Akron General LifeStyles. Member Survey Results. Akron, OH: Akron General Health System; 1996, 1997, 1998, 1999, 2000.

Akron General LifeStyles. Membership Demographic Statistics. Akron, OH: Akron General Health System; 1996, 1997, 1998, 1999, 2000.

Akron General LifeStyles. Responsibility Summaries. Akron, OH: Akron General Health System; 1996, 1997, 1998, 1999, 2000.

International Health, Racquet and Sports Association (IRHSA). Industry Survey. Boston: IRHSA; 2000.

CHAPTER 47

Relationship-Centered Service: St. Charles Medical Center

Nancy S. Moore

OVERVIEW

St. Charles Medical Center is a 181-bed regional-referral tertiary care hospital. It is the largest hospital in Oregon east of the Cascade Mountains with a 25,000-square-mile service area and receives all types of patients. The hospital provides heart surgery and cardiac care; trauma care for the region, including the services of an air ambulance; and rehabilitation. Smaller hospitals refer their complex patients to St. Charles. The only type of intervention that is not provided is organ transplantation.

A decade ago, like many hospitals the executive team at the medical center conducted an environmental assessment and realized the need to restructure the services that the hospital provided. Health care was becoming too expensive. The leadership began to analyze ways in which services could reorganize to improve cost-effectiveness and patient outcomes while enhancing the organization's mission.

Nancy S. Moore, RN, MS, PhD, is vice president and one of the founders of Healing Health Services at St. Charles Medical Center in Bend, Oregon. Her educational background includes degrees in nursing and in counseling and a PhD from Greenwich University, having studied under Leland Kaiser. She is also a member of Kaiser Consulting Services. With more than three decades of experience as a practicing hospital nurse and administrator, she has both experiential and theoretical knowledge of health care in this country. Ms. Moore is listed in the *National Distinguished Registry in Nursing* (1988) and *Who's Who in American Nursing* (1990–1993), and she is coauthor of *Patient-Focused Healing* (Jossey-Bass, 1993).

The efforts of the hospital to maximize services appear to be making a difference. A recent Press, Ganey survey (2000) indicated exceptionally high levels of patient satisfaction. In addition, hospital costs have dropped. St. Charles continues to be a good investment for its community (Center for Healthcare Industry Performance Studies, 1995–2000).

- The medical center is now one of the lowest-cost hospitals in the nation.
- In 1999, St. Charles was in the top 3% of patient ratings among more than 500 U.S. hospitals in terms of both satisfaction and overall rating (Press, Ganey, 2000).
- The medical center provides community-focused services. For example, following the initiation of a program to increase prenatal care, in 1999, only 5 mothers of 1,270 who delivered at St. Charles were lacking prenatal care (St. Charles Medical Center, 2000).

SUPPORTING THE PROVIDERS

Maximizing the Service Ethic

The focus of service improvement is the enhancement of the hospital's healing mission and the development of the healing health care philosophy. We evaluated a great deal of research focused on outcomes—on what works. A team from the hospital went on site visits, performed literature reviews, and looked at other types of programs, such as the Planetree model. The team visited California Pacific Medical Center in San Francisco and saw its new integrative clinic and resource library. Visits were made to other medical centers that were applying an integrative model. Inspiration and ideas were drawn from these programs and from the research and applied to the medical center.

One of the most unique aspects of St. Charles as an organization involves its emphasis on the quality of patient care. A primary way this is achieved is through investment in the personal growth and development of the care providers. We realized early on that, fundamentally, we are a *human* service. The hospital is very conscious that it is an organization in which services are provided *to* people *by* people. Who we are and how we work together are what our patients receive. Consequently, we invest a great deal in the quality of relationships—provider to patient, provider to provider, and hospital to community (Tresolini, 1994).

We have created an intentional culture that is relationship-based by providing:

- workshops—People-Centered Teams: Healing the Workplace™
- one-on-one coaching
- structured processes that build these concepts into the day-to-day work life of each department.

Everyone in the organization is considered a caregiver. Clearly, the nurses and the care associates are the closest to the patient. However, even the Chief Executive Officer is viewed as a caregiver because, ultimately, his efforts affect patient care. If his efforts are not intended to support patient healing, the organization will be less successful in addressing its mission.

We came to realize this phenomenon early on. I was working with a hospital task force to design patient services when one of the nurses raised her hand and said, "What about us?" My first thought was "Oh, we'll get to us, but first we have to take care of the patients." Over time, it became very clear through the dialogue in health care that it would not matter what we created for patients if we did not heal ourselves and our relationships in the process. It would not

matter whether we studied what patients needed and designed ideal care teams. Organizational changes would be an empty shell if we did not have staff members who were themselves cared for in the process.

Staff nurturing and team cohesion also affect patient outcomes. Research (Knaus et al, 1986) indicates that patients' lives may depend on the quality of the collaborative relationships between nurses and physicians reflected in the continuity of care. Researchers at George Washington University Medical Center, in Washington, DC, studied the treatment and outcome of 5,030 patients in intensive care units at 13 tertiary care hospitals. Outcomes were predicated on a number of variables, including scores from the APACHE (Acute Physiology and Chronic Health Evaluations), which predict the chances of each patient's survival. The research found that the accuracy of this prediction varied depending on the patient's assignment of hospital location. In the units with the greatest rates of survival, 55% more patients lived than had been predicted. In those with the worst survival rates, 58% more patients died than anticipated. After careful study of these surprising findings, the researchers concluded that the significant variables between the most and least effective units were the collaborative relationships between nurses and physicians, based on mutual respect and trust, as well as staff autonomy and the continuity of care.

DEVELOPING TEAM TRAINING

Out of this approach, two-and-one-half-day seminars were developed, *People-Centered Teams: Healing the Workplace*. Initially, our caregivers were not accustomed to this focus, so the project gathered momentum slowly. However, we found that the seminars touched a deep need for those who work in health care. Over time, the seminars became known in the medical community, and eventually we had an enormous waiting list. People were eager to have the opportunity to develop themselves. We created healing health care coaches who assisted people in use of these skills when they returned to the workplace. We found that they were using the skills not only in patient care and in their team relationships, but also with their family and their children. At this point, our entire hospital staff has participated in this approach, including approximately 30% of our physicians.

This workshop process involves small groups and large groups, training, and information sharing. The workshops are built on the perspective that everyone in the organization is a caregiver. The hierarchy of the workplace is suspended in the workshops. In the philosophy and in the actual workshop, everyone is viewed as a caregiver. The workshop is conducted with staff that includes people from different levels of organizational authority participating side by side. Consequently a mix of management, physicians, nurses, housekeepers, and others all participate together in any given workshop. This is impor-

tant—it helps people to see people as people and not just their job titles. We see people as human beings who are all vulnerable, feel insecure sometimes, and make mistakes. This aspect of the process has been very powerful in helping the organization move away from the "us-versus-them" mentality.

To create the right emotional and psychological environment, we have found that staff need a range of capabilities focused on processes for personal empowerment, gaining a greater sense of control, and increasing accountability:

- some enhancement of skills, particularly communication skills
- time to explore values and vision
- awareness of ways to develop one's own consciousness
- additional skills in group process
- personal time for healing.

WORKSHOPS FOR PEOPLE-CENTERED TEAMS

WORKSHOP CONTENT

Organizational Overview

- *Shifting Organizational Standards*—Creating a context from historical patterns.
- *Social Context*—Reflections on moving from agrarian to industrial to information/service age, viewing the organization in the context of national consciousness.

Personal Values and Vision

- *Personal Vision Development*—Designing our future and aligning with organizational vision as a vehicle for success.
- *Stages of Change*—A road map for navigating our ever-changing lives.

Awareness and Attitude

- *Internal Drivers*—Identifying underlying intentions: To avoid pain or to learn and grow (seek pleasure or happiness). Short-term versus long-term vision: How do we strengthen our capacity to be involved for the long term and be responsive in the moment. Choice is in the present moment, yet the outcome is a long-term one.
- *Comfort Zone*—Building a strategy for learning and growing: How to develop learning in the "safe zone of discomfort."

continues

Workshop Content *continued*

- *Levels of Accountability*—How to recognize these levels and realign intentions: Is my current action supporting my desired outcome?
- *The Awareness Wheel*—A focus on differentiation, which includes clarifying our internal experience and communicating more effectively: Skills for decreasing reactivity and keeping people in the place of choice.
- *Drama Triangle*—How we play and how we stop this dynamic that can be highly destructive to relationships and organizations.
- *Mind Traps*—Recognizing common traps of habitual thinking: How they keep us from getting what we want and rob us of the gift of presence.
- *Assumptions and Choices*—How we can learn to see opportunities in what initially appear to be threats or challenges.

Communication Skills

- *Compassionate Listening*—The power of therapeutic presence, which is one of our most powerful tools for healing. Listening not just to the content but also for the meaning and checking for clarity and the intention.
- *Conflict Resolution*—Skill enhancement for dealing with conflict and mistakes.
- *Appreciation Exercise*—Noticing what is right and using gratitude to build team capacity.

Group Development

- *Myers-Briggs Type Indicator*—Understanding differences and appreciating diversity on a team.
- *Group Differentiation*—Where groups get stuck and how to get them moving again.
- *Group Development*—Predictable stages groups go through in becoming interdependent and how to support positive growth and development: The importance of personal leadership of all group members in the functioning of the group.
- *Decision Model*—Clarifying how decisions are made in organizations: Assumptions around decisions are one of the major destroyers of trust on teams and in organizations.
- *Group Values Clarification*—Defining group values: How will we work together? What are our shared beliefs and desires?
- *Group Process*—Exercises in a small group.

SETTING SERVICE STANDARDS

Relating Vision and Training to Performance

We also created structured processes to support the use of the skills and attitudes of a relationship- and accountability-based culture. We used IMPAQ Accountability-Based Improvement Systems to support this process (Samuel, 2000). Each department defines its:

- vision and assesses how it fits into the overall vision of the hospital.
- success factors that describe how all areas of the department will look when it is achieving its vision

• interaction agreement—to set a consensus statement of its intention for the team and how they will work together to accomplish it.

Programs That Operationalize Values

Ongoing Team Support. Within every patient care area, there are nurses who are identified as healing health care resources. This approach developed out of recommendations by a quality improvement team for pain management (St. Charles Medical Center, 1998). The resource person receives intensive education in providing guided imagery, therapeutic touch, and relaxation, using breathing techniques and therapeutic presence. Many are trained in therapeutic touch as well as how to assess the sensory environment and its healing properties. They will serve as resources within their patient care area to teach other staff members, coach them, and support them in learning these skills.

Service-Focused Performance Appraisal. We have developed service standards around these relationship skills, which are built into the performance appraisal process (see Exhibit 47–1), focused in four areas:

• safety
• therapeutic presence
• excellence
• healing environment.

Community Workshops. We now also offer the workshops in the community. One of our largest medical clinics requires that all new doctors participate in this consciousness-raising seminar. We have found that other organizations are interested in the seminars. St. Charles staff provide workshops to other hospitals and communities, as well as train trainers to provide them.

RESOURCES FOR PATIENTS

The Planetree philosophy has influenced the way in which the hospital and its staff view patient-centered care and the involvement of the family.

A Range of Therapeutic Approaches

Accommodations. For the families of patients who are here for a long stay, rooms have been remodeled so that families can stay with patients and learn their care while providing emotional support.

Using the Environment as a Tool for Healing. We have sought to integrate these approaches into the environment. One of the principles that guides our awareness is that everything in the environment has an effect on healing—it can either enhance or impair. Very little is just neutral. Consequently, our intention is very important, whatever our sphere of influence, in the process of enhancing the healing potential of the environment. This can be as simple as picking up trash from the floor or selecting a soothing color of paint for the walls.

Music. We have also explored the healing qualities of music. Music systems that can be purchased by hospitals include audio and video components available for television transmission. This is called the Continuous Ambient Relaxation Environment (the CARE channel, Healing Health Care Systems) (Mazer and Smith, 1995). Years ago, nurses used a variation of this. When patients could not sleep, nurses would turn on a weather channel or pop music. Now there is a video channel designed to meet that need that has music programmed for the day-night cycle. At night, it provides a star scene with very peaceful music. The music and visuals are more stimulating during the day, featuring an ocean or some other type of natural scene.

Other Forms of Creativity. The health system uses other forms of creativity and art in the hospital. We found that once people learned that we were open to this creative approach, many people from the community came forward to

Exhibit 47–1 St. Charles Medical Center Caregiver Service Standards

Values in Action

Indicate the percent of time the caregiver met the standard. (Example: 0% not met standard and 100% always met standard)

	0–20%	20–40%	40–60%	60–80%	80–100%

Safety—To protect the physical, emotional, mental, and spiritual well-being of SCMC patients, guests, and caregivers.

1. I maintain an environment that protects patients, guests, and caregivers from harm.
2. I protect the confidentiality of patients, guests, and caregivers.
3. I assist patients/families in making informed choices about care.

Therapeutic Presence—To be present for others with an intention of healing or enhancing healing, respecting the sacredness of life and uniqueness of each person.

1. I introduce myself to patients, guests, and other caregivers.
2. I ask patients, guests, and other caregivers how they wish to be addressed.
3. I listen for meaning as well as content, and ask questions or repeat information for clarification.
4. I represent SCMC in a caring professional manner with my personal appearance and behavior.
5. I do not involve patients or guests in internal issues.

Excellence—To demonstrate improvement with the intention to learn and grow as individuals, and as an organization.

1. When presented with a problem or request, I personally take care of it. If I must transfer the request to someone else, I stay in touch with the patient, guest, or caregiver and follow up to make sure the request is being dealt with.
2. I do what I agree to do, and communicate about delays to patients, guests, and caregivers.
3. I anticipate and respond to patient, guest, and caregiver needs.
4. I honor patient, guest, and caregiver preferences.

Healing Environment—To create physical surroundings that promote healing through sight, sound, smell, taste, and touch.

1. I protect and maintain the privacy of patients, guests, and caregivers.
2. I assist in maintaining a clean environment throughout the hospital campus.
3. I ensure activities, processes, and procedures are convenient for patients, guests, and caregivers.
4. I demonstrate awareness and maintenance of the healing potential of the sense environment (sight, sound, smell, taste, touch).

Courtesy of St. Charles Medical Center, Bend, Oregon.

volunteer. We have professional clowns who provide humor. We have invited compassionate performers who make rounds and visit patients with their repertoire: Patients can choose poetry or song. We even have harpists. In some cases, we have invested in the education of performers, such as the Chalice of Repose, which provides music to facilitate the dying process.

End-of-Life Care. St. Charles Medical Center leads a community-based quality end-of-life care coalition. This coalition includes hospitals, physicians, hospices, long-term care, and community members. The coalition provides education to providers and the public, enhancing awareness of the needs of people in the dying process. As a result of the coalition's recommendation, St. Charles provides a comfort care team and a comfort care unit. The team includes a nursing case manager, pharmacist, social worker, pastoral care, hospice staff, and nursing. The case manager ensures the continuity of care for patients throughout the hospital and, once they return home, under the care of the hospice. The team provides pharmaceuticals as well as therapeutic presence, the life story process, and spiritual care. The accomplishments of the team are encouraging. Our region was cited on Oregon Public Broadcasting (OPBS) as having the most supportive programs for the dying process in the country.

Cancer Support. The cancer services program has worked closely with community volunteers. Their efforts have evolved into a project named after a teacher in our community, Sara Fisher, who died of breast cancer. People wanted to do something to memorialize her, so volunteers came together and developed a comprehensive program. *The Sara Fisher Project* offers free mammography for low-income women and education in the public schools. As the project evolved, they were able to obtain grant funding from the Coleman Foundation. They developed a coalition among the seven counties in their service area, county health departments, and community members to form the women's health coalition.

Currently, for our service area, our detection of cancer at the early stage is 73% and has been as high as 84% (St. Charles Medical Center, 1996–2000). The U.S. average is 49%, so we continue to provide the national benchmark for the early detection of breast cancer. This program is a tremendous reflection of partnerships focused on education and prevention—relationships between physicians, community members, and the community health departments. The women who are involved in this project are highly dedicated. Through their volunteer efforts, they have doubled the success rate in our region.

The Health Coach. In this program, health coaches meet with clients, in collaboration with their primary care physician. The coaches are registered nurses who have extensive training and experience in clinical nursing, wellness education, and group facilitation, and provide assistance in:

- identifying health problems, concerns, and risk factors
- identifying areas in clients' lives that may be out of balance
- developing personal action goals
- creating a health action plan to assist clients in meeting goals, including follow-up, support, and referrals, as needed or desired.

Life Choice Seminar. This one-day seminar is intended to increase awareness of how day-to-day choices impact health and well-being, based on the concepts of the mind-body-spirit connection. Participants define personal health, identify the life patterns that get in the way of having the health they want, and target ways in which to overcome those barriers and become more accountable in creating personal health.

HealthyStart. Our HealthyStart program reflects similar partnership principles. Prenatal care is now a priority for every health care professional and agency in this medical community: The physicians, the public health department, and the hospital have all joined forces to improve prenatal care. As a result, in 1999, only 5 mothers of 1,270 who delivered at St. Charles were lacking prenatal care.

THE MEDICAL SYMPTOM REDUCTION PROGRAM

The Medical Symptom Reduction Program is a course for patients or members of the community, developed to assist in the management of symptoms associated with chronic conditions such as diabetes, heart disease, hypertension, chronic pain, panic disorder, digestive disorders, fibromyalgia, insomnia, or hyperlipidemia. It is designed after a similar program initially developed by the Harvard Mind-Body Medicine Program.

The program is intended for clients who desire assistance with:

- management of medical symptoms
- decreased need for medications or improved response to medications
- health-promoting behaviors.

Participants may enter the program either through self-referral or by referral from their physician. Participants are evaluated using the Personal Wellness Profile, which is also communicated to their primary care physicians with their permission. The intention of the program is to work in collaboration with the primary care provider to promote greater continuity and quality of care.

All participants receive a comprehensive assessment and health history that is administered by a nurse and reviewed by an interdisciplinary team that includes a physician. The Personal Wellness Profile is used as part of the assessment process. No pharmaceutical prescriptions are given through the program, and any medication changes are handled through the participant's primary care providers.

Program Timeline

The program is held for 10 weeks. At the beginning and end of the series, a comprehensive Personal Wellness Profile is completed. Laboratory tests are performed at weeks 1 and 10 to evaluate levels of lipid profiles and fasting glucose.

During the course, participants meet once a week for three hours. A weekly progress report is completed by the participant at each session and reviewed by the health coach and the medical director. Progress reports include symptoms experienced during the week; use of drugs, alcohol, and cigarettes; exercise (type of exercise and how much); stress perception (triggers and resulting behaviors); use of relaxation techniques; weight; blood pressure; and pulse. Participants keep a workbook that helps them to track health-related goals at each session.

Each three-hour session includes the following:

- general health and wellness
- health and the mind-body-spirit connection
- stress mastery
- social support and communication
- spirituality and life purpose
- maintaining changes
- nutrition
- exercise and physiology
- movement/exercise
- yoga and T'ai chi
- relaxation response
- small group process

Most insurance companies reimburse for this program, and billing is performed through St. Charles Medical Center. Profits go directly to the Center for Health and Medicine at St. Charles. The goal is to provide this program three times a year.

OUTCOMES

St. Charles Medical Center uses a variety of methods to measure the outcomes of its programs. As the major tertiary medical center for all of central and much of eastern Oregon, we serve a diverse population and receive many complex cases (MECON, 1999). For 2000, our case mix index (CMI) is comparatively high at 1.41, and our total costs per adjusted discharge and adjusted for case mix (CMA) is $4,928, lower than most hospitals. Since we initiated this series of approaches, patient accidents have dropped 33% (St. Charles Medical Center, 1999). Employee lost time accidents have dropped. In 1997, St. Charles Medical Center won the Oregon Quality Award. In that same year, an outside research group performed customer research in the community and found that more than 90% of respondents indicated high confidence in our services (Endresen Research, 1999). In recent years, we have twice been recognized in the top 100 hospitals by HCIA (HCIA and Mercer Management Consulting, 1993, 1994). Our hope is that the data and the awards indicate that we are on the right track.

REFERENCES

Center for Healthcare Industry Performance Studies. *Operating Performance Report, St. Charles Medical Center, Bend, Oregon.* Columbus, OH, 1995–2000.

Endresen Research. *St. Charles Medical Center, Bend, Oregon, Survey of Community Residents.* Final Report. Seattle, WA, 1/1999.

HCIA and Mercer Management Consulting. *100 Top Hospitals: Benchmarks for Success.* Baltimore, MD, and New York, 1993, 1994.

Knaus W, Draper E, Wagner D, Zimmerman J. An evaluation of outcome from intensive care in major medical centers. *Ann Intern Med.* 1986;104(3):410–418.

Mazer S, Smith D. Continuous Ambient Relaxation Environment (CARE) Channel, Healing HealthCare Systems, Reno, NV; 1995.

MECON. Assessment of Comparative Performance and Labor Productivity Improvement Opportunity. San Ramon, CA; 1999.

Moore N, Komras H. *Patient-Focused Healing.* San Francisco: Jossey-Bass, Publishers; 1993.

Press, Ganey Associates. *Press, Ganey Satisfaction Measurement, St. Charles Medical Center, Bend, Oregon, 1/1/200–3/31/2000.* South Bend, IN; 2000.

St. Charles Medical Center. *HealthyStart Prenatal Service Quarterly Report.* Bend, OR; 2000.

St. Charles Medical Center. *Pain Management Performance Excellence Process Team, Performance Process Committee Report.* Bend, OR; 1998.

St. Charles Medical Center. *Performance Excellence Process (PEP) Committee, Quality Satisfaction Indicators (Patient Accidents).* Bend, OR; 1999.

St. Charles Medical Center, Tumor Registry, Central Oregon Cancer Database, Bend, OR; 1996–2000.

Samuel M. *The Accountability Revolution: Achieving Breakthrough Results in Half the Time.* Orange, CA: IMPAQ® Publishing; 2000.

Tresolini CP, Pew-Fetzer Task Force. *Health Professions Education and Relationship-Centered Care.* San Francisco, CA: Pew Health Professions Commission, 1994.

CHAPTER 48

Reinventing the Health Improvement Company: Riverside Health System

M. Caroline Martin with Nancy Faass

REDEFINING THE HEALTH SYSTEM

The Riverside Health System began as a single hospital in 1916. The health system currently includes three acute care hospitals, a physical rehabilitation hospital, a psychiatric hospital, a number of nursing homes, six wellness and fitness centers, a physician organization, ambulatory services such as dialysis units, and a freestanding day surgery center. The system is an integrated delivery network that serves the peninsula of southeastern Virginia.

In recognition of the innovative efforts of Riverside to improve access to care in the community, in 1999 the health system received the Community Benefit Award, presented by National Health, Inc. This honor provides a benchmark of the institution's efforts over more than a decade to develop practical tools that improve community health, which include:

- a health self-assessment profile that has been taken by more than 37,000 people in the community

M. Caroline Martin, RN, MHA, is the president/CEO of Riverside Regional Medical Center and executive vice president of Riverside Health System, one of the largest nonprofit health care systems in Virginia. She earned her degree in nursing, Phi Beta Kappa, from the University of Maine and a graduate degree in health care administration from the Medical College of Virginia. Her career includes extensive experience in hospital and health care administration, and she has served in a leadership capacity within Riverside Health System since 1986. Mrs. Martin is a diplomate of the American College of Healthcare Executives, a board member of the Virginia Hospital Association, and has been an active board member of numerous other health care, community, and charitable organizations.

Courtesy of Riverside Regional Medical Center, Newport News, Virginia.

- self-care resource manuals that have been distributed to more than 68,000 people
- a telephone resource center that has provided more than 1.1 million responses to callers over the past 11 years
- a support group process that is relevant to clients at risk, as well as those in need of disease management.

The system's commitment to community access is also reflected in its programs:

- Wellness/fitness centers that serve more than 20,000 members
- Health screenings—over 32,000 are provided annually throughout the system and by mobile van
- Hundreds of health education classes and programs that reach out to families and individuals throughout the region
- Innovative programs, such as the new biofeedback center, which serves the needs of clients with attention deficit–hyperactivity disorder (ADD/ADHD) and their families; asthma camp for children; and support groups for families at risk
- A range of other targeted programs designed to improve community health and create greater self-responsibility

DEVELOPING A SYSTEMWIDE STRATEGY

Expanding the Continuum of Care

Over the years, Riverside has evolved from a traditional delivery system into a multifaceted health system. With the expansion of our organization into wellness centers and physician groups, our mission now extends beyond caring for the sick. When we realized that the scope of our services had expanded, it became clear that we had to redefine ourselves as an organization. This spurred a reevaluation of our mission and, ultimately, the redefinition of our organization as "the health improvement company."

If Our Mission Extends beyond Caring for Those Who Are Ill, How Do We Define the Health System?

A Communitywide Needs Assessment. We performed an organizationwide needs assessment to evaluate our service delivery and identify gaps in the services we offer to people in the community.

Serving a Broader Population. When we evaluated the disease management component, it was clear that we provide well-developed models of care for those who are ill. However, when we moved up the continuum to those with less intensive needs, we found that our care management processes and protocols were not as well developed. To expand the continuum of care, we realized that we wanted to increase services to additional populations:

- People in the early stages of the disease process with minor symptoms
- Those at risk
- Those who were well but interested in preventive activities

If Our Charge Is To Help Our Clients Improve Their Health, How Do We Accomplish That?

Redefining Service Delivery. This new identity raised additional questions. At Riverside, we have responded to client needs through the identification and the reduction of health-related risk. This essentially involves risk management. In a risk-management model, the first step is to provide preventive services. To successfully and economically manage the incidence of disease in a large population, this is accomplished through

health promotion and risk reduction. When these are not sufficient, the next step is to improve access to care and disease management.

Including a Focus on Health. Our mission to serve the community has expanded from our traditional role as a hospital to include services to those who are well. This process initially involved defining our role more clearly. For our health system, preventive programming means facilitating self-responsibility in our clients. In this process, we found that, like most health care delivery systems, we had not yet fully developed the tools necessary to serve as a resource to the community for prevention and health promotion. Consequently, an important component of this program has been the development of mission statements and tools designed to be utilized by providers at the community level who work with targeted populations in both prevention and risk reduction.

Redefining Health and Health Care. To expand our mission, we also had to redefine the terms *health, health care provider, and customer*. In addition, this has meant identifying and defining who is in charge at different stages of health and disease management and evaluating the strengths and weaknesses of a variety of approaches. We had to redefine the term *health care facility*. Is a fitness center a health care facility? Is the institution reflected only in a bricks-and-mortar facility? Or does it also encompass programs such as support groups in a community setting?

The Role of the Individual. We recognize that even in a well-developed system, the individual ultimately must assume responsibility for his or her own health and health improvement. Our goal is to be the hand on the shoulder—we view ourselves as a limited partner. The individual (formerly the patient) would be the managing partner. The idea that we are facilitators is very important to us. Within our organization, we emphasize the value of empowerment. We provide resources to support the confidence and competence that enable community members to take greater charge of their own health.

Risk Identification. Once we expanded the model to include a clear focus on risk reduction, we also spent a great deal of time developing a model of prevention, access, and management (Exhibit 48–1). We have created a process by which people can identify their risks and access the tools to modify those risks. This perspective involves four steps to risk reduction focused on the individual, but which can be applied to the community as a whole, to determine what needs to be accomplished.

PROGRAMS IN RISK REDUCTION

Well Care Management

Riverside also provides resources to the community to help people reduce their health risks through programs described as well care management. This approach utilizes support groups, health management, and disease management processes. The targeted populations reflect a range of needs that includes specific diseases (diabetes, for example), life stages (such as aging), and psychosocial needs (such as families or teens at risk). The program uses identified

Exhibit 48–1 A Four-Step Process to Risk Reduction

RIVERSIDE S FOUR STEPS TO CLIENT SELF RESPONSIBILITY

1. *Know your risk factors.* Riverside provides annual health risk appraisals free of charge. More than 37,000 members of the community have now taken these appraisals. A summary of the results is forwarded to the community members, their primary care physician, and a resource person within the health system (the well care manager). We consider it vital that community members recognize and understand their own health profiles. The health system pays for the appraisal process as part of its contribution to community members to improve their health.

2. *Use self-care resources at home.* The use of resources is facilitated through in-depth self-care resource manuals, distributed at no cost to community members. To date, more than 68,000 manuals have been provided in our service area, through the 24-hour call center, physician practices, local employers, and by Riverside's own employees, community health events, and civic events, and the manual is distributed in places of worship, through our Parish Nurse Program. Follow-up calls are made 4 months after receipt of the manual to respond to questions and be sure people in the community know how to access the resources provided in the book. Our primary intention is to benefit members of the community. The self-care manuals are also a good form of promotion for the health system's programs and services.

3. *Consult with a health advisor through the call center (Ask-a-Nurse) or a health advisor (well care managers).* Riverside's Ask-A-Nurse telephone resource is now in its 11th year of operation and has provided more than 1.1 million responses to community members, giving health information and referrals. Health advisors facilitate programs and disease management support groups sponsored by the health system to meet a range of needs, from normal pregnancy and parenting to diabetes and heart disease.

4. *Establish a relationship with a physician.* Information provided to the community stresses the importance of working with a primary care physician to maximize continuity of care and minimize use of the emergency room for nonemergent conditions. Referrals to physicians are available through the call center, which includes an extensive database of health care providers categorized by factors such as location, gender, and specialty.

Courtesy of Riverside Regional Medical Center, Newport News, Virginia.

care guidelines and a broad range of resources to assist clients in managing their health conditions and individual needs. Well care management takes a very behavioral approach; clients set specific goals and work toward tangible positive outcomes. The program seeks to provide the resources that individual participants require, whether those are support, health care, or community resources to meet clinical and psychosocial needs (Figure 48–1).

Within the target group, the program is further individualized to the specific needs of each client. For example, in groups focused on diabetes management, participants are provided information on how to eat the right foods, exercise with their particular conditions in mind, and manage their insulin use and regulation. The practical goal in this particular population is to stabilize blood sugar, avoid a crisis lifestyle, and overcome the chronic side effects of poor disease management. For all groups, the ultimate goals are enhanced health and quality of life.

Our goal is also to make available support and advice from the person who is most appropriate (such as the nurse advisors in the call center), and least costly. Practical tools are provided such as the self-evaluation form and the handbook. A foundation of support is provided through resources such as the call center, nurse health advisors, and a range of services within the health system. To streamline the self-assessment process, we have developed and recently licensed a software product in well care management.

Health Promotion for Patients with Chronic Illness

We have found that well care management is an important philosophy that can be utilized no matter where people are on the age or health continuum. We currently have a well care management program within our six dialysis units. Dialysis patients tend to be quite physically compromised, yet we have found that we can do a great deal to improve their health—physically, mentally, and spiritually—regardless of their physiological state. Due to the success of programs of this type, we are now focusing on well care management not only on the individual level but also for targeted populations. It has become apparent that there may still be opportunities to provide health enhancement services for patients with chronic illnesses, such as diabetes or congestive heart failure. Programs designed around a support group model maximize both psychosocial benefit and cost-effectiveness.

Support Groups

The group process draws on the well care management philosophy, but we also ensure that the group facilitators have the clinical expertise to deal with chronic disease. "Living healthy" programs are conducted in a group that serves clients with a particular diagnosis, such as diabetes. In addition to the well care management component, we look at the specific risks associated with their conditions. For example, with diabetes, there is the need for good foot care and an annual retinal exam. The group also provides psychosocial support. When applied to the needs of clients with chronic illness, well care management also incorporates the principles of effective disease management.

PHASING IN INTEGRATIVE MEDICINE

The Institute of Integrative Healing Arts

Programs in Complementary Medicine. Several years ago, Riverside began looking at opportunities to provide complementary medicine in the community and in our traditional medical care system. The health system's advisory committees worked collaboratively to define and describe integrative medicine and its relevance for Riverside's broad range of clients. Through this process, we identified the complementary services we already offer and those that people in the community most rely on. We then reevaluated the gaps in preventive services identified in our needs assessment and considered which forms of complementary medicine would best meet these needs. The evaluation of new

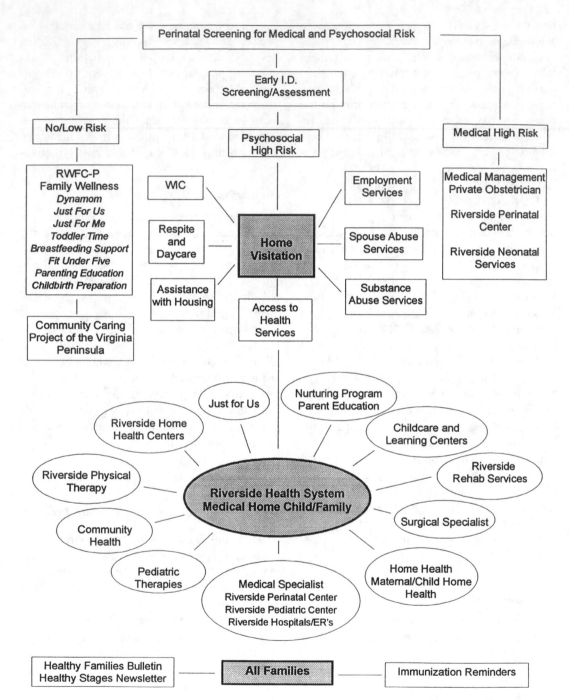

Figure 48–1 The Healthy Families Model. Courtesy of Riverside Regional Medical Center, Newport News, Virginia.

programs and therapies is an ongoing process. Riverside recently initiated the Institute of Integrative Healing Arts through community education programs.

Biofeedback Services. As one of the first initiatives of the Institute, the health system has developed a program of neurotherapy services that will provide biofeedback to the community. Initially, this center focuses on the needs of children and adults with ADD and ADHD. Services include intake and assessments; neurotherapy (including enhancement of academic skills); family support, family education, counseling, and mentoring; and dietary intervention. This approach is also relevant to the needs of clients with epilepsy, head injury, labile affect, depression, and panic attacks.

PROGRAMS IN HEALTH PROMOTION

Fitness Centers

Riverside became involved in the fitness program in 1982 when the opportunity arose to purchase a racquetball club. The wellness/fitness centers have been highly successful, and the health system now owns six centers with more than 20,000 members. Initially, there were concerns that a fitness facility might drain funds from clinical programs. However, the fitness centers have proven to be self-supporting from their inception. The need for medical oversight, initially another issue, has been addressed by providing a medical advisory committee that oversees the program. The fitness facilities provide a tangible bridge between the health system and the community. By offering wellness programming, screenings, and assessments within a fitness facility, Riverside encourages its clients to play a more active role in developing their own personal health.

Health Assessment Services: The Mobile Medical Unit

In addition to its other community outreach efforts (Exhibit 48–2), another aspect of the health system's mission is to maximize access to services and identify clients at risk. The mobile medical unit provides an opportunity to address these needs within the community. Health screenings are provided on site in a motorized 42-foot vehicle staffed by registered nurses. This vehicle makes it possible to respond to the needs of a service area that covers more than 2,000 square miles. The unit is in operation six days a week, providing services at day care centers, schools, libraries, malls, shopping centers, churches, medical clinics, fitness centers, health fairs, community centers, and special events, at two or three sites a day. People in the community can receive free glucose and cholesterol screening and a personal wellness profile. Nursing staff in the mobile unit provide assessment, individualized health education, and referrals on site. The unit also provides blood pressure checks, flu and pneumonia vaccines, free immunizations, information resources, and referrals.

REGIONAL COLLABORATION

To improve the health and quality of life of the community as a whole, we have also created five community health and wellness councils, with representatives from all major departments of the health system, as well as the agencies that provide care to clients at different levels of the continuum. These councils are coordinated by Riverside's department of Community Health Improvement and serve the Virginia Peninsula, the Middle Peninsula, the Northern Neck, Williamsburg, and Smithfield areas. The councils function as multidisciplinary teams, with participants from long-term care, ambulatory and hospital care, outpatient services, rehabilitation, and care management. Together, we evaluate the needs and resources in the community to identify other organizations with similar purpose and to determine how we can collaborate, efficiently and effectively, to improve the quality of health in the community.

Through the coordinated efforts of the councils, we have invested in performance-based planning for improved community health outcomes.

Exhibit 48–2 Community Outreach

Riverside has expanded the population that it considers to be its clients or customers to include all of the 550,000 people within its service area. Some of the services offered annually include:

- *Fitness.* Riverside's six wellness and fitness centers serve more than 20,000 members in rural, suburban, and urban parts of Virginia. The fitness centers have over 16 years of experience and a return of better than 15% on investment.
- *On-site access to health screenings.* A mobile unit annually provides more than 32,000 free screening and health education services to underserved clients in their communities.
- *Telephone call center.* Ask-A-Nurse, a telephone resource, fielded more than 300,000 calls in 1999. Overall, the Health Communications call center at Riverside has responded to more than 1.1 million callers.
- *Personal assessment.* To date, more than 37,000 Personal Wellness Profiles have been distributed.
- *Resource handbooks.* Over 58,000 *Healthwise* handbooks have been provided to community members. Based on a study of the population using the handbook, an average $700,000 in annual cost savings was realized for the health system, due to decreased utilization of the emergency department, urgent care centers, and other physician services (Riverside Health System, 1998).
- *Resource handbook for seniors.* Approximately 10,000 copies of *Healthwise for Life*, a large-print version of the handbook, have been distributed.
- *Family services.* Riverside's Partners in Family Health screens 300 families monthly for appropriate interventions related to child abuse and neglect. The Well Care Management program serves an average of 20 families each month who are referred for intensive, in-home support services and the support groups. Of the families who are referred for support services, 100% elect participation.
- *Health improvement in the schools.* Partnerships with school systems in our region have led to health improvement initiatives touching the lives of more than 5,000 students, including the provision of health education, community speakers, and, in one system, a school-based community health clinic.
- *Health in faith communities.* An ongoing parish nursing program has now graduated dozens of registered nurses who provide health services and outreach in their parishes and communities.
- *Well care management.* Currently, more than 900 individuals are enrolled in support groups that provide wellness, risk reduction, or disease management in areas such as diabetes, cancer, and bereavement, based on the needs of the participants.
- *Community-based initiatives.* Initiatives such as a free clinic are supported by donations and volunteer health care professionals.
- *Transportation.* Riverside's transportation services provide an average of 1,850 services per month to community members.
- *Insurance savings.* Health insurance premiums for Riverside employees have not increased in five years, and in 1998, employees received two months of free premiums as a result of well-controlled insurance claims.

Courtesy of Riverside Regional Medical Center, Newport News, Virginia.

This involves a number of key processes:

- defining the mission and desired outcome (performance improvement methodology)
- linking budget or use of resources closely to performance
- reporting results and holding departments and facilities accountable for results.

With each project, partnership, or initiative, the action plan is examined, updated, and adapted regularly to reflect actual performance, new learning, and any changes in the environment of the project or initiative. This is accomplished through quarterly meetings of the councils. We also perform an audit of the community-based activities provided by all of the health system's departments and facilities. This allows us to annually qualify and quantify our contributions to the community that benefit our constituents and maintain our tax-exempt status. The challenge is the continued restructuring toward preventive and community-based health care. Performance-based planning and quality relationships are the keys to our success.

REFERENCE

Riverside Health System. *Health Utilization Survey*. Riverside Health System Health Communications Department, Newport News, VA; 1998.

CHAPTER 49

Cost Savings through Work Site Health Promotion

Ron Z. Goetzel, Bert H. Jacobson, Steven G. Aldana, Kris Vardell, and Leslie Yee

Total and lifestyle-related medical care costs for employees of a major corporation participating in a work site health promotion program over a three-year period were compared with the costs for nonparticipants in a cross-sectional study. In the third year of the program, the 3,993 participants had significantly lower health care costs ($392 per person), when compared with the 4,341 nonparticipants. Similarly, in the third year of the program, participants had significantly lower inpatient costs, fewer hospital admissions, and fewer hospital days of care, when compared with nonparticipants. Although the study design does not allow for inference on causality, the strong association between work site health promotion participation and lower health care costs found in this research has been noted with some consistency previously. In this particular study, the reduction in direct health care costs in the third year totaled $1.56 million.

The dramatic rise in health care cost has increased exponentially for the past four decades and has grown beyond the prudent financial capabilities of many businesses. Corporate expenses for employee health care are nearly $250 billion annually and account for approximately 50% of corporate after-tax profits (Health Insurance Association of America, 1993).

For more than a decade, increased attention has been directed at health promotion and dis-

ease prevention initiatives in employer and managed care settings (O'Donnell, 1988). Motivation for implementing work site health promotion programs includes a commitment to optimizing employee health, job satisfaction, and productivity, as well as a desire to reduce health care costs, accidents, and absenteeism (Gebhardt and Crump, 1990; Bly et al, 1986). In reviews of the literature focused on cost savings associated with health promotion, Pelletier (1993, 1999) reported that many studies provided evidence supporting the implementation of this approach, although several contained serious methodologic flaws. Previous studies have shown the related reduction of several modifiable risk factors, all of which are fundamentally related to health care costs (Donatelle and Hawkins, 1989; Cole et al, 1987; Goodspeed, 1990; Browne et al, 1984; Aldana et al, 1993; Goetzel et al, 1996).

The purpose of this study is to compare retrospectively the total and lifestyle-related medical care utilization and costs between participants and nonparticipants in the Procter and Gamble Company's (P&G) work site health promotion program, Health Check.

DEMOGRAPHICS

The subjects for this cross-sectional study were restricted to active P&G employees who were continuously employed between January 1990 and December 1992 and who were eligible for the company's medical benefits plan administered by Metropolitan Life. Participants in the P&G Health Check program (N = 3,993) were defined as those who voluntarily com-

Ron Z. Goetzel, PhD, is a member of The MEDSTAT GROUP in Washington, DC.

Source: Reprinted with permission from Goetzel et al, Health Care Costs of Worksite Health Promotion Participants and Non-participants, *Journal of Occupational and Environmental Medicine*, Vol. 40, No. 4, © 1998, Lippincott Williams and Wilkins.

pleted an optical scan Health Check health profile questionnaire administered by Johnson & Johnson Health Care Systems at any time during the three-year study period and who also participated in follow-up high-risk interventions. Nonparticipants (N = 4,341) were employees who did not participate in any aspect of the health promotion program during the study period.

Of the total cohort (N = 8,334), 53% were males and 48% were female. Employees between the ages of 25 and 54 comprised the majority of the subject pool (87%). Six percent of the participants were over 55 years of age, and 7% were under the age of 25 years; 81% were white, 13% were black, and 6% were Native American, Asian, Hispanic, or other ethnicity. Fifty-five percent had some college education, college degree, or graduate school education; 1% were without high school degrees; and the remainder had high school degrees and/or vocational training. Participants were predominantly clerical workers (28%), those in sales/marketing (23%), or professional/technical workers (22%).

RISK REDUCTION AND MONITORING

After completion of a Health Profile Questionnaire, participants received individualized reports outlining their health status in relation to specific risk areas: elevated blood pressure, elevated cholesterol, cigarette smoking, poor diet, lack of activity, stress, and multiple risks. Participants in the program who were determined to be at high risk were provided one-to-one counseling and behavior change support by P&G clinical staff. Additionally, quarterly follow-ups were conducted by health professionals.

The program also focused on disease prevention and the identification and reduction of health risk factors. Risk factors associated with heart disease or other risk categories were communicated to participants. High-risk individuals were referred to clinicians, when appropri-

ate, and a health improvement action plan was designed. Ancillary health support programs included fitness flex time, after-work on-site aerobics, noon aerobics, diet/weight management programs, cholesterol and blood pressure education, smoking cessation programs, brown-bag educational programs, annual mammography screening, voluntary health screening, and exercise incentives, such as participation prizes. All employees were given equal access to all facets of the program. No attempt was made to ascertain personal decisions for participation or nonparticipation.

Cost experience data were collected from Metropolitan Life Medical Claims computerized database for the total study population. The analysis focused on claims incurred for a continuous three-year period. Claims were aggregated and categorized as inpatient and outpatient. Claims were further classified as either potentially lifestyle-related (resulting from modifiable risk factors) or non–lifestyle-related medical care conditions. Lifestyle-related health care costs included health care expenditures from diseases likely to be related to individuals' behaviors and lifestyles. Claims with a potential lifestyle-related diagnosis were categorized in one of the 46 Lifestyle Diagnosis Groups. Data analysis consisted of descriptive statistics of medical care costs and utilization by participants and nonparticipants by year. All data were adjusted for age and gender.

RESULTS

At the conclusion of the third year of study:

- Nonparticipants' total medical costs were 29% higher than those of health promotion participants.
- The difference in health care expenditures averaged $1,731 for nonparticipants vs. $1,339 for participants.
- During the first two years of the program, lifestyle-related costs were comparable between the groups.

- Nonparticipant annual *lifestyle-related medical costs* were also significantly higher—a 36% greater expenditure
- At the end of the third year, nonparticipants averaged $604 lifestyle-related medical costs vs. $445 for participants.

On average, lifestyle-related medical costs accounted for approximately 35% of P&G's total medical costs over the three-year period ($2.3–$3 billion per year). A comparison of lifestyle-related medical costs between the average of the first two years and the third year indicated a 7% increase for the participants, contrasted with a 43% increase for the nonparticipants.

DISCUSSION

Employee lifestyle-related health care costs have been strongly associated with behaviors such as smoking (Penner and Penner, 1990), obesity (Bertera, 1991), hypertension (Bertera, 1991), poor fitness (Aldana et al, 1993; Tucker et al, 1990), and high stress (Donatelle and Hawkins, 1989; Cole et al, 1987; Goodspeed, 1990), all of which have a modifiable component. The results of the present study suggest a significant relationship between reduced health care utilization and costs and active participation in a health promotion program.

Self-selected participants in the program experienced lower total and lifestyle-related health care costs in the third year after program initiation, when compared with nonparticipants. Careful evaluation of the current results reveals that health care cost reduction was minimal until the third year of program implementation and that the cost differential between participants and nonparticipants expanded from the first year to the third year of participation. This trend is consistent with other studies (Bly et al, 1986; Aldana et al, 1994; Kingery et al, 1994; Warner et al, 1988; Hatziandreu et al, 1988). Because significant health care cost reductions were evident only in the third year of participation, the commitment to a health promotion program needs to be made on a long-term basis to establish a positive benefit/cost ratio. Because many latent diseases may result from long-term unhealthy behavior, the three years examined in the present study represent a minimum time period necessary to recognize the impact that lifestyle factors have on hospital utilization and costs.

The aspect of self-selection in the study design suggests that participants may have been more motivated and willing to change their health risk behaviors than were their nonparticipant counterparts. However, no meaningful differences in the cost of health care used by participants and nonparticipants were evident at the onset of the study.

Participants and nonparticipants began the study at about the same baseline costs (approximately $1,100 per year). Over time, costs for participation grew at a much slower pace than did those of nonparticipants, and, in fact, costs between the two groups diverged significantly. Thus, it seems plausible to suggest that participation in health promotion did contribute to improved health status and reduced cost. This study supports prior research that has shown a positive relationship between well-executed, targeted health promotion programs and health care cost reduction. In summary, at the outset, health care expenditures for the two groups were approximately 2% apart. After three years, their total costs were 29% apart. Although causality cannot be ascribed, due to the study design, the finding of approximately $400 decrease in expenditure per participant (mean $392), compared with nonparticipants, suggests the value in additional monitoring and evaluation.

Additional research is needed to identify the aspects of intervention that contribute most to cost reductions and which categories of illness are most affected by the intervention. Furthermore, research is needed to assess whether similar outcomes may be observed in other benefit areas and overall productivity (eg, absenteeism, turnover, and productivity) and whether the cost savings can be sustained over time.

REFERENCES

Aldana SG, Jacobson BH, Harris CJ. Influence of a mobile work site health promotion program on health care costs. *J Prev Med.* 1994;9:378–382.

Aldana SG, Jacobson BH, Kelly PL. Mobile work site health promotion programs can reduce selected employee health risks. *J Occup Med.* 1993;35:922–928.

Bertera RL. The effects of behavioral risks on absenteeism and health-care costs in the workplace. *J Occup Med.* 1991;33:1119–1124.

Bly J, Jones R, Richardson J. Impact of worksite health promotion on health care costs and utilization: Evaluation of Johnson & Johnson's LIVE FOR LIFE program. *JAMA* 1986;256:3235–3240.

Browne DW, Russell ML, Morgan JL, Optenberg SA, Clarke AE. Reduced disability and health care costs in an industrial fitness program. *J Occup Med.* 1984;26:809–815.

Cole GE, Tucker LA, Friedman GM. Absenteeism data as a measure of cost effectiveness of stress management programs. *Am J Health Promotion.* 1987;1:12–15.

Donatelle RJ, Hawkins MJ. Employee stress claims: Increasing implications for health promotion programming. *Am J Health Promotion.* 1989;3:19–25.

Gebhardt DL, Crump C. Employee fitness and wellness programs in the workplace. *Am Physiol.* 1990;45:262–272.

Goetzel RZ, Kahr TY, Aldana SG, Kenny GM. An evaluation of Duke University's LIVE FOR LIFE health promotion program and its impact on employee health. *Am J Health Promotion.* 1996;10:340–342.

Goodspeed RB. Stress reduction at the worksite: An evaluation of two methods. *Am J Health Promotion.* 1990;4:333–337.

Hatziandreu EI, Koplan JP, Weinstein MC, Caspreson CJ, Warner KE. A cost-effectiveness analysis of exercise as a health promotion activity. *Am J Public Health.* 1988;78:1417–1421.

Health Insurance Association of America and American Council of Life Insurance. *Wellness at the Worksite.* Washington, DC: Health Insurance Association of America; 1993.

Kingery PM, Ellsworth CG, Corbett BS, Bowden RG, Brizzolara JA. High-cost analysis: A closer look at the case for work site health promotion. *J Occup Med.* 1994;36:1341–1347.

O'Donnell MP. Definition of health promotion. *Am J Health Promotion.* 1988;1:4–5.

Pelletier KR. A review and analysis of the clinical and cost-effectiveness studies of comprehensive health promotion and disease management programs at the worksite: 1995–1998 update (IV). *Am J Health Promotion.* 1999;13(6):333–345, iii.

Pelletier KR. A review and analysis of the health and cost-effective outcome studies of comprehensive health promotion and disease prevention programs at the worksite: 1991–1993 update. *Am J Health Promotion.* 1993;8:50–61.

Penner M, Penner S. Excess insured health care costs from tobacco-using employees in a large group plan. *J Occup Med.* 1990;32:521–523.

Tucker LA, Aldana SG, Friedman GM. Cardiovascular fitness and absenteeism in 8,301 employed adults. *Am J Health Promotion.* 1990;5:140–145.

Warner KE, Wickizer TM, Wolfe RA, Schildroth J. Economic implications of workplace health promotion program: Review of the literature. *J Occup Med.* 1988;30:106–112.

INTEGRATIVE DISCIPLINES

Acupuncture

CHAPTER 50

The Discipline of Acupuncture

50.1 Utilization Data: Acceptance of Acupuncture in the United States

Acupuncture and Oriental Medicine Alliance

Acupuncture and Oriental medicine comprise one of the fastest growing forms of health care in the United States. This expansion is due to the recognition by consumers and regulators of the safety, effectiveness, and low cost of this form of health care. Below are listed highlights of the growing utilization data for acupuncture.

- Forty-one states and Washington, DC, have recognized the practice of acupuncture and Oriental medicine. Legislation has been introduced in an additional eight states.

The Acupuncture and Oriental Medicine Alliance is a national membership organization composed of acupuncture and Oriental medicine practitioners, consumers, students, colleges, vendors, and other health care providers who support the practice of acupuncture and Oriental medicine. A 501(c)(4) public welfare organization, the alliance works for sound standards of competency for all practitioners and provides information to consumers, legislatures, and the media; a quarterly newsletter; a conference the first weekend each May; and referrals to over 10,000 state-licensed or national, board-certified practitioners. AOMA can be contacted at <www.AcupunctureAlliance.org>.

Courtesy of National Acupuncture and Oriental Medicine Alliance, Olalla, Washington.

- The Food and Drug Administration estimated in May 1993 that there were 9 to 12 million patient visits each year for acupuncture.
- The World Health Organization has cited acupuncture as an appropriate treatment for more than 43 conditions including allergies, asthma, back pain, carpal tunnel syndrome, colds and flu, constipation, depression, gynecological disorders, headaches, heart problems, infertility, insomnia, premenstrual syndrome, sciatica, sports injuries, tendonitis, and stress.
- The U.S. Department of Education recognizes the Accreditation Commission for Acupuncture and Oriental Medicine (ACAOM). Acupuncture is a 3-year master's-level program. Oriental medicine is a 4-year master's-level program. Over 40 colleges are accredited or in candidacy status.
- Acupuncture is used in over 800 drug-dependency programs. Successful outcomes frequently range from 60% to 90%.
- The 1997 National Institutes of Health Consensus Conference on Acupuncture stated,

"The data in support of acupuncture are as strong as those for many accepted Western medical therapies" (NIH, 1997).

- The National Institutes of Health Consensus Conference on Acupuncture recognized the effectiveness of acupuncture in the treatment of several diseases and stated that "one of the advantages of acupuncture is that the incidence of adverse effects is substantially lower than that of many drugs and other accepted medical procedures used for the same conditions" (NIH, 1997).

- The *Western Journal of Medicine* in 1998 reported that a 1996 Kaiser study found that 57.2% of primary care physicians in Northern California used or recommended acupuncture in the last 12 months.

- A study in six clinics in five states showed the efficacy and cost savings of acupuncture. Of the patients treated with acupuncture, 91.5% reported disappearance or improvement of symptoms; 84% said they see their physicians less, 79% said they use fewer prescription drugs, and 70% of those to whom surgery had been recommended said they avoided it.

- The number of licensed acupuncturists in the United States has doubled between 1992 and 1998, rising from 5,525 in the fall of 1992 to 10,512 in 1998.

- Controlled clinical trials in the United States have evaluated the use of acupuncture combined with standard stroke protocol for the treatment of paralysis due to stroke. Effective or markedly effective results were found for over 80% of the patients receiving acupuncture, with an average cost savings of $26,000 per patient.

- The National Certification Commission for Acupuncture and Oriental Medicine (NCCAOM) offers three independent certification programs: Acupuncture, Chinese Herbology, and Oriental Bodywork Therapy. The NCCAOM has certified over 9,000 practitioners in 47 states and 18 foreign countries.

- In Miami-Dade County, drug offenders have a choice of acupuncture or jail.

- Clinical studies indicate that acupuncture is effective in treating headache, dysmenorrhea, fibromyalgia, stroke, substance abuse, menopause syndrome, depression, female infertility, back pain, low-back pain, osteoarthritis, morning sickness, respiratory disease, urinary dysfunction, tennis elbow, and facial pain.

BIBLIOGRAPHY

Birch S, Hammerschlag R. *Acupuncture Efficacy: A Summary of Controlled Clinical Trials*. Tarrytown, NY: National Academy of Acupuncture and Oriental Medicine. 1996.

Cassidy CM. Chinese medicine users in the United States: Part I: utilization, satisfaction, medical plurality. *Journal of Alternative and Complementary Medicine*. 1998; 4(1):17–27.

Culliton P. Current utilization of acupuncture by U.S. patients. Paper presented at NIH Consensus Development Conference on Acupuncture. November 3, 1997.

Gordon NP, Sobel DS, Tarazona EZ. Use of and interest in alternative therapies among adult primary care clinicians and adult members in a large health maintenance organization. *WMJ*. 1998 Sept;169(3):153–161.

Johansson K, Lindgren I, Widner H, Wiklund I, Johansson BB. Can sensory stimulation improve the functional outcome in stroke patients? *Neurology*. 1993; 43: 2189–2192.

Lytle CD. *An Overview of Acupuncture*. Washington, DC: United States Department of Health and Human Services, Health Sciences Branch, Division of Life Sciences, Office of Science and Technology, Center for Devices and Radiological Health, Food and Drug Administration. 1993.

Mitchell B. *Acupuncture and Oriental Medicine Laws*. Gig Harbor, WA: National Acupuncture Foundation. 1999.

National Commission for Certification in Acupuncture and Oriental Medicine (NCCAOM). <http://www.nccaom.org>. Accessed 5/15/00.

National Institutes of Health Consensus Panel. *Acupuncture. National Institutes of Health Consensus Development Statement* (Bethesda, MD, November 3–5, 1997). Sponsors: Office of Alternative Medicine and Office of Medical Applications of Research. Bethesda, MD: National Institutes of Health; 1997.

World Health Organization. *Viewpoint on Acupuncture.* Geneva, Switzerland: World Health Organization; 1979.

50.2   Overview of Clinical Acupuncture

Efrem Korngold and Nancy Faass

ACCESS TO TRADITIONAL CHINESE MEDICINE

In the United States, there are approximately 10,000 certified or licensed practitioners of acupuncture and herbal medicine. There are more than two dozen schools of Chinese medicine that offer 3- and 4-year programs that graduate hundreds of new practitioners annually. There are also numerous state and national organizations of Chinese medicine professionals, researchers, and educators. The following overview identifies organizations, institutions, and other resources that provide information, services, and products related to Chinese medicine.

Efrem Korngold, LAc, OMD, has been practicing and teaching Chinese traditional medicine since 1973, and has traveled to China on three occasions for advanced study. A founding faculty member of the San Francisco College of Acupuncture and Oriental Medicine in 1980, he is currently adjunct faculty at the American College of Traditional Chinese Medicine, and a certification and examination consultant to the National Certification Commission for Acupuncture and Oriental Medicine (NCCAOM). He is co-author with Harriet Beinfield, LAc, of the book *Between Heaven and Earth: A Guide to Chinese Medicine* and maintains a private practice at his San Francisco center, Chinese Medicine Works.

Nancy Faass, MSW, MPH, is a writer and editor in San Francisco who provides book and project development in integrative medicine and the social sciences.

Courtesy of Efrem Korngold, OMD, and Nancy Faass, MSW, MPH, San Francisco, California.

ORIGINS

Acupuncture is based on a comprehensive body of theory and practice. The same procedures and acupuncture points are used throughout China and the world. The location of the points is extremely precise, and acupuncture treatment, although individualized, is highly systematic. An extensive body of literature has developed in Chinese medicine over the past 2,000 years. Ancient texts still exist that identify acupuncture points in continuous use for centuries and even millennia, now part of standard practice. Currently, the medical journals indexed by the National Institutes of Health (NIH) National Library of Medicine include more than 7,000 articles from the world literature on acupuncture.

THEORY

Acupuncture is a system of healing that activates the body's ability to strengthen and regulate itself. It is based on the theory that life force (Qi, or *chi*, pronounced "chee") flows continuously in the body, through a network of channels called meridians. The meridian pathways may develop blockages or become congested. Each meridian is associated with a particular internal organ and organ system. Any dysfunction, either in the meridian itself or in the associated organ system, can result in physical disturbances or disease. These dysfunctions can also produce symptoms or disorders elsewhere in the body.

Acupuncture treatment is intended to remove blockages, restoring circulation and coherence to the system. The acupuncturist must determine the significant areas of congestion or depletion in order to most effectively treat the patient. This involves activating the relevant acupuncture points to move the Qi, thereby increasing circulation in the meridian to restore a homeo-dynamic condition.

DIAGNOSIS

The practice of acupuncture is holistic; it incorporates a patient's symptoms, history, life situation, and environmental context. Acupuncturists view each patient as a distinct individual. As part of the patient examination, a unique method of pulse diagnosis is used to obtain information regarding the level of vitality or weakness and the functional status of the organ systems. The patient's health is also evaluated by inspecting the tongue (tongue diagnosis) and through general observations of posture, demeanor, facial skin color, and other observable reflections of internal vitality. The practitioner develops skill in acute observation to evaluate the degree of dysfunction and to monitor the patient's subsequent responses to treatment.

TREATMENT

In treatment, the goal is to modulate the flow of Qi, to intensify or diminish it, thereby improving circulation and correcting imbalances. This is achieved by inserting fine, hair-thin sterile needles at specific points along the meridian pathways. In some cases, low-intensity electrostimulation is applied to the needles to amplify the effect. Other interventions may include modification of the patient's lifestyle such as diet, exercise, or daily habits, and, when appropriate, prescribing medicinal herbs in the form of teas, liquid extracts, powders, or tablets. Chinese herbs are low in toxicity, and the guidelines for their use have been established over many centuries. Interventions also include the use of a specific form of heat therapy known as moxibustion.

Auricular Acupuncture

Acupuncture detoxification is a modern application of these techniques, pioneered in the United States by Dr. Michael Smith in New York. This approach uses a simple form of acupuncture applied to points on the ear, to ease the stress of drug withdrawal and regulate the metabolism (Smith, 1988a). This modality has achieved exceptional success, even for people who have had problems with drugs or alcohol for years; this form of treatment is associated with very low rates of recurrence. (Please see Acupuncture Resources at the end of this chapter for contact information.)

Auricular therapy uses specific acupuncture points on the external ear, rather than the body, to alleviate pain, dysfunction, or disease. There is now a substantial amount of research that documents the effectiveness and safety of this approach in the treatment of addictive disorders. Currently, there are more than 750 practitioners across the United States certified to provide treatment for substance abuse with auricular acupuncture (Renaud, 2000). Auricular therapy has documented outcomes of successful addiction treatment ranging from 50% to better than 80%. It is an effective intervention to promote recovery through detoxification, stress reduction, and relapse prevention. Auricular treatment undermines addiction by reducing withdrawal symptoms, cravings, anxiety, and sleep disorders. It enhances health by strengthening immune function, regulating hormonal secretions, and enhancing the production of endorphins. This type of acupuncture treatment also has very positive success rates in the treatment of pregnant women with addictions (Smith, 1988b). Rates of relapse are unusually low, even in 2-year follow-up studies.

Acupressure

Acupressure therapy is based on the same principles as acupuncture. However, treatment is provided manually without the use of needles. Blockages along meridians and at acupuncture points are dispersed through massage or finger pressure. This modality has been integrated into various systems of physical medicine through the treatment of *trigger* points by physical therapists, physiatrists, osteopaths, and chiropractors and is combined with other forms of body work.

Additional Therapies

Additional therapies used in conjunction with acupuncture include:

- *Cupping,* which utilizes a glass or bamboo cup to create suction on the skin over a painful muscle or acupuncture point
- *Electroacupuncture,* which is the mild, low current low-voltage electric stimulation of acupuncture points with or without needles
- *Moxibustion,* which is the application of heat to an acupuncture point by burning an herb called moxa (*Artemisia vulgaris*) near the skin
- *Laser-Puncture,* which is the use of low-intensity, "cool" lasers to stimulate acupuncture points on the body and the ear; this technique is especially useful in pediatrics.

REFERENCES

Renaud J, editor and publisher of *Guidepoints: Acupuncture in Recovery*. Written communication; 5/15/00.

Smith MO. Acupuncture treatment for crack cocaine; clinical survey of 1,500 patients. *American Journal of Acupuncture*. 1988a;16(3):241–247.

Smith MO. Acupuncture as a treatment for drug-dependent mothers. Testimony presented to the New York City Council, New York, NY. April 11, 1988b.

50.3   Resources: Acupuncture

Efrem Korngold and Nancy Faass

RESEARCH

One of the primary public information resources available for information on acupuncture is the MEDLINE database of the U.S. National Library of Medicine. The MEDLINE literature lists more than 7,000 journal articles on acupuncture, dating from 1966 to the present. More than 300 are review articles that evaluate numerous conditions and originate in medical institutions worldwide. While skepticism is reflected in some of the literature, the majority of the meta-analyses are positive. There are few reports of adverse outcomes. MEDLINE can be accessed on the World Wide Web at www.ncbi.nlm.nih.gov. Additional information on searching MEDLINE can be obtained through the MEDLARS help desk at (888) 346-3656.

The National Center for Complementary and Alternative Medicine (NCCAM) at the NIH currently sponsors acupuncture research (see below). Their Web site on the Internet contains extensive in-depth information and can be searched at http://nccam.nih.gov. The clearinghouse of NCCAM can be reached by telephone at (888) 644-6226.

An overview of more than 20 of the highest quality studies on acupuncture can be found in a review of clinical research used to document the

Courtesy of Efrem Korngold, OMD, and Nancy Faass, MSW, MPH, San Francisco, California.

successful petition that gained Food and Drug Administration (FDA) approval of acupuncture needles as a medical device. The 75-page report, *Acupuncture Efficacy: A Compendium of Controlled Clinical Studies*, can be ordered from the Acupuncture Alliance (AAOM) at (206) 851-6895 in Washington state.

Information on the clinical applications of acupuncture is available through programs of the NCCAOM (see "National Associations and Organizations" below).

INSURANCE COVERAGE

Currently, primary sources of coverage for acupuncture services include:

- Specific managed care plans in which acupuncture may be authorized by a primary care physician or medical specialist. Physicians typically refer patients to acupuncture treatment for conditions such as acute and chronic pain.
- Workers' compensation coverage in certain states. In workers' compensation, the diagnoses most often covered involve the treatment of musculoskeletal conditions and other types of injuries.
- Specific programs for the treatment of addictions using the services of specially trained practitioners.

The number of third-party payers now covering acupuncture has grown significantly. For example, the Federal Medical Expense Reimbursement Account allows the use of tax-free money to pay for almost all medical expenses incurred by the subscriber and his or her family that are not already covered by an insurance policy. Under this plan, acupuncture services are allowable expenses.

NATIONAL ASSOCIATIONS AND ORGANIZATIONS

Associations that provide certification or serve professional membership include:

- organizations involved in training, certification, and licensure
- professional membership organizations
- professional organizations with a specific mission

Licensing and Certification

In the United States, licensing requirements for acupuncturists are defined by state and vary significantly from one state to the next. Educational requirements are also defined and specified in state law and regulatory requirements. For specific information on a state's individual licensing and academic requirements, contact the appropriate state agency. (See Chapter 17 for examples of law on acupuncture scope of practice in three states.)

Certification

National Certification Commission for Acupuncture and Oriental Medicine (NCCAOM)

11 Canal Center Plaza, Suite 300
Alexandria, VA 22314
Phone: (703) 548-9004; fax: (703) 548-9079
E-mail: info@NCCAOM.org
Web site: http://www.NCCAOM.org

The NCCAOM was established by the profession in 1982 to develop and implement nationally recognized standards of competence for the practice of acupuncture and Oriental medicine. The NCCAOM is a member of the National Organization for Competency Assurance and accredited by the National Commission for Certifying Agencies. Testing is provided nationwide by Assessment Systems, Inc. The NCCAOM currently administers both written and practical certification examinations in acupuncture (more than 6,800 diplomates certified), Chinese herbology (1,800 certified), and a new certification program in Oriental bodywork.

At this writing, 37 states have practice standards in acupuncture and of those, 34 require NCCAOM certification. However, it is important to check the licensing requirements of each state regarding examinations and requirements. A few states provide their own examination or require additional testing on clinical competence.

Accredited Training for Acupuncturists

Accreditation Commission for Acupuncture and Oriental Medicine (ACAOM)

1010 Wayne Avenue, Suite 1270
Silver Spring, MD 20910
Phone: (301) 608-9680; fax: (301) 608-9576
E-mail: 733522467@CompuServe.com

Many states require that the practitioner have training from an accredited institution. Schools of acupuncture are accredited by the ACAOM, a peer-review group recognized by the U.S. Department of Education Council for Higher Education Accreditation and the Commission on Recognition of Postsecondary Accreditation. Formed in 1982 for the purpose of advancing the profession, ACAOM has developed academic and clinical guidelines and core curriculum requirements for master's level programs in acupuncture and Oriental medicine, as well as for doctoral level programs. Information on the accreditation or candidacy status of any particular program can be obtained directly from the ACAOM. State requirements on training and education can vary significantly. For example, in the state of California, training from diploma-level programs is not accepted and a master's level program required for licensure. Additionally, California does not accept NCCAOM certification as a basis for licensure but requires its own more stringent exam.

The Council of Colleges of Acupuncture and Oriental Medicine (CCAOM)

1010 Wayne Avenue, Suite 1270
Silver Spring, MD 20910
Phone: (301) 608-9175; fax: (301) 608-9576
Web site: http://www.CCAOM.org

The CCAOM provides a list of accredited training programs and a course on clean-needle technique. Accreditation information is particu-

larly important. For example, some states will not license practitioners who have been trained at institutions located outside the United States. Others license graduates of a few specific non-U.S. institutions. In California, only two international schools are accepted—one California school that has a branch in Japan, the other with a branch in England.

Professional Membership Organizations

Association of Acupuncture and Oriental Medicine (AAOM, formerly AAAOM)

433 Front Street
Catasauqua, PA 18032
Phone: (610) 433-2448; fax: (610) 264-2768
E-mail: aaom1@aol.com
Web site: http://www.aaom.org

The AAOM provides public information and referrals to board-certified acupuncturists and practitioners of Oriental medicine in most parts of the country. For members, they provide client referrals over the phone, and on their Web site, they provide information on malpractice insurance; discounted telephone service; practice information; a journal; discounted rates on books, publications, and conferences; educational materials for patients; and a directory of members.

Acupuncture and Oriental Medicine Alliance (AOMA)

14637 Starr Road S.E.
Olalla, WA 98359
Phone: (253) 851-6896; fax: (253) 851-6883
Web site: http://www.AcuAll.org

The AOMA is a nonprofit professional association (501(c)(4)) with membership nationwide that was founded in 1993 to represent the diversity of practitioners of acupuncture and Oriental medicine in the United States. AOMA publishes a quarterly newsletter containing clinical articles, legislative updates, and discussions within the field; sponsors an annual conference the first weekend each May; and maintains a referral service of over 10,000 state-licensed or national board-certified practitioners. Membership is open to licensed acupuncturists, Chinese herbalists, Oriental bodywork therapists, acupuncture detoxification specialists, students, consumers, colleges, state associations, vendors, and other health care providers interested in the advancement of acupuncture and Oriental medicine.

National Acupuncture Foundation (NAF)
PO Box 2271
Gig Harbor, WA 98335-4271
Phone: (253) 851-6538; fax: (253) 851-6883

The NAF publishes *Acupuncture and Oriental Medicine Law, Clean Needle Technique Manual,* and *Legislative Handbook* (see below under "Information Resources"). The NAF was pivotal in the FDA Needle Reclassification Petition and conducted the research that has provided the basis for the herbal certification program of the NCCAOM. The NAF also maintains a national database of acupuncture and Oriental medicine practitioners, state associations, colleges, and state regulatory boards.

National Acupuncture Detoxification Association (NADA)
NADA Office
PO Box 1927
Vancouver, WA 98668-1927
Phone: (360) 254-0186; fax: (360) 260-8620
E-mail: NADAClear@aol.com

NADA is an international organization with 750 active members in the United States that conducts a training program for health professionals in the use of acupuncture as an adjunctive treatment for addictions. This method is currently used worldwide in more than 1,000 comprehensive addiction treatment programs. Founded in 1985, the association also publishes reference materials in the subject area and conducts an annual meeting open to all interested persons. NADA is affiliated with the publication of *Guidepoints*, a newsletter written for both administrators and clinicians. Content includes objective reportage on clinical aspects, funding, public policy, and research issues.

Acupuncture Research Programs
Hennepin County Medical Center
Alternative Medicine Division
825 S. 8th Street, Suite 1106
Minneapolis, MN 55404
Phone: (612) 347-6238; fax: (612) 373-1882
E-mail: aamc@winternet.com

The Division has conducted research for more than 20 years on the use of acupuncture in the treatment of addictions, and published generalized outcomes research on the demographics of acupuncture utilization and on the effectiveness of acupuncture for the treatment of chronic pain. Currently, the research program focuses on the study of acupuncture through randomized controlled clinical trials. The Division serves as a resource to hospitals, insurance companies, and agencies interested in the development of integrative medicine programs and research initiatives.

NIH NCAAM Research Center—Pain Research
University of Maryland, Center for CAM
Complementary Medicine Program (CMP), The Mansion House
2200 Kernan Drive
Baltimore, MD 21207
Phone: (410) 448-6871; fax: (410) 448-6875
Web site: http://
    www.compmed.UMMC.UMaryland.edu

CMP was one of the first NIH alternative medicine centers. It provides research, education, and clinical care, with a focus on the treatment of chronic pain conditions. CMP has also been awarded NIH status as a specialized center of research in alternative medicine for arthritis and related disorders. In addition, the program is a coordinating center of the Cochrane Collaboration, an international effort to prepare and disseminate systematic reviews of randomized, controlled clinical trials. In this endeavor, the program serves as a repository for complementary medicine research.

The Quan Yin Healing Arts Center
455 Valencia
San Francisco, CA 94103
Phone: (415) 861-4964; fax: (415) 861-0579
E-mail: qyhac@aol.com

The center is a 16-year-old, nonprofit, integrative medicine clinic specializing in acupuncture, herbal medicine, massage, Qigong, and nursing services, with a focus on chronic health issues, HIV, hepatitis C, cancer support, stroke, brain injury, addictions, asthma programs, and general health. Reimbursement is accepted from MediCal, Medicare, private insurance, sliding-scale fees, workers' compensation, and personal injury coverage. Quan Yin Healing Arts Center is committed to providing quality services to the community, regardless of income.

The AIDS and Chinese Medicine Institute
455 Valencia
San Francisco, CA 94103
Phone: (415) 861-4964; fax: (415) 861-0579
E-mail: qyhac@aol.com

The Institute is a program of Quan Yin Healing Arts Center, a 501(C)3 nonprofit founded to promote collaboration among Chinese medicine practitioners who work in the public health sector providing services for patients with HIV and AIDS. The primary missions of the Institute are education and research.

Immune Enhancement Project (IEP),
  San Francisco
3450 16th Street
San Francisco, CA 94114
Phone: (415) 252-8711; fax: (415) 252-8710
Web site: http://www.iepclinic.com

American Acupuncture Council
1851 First Street, Suite 1160
Santa Ana, CA 92705
Phone: (800) 838-0383

The council offers malpractice insurance for acupuncturists.

INFORMATION RESOURCES

Books on acupuncture can be purchased by phone, Internet, and/or mail from the following vendors.

Blue Poppy Press
5441 Western Avenue, Suite #2
Boulder, CO 80301
Phone: (800) 487-9296
Web site: http://www.bluepoppy.com

Redwing Book Co.
44 Linden Street
Brookline, MA 02445
Phone: (800) 873-3946
Fax: (617) 738-4620
Web site: http://www.redwingbooks.com

Regulatory Information

National Acupuncture Foundation books
Available through Bookmasters
Phone: (800) 247-6553

- Mitchell B. *Acupuncture and Oriental Medicine Laws.* Washington, DC: National Acupuncture Foundation; 1997. A summary of the laws in each state for the practice of acupuncture.
- Mitchell B. *The Legislative Handbook for Practicing Acupuncture.* Washington, DC: National Acupuncture Foundation; 1995.
- National Acupuncture Foundation. *Clean Needle Technique Manual.* 4th ed. Washington, DC: National Acupuncture Foundation; 1997. Also available in two foreign language editions in Chinese and in Korean from the Acupuncture and Oriental Medicine Alliance by calling (253) 851-6895.
- Kailin DC. *Acupuncture Risk Management.* CMS Press; 1997. Available from Convergent Medical Systems, Inc, PO Box 2115, Corvallis, OR 97339. A valuable reference on practice standards and regulatory compliance. Order by phone: (541) 757-8601; e-mail: kailin@convergentmedical.com

Clinical Bibliography

The following books on acupuncture are used as the basis for the state of California acupuncture-licensing exam.

Ellis A, Wiseman N, et al. *Fundamentals of Chinese Acupuncture*. R. Felt, ed. St. Paul, MN: EMC-Paradigm Publishing; 1991.

Maciocoa G. *Foundations of Chinese Medicine*. New York: Churchill Livingston; 1989.

Maciocoa G. *Tongue Diagnosis in Chinese Medicine*. Rev ed. Seattle, WA: Eastland Press; 1994.

Rui CJ. *Acupuncture Case Histories from China*. Seattle, WA: Eastland Press; 1988.

Shanghai College of Traditional Chinese Medicine. *Acupuncture: A Comprehensive Text*. Chicago: Eastland Press; 1983.

Xinnong C, ed. *Chinese Acupuncture and Moxibustion: The New Essentials*. Beijing, China: Foreign Languages Press; 1990.

Additional Professional Bibliography

Beinfield H, Korngold E. *Between Heaven and Earth*. New York: Ballantine Books; 1991. One of the definitive classics in this field.

Birch S, Hammerschlag R. *Acupuncture Efficacy: A Summary of Controlled Clinical Studies*. Tarrytown, NY: National Academy of Acupuncture and Oriental Medicine; 1996. Order through Redwing Book Company, Brookline, MA at (800) 873-3946.

Brumbaugh AG. *Transformation and Recovery: A Guide for the Design and Development of Acupuncture-Based Chemical Dependency Treatment Programs*. New York: Stillpoint Press; 1994.

Cohen M. *The HIV Wellness Sourcebook*. New York: Henry Holt; 1998.

Hammerschlag R, Stux G, eds. *Clinical Acupuncture: Scientific Basis*. Berlin: Springer-Verlag; 2000.

Huan ZY, Rose K. *Who Can Ride the Dragon? An Exploration of the Cultural Roots of Traditional Chinese Medicine*. St. Paul, MN: EMC-Paradigm Publishing; 1999.

Johns R. *The Art of Acupuncture Techniques*. Berkeley, CA: North Atlantic Books; 1996. Written for the practitioner in the vocabulary of Chinese medicine, with sample case histories.

Kaptchuk T. *The Web That Has No Weaver: Understanding Chinese Medicine*. New York: Congdon and Weed; 1992. Another classic.

Maciocoa G. *The Practice of Chinese Medicine*. New York: Churchill Livingston; 1994.

Pomerantz B, Stutz G, eds. *The Scientific Bases of Acupuncture*. New York: Springer-Verlag; 1988.

Stux G, Pomeranz B. *The Basics of Acupuncture*. 3rd ed. New York: Springer Verlag; 1996. Written by a physician in the vocabulary of Western medicine for other physicians and medical students.

Overviews of Acupuncture

Cargill M. *Acupuncture: A Viable Medical Alternative*. Portsmouth, NH: Butterworth Trade; 1994. An overview and history of acupuncture from a Western medical perspective.

Birch S, Felt R. *Understanding Acupuncture*. New York: Harcourt Health Sciences; 1999.

Mitchell ER. *Fighting Drug Abuse with Acupuncture: The Treatment That Works*. Berkeley, CA: Pacific View Press; 1995.

Williams T. *The Complete Illustrated Guide to Chinese Medicine*. Rockport, MA: Element Books, Inc; 1996. An broad overview of Chinese medicine.

Journals

American Journal of Acupuncture. A quarterly academic/scholarly publication
Phone: (408) 475-1700; fax: (408) 475-1439

American Journal of Chinese Medicine: Comparative Medicine East and West. Three issues per year, sponsored by the Institute for Advanced Research in Asian Science and Medicine.

Web sites: http://www.allenpress.com; http://www.ajcm.org

E-mail: orders@allenpress.com; editor's e-mail: kao@ajcm.org

Phone: (415) 831-4289; fax: (415) 831-4248

Clinical Acupuncture and Oriental Medicine
Harcourt Publishers, Ltd, editor Ken Rose
An international journal covering topics in clinical treatment, physiology, theory, and research.
Subscriptions, Edinburg, Scotland
Phone: 011-44-131-556-2424; fax: 011-44-131-459-1177

Guidepoints: Acupuncture in Recovery. An independent monthly subscription newsletter for professionals concerned with acupuncture in treating addictive and mental disorders.
J&M Reports
7402 NE 58th Street
Vancouver, WA 98662-5207
Phone: (888) 276-9978; fax: (888) 211-8830
E-mail: AcuDetox@AOL.com
Web site: http://www.acudetox.com

Journal of Chinese Medicine. An academic and scholarly publication with three issues per year.
Fax: 44-1273-7485888
Web site: http://www.jcm.co.uk
Editor's e-mail: jcm@pavilion.co.uk

Web Sites

Academy of Medical Acupuncture: http://www.medicalacupuncture.org

The Chinese Medicine Sampler: http://www.chinesemedicinesampler.com

Current Bibliographies in Medicine (acupuncture research titles): http://www.nlm.nih.gov/pubs/resources.html. Click on 1997, where you will see a listing for "Acupuncture, 230 citations, January 1970–October 1997."

HealthWorld Online: Acupuncture: http://www.healthy.net/clinic/therapy/acupuncture/index.asp

Institute for Traditional Medicine: http://www.itmonline.org

Redwing Book Company—Chinese medicine and acupuncture books: http://www.redwingbooks.com

WholeHealthmd Advisor: http://www.americanwholehealth.com/library/acupuncture/tcm.htm

Databases

MEDLINE. The MEDLINE database of the National Library of Medicine at NIH (PubMed) at http://www.ncbi.nlm.nih.gov. Free user support is available from the MEDLARS help desk at (888) 346-3656.

50.4   Research Data: Cost-Effectiveness of Acupuncture

Acupuncture and Oriental Medicine Alliance and
Richard Hammerschlag

BENEFITS AND COST SAVINGS ASSOCIATED WITH ACUPUNCTURE

Avoidance of Surgery

In this study (Christensen et al, 1992), 29 patients with severe osteoarthritis of the knee, each awaiting arthroplasty surgery, were randomized to receive a course of acupuncture treatment or be placed on a waiting list to receive similar acupuncture treatment starting 9 weeks later. Of the 29 patients, 7 were able to cancel their scheduled surgeries. The cost savings were $9,000 per patient.

Decreased Days in Hospital or Nursing Home

Half of 78 stroke patients receiving standard rehabilitative care were randomly assigned to receive adjunctive acupuncture treatment (Johansson et al, 1993). Patients given acupuncture recovered faster and to a greater extent. Those who received acupuncture spent, on average, 88 days per patient in the hospital and nursing home compared to 161 days per patient for standard care alone. The cost savings averaged $26,000 per patient.

Richard Hammerschlag, PhD, is Research Director at the Oregon College of Oriental Medicine in Portland and also serves as President of the Society for Acupuncture Research. <www.acupunctureresearch.org>

The Acupuncture and Oriental Medicine Alliance (AOMA) is a national membership organization composed of acupuncture and Oriental medicine practitioners, consumers, students, colleges, vendors, and other health care providers who support the practice of acupuncture and Oriental medicine. <www.acupuncturealliance.org>

Courtesy of National Acupuncture and Oriental Medicine Alliance, Olalla, Washington.

Quicker Return to Physical Labor

Fifty-six patients at a workers' compensation clinic were randomized to receive either physical therapy/occupational therapy/exercise or the standard care plus acupuncture (Gunn et al, 1980). Of the 29 treated with acupuncture, 18 returned to their original or equivalent jobs, and 10 returned to lighter employment. Of the 27 who received only standard therapy, 4 returned to their original or equivalent jobs and 14 to lighter employment.

Avoidance of Surgery, Fewer Hospital Visits, and Greater Return to Employment

Sixty-nine patients with severe angina pectoris received 12 acupuncture treatments in 4 weeks (Ballegaard et al, 1996). Patients were also instructed to perform shiatsu 2 times per day and received counseling in stress reduction, exercise, and diet. Of the 49 patients who were candidates for coronary bypass or balloon angioplasty surgery, at the 2-year follow-up, 30 had surgery postponed due to clinical improvement. The cost savings were $13,000 per patient. There was a decrease in the number of in-hospital days for all 69 patients: 79% reduction in the first year posttreatment, 95% reduction in the second year posttreatment. There was also a reduction in the number of outpatient visits: 60% and 87%, respectively. Additional cost savings resulted from the increase in percent of patients able to work from 11% prior to treatment, to 60% at 2 years posttreatment. Estimated savings in annual sick pay were $18,000 per patient.

For more details, see Chapter 52, *Acupuncture Efficacy: A Summary of Controlled Clinical Trials*.

REFERENCES

Ballegaard S, et al. Cost-benefit of combined use of acupuncture, shiatsu and lifestyle adjustment for treatment of patients with severe angina pectoris. *Acupunct Electro-Ther Res*. 1996;21:187–197.

Christensen BV, et al. Acupuncture treatment of severe knee osteoarthrosis: A long-term study. *Acta Anesthesiol Scand*. 1992;36:519–525.

Gunn CC, et al. Dry needling of muscle motor points for chronic low-back pain. *Spine*. 1980;5:279–291.

Johansson K, et al. Can sensory stimulation improve the functional outcome in stroke patients? *Neurology*. 1993;43:2189–2192.

CHAPTER 51

Chinese Medicine in the United States: Utilization and Satisfaction

Claire M. Cassidy

INTRODUCTION

Chinese medicine, although barely known outside of Asian-American communities before the 1970s, experienced a rapid rise in interest in the United States after James Reston's report in 1971 (Reston, 1971). Today there are 35 accredited schools (Accreditation Commission for Acupuncture and Oriental Medicine, 2000) and more than 10,000 practitioners (Mitchell, 1999) who serve an estimated 1 million patients yearly (Culliton, 1997).

There has been limited research focused on characterizing users or understanding the reasons for purchasing Chinese medicine care—factors relevant to both referral and health care policy planning. A handful of ethnographic studies (Hare, 1992, 1993; Emad, 1994) has provided detailed perceptions of small groups of patients. One survey compared users of biomedicine (family practice), chiropractic, and Chinese medicine (Anderson, 1991); another reported user demographic and complaint patterns for a hospital-based alternative medicine clinic (Bullock et al, 1997).

This chapter reports quantitative data from the first in-depth survey of acupuncture users.

Claire M. Cassidy, PhD, is a medical anthropologist and acupuncture intern with a specialty in comparative medicine and professional interest in the development of appropriate research methods for studying alternative medical systems. She heads her own consulting firm, served for 6 years as research director at a premier U.S. acupuncture school, and taught at universities for over 15 years. She has an extensive publication list and currently serves on the editorial boards of two leading CAM journals.

Courtesy of Claire Cassidy, Ph.D., Bethesda, Maryland.

It was conducted among patients of six large clinics in five states using a mixed qualitative-quantitative written questionnaire format. The final sample size consisted of 575 respondents to the quantitative segment of the research questionnaire. In addition, 460 participants responded to requests for written narrative (Chinese Medicine Users, 1998). The study gathered data on the following issues: Who attends these clinics? What complaints do they bring for care? What is their self-reported response to Chinese medicine care? What other form of health care do they use? How satisfied are they with Chinese medicine care?

The answers to these questions can stand alone as descriptors of utilization, but can also be used to explore why Chinese medicine is popular, an issue that matters both to practitioners and at the national policy planning level. Thus, it is also important to understand what values cause patients to seek Chinese medicine care in the first place, and what motivates them to continue its use and (usually) pay for it out of their own pockets afterwards.

In the following study, statistical data are used to describe users in terms of sociodemographics, conditions brought for care, response to care, and satisfaction with care. Additionally, data are presented indicating that users of Chinese medicine often employ a variety of different medicines, and suggest that this use is not necessarily additive, but selective. The data from this study, paired with a review of respondent reports that identified qualitative factors, indicate that users of Chinese medicine in the United States are astute selective consumers in a pluralist national health care environment.

The goal of the research was to characterize people who used Chinese medicine by gathering descriptive and perceptual data. The respondents were patients currently using general service clinics and "whole body" Chinese medicine care. Accordingly, no applied health care hypothesis was tested, no users of specialty clinics or specialty styles of acupuncture care were surveyed, and no effort was made to survey former users of Chinese medicine care.

A mixed qualitative-quantitative questionnaire was developed based on in-depth interviews of 65 current and former acupuncture patients, and two pilot tests (Bernard, 1992; Cassidy, 1994a, 1994b). The quantitative portion of the questionnaire included questions using both check boxes and Likert scales, as appropriate. These questions solicited information on Chinese medicine modalities used, relation to practitioner, sociodemographics, complaints brought for Chinese medicine care, response to care, other forms of health care costs in the previous 3 months, recall of health care costs in the previous 3 months, and satisfaction with Chinese medicine care. Six quantitative questions solicited additional information in the form of an open-ended question requiring a handwritten answer. All questions that solicited perceptions of Chinese medicine care provided opportunity to report negative as well as positive results and opinions.

Participant clinics were selected according to criteria including the provision of comprehensive care, location in urban/suburban centers of Chinese medicine usage, "large" patient flow rate of 80 or more patients per week, staffing by licensed professional Chinese medicine practitioners, and willingness to participate.

The six clinics that participated included two school clinics (Northwest Institute of Acupuncture and Oriental Medicine, Seattle, Washington; New England School of Acupuncture, Watertown, Massachusetts), and four private clinics (Chinese Medicine Works, San Francisco, California; Gipson Specialty Center, Memphis, Tennessee; Ruscombe Mansion, Baltimore, Maryland; and The Centre for Traditional Acupuncture, Columbia, Maryland). The clinics are multipractitioner sites except for the Gipson Specialty Center, which is an orthopedic clinic with one Chinese medicine practitioner on staff.

Final sample size for the whole questionnaire was 575, with a response rate of 45.9%. Within clinic sites, survey participants did not differ from nonparticipants with regard to sex or the length of time they had used Chinese medicine. Complaint, response, and satisfaction levels did not differ significantly by site, and data from all six sites are combined in this report.

SOCIODEMOGRAPHICS OF THE RESPONDENTS

More women than men used Chinese medicine care; the highest usage was among people between the ages of 30 and 60; most users self-identify as "white." There were few low-income patients, reflecting the fact that most Chinese medicine patients pay for their care out of their own pockets (although 88% of the sample had reimbursement coverage for biomedical care, only 22% had any for acupuncture care). Respondents were well educated. Of those employed, a majority had professional or technical occupations, and an additional large proportion were self-employed in creative or entrepreneurial occupations.

School sites charge lower fees because they utilize supervised trainee practitioners. These sites had significantly more respondents with lower incomes ($p < 0.001$), under 30, with high school or trade-school educations in clerical/laborer and unsalaried occupations, and self-describing as nonwhite.

The demographic picture of the majority of users reflects a population that is educated, employed, and professional (see Table 51–1). This pattern is similar to that reported from other clinic-based surveys of alternative medicine users (Bullock et al, 1997; Cassileth et al, 1984; Clinical Oncology Group, 1987; Eisenberg et al, 1993; James et al, 1983; McGinnis, 1991; McGuire, 1988; Thomas et al, 1991; Verhoef et al, 1990).

Table 51–1 Demographics

Sample Characteristic	Sample Size (N = 575)*	Percent of Total Sample
Gender		
Female	411	72.1
Male	158	27.9
Age (years)		
11–20	9	1.6
21–30	61	10.8
31–40	150	26.5
41–50	214	37.8
51–60	82	14.5
61–70	36	6.4
71–80	14	2.5
Origin		
White	501	89.3
Black	12	2.1
Asian	16	2.9
Other	32	5.7
Civil Status		
Single	153	26.9
Separated, divorced, widowed	87	15.3
Partnered, not married	99	17.4
Married	230	40.4
Education		
Less than high school diploma	8	1.4
High school diploma	26	4.6
Some college or trade school	117	20.6
Bachelor's degree	127	22.3
Some graduate school	98	17.2
Graduate degree	193	33.9
Annual Household Income		
< $20,000	129	23.7
$20,000 < $40,000	132	24.3
$40,000 < $60,000	98	18.0
$60,000 < $80,000	70	12.9
> $80,000	115	21.1
Occupation		
Professional, technical	216	37.9
Entrepreneurial, creative	78	13.7
Business management, sales	65	11.4
Clerical, service, laborer	55	9.6
Not employed[†]	156	27.4

*Sample total is 575; within cells total may not sum to 575 because of missing answers.
[†]Category includes students, 9.5%; retirees, 6.7%; homemakers, 6.1%; and disabled and unemployed, 5.1%.
Courtesy of Claire Cassidy, Ph.D., Bethesda, Maryland.

USE OF CHINESE AND BIOMEDICINE MODALITIES

Survey respondents ranged from novices to others who had years of experience with Chinese medicine care. Almost all (99%) of respondents had received acupuncture care, 59.7% had received moxibustion (warming of acupuncture sites with mugwort herb *Artemesia vulgaris*), and 35.5% had received Chinese herbs. Disposable acupuncture needles alone were used 85.3% of the time, and reusable needles alone in 8.4% of cases; electroacupuncture was used by 3.5% of the sample, but only in combination with manual needling. More than one type of needle was used 5.2% of the time. No respondent reported experiencing important adverse events from the needles.

Primary Health Complaints Treated

At all sites, the top three reasons respondents sought Chinese medicine care were for relief of pain, relief from unstable mood, and maintenance of well-being or good health (see Table 51–2). Other important reasons were for respiratory, digestive, and head and neck complaints. Among these, the most common specific complaints were allergies, asthma, and headaches as well as autoimmune disorders. The most common infections that respondents reporting having treated with Chinese medicine care were colds, sinusitis, hepatitis, and human immunodeficiency virus (HIV) infection. In this middle-class population, none reported seeking detoxification for recreational drugs, and only a few for alcohol or nicotine, but many reported seeking help for reducing dependency on prescription drugs including steroids, sympathomimetics, antidepressants, and nonsteroidal anti-inflammatory drugs (NSAIDs).

Response to Chinese Medicine Care

In reports on past treatment, respondents indicated symptoms or complaints for which they had sought Chinese medicine care. In response to this question, 91.5% reported symptoms or conditions that had "resolved" or "improved," 7.5% reported on a condition that had "not changed," and 0.7% reported a symptom that had "worsened." See Table 51–3.

Respondents also reported improvements in general measures of quality of life (Table 51–3). Additionally, a majority claimed that their use of non-Chinese care had decreased since they began receiving Chinese medicine care. Although unquantified in this survey, these decreases represent potentially large biomedical care cost savings, particularly for surgery avoided (see Table 51–4).

Other Forms of Health Care Used

Survey respondents used a wide range of health care in addition to Chinese medicine, including a variety of self-care activities as well as use of professional health care other than Chinese medicine. Biomedicine was the most used system after Chinese medicine, medical doctors having been consulted by 54.4% of respondents in the 3 months preceding the survey. Findings indicated that only 15% of respondents depended on acupuncture alone; most respondents were using multiple systems of care. In fact, the average number of professionalized systems used in addition to Chinese medicine was 2.2 (17 choices offered; respondents used 1 to 10 other modalities concurrently).

Satisfaction with Chinese Medicine

When asked in a five-point Likert scale question to say "what made the difference" in their health, a majority said it was "definitely" or "probably" Chinese medicine, and this response pattern predominated even when respondents reported using several forms of health care (Table 51–5; $p < 0.03$). This counterintuitive result deserves further exploration. For the moment, it indicates that Chinese medicine care has high face value—that is, users find it convincing even when they compare it with other forms of health care that they have tried.

Table 51–2 Complaints and Resolution

Reasons*			Response†				
			Condition Resolution	Improved	Same	Worse	
Condition‡	N	%	%	%	%	%	N
Stress, anxiety, depression, fatigue, including chronic fatigue	381	66.3	10.7	82.7	6.2	0.4	243
Well care	362	63.0	7.1	91.1	—	1.8	56
Musculoskeletal system	321	58.8	15.1	74.6	9.9	0.4	232
Respiratory system	231	40.2	17.6	68.2	7.1	—	85
Head and neck	182	31.7	17.5	76.3	5.0	1.3	80
Digestive system	129	22.4	7.5	85.1	7.5	—	67
Urinary and male reproductive system	117	20.3	11.8	58.8	29.4	—	17
Female reproductive system	100	17.4	13.3	78.3	6.7	1.7	60
Infectious illness	77	13.4	43.2	54.1	2.7	—	37
Autoimmune dysfunctions	72	12.5	9.5	66.7	23.8	—	21
Weight problems	62	10.8	—	61.1	33.3	5.6	18
Other	254	44.2	12.8	82.6	3.7	0.9	109
Total size of sample (N)	575		139	782	79	7	1,007
Total percentage of sample			13.8	77.7	7.8	0.7	100.0

*Using a menu of 30 items, respondents marked any for which they had ever received Chinese medicine. Table 53–2 lists separately reasons that were mentioned by more than 10%.

†Respondents could choose to report up to four changes in symptoms or conditions; 95 people did not answer the question; 478 named one symptom; 303 named two symptoms; 167 named three symptoms; 58 named four symptoms. Choices included symptoms that disappeared, improved, did not change, or got worse, which appear in headings "Resolved," "Improved," "Same," and "Worse."

‡Conditions***

- Fatigue or stress category includes all reports of mood support; those seeking Chinese medicine care to relieve stress, anxiety, fatigue, depression; and those reporting "chronic fatigue syndrome."
- Well care category includes all reports of using Chinese medicine care for maintaining well-being and health, as well as illness prevention.
- Musculoskeletal system category includes all reports of pain and other disability in bones, muscles, joints, and ligaments.
- Head and neck category includes all reports of headache, chronic neck or head pain of all forms, learning disabilities, and epilepsy and insomnia; it excludes cancers.
- Respiratory system category includes all reports of asthma, allergies, rhinitis, emphysema, and multiple chemical sensitivities; it excludes respiratory infections and cancers.
- Digestive system category includes all reports of painful and nonpainful, noninfectious, digestive system conditions.
- Urinary and male reproductive system category includes all reports relative to the urinary system as well as the male reproductive system.
- Female reproductive system category includes all reports of menstrual pain or discomfort, menopausal symptoms, infertility, endometriosis, uterine fibroids, and other reproductive system complaints.
- Infectious illness category includes all reports of infections, including colds, sinusitis, pneumonia, cystitis, hepatitis (N = 7), and HIV (N = 10).
- Autoimmune dysfunctions category includes all reports of immune dysfunctions including diabetes (N = 8), thyroiditis (N = 5), multiple sclerosis (N = 3), lupus erythematosus (N = 3); it excludes reproductive system complaints.
- Weight problems category includes all reports of anorexia, bulimia, low weight, and high weight.
- "Other" category includes all conditions with fewer than 10% of sample reporting the complaint category including circulatory (N = 53); eye and ear (N = 48); skin (N = 45); substance abuse (N = 43); mouth or jaw (N = 30); sleep disturbance (N = 21, a respondent-created category); cancer and radiation chemotherapy (N = 14); and complaints phrased in Chinese medical terms (N = 10; a respondent-created category).

Courtesy of Claire Cassidy, Ph.D., Bethesda, Maryland.

Table 51–3 Quality of Life Changes in Response to Receipt of Chinese Medicine Care

Statement	Number of Respondents (N = 575)	Percentage			
		None of the Time	A Little of the Time	Some of the Time	Most of the Time
Feel better	478	0.4	2.3	21.1	76.2
Miss fewer workdays	331	9.4	3.0	16.6	71.0
Get along better with others	394	2.3	4.8	24.1	68.8
Have less pain	423	1.9	5.9	28.4	63.8
Can work better	440	1.6	4.5	30.2	63.6
Have more energy	452	1.1	6.4	34.3	58.2
Am more focused	433	1.2	7.4	33.3	58.2

Courtesy of Claire Cassidy, Ph.D., Bethesda, Maryland.

AN INFORMED PLURALITY OF MEDICAL USAGE

Although not rejecting biomedicine, respondents may be learning to use this medical system selectively, rather than as a generic or "normative" system to which they refer all problems. Remarks respondents offered spontaneously in their written reports indicate that they evaluated practices and used them "for what they do best," sometimes creating teams of practitioners of different medicines to serve personal needs. While this finding may yet be surprising on the American scene, in settings where medical plurality is normative, it has long been established that consumers are astute at distinguishing among options and using them wisely (Anderson, 1996; MacLean, 1978; O'Connor, 1995; Welsch, 1983; Young, 1981).

DISCUSSION

The survey reported here is the first in-depth and large-scale survey of Chinese medicine users in the United States. As such, it is exploratory, and provides an initial database on

Table 51–4 Respondent Reports of Other Health Care Utilization While Receiving Chinese Medicine Care

Changes in Utilization of Other Health Care Services	Number Question Applied to (N = 575)	Number Who Responded Positively	Responded Positively (Percent)
Reduced office visits to medical doctors	334	281	84.1
Reduced use of prescription drugs	299	236	78.9
Reduced use of physical therapist	169	131	77.5
Reduced insurance claims	191	147	77.0
Avoided surgery	97	68	70.1
Reduced use of psychotherapy	200	117	58.5

Courtesy of Claire Cassidy, Ph.D., Bethesda, Maryhland

Table 51–5 Respondents' Perception of What Made the Difference in Their Health*

Intervention	Percent Probable Source of Improvement	Percent Unclear as to Source of Improvement	Response: A Combination of Factors
Used Chinese medicine (CM) only	89.3	5.4	5.3†
Used CM and biomedicine only	82.4	7.8	9.8
Used CM and other biomedical care only	75.0	7.4	17.6
Used CM, biomedicine, and other nonbiomedical care	73.9	3.9	22.2

*Data collected in response to a question phrased: "If you have experienced a change in your health since beginning acupuncture care, do you think it is acupuncture that made the difference?" The original Likert scale included five choices, combined in the above table: Probable = "Definitely" plus "Probably"; Unclear = "Unclear" plus "Probably Not"; Combination = "A Combination of Factors."

†Data may reflect a response indicating self-care in addition to professional care.

Courtesy of Claire Cassidy, Ph.D., Bethesda, Maryland.

which future research can draw and build. It also provides insight into causes for the rising popularity of Chinese medicine.

The demographic picture is one of middle-class, educated users in relatively self-determining occupations who are willing to risk trying a new (to the United States) form of health care, and with sufficient income to pay out of pocket for their care. As noted, this pattern matches demographic images from earlier research. However, as third-party reimbursement for Chinese medicine care becomes more common in the United States, it is probable that we will see a shift to a demographic picture more nearly mirroring the United States population at large, that is, a broader age range, and full occupational and educational range.

The utilization pattern that emerged from this research indicates that when respondents are given free rein to express their own goals for use of health care, symptom relief is an important issue, but mood care and preventive care emerge as equally important.

Relief of symptoms was reported by 91.5% of respondents, even when offered the option of reporting no change or worsening. A majority also reported improvements in quality of life. Among respondents using other forms of care, a majority of acupuncture users reported decreased use of pharmaceuticals, surgery, and the services of a range of biomedical practitioners (Table 51–4).

The unique data presented here concerning decreased use of prescription drugs and avoidance of surgical procedures suggest a high potential for cost savings. Since this research was not experimental, it is not possible to formally link patient reports of treatment effectiveness and cost savings to physiological change and measured improvement in health status; these are not cost-effectiveness data. Combined with the satisfaction data, however, and by the measures used, it is clear that users perceive and report improved health and well-being. In sum, many users are highly satisfied with their Chinese medicine care.

REFERENCES

Accreditation Commission for Acupuncture and Oriental Medicine (ACAOM). Accredited and candidate programs. [Fact Sheet]. Silver Spring, MD: ACAOM, May 9, 2000.

Anderson R. An American clinic for traditional Chinese medicine: Comparisons to family medicine and chiropractic. *J Manipulative Physiol Ther.* 1991;14:462–465.

Anderson R. *Magic, Science and Health, the Aims and*

Achievements of Medical Anthropology. Fort Worth, TX: Harcourt Brace College Publishers; 1996.

Bernard HR. *Research Methods in Cultural Anthropology.* 2nd ed. Thousand Oaks, CA: Sage Publications; 1992.

Bullock M, Pheley A, Kiresuk R, Lenz S, Culliton P. Characteristics and complaints of patients seeking therapy at a hospital-based alternative medicine clinic. *J Altern Complement Med.* 1997;3:31–37.

Cassidy CM. Walk a mile in my shoes: Culturally sensitive food-habit research. *Am J Clin Nutr.* 1994a;59(suppl): 190s–197s.

Cassidy CM. Unraveling the ball of string: Reality, paradigms, and the study of alternative medicine. *J Mind-Body Health.* 1994b:10:5–31.

Cassileth B, et al. Contemporary unorthodox treatments in cancer medicine. *Ann Intern Med.* 1984;101:105–112.

Chinese medicine users in the United States. Part II: Preferred aspect of care. *J Altern Complement Med.* 1998;4(2):189–202. Review.

Clinical Oncology Group. New Zealand cancer patients and alternative medicine. *N Z Med J.* 1987;100:110–113.

Culliton P. Current utilization of acupuncture by U.S. patients. Paper presented at NIH Consensus Development Conference on Acupuncture; November 3, 1997.

Eisenberg D, Kessler R, Norlock F, Dlakins D, Delbanco R. Unconventional medicine in the United States, prevalence, costs and patterns of use. *N Engl J Med.* 1993; 328:246–252.

Emad M. Does acupuncture hurt? Cultural shifts in experiences of pain. *Proc Soc Acupunct Res.* 1994;2: 129–140.

Hare M. 1992. *East-Asian Medicine Among Non-Asian New Yorkers: A Study in Transformation and Translation.* Dissertation available from Michigan Microfilms, Ann Arbor, MI.

Hare M. The emergence of an urban U.S. Chinese medicine. *Med Anthropol Q.* 1993;7:30–49.

James R, Fox M, Taheri G. Who goes to a natural therapist? Why? *Aust Fam Physician.* 1983;12:383–386.

MacLean U. Choices of treatment among the Yoruba. In: Morley P, Wallis R, eds. *Culture and Curing, Anthropological Perspectives on Traditional Medical Beliefs and Practices.* Pittsburgh, PA: University of Pittsburgh Press; 1978:152–167.

McGinnis D. Alternative therapies: An overview. *Cancer.* 1991;67:1788–1792.

McGuire M. *Ritual Healing in Suburban America.* New Brunswick, NJ: Rutgers University Press; 1988.

Mitchell B. *Acupuncture and Oriental Medicine Laws.* Gig Harbor, WA: National Acupuncture Foundation, 1999.

O'Connor BB. *Healing Traditions, Alternative Medicine and Health Professions.* Philadelphia: University of Pennsylvania Press; 1995.

Reston J. Now about my operation in Peking. *New York Times.* July 26, 1971:1, 6.

Thomas K, Carr J, Westlake L, Williams B. Use of non-orthodox and conventional health care in Great Britain. *BMJ.* 1991;302:207–210.

Verhoef M, Sutherland L, Birkich L. Use of alternative medicine by patients attending a gastroenterology clinic. *Can Med Assoc J.* 1990;142:121–125.

Welsch RL. Traditional medicine and Western medical options among the Ningerum of Papua New Guinea. In: Romanucci-Ross L, Moerman DE, Tancredi LR, eds. *The Anthropology of Medicine, from Culture to Method.* South Hadley, MA: JF Bergin Publishers; 1983:32–53.

Young JC. *Medical Choice in a Mexican Village.* New Brunswick, NJ: Rutgers University Press; 1981.

CHAPTER 52

The Clinical Research on Acupuncture

52.1 Acupuncture Efficacy: A Summary of Controlled Clinical Trials

Stephen Birch and Richard Hammerschlag

A review of the clinical research on acupuncture affirms the value of acupuncture in the treatment of a variety of illnesses. While far from perfect or exhaustive, these studies clearly indicate that acupuncture, properly done and applied, can aid in the alleviation of pain and discomfort. In addition, the overwhelmingly convincing conclusion that can be drawn from the research is that acupuncture must be done in a manner which is informed by its own body of theory, and appropriate to the overall therapeutic approach.

The literature clearly highlights the need for more research into the clinical applications of correctly performed acupuncture and leads to inquiries about the possibilities that acupuncture presents if it were more readily available. While acupuncture is little used in inpatient settings in this country, the evidence indicates that it could offer much to hospital patients in alleviat-

---

Richard Hammerschlag, PhD, is currently research director at the Oregon College of Oriental Medicine in Portland and also serves as president of the Society for Acupuncture Research, an organization whose mission is to increase the quality, scope, and awareness of acupuncture research.

The Oregon College of Oriental Medicine is a nationally-accredited college offering a master's degree in Acupuncture and Oriental Medicine. Students receive academic and clinical training in all modalities of Oriental medicine and upon graduation are qualified to take national licensing examinations. The research program at the college includes studies on acupuncture and Chinese herbal therapies, and participation in federally-funded collaborative research with Oregon Health Sciences University, Kaiser Permanente Center for Health Research, the National College of Naturopathic Medicine, Western States Chiropractic College, and the Oregon School of Massage.

Stephen Birch, PhD, is coauthor of a number of books on acupuncture: *Understanding Acupuncture* with Robert Felt (New York: Harcourt Health Sciences, 1999), *Chasing the Dragon's Tail, Extraordinary Vessels, Essentials of Japanese Acupuncture*, and with Richard Hammerschlag, the report *Acupuncture Efficacy: A Compendium of Controlled Clinical Studies*. He has been a practicing clinician for more than a decade. Active in acupuncture research, he is cofounder and past president of the Society for Acupuncture Research, has been research director of the New England School of Acupuncture, has also performed acupuncture research at Yale University, and chaired the 1994 Workshop on Acupuncture, sponsored by the Office of Alternative Medicine at the National Institutes of Health.

ing pain and postoperative discomfort, and in improving the speed and quality of recovery.

ACUTE AND CHRONIC PAIN

Pain management is the most widely investigated use of acupuncture (Birch et al, 1996). The explosion of interest in acupuncture in the West, triggered by James Reston's article in the *New York Times* and Richard Nixon's trip to China in the early 1970s, focused almost entirely on the use of the needles to produce analgesia. Not only were numerous clinical trials conducted, but many studies investigated the mechanisms by which acupuncture alleviates pain. The initial progress in explaining the analgesic action in Western scientific terms provided a measure of credibility for acupuncture within the biomedical community. But it also had the inappropriate effect of focusing the clinical testing on acupuncture largely within the framework of the drug model.

Slow in coming were the realizations that, in many of the clinical trials for pain, what were designed as "placebo acupuncture" treatments were causing significant nonplacebo effects. Needling of supposed nonpoints ("irrelevant acupuncture") as a sham control was often producing effects intermediate between placebo responses and the effects of true needling. The design of clinical trials of acupuncture has only recently begun to receive the necessary attention to ensure that it is tested by methods that on the one hand are rigorous enough to satisfy scientific standards, while on the other, do not distort the diagnostic and treatment principles that are unique to this therapeutic tradition.

The best designed and most clinically promising studies in the use of acupuncture for relief of acute and chronic pain reflect a wide range of pain conditions for which acupuncture has been effectively applied (see Chapter 52.2). These conditions include headache, facial, dental, neck and low-back pain, tennis elbow, osteoarthritis, renal colic, dysmenorrhea, fibromyalgia, athletic injury, endoscopy-associated pain, and postsurgical pain. In a number of the clinical trials, acupuncture proved as good or better than current standard care (eg, Junnila, 1982; Ahonen et al, 1983; Johansson et al, 1991) and usually without the side effects commonly associated with the standard therapies (eg, Wang et al, 1992; Hesse et al, 1994).

The cumulative evidence suggests that acupuncture represents a therapeutically beneficial, cost-effective treatment option for a broad spectrum of acute and chronic pain conditions. Patients unwilling to accept, unable to tolerate, or nonresponsive to standard therapies for pain management should especially be offered the opportunity to receive an adequate course of acupuncture treatment for their conditions.

NAUSEA AND VOMITING

These conditions are regularly experienced following general anesthesia and cancer chemotherapy. While partial success in moderating unpleasant side effects is usually achieved with antiemetic drugs, medication frequently provides inadequate relief if anesthesia is prolonged or if chemotherapy is in the high-dose range. This has encouraged the testing of acupuncture as an alternative, and as a supplement, to standard antiemetic care (Parfitt, 1996; Vickers, 1996).

These clinical trials are unique since emesis is the one condition for which acupuncture has been consistently tested at only a single point. The collective evidence from the studies listed in Chapter 52.2 indicate that stimulation of the acupuncture point called Neiguan or P6, located on the inner side of the wrist, provides effective therapy for postoperative and cancer/chemotherapy-related emesis. In several of the studies, P6 stimulation provided significantly better relief from nausea and vomiting than stimulation at a "dummy" point (Dundee et al, 1989a, 1989b), while in others, P6 therapy was at least as beneficial as antiemetic drugs (Ghaly et al, 1987; Dundee et al, 1989a; Ho et al, 1990) or was an effective adjunct to medication (Dundee et al, 1989b; Dundee and Yang, 1990; Aglietti et al, 1990).

Acupressure at P6, provided manually or by wearing the commercially available Sea Bands, was also found to suppress nausea and vomiting beyond the level of placebo (Barsoum et al, 1990) and to prolong the effectiveness of acupuncture (Dundee and Yang, 1990). Additional studies found that acupressure at P6 was effective as a nondrug alternative for alleviating nausea and vomiting of pregnancy-related morning sickness and visually induced motion sickness. Advantages of acupressure are that it requires only a brief instruction period and can be applied as needed by the patient without additional office or clinic visits.

STROKE

The efficacy of acupuncture for the treatment of paralysis due to stroke has been examined in five controlled clinical trials (p. 526). Randomized trials based in the United States, Sweden, Taiwan, and Norway tested acupuncture as a supplement to physical therapy. Another study, from China, compared an acupuncture group to a previously treated group given medication. (No stroke studies have tested acupuncture in comparison, or as adjunctive, to the recently approved clot-dissolving drugs.) All five studies showed a positive outcome for acupuncture.

Additional information was generated on the value of neurological function tests and CT scans for predicting which patients were most likely to benefit from acupuncture. Of particular interest is that acupuncture was shown to increase the effectiveness of physical therapy when treatment was provided as soon as patients were medically stabilized (within 1 to 10 days of stroke). The research also found benefits even when treatment was not begun until 1 to 3 months poststroke, but not as great as that obtained through early intervention.

RESPIRATORY DISEASE

Clinical trials of acupuncture for the treatment of respiratory diseases have been extensively reviewed (Jobst, 1995). A major reason for assess-

ing the benefits of acupuncture for such chronic conditions as asthma and disabling breathlessness is that long-term use of corticosteroids and other commonly prescribed inhalants can result in a variety of adverse side effects (Lane and Lane, 1991). In the studies reviewed, acupuncture was found to be effective for reversing the acute effects of bronchoconstriction induced by either pharmacological means or exercise. It was also found to alleviate the chronic effects of asthma.

In two of the studies, acupuncture was performed at a standard set of points, while in the third study, patients were needled at individualized sets of points chosen on the basis of traditional Chinese medicine diagnosis. Control needling was always matched to acupuncture in terms of number of needles, region of the body needled, and frequency and duration of treatments. In all three blinded studies, acupuncture significantly outperformed control needling under conditions designed to keep the patients as well as the treatment assessors unaware of whether true or control points had been needled.

SUBSTANCE ABUSE

At present in the United States, acupuncture is used in more than 300 government-supported and private clinics as adjunctive therapy for the treatment of persons dependent on opiates, cocaine, tobacco, alcohol, and other substances (Brewington et al, 1994). Acupuncture treatment programs are also being increasingly instituted in the legal and prison systems (Brumbaugh, 1993). Despite the growth of acupuncture as a viable treatment option for substance abuse (Culliton and Kiresuk, 1996), and the formation of the National Acupuncture Detoxification Association that promotes acupuncture for treating addictions, relatively few clinical trials have examined this aspect of acupuncture use. However, trials have been performed with a focus on chronic cigarette smoking, alcoholism, and cocaine dependence. Research found that in a study of nicotine addiction, acupuncture and nicotine gum achieved a similar modicum of success in enabling chronic smokers to abstain from cigarettes (Clavel et al, 1985). Chronic alcohol consumption, the focus of a 1989 study published in *Lancet*, galvanized interest in the use of acupuncture to treat chemical dependency (Bullock et al, 1989). Acupuncture therapy compared favorably to a previous trial of medication for treating methadone-maintained cocaine addicts (Margolin et al, 1993). Acupuncture also outperformed control needling for decreasing cocaine use, as determined by urinalysis (Lipton et al, 1994). Several United States-based multicenter trials currently in progress are likely to help clarify the efficacy of acupuncture for substance abuse problems.

PROBLEMS IN THE DESIGN AND REPORTING OF ACUPUNCTURE RESEARCH

In reviewing clinical trials of acupuncture, five problems were identified that can create difficulties when assessing results of the studies (see also Hammerschlag, 1998). These problems are pointed out, where relevant, in the summaries of the individual studies.

First is a lack of information on the training of the acupuncturist(s). Since, in some medical circles, acupuncture is regarded, inappropriately, as a "technique" that can be learned in several short sessions, insufficient training may be an inadvertent factor contributing to a negative outcome.

Second is the inadequate description of the points needled or the frequency and duration of acupuncture treatment. Without sufficient information on the nature of the treatment, it is difficult to assess whether a negative outcome indicates that the acupuncture treatment was truly ineffective or was, instead, inadequately provided.

Third is the implicit assumption that needling at control points equates to a placebo treatment. However, invasive needling at points inappropriate to the treatment is likely to produce nonspecific effects as well as placebo effects. Such nonspecific effects include local responses to the microtrauma of needling (Kendall, 1989) as well as neurally mediated responses to noxious stimuli (Le Bars et al, 1991). As a result, control needling often produces effects that are intermediate between those of real acupuncture and no treatment (Vincent and Lewith, 1995).

Fourth is the underenrollment of patients. Dropouts can reduce group size to an extent where statistical significance of treatment is lost, particularly in studies involving treatment of outpatients.

Fifth is that some studies administered acupuncture at a fixed set of treatment points (following a Western medicine-style research design) while in others, acupuncture points were chosen on an individualized basis (in keeping with traditional Chinese medicine diagnostic principles). Ulcers, for example, in an acupuncturist's view can arise from at least a half dozen different underlying conditions, each requiring a distinctly different treatment plan (Kaptchuk, 1983). Unless the fixed-protocol patients have been preselected for the same Chinese medicine diagnosis, such a study design may contribute to a poor treatment outcome. This variable of fixed versus individualized treatment plans is a particular problem when attempting to compare results from different clinical trials.

Despite the above problems, the author concurs with the Food and Drug Administration that "the clinical studies and preclinical animal studies included in the petitions constitute valid scientific evidence in support of clinical effectiveness of acupuncture needles for the performance of acupuncture treatment" (FDA, 1996). This review of the research supports this conclusion.

REFERENCES

Birch S, Hammerschlag R, Berman BM. Acupuncture in the treatment of pain. *J Alt Compl Med.*1996;2:101–124.

Food and Drug Administration (FDA), Public Health Service, U.S. Department of Health and Human Services.

Reclassification Order: Docket No. 94P-0443. Acupuncture needles for the practice of acupuncture. March 29, 1996.

Hammerschlag R. Methodological and ethical issues in clinical trials of acupuncture. *J Altern Complement Med.* 1998;4:159–171.

Kendall DE. A scientific model for acupuncture. *Am J Acupunct.* 1989;17:251–268.

Kaptchuk TJ. The Web That Has No Weaver. New York: Congden and Weed. 1983, pp. 4–6.

Le Bars D, Villaneuva L, Willer JC, Bouhassira D. Diffuse noxious inhibitory control (DNIC) in man and animals. *Acupunct Med.* 1991;9:47–57.

Reston J. Now let me tell you about my appendectomy in Peking. *New York Times.* July 26, 1971: 1, 16.

Vincent C, Lewith G. Placebo controls for acupuncture studies. *J Roy Soc Med.* 1995:88:199–202.

Note: For references to specific clinical trials, see Chapter 52.2.

52.2   Annotated Bibliography

Stephen Birch and Richard Hammerschlag

The primary criterion for selecting a study for review was that acupuncture had been compared to some form of control treatment (de la Torre, 1993; Vincent and Lewith, 1995; Birch, 1995). This means that patients were randomly assigned to one group that would receive acupuncture or to a second group that would receive a control treatment. Most commonly, the second group was treated either with control needling (usually at points inappropriate to the condition being studied), an inactive surface-electrode device (TENS unit), or standard care (medication, a medical device or physiotherapy). A few studies used delayed treatment (wait-list control). For acupuncture to be considered effective, it must have produced significantly better results than control needling, inactive TENS or no treatment, or it must have performed at least as well as effective standard care.

Additional selection criteria were that the studies are full papers (not abstracts), published in English, in journals listed in MEDLINE, EMBASE, or AMED medical citation indices. In most of the studies selected, the acupuncture treatment involved insertion of needles, with or without mild electrical stimulation applied through the needles (electroacupuncture). A few

studies were included in which points were stimulated by either acupressure or moxibustion (a form of heat therapy) since these techniques fall within the scope of practice of acupuncture in most states. Studies in which acupuncture points were stimulated by other methods, such as surface electrodes or laser, were not considered.

ACUTE AND CHRONIC PAIN

Headache and Migraine

Ahonen E, Hakumaki M, Mahlamaki S, Partanen J, Riekkinen P, Sivenius J. Acupuncture and physiotherapy in the treatment of myogenic headache patients: pain relief and EMG activity. *Adv Pain Res Ther.* 1983;5:571–576.

Carlsson J, Fahlcrantz A, Augustinsson LE. Muscle tenderness in tension headache treated with acupuncture or physiotherapy. *Cephalalgia.* 1990;10:131–141.

Hesse J, Mogelvang B, Simonsen H. Acupuncture versus metroprolol in migraine prophylaxis: a randomized trial of trigger point inactivation. *J Intern Med.* 1994;235:451–456.

Loh L, Nathan PW, Schott GD, Zilkha KJ. Acupuncture versus medical treatment for migraine and muscle tension headaches. *J Neurol Neurosurg Psychiatr.* 1984;47:333–337.

Courtesy of Richard Hammerschlag, PhD, Portland, Oregon.

Vincent CA. A controlled trial of the treatment of migraine by acupuncture. *Clin J Pain*. 1989; 5:305–312.

Vincent CA. The treatment of tension headache by acupuncture. A controlled single-case design with time series analysis. *J Psychosomatic Res*. 1990;34:553–561.

Facial Pain

Hansen PE, Hansen JH. Acupuncture treatment of chronic facial pain: a controlled cross-over trial. *Headache*. 1983;23:66–69.

Johansson A, Wenneberg B, Wagersten C, Haraldson T. Acupuncture in treatment of facial muscular pain. *Acta Odontol Scand*. 1991;49: 153–158.

List T, Helkimo M. Acupuncture and occlusal splint therapy in the treatment of craniomandibular disorders, part II: a one year follow-up study. *Acta Odontol Scand*. 1992;50:375–385.

List T, Helkimo M, Andersson S, Carlsson GE. Acupuncture and occlusal splint therapy in the treatment of craniomandibular disorders, part I: a comparative study. *Swed Dent J*. 1992;16: 125–141.

Raustia AM, Pohjola RT, Virtanen KK. Acupuncture compared with stomatognathic treatment for TMJ dysfunction, part I: a randomized study. *J Prosthet Dent*. 1985;54: 581–585.

Dental Pain

Lao L, Bergman S, Langenberg P, Wong RH, Berman B. Efficacy of Chinese acupuncture on postoperative oral surgery pain. *Oral Surg Oral Med Oral Pathol Oral Radiol Endod*. 1995;79:423–428.

Sung YF, Kutner MH, Cerine FC, Frederickson EL. Comparison of the effects of acupuncture and codeine on postoperative dental pain. *Anesth Analag Curr Res*. 1977;56:473–478.

Neck Pain

Coan R, Wong G, Coan PL. The acupuncture treatment of neck pain: a randomized controlled study. *Am J Chin Med*. 1982;9: 326–332.

Loy TT. Treatment of cervical spondylosis—electroacupuncture versus physiotherapy. *Med J Aust*. 1983;2:32–34.

Petrie JP, Langley GB. Acupuncture in the treatment of chronic cervical pain: a pilot study. *Clin Exp Rheumatol*. 1983;1:333–336.

Low-Back Pain

Coan RM, Wong G, Ku SL, et al. The acupuncture treatment of low back pain: a randomized controlled study. *Am J Chin Med*. 1980;8: 181–189.

Fox EJ, Melzack R. Transcutaneous electrical stimulation and acupuncture: comparison of treatment for low-back pain. *Pain*. 1976;2: 141–148.

Gunn CC, Milbrandt WE, Little AS, Mason KE. Dry needling of muscle motor points for chronic low-back pain. *Spine*. 1980;5: 279–291.

Laitinen J. Acupuncture and transcutaneous electric stimulation in the treatment of chronic sacrolumbalgia and ischialgia. *Am J Chin Med*. 1976;4:169–175.

MacDonald AJR, Macrae KD, Master BR, Rubin AP. Superficial acupuncture in the relief of chronic low-back pain. *Ann Roy Coll Surg Eng*. 1983;65:44–46.

Thomas M, Lundberg T. Importance of modes of acupuncture in the treatment of chronic nociceptive low-back pain. *Acta Anaesthesiol Scand*. 1994;38:63–69.

Tennis Elbow

Brattberg G. Acupuncture therapy for tennis elbow. *Pain*. 1983;16:285–288.

Haker E, Lundeberg T. Acupuncture treatment in epicondylalgia: a comparative study of two acupuncture techniques. *Clin J Pain.* 1990;6: 221–226.

Molsberger A, Hille E. The analgesic effect of acupuncture in chronic tennis elbow pain. *Br J Rheumatol.* 1994;33:1162–1165.

Osteoarthritis

Christensen BV, Iuhl IU, Vilbek H, Bulow HH, Dreijer NC, Rasmussen HF. Acupuncture treatment of severe knee osteoarthritis: a long-term study. *Acta Anaesthesiol Scand.* 1992;36:519–525.

Dickens W, Lewith GT. A single-blind, controlled and randomized clinical trial to evaluate the effect of acupuncture in the treatment of trapezio-metacarpal osteoarthritis. *Compl Med Res.* 1989;3:5–8.

Junnila SYT. Acupuncture superior to Piroxicam™ in the treatment of osteoarthritis. *Am J Acupunct.* 1982;10:341–346.

Thomas M, Eriksson SV, Lundberg T. A comparative study of diazepam and acupuncture in patients with osteoarthritis pain: a placebo-controlled study. *Am J Chin Med.* 1991;19: 95–100.

Renal Colic

Lee YH, Lee WC, Chen MT, Huang JK, Chung C, Chang LS. Acupuncture in the treatment of renal colic. *J Urol.* 1992;147:16–18.

Dysmenorrhea

Helms JM. Acupuncture for the management of primary dysmenorrhea. *Obstet Gynecol.* 1987; 69:51–56.

Fibromyalgia

Deluze C, Bosia L, Zirbs A, Chantraine A, Vischer TL. Electroacupuncture in fibromyalgia: results of a controlled trial. *Br Med J.* 1992;305:1249–1252.

Athletic Injury

Wang L, Wang A, Zhang S. Clinical analysis and experimental observation on acupuncture and moxibustion treatment of patellar tendon terminal disease in athletes. *J Tradit Chin Med.* 1985;5:162–166.

Endoscopy-Associated Pain and Discomfort

Cahn AM, Carayon P, Hill C, Flamant R. Acupuncture in gastroscopy. *Lancet.* 1978;i: 182–183.

Wang HH, Chang YH, Liu DM. A study in the effectiveness of acupuncture analgesia for colonoscopic examination compared with conventional premedication. *Am J Acupunct.* 1992;20:217–221.

Postoperative Pain

Christensen PA, Noreng M, Andersen PE, Nielsen JW. Electroacupuncture and postoperative pain. *Br J Anaesth.* 1989;62: 258–262.

Martelete M, Fiori AMC. Comparative study of the analgesic effect of transcutaneous nerve stimulation (TNS), electroacupuncture (EA) and meperidine in the treatment of postoperative pain. *Acupunct Electro-Ther Res Int J.* 1985;10:183–193.

NAUSEA AND VOMITING

Parfitt A. Acupuncture as an antiemetic treatment. *J Alt Compl Med.* 1996;2:167–173.

Vickers A. Can acupuncture have specific effects on health? A systematic review of acupuncture antiemesis trials. *J Roy Soc Med.* 1996;89:303–311.

Anesthesia (Postoperative)

Barsoum G, Perry EP, Fraser IA. Postoperative nausea is relieved by acupressure. *J Roy Soc Med.* 1990;83:86–89.

Dundee JW, Ghaly RG, Bill KM, Chestnutt WN, Fitzpatrick KTJ, Lynas AGA. Effect of stimulation of the P6 antiemetic point on postoperative nausea and vomiting. *Br J Anaesth*. 1989a;63:612–618.

Ghaly RG, Fitzpatrick KTJ, Dundee JW. Antiemetic studies with traditional Chinese acupuncture: a comparison of manual needling with electrical stimulation and commonly used antiemetics. *Anaesthesia*. 1987;42: 1108–1110.

Ho RT, Jawan B, Fung ST, Cheung HK, Lee JH. Electro-acupuncture and postoperative emesis. *Anaesthesia*. 1990;45:327–329.

Chemotherapy

Aglietti L, Roila F, Tonato M, et al. A pilot study of metoclopramide, dexamethasone, diphenhydramine and acupuncture in women treated with cisplatin. *Cancer Chemother Pharmacol*. 1990;26:239–240.

Dundee JW, Ghaly RG, Fitzpatrick KTJ, Abram WP, Lynch GA. Acupuncture prophylaxis of cancer chemotherapy-induced sickness. *J Roy Soc Med*. 1989b;82:268–271.

Dundee JW, Yang J. Prolongation of the antiemetic effect of P6 acupuncture by acupressure in patients having cancer chemotherapy. *J Roy Soc Med*. 1990;83:360–362.

Morning Sickness

De Aloysio D, Penacchioni P. Morning sickness control in early pregnancy by Neiguan point acupressure. *Obstet Gynecol*. 1992;80: 852–854.

Dundee JW, Sourial FBR, Ghaly RG, Bell PF. P6 acupressure reduces morning sickness. *J Roy Soc Med*. 1988;81:456–457.

Hyde E. Acupressure therapy for morning sickness: a controlled clinical trial. *J Nurse-Midwifery* 1989;34:171–178.

Motion Sickness

Hu S, Stritzel R, Chandler A, Stern RN. P6 acupressure reduces symptoms of vection-induced motion sickness. *Aviat Space Environ Med*. 1995;66:631–634.

STROKE

Hu HH, Chung C, Liu TJ, et al. A randomized controlled trial on the treatment of acute partial ischemic stroke with acupuncture. *Neuroepidemiology*. 1993;12:106–113.

Johansson K, Lindgren I, Widner H, Wiklund I, Johansson BB. Can sensory stimulation improve the functional outcome in stroke patients? *Neurology*. 1993;43:2189–2192.

Naeser MA, Alexander MP, Stiassny-Eder D, Galler V, Hobbs J, Bachman D. Real versus sham acupuncture in the treatment of paralysis in acute stroke patients: a CT scan lesion site study. *J Neurol Rehabil*. 1992;6:153–173.

Sallstrom S, Kjendahl A, Osten PE, Stanghelle JH, Borchgrevink CF. Acupuncture in the treatment of stroke patients in the subacute stage: a randomized, controlled study. *Compl Ther Med*. 1996;4:193–197.

Zhang W, Li S, Chen G, Zhang Q, Wang Y. Acupuncture treatment of apoplectic hemiplegia. *J Tradit Chin Med*. 1987;7:157–160.

RESPIRATORY DISEASE

Fung KP, Chow OKW, So SY. Attenuation of exercise-induced asthma by acupuncture. *Lancet*. 1986;2:1419–1422.

Jobst K, Chen JH, McPherson K, et al. Controlled trial of acupuncture for disabling breathlessness. *Lancet*. 1986;2:1416–1419.

Jobst KA. A critical analysis of acupuncture in pulmonary disease: efficacy and safety of the acupuncture needle. *J Alt Compl Med*. 1995; 1:57–85.

Lane DJ, Lane TV. Alternative and complementary medicine for asthmas. *Thorax*. 1991;46: 787–797.

Tashkin DP, Bresler DE, Kroening RJ, Kerschner H, Katz RL, Coulson A. Comparison of real and simulated acupuncture and isoproterenol in methacholine-induced asthma. *Ann Allergy*. 1977;39:379–387.

SUBSTANCE ABUSE

Brewington V, Smith M, Lipton D. Acupuncture as a detoxification treatment: an analysis of controlled research. *J Subst Abuse Treatment.* 1994;11:289–307.

Brumbaugh AG. Acupuncture: new perspectives in chemical dependency treatment. *J Subst Abuse Treatment.* 1993;10:35–43.

Bullock ML, Culliton, PD, Olander RT. Controlled trial of acupuncture for severe recidivist alcoholism. *Lancet.* 1989;1:1435–1439.

Bullock ML, Umen AJ, Culliton PD, Olander RT. Acupuncture treatment of alcoholic recidivism, a pilot study. *Alcohol: Clin Exp Res.* 1987;11:292–295.

Clavel F, Brenhamou S, Company-Huertas A, Flamant R. Helping people to stop smoking: randomized comparison of groups being treated with acupuncture and nicotine gum with control group. *Br Med J.* 1985;291:1538–1539.

Culliton PD, Kieresuk TJ. Overview of substance abuse acupuncture treatment research. *J Alt Compl Med.* 1996:149–159.

Lipton DS, Brewington V, Smith M. Acupuncture for crack-cocaine detoxification: experimental evaluation of efficacy. *J Subst Abuse Treatment.* 1994;11:205–215.

Margolin A, Avants SK, Chang P, Kosten TR. Acupuncture for the treatment of cocaine dependence in methadone-maintained patients. *Am J Addict.* 1993;2:194–201.

52.3   Controlled Clinical Trials of Acupuncture: An Annotated Bibliography

Jeffrey A. Weih

Each condition listed in this bibliography is the subject of at least one controlled trial that demonstrated the effectiveness of acupuncture treatment. All available controlled clinical trials of acupuncture published in English since 1966 are reviewed to portray the full range of outcomes obtained. Studies published since 1995 are reviewed from their English language abstracts in the MEDLINE database (PubMed) of the National Library of Medicine, National Institutes of Health (http://www.ncbi.nlm.nih.gov), even if they were not originally published in English. To avoid redundancy, no studies are included that were cited in Chapter 52.2.

Assessment of each trial's outcome is based solely on its own report of results. Methodologic quality varies greatly from trial to trial and is not assessed in this review.

For additional information or interpretation, the reader is advised to consult critical reviews of acupuncture research methodology by Hammerschlag and Morris (1997), Birch and Hammerschlag (1996), Vincent and Richardson (1986), and ter Riet et al (1990a, 1990b). In most of the studies, subjects in the acupuncture intervention group received treatment via acupuncture needles placed at acupuncture points or via

Jeffrey Weih, PA, LAc, is a graduate of the University of Iowa Physician's Assistant Program and of the Oregon College of Oriental Medicine. For more than a decade, he has worked as a physician's assistant in Physiatry at Kaiser Permanente in Portland, Oregon, and, for the last 7 years, has also provided acupuncture treatment for workers' compensation patients in that setting. He serves as medical director of Complementary Healthcare Plan's AcuMedNet, a preferred provider organization for acupuncturists in the Pacific Northwest.

electrical stimulation through inserted needles (electroacupuncture) at such points. In some studies, related methods were used in the treatment group and were applied to acupuncture points in lieu of needling. These various techniques included focused manual pressure (acupressure), transcutaneous electric nerve stimulation, laser light, or heat (moxibustion). Uncommonly used techniques included dry needling at trigger points or glucose injection; in a few studies, subjects received medication in addition to acupuncture. Control treatments included some of the acupuncture-related techniques listed above, as well as a variety of placebo procedures.

If a study included a variety of diagnoses in its groupings, the included diagnoses are listed in parentheses following its citation. Studied conditions are categorized with the understanding that there are often many possible etiologies for any given condition. The bibliography is organized in the following format:

- **TYPES OF CONDITIONS** (by physio-anatomic classification)
- **Body Regions and/or Symptoms** (by affected location and/or subjective complaint)
- *Diagnoses* (by etiologic assessment)

ACUTE NEUROMUSCULOSKELETAL PAIN

Acute Low-Back Pain

Hackett GI, Seddon D, Kaminski D. Electroacupuncture compared with paracetamol for acute low back pain. *The Practitioner*. 1988; 232:163–164. Acupuncture was found to be significantly more effective than control.

CHRONIC NEUROMUSCULOSKELETAL PAIN

Godfrey CM, Morgan P. A controlled trial of the theory of acupuncture in musculoskeletal pain. *J Rheumatol*. 1978;5:121–124. (Degenerative disc disease, osteoarthritis, lumbosacral strain, cervical strain, tennis elbow, bursitis, eight other diagnoses unspecified.) Acupuncture was found to be nonsignificantly more effective than control.

Grewal JK, Iyer NKN, Sim MK. Effects of acupuncture and biofeedback on EMG and symptom severity in chronic pain patients. *Am J Acupunct*. 1989;17:219–224. (Joint pain, headache, backache.) Acupuncture and control were both found to be significantly effective per first of three measures.

Lee PK, Andersen TW, Modell JH, Saga SA. Treatment of chronic pain with acupuncture. *JAMA*. 1975;32:1133–1135. (Osteoarthritis, rheumatoid arthritis, low-back pain, headache, spondylitis, postherpetic neuralgia, trigeminal neuralgia, miscellaneous other diagnoses.) Acupuncture and control were both found to be significantly effective.

Man PL, Chen CH. Acupuncture for pain relief, a double-blind, self-controlled study. *Michigan Med*. 1974;73:15–24. (Trigeminal neuralgia, postherpetic neuralgia, traumatic intercostal neuralgia, occipital neuralgia, low-back pain, arthritis, hysterical headaches, tennis elbow, post–cancer operation pain, paraplegia with pain, carpal tunnel syndrome.) Acupuncture was found to be more effective than control; significance was not specified.

Chronic Facial Pain

Orofacial Muscle Pain

Widerstrom-Noga E, Dryehag LE, Borglum-Jensen L, Aslund PG, Wenneberg B, Andersson SA. Pain threshold responses to two different modes of sensory stimulation in patients with orofacial muscular pain: psychologic considerations. *J Orofac Pain*. 1998; 12:27–34. Acupuncture was found to be significantly more effective than control.

Trigeminal Neuralgia

Spacek A, Hanl G, Groiss O, Koinig H, Kress HG. Acupuncture and ganglionic local opioid analgesia in trigeminal neuralgia [In German]. *Win Med Wochenschr*. 1998;148: 447–449. In one of two acupuncture groups, acupuncture was found to be significantly more effective than control.

Zhang Z. Observation on therapeutic effects of blood letting puncture with cupping in acute trigeminal neuralgia. *J Tradit Chin Med*. 1997; 17:272–274. Acupuncture was found to be significantly more effective than control over the long term.

Chronic Jaw Pain

Masseter/Temporalis Myofascial Pain

McMillan AS, Nolan A, Kelly PJ. The efficacy of dry needling and procaine in the treatment of myofascial pain in the jaw muscles. *J Orofac Pain*. 1997;11(4):307–314. Acupuncture and controls were both found to be significantly effective.

Temporomandibular Joint Disorder

Elsharkawy TM, Ali NM. Evaluation of acupuncture and occlusal splint therapy in the treatment of temporomandibular joint disorders. *Egypt Dent J*. 1995;41(3):1227–1232. Acupuncture was found to be more effective than were two of three controls; significance was not specified.

Chronic Headache

Jensen LB, Melsen B, Jensen SB. Effect of acupuncture on headache measured by reduction in number of attacks and use of drugs. *Scand J Dent Res*. 1979;87:373–380. Acupuncture was found to be significantly more effective than control per each measure.

Wylie KR, Jackson C, Crawford PM. Does psychological testing help to predict the response to acupuncture or massage/relaxation therapy in patients presenting to a general neurology clinic with headache? *J Tradit Chin Med*. 1997; 17(2):130–139. Acupuncture and control were both found to be significantly effective.

Muscle Tension Headache

Hansen PE, Hansen JH. Acupuncture treatment of chronic tension headache: a controlled cross-over trial. *Cephalalgia*. 1985;5:137–142. Acupuncture was found to be significantly more effective than control.

Tavola T, Gala C, Conte G, Invernizzi G. Traditional Chinese acupuncture in tension-type headache: a controlled study. *Pain*. 1992;48: 325–329. Acupuncture was found to be non-significantly more effective than control.

Migraine Headache

Dowson DI, Lewith GT, Machin D. The effects of acupuncture versus placebo in the treatment of headache. *Pain*.1985;21:35–42. Acupuncture was found to be nonsignificantly more effective than control.

Lenhard L, Waite PME. Acupuncture in the prophylactic treatment of migraine headaches: pilot study. *NZ Med J*. 1983;96:663–666. Acupuncture and control were both found to be significantly effective.

Shuyuan G, Donglan Z, Yanguang X. A comparative study on the treatment of migraine headache with combined distant and local acupuncture points versus conventional drug therapy. *Am J Acupunct*. 1999;27(1–2):27–30. Acupuncture was found to be significantly more effective than control.

Childhood Migraine

Pintov S, Lahat E, Alstein M, Vogel Z, Barg J. Acupuncture and the opioid system: implications in management of migraine. *Pediatr Neurol*. 1997;17(2):129–133. Acupuncture was found to be significantly more effective than control.

Chronic Neck Pain

David J, Modi S, Aluko AA, Robertshaw C, Farebrother J. Chronic neck pain: a comparison of acupuncture treatment and physiotherapy.

Br J Rheumatol. 1998;37(10):1118–1122. Acupuncture and control were both found to be effective; significance was not specified.

Petrie JP, Hazleman BL. A controlled study of acupuncture in neck pain. *Brit J Rheumatol*. 1986;25(3):271–275. Acupuncture and control were both found to be ineffective.

Myofascial Neck Pain

Birch S, Jamison RN. Controlled trial of Japanese acupuncture for chronic myofascial neck pain: assessment of specific and nonspecific effects of treatment. *Clin J Pain*. 1998;14(3): 248–255. Acupuncture was found to be significantly more effective than control.

Chronic Back/Spine Pain

Giles LG, Muller R. Chronic spinal pain syndromes: a clinical pilot trial comparing acupuncture, a nonsteroidal anti-inflammatory drug, and spinal manipulation. *J Manipulative Physiol Ther*. 1999;22(6):376–381. Acupuncture and the first control were found to be equally ineffective; acupuncture was found to be significantly less effective than the second control.

Grant DJ, Bishop-Miller J, Winchester DM, Anderson M, Faulkner S. A randomized comparative trial of acupuncture versus transcutaneous electrical nerve stimulation for chronic back pain in the elderly. *Pain*. 1999;82(1): 9–13. Acupuncture was found to be significantly more effective than control per one of three measures.

Ankylosing Spondylitis

Emery P, Lythgoe S. The effect of acupuncture on ankylosing spondylitis. *Brit J Rheumatol*. 1986;25(1):132–133. Acupuncture was found to be significantly effective in the short term by one of three measures; the effectiveness of the control was not specified.

Chronic Low-Back Pain

Edelist G, Gross AE, Langer F. Treatment of low back pain with acupuncture. *Can Anaesth*

Soc J. 1976;23(3):303–306. No significant difference was found in effectiveness between acupuncture and control; relative effectiveness was not unspecified.

Lehmann TR, Russell DW, Spratt KF, Colby H, Liu YK, Fairchild ML, Christensen S. Efficacy of electroacupuncture and TENS in the rehabilitation of chronic low back pain patients. *Pain*. 1986;26:277–290. Acupuncture was found to be nonsignificantly more effective than each control.

Mendelson G, Selwood TS, Kranz H, Loh TS, Kidson MA, Scott DS. Acupuncture treatment of chronic back pain. *Am J Med*. 1983;74: 49–55. Acupuncture was found to be nonsignificantly more effective than control.

Selwood TS, Kidson MA, Kranz H, Loh ST, Mendelson G, Scott DF. Evaluation of acupuncture treatment for chronic low back pain. In: Peck, ed. *Problems in Pain*. Sydney: Pergamon; 1980:179–187. Acupuncture was found to be significantly more effective than control.

Low-Back Strain

Garvey TA, Marks MR, Wiesel SW. A prospective, randomized, double-blind evaluation of trigger-point injection therapy for low-back pain. *Spine*. 1989;14(9):962–964. Acupuncture was found to be nonsignificantly more effective than two of three controls.

Chronic Shoulder Pain

Rotator Cuff Lesion

Berry H, Fernandez L, Bloom B, Clark RJ, Hamilton EBD. Clinical study comparing acupuncture, physiotherapy, injection and oral anti-inflammatory therapy in shoulder-cuff lesions. *Curr Med Res Opin*. 1980;7(2): 121–126. No significant difference was found in effectiveness between acupuncture and all controls; relative effectiveness was not specified.

Rotator Cuff Tendonitis

Kleinhenz J, Streitberger K, Windeler J, Gusbacher A, Mavridis G, Martin E. Randomized clinical trial comparing the effects of acupuncture and a newly designed placebo needle in rotator cuff tendonitis. *Pain*. 1999;83(2): 235–241. Acupuncture was found to be significantly more effective than control.

Chronic Knee Pain

Arichi S, Arichi H, Toda S. Acupuncture and rehabilitation (III) effects of acupuncture applied to the normal side on osteoarthritis deformans and rheumatoid arthritis of the knee and on disorders in motility of the knee joint after cerebral hemorrhage and thrombosis. *Am J Chin Med*. 1983;11(1–4):146–149. (Osteoarthritis deformans, rheumatoid arthritis, disorders of knee joint mobility post cerebral hemorrhage or thrombosis.) Acupuncture was found to be significantly more effective than each control.

Osteoarthritic Knee Pain

Berman BM, Singh BB, Lao L, Langenberg P, Li H, Hadhazy V, Bareta J, Hochberg M. A randomized trial of acupuncture as an adjunctive therapy in osteoarthritis of the knee. *Rheumatology (Oxford)*. 1999;38(4):346–354. Acupuncture was found to be significantly more effective than control.

Takeda W, Wessel J. Acupuncture for the treatment of pain of osteoarthritic knees. *Arthritis Care Res*. 1994;7(3):118–122. Acupuncture was found to be nonsignificantly more effective than control.

Rheumatoid Arthritic Knee Pain

Man SC, Baragar FD. Preliminary clinical study of acupuncture in rheumatoid arthritis. *J Rheumatol*. 1974;1(1):126–129. Acupuncture was found to be significantly more effective than control.

Chronic Extremity Pain

Kreczi T, Klinger D. A comparison of laser acupuncture versus placebo in radicular and pseudoradicular pain syndromes as recorded by subjective responses of patients. *Acupunct Electrother Res*. 1986;11:207–216. (Cervical radicular pain, lumbar radicular pain, pseudoradicular pain.) Acupuncture was found to be significantly more effective than control.

Extremity Pain of Sickle Cell Crisis

Co LL, Schmitz TH, Havdala H, Reyes A, Westerman MP. Acupuncture: an evaluation in the painful crises of sickle cell anemia. *Pain*. 1979; 7:181–185. Acupuncture was found to be nonsignificantly more effective than control.

Chronic Distal Extremity Pain

Longobardi AG, Clelland JA, Knowles CJ, Jackson JR. Effects of auricular transcutaneous electric nerve stimulation on distal extremity pain: a pilot study. *Phys Ther*. 1989;69(1): 10–17. Acupuncture was found to be significantly more effective than control per the first of two pain assessment instruments.

Reflex Sympathetic Dystrophy

Fialka V, Korpan MI, Nikoliakis P, Dezu IU, Schneider I, Leita T. Acupuncture in the treatment of a posttraumatic pain syndrome [In Ukrainian]. *Lik Sprava*. 1998;7:152–154. Acupuncture and control were both found to be effective; significance was not specified.

Korpan MI, Dezu Y, Schneider B, Leitha T, Fialka-Moser V. Acupuncture in the treatment of posttraumatic pain syndrome. *Acta Orthop Belg*. 1999;65(2):197–201. No significant difference in effectiveness was found between acupuncture and control; relative effectiveness was not specified.

Chronic Joint Pain

Osteoarthritis

Gaw AC, Chang LW, Shaw LC. Efficacy of acupuncture on osteoarthritic pain. *N Engl J Med*. 1975;293(8):375–378. (Osteoarthritis of knee, hip, lumbar, thoracic, cervical or finger joints.) Acupuncture was found to be nonsignificantly more effective than control.

Zherebkin VV. The use of acupuncture reflex therapy in the combined treatment of osteoarthrosis patients [In Russian]. *Lik Sprava*. 1998;8:149–151. Acupuncture was found to be significantly more effective than control.

Chronic Gouty Polyarthritis

Zherebkin VV. The use of acupuncture reflexotherapy in the combined treatment of patients with chronic gouty polyarthritis [In Russian]. *Lik Sprava*. 1998;2:151–153. Acupuncture was found to be significantly more effective than control.

Chronic Muscle Pain

Myalgia

Lundeberg T. A comparative study of the pain alleviating effect of vibratory stimulation, transcutaneous electrical nerve stimulation, electroacupuncture and placebo. *Am J Chin Med*. 1984;12(1–4):72–79. Acupuncture and the first two controls were each found to be effective, all being more effective than the third control; significance was not specified.

Fibromyalgia

Sprott H, Franke S, Kluge H, Hein G. Pain treatment of fibromyalgia by acupuncture. *Rheumatol Int*. 1998;18(1):35–36. Acupuncture was found to be significantly more effective than control.

ORGANIC PAIN

Stable Angina Pectoris

Ballegaard S, Meyer CN, Trojaborg W. Acupuncture in angina pectoris: does acupuncture have a specific effect? *J Intern Med*. 1991; 229:357–362. Acupuncture and control were both found to be significantly effective.

Moderate Angina Pectoris

Ballegaard S, Pedersen F, Pietersen A, Nissen VH, Olsen NV. Effects of acupuncture in moderate, stable angina pectoris: a controlled study. *J Intern Med*. 1990;227:25–30. Acupuncture was found to be nonsignificantly more effective than control.

Severe Angina Pectoris

Ballegaard S, Jensen G, Pedersen F, Nissen VH. Acupuncture in severe, stable angina pectoris: a randomized trial. *Acta Med Scand*. 1986; 220:307–313. Acupuncture was found to be nonsignificantly more effective than control.

Ballegaard S, Johannessen A, Karpatschof B, Nyboe J. Addition of acupuncture and self-care education in the treatment of patients with severe angina pectoris may be cost beneficial: an open, prospective study. *J Alt Compl Med*. 1999;5(5):405–413. Acupuncture was found to be more effective than control per two measures; significance was not specified.

Ballegaard S, Norrelund S, Smith DF. Cost-benefit of combined use of acupuncture, shiatsu and lifestyle adjustment for treatment of patients with severe angina pectoris. *Acupunct Electrother Res*. 1996;21(3–4):187–197. Acupuncture was found to be more effective than control per one of two measures; significance was not specified.

Richter A, Herlitz J, Hjalmarson A. Effect of acupuncture in patients with angina pectoris. *Eur Heart J*. 1991;12:175–178. Acupuncture was found to be significantly more effective than control.

Pain of Childbirth

Ternov K, Nilsson M, Lofberg L, Algotsson L, Akeson J. Acupuncture for pain relief during childbirth. *Acupunct Electrother Res*. 1998; 23(1):19–26. Acupuncture was found to be significantly more effective than control.

PROCEDURAL PAIN

Colonic Endoscopy Pain

Wang HH, Chang YH, Liu DM, Ho YJ. A clinical study on physiological response in electroacupuncture analgesia and meperidine analgesia for colonoscopy. *Am J Chin Med*. 1997;

25(1):13–20. Acupuncture was found to be significantly more effective than control per one of two measures.

INTRAOPERATIVE PAIN

Intraoperative Ophthalmic Pain

Masuda A, Miyazaki H, Yamazaki M, Pintov S, Ito Y. Acupuncture in the anesthetic management of eye surgery. *Acupunct Electrother Res*. 1986;11:259–267. Acupuncture was found to be significantly more effective than control.

Intraoperative Abdominal Pain

Kho HG, Eijk RJR, Kapteijns WMMJ, van Egmond J. Acupuncture and transcutaneous stimulation analgesia in comparison with moderate-dose fentanyl anaesthesia in major surgery. *Anaesthesia*. 1991;46:129–135. Acupuncture was found to be significantly more effective than control.

Pain During Anterior Cervical Discectomy

Li SR, Guo ZR, Liu Y. Clinical study of combined acupuncture-drug anesthesia for anterior approach cervical discectomy [In Chinese]. *Chung Kuo Chung Hsi I Chieh Ho Tsa Chih*. 1997;17(3):148–149. Acupuncture was found to be more effective than control per two of three measures; significance was not specified.

Intraoperative Cranial Pain

Gao LD, He NQ, Jin DF, Zhou RX, Xue ZN, Yang SR. Electro-acupuncture anesthesia in pituitary adenoma extirpation. *Chin Med J*. 1983;96(6):469–474. Acupuncture and control both found to be nonsignificantly effective.

POSTOPERATIVE PAIN

Grabow L. Controlled study of the analgesic effectivity of acupuncture. *Arzneim Forsch/ Drug Res*. 1994;44(4):554–558. (Thoracic,

abdominal or spinal surgery.) Acupuncture was found to be less effective than two of three controls; significance was not specified.

Postoperative Dental Pain

Ekblom A, Hansson P, Thomsson M, Thomas M. Increased postoperative pain and consumption of analgesics following acupuncture. *Pain*. 1991;44:241–247. Acupuncture was found to be less effective than control in both of two groups receiving acupuncture.

Lao LX, Bergman S, Anderson R, Langenberg P, Wong RH, Berman B. The effect of acupuncture on post-operative oral surgery pain: a pilot study. *Acupunct Med*. 1994;12(1):13–17. Acupuncture was found to be nonsignificantly more effective than control.

Lao L, Bergman S, Hamilton GR, Langenberg P, Berman B. Evaluation of acupuncture for pain control after oral surgery: a placebo-controlled trial. *Arch Otolaryngol Head Neck Surg*. 1999;125(5):567–572. Acupuncture was found to be significantly more effective than control.

Postoperative Lower Abdominal Pain

Wang B, Tang J, White PF, et al. Effect of the intensity of transcutaneous acupoint electrical stimulation on the postoperative analgesic requirement. *Anesth Analg*. 1997;85(2): 406–413. Acupuncture was found to be significantly more effective than each control.

Postoperative Gynecologic Pain

Chen L, Tang J, White PF, Sloninsky A, Wender RH, Naruse R, Kariger R. The effect of location of transcutaneous electrical nerve stimulation on postoperative opioid analgesic requirement: acupoint versus nonacupoint stimulation. *Anesth Analg*. 1998;87(5): 1129–1134. Acupuncture was found to be significantly more effective than two of three controls.

Pain Following Laparoscopy

Chiang MH, Wong JO, Chang DP, et al. The effect of needleless electroacupuncture in general anesthesia during laparoscopic surgery [In Chinese]. *Acta Anaesthesiol Sin.* 1995;33(2):107–112. Acupuncture was found to be significantly more effective than control.

Pain after Mammary Oncologic Surgery

He JP, Friedrich M, Ertan AK, Muller K, Schmidt W. Pain-relief and movement improvement by acupuncture after ablation and axillary lymphadenectomy in patients with mammary cancer. *Clin Exp Obstet Gynecol.* 1999;26(2):81–84. Acupuncture was found to be significantly more effective than control.

NUTRITIONAL DISORDERS

Obesity Associated with Excessive Appetite

Richards D, Marley J. Stimulation of auricular acupuncture points in weight loss. *Aust Fam Physician.* 1998;27:S73–S77. Acupuncture was found to be significantly more effective than control.

DERMATOLOGIC CONDITIONS

Psoriasis

Jerner B, Skogh M, Vahlquist A. A controlled trial of acupuncture in psoriasis: no convincing effect. *Acta Dermatol Venereol.* 1997; 77(2):154–156. Acupuncture and control both significantly effective.

OTORHINOLARYNGOLOGIC CONDITIONS

Upper Respiratory Tract Infection

Takeuchi H, Jawad MS, Eccles R. The effects of nasal massage of the "yingxiang" acupuncture point on nasal airway resistance and sensation of nasal airflow in patients with nasal congestion associated with acute upper respiratory tract infection. *Am J Rhinol.* 1999;13: 77–79. Acupuncture was found to be nonsignificantly more effective than control.

Nonallergic Rhinitis

Davies A, Lewith G, Goddard J, Howarth P. The effect of acupuncture on nonallergic rhinitis: a controlled pilot study. *Altern Ther Health Med.* 1998;4(1):70–74. Acupuncture was found to be nonsignificantly more effective than each control.

Allergic Rhinitis

Chari P, Biwas S, Mann SBS, Sehgal S, Mehra YN. Acupuncture therapy in allergic rhinitis. *Am J Acupunct.* 1988;16(2):143–147. Acupuncture and control were both found to be significantly effective.

Wolkenstein E, Horak F. Protective effect of acupuncture on allergen provoked rhinitis [In German]. *Win Med Wochenschr.* 1998; 148(19):450–453. Acupuncture was found to be nonsignificantly more effective than control.

Rhinitis Accompanying Asthma

Zhou RL, Zhang JC. An analysis of combined desensitizing acupoints therapy in 419 cases of allergic rhinitis accompanying asthma [In Chinese]. *Chung Kuo Chung Hsi I Chieh Ho Tsa Chih.* 1997;17(10):587–589. Acupuncture was found to be significantly more effective than control.

Sinusitis

Lundeberg T, Laurell G, Thomas M. Effect of acupuncture on sinus pain and experimentally induced pain. *Ear Nose Throat J.* 1988;67: 565–575. (Maxillary or frontal sinusitis.) Acupuncture was found to be more effective than two of four controls; significance was not specified.

Chronic Maxillary Sinusitis

Pothman R, Yeh HL. The effects of treatment with antibiotics, laser and acupuncture upon chronic maxillary sinusitis in children. *Am J Chin Med.* 1982;10(1–4):55–58. Acupuncture was found to be significantly more effective than either control.

Laryngospasm Following Extubation

Lee CK, Chien TJ, Hsu JC, Yang CY, Hsiao JM, Huang YR, Chang CL. The effect of acupuncture on the incidence of postextubation laryngospasm in children. *Anaesthesia*. 1998;53(9):917–920. Acupuncture was found to be significantly more effective than control.

RESPIRATORY CONDITIONS

Exercise-Induced Asthma

Morton AR, Fazio SM, Miller D. Efficacy of laser-acupuncture in the prevention of exercise-induced asthma. *Ann Allergy*. 1993;70(4):295–298. Acupuncture and two of three controls were each found to be ineffective.

Pediatric Exercise-Induced Asthma

Chow OKW, So SY, Lam WK, Yu DYC, Yeung CY. Effect of acupuncture on exercise-induced asthma. *Lung*. 1983;161:321–326. Acupuncture and control were both found to be ineffective.

Bronchial Asthma

Dias PLR, Subramanium S, Lionel NDW. Effects of acupuncture in bronchial asthma: preliminary communication. *J Roy Soc Med*. 1982;75:245–248. Acupuncture was found to be less effective than control; significance was not specified.

Mild Bronchial Asthma

Medici TC. Acupuncture and bronchial asthma [In German]. *Forsch Komplementarmed*. 1999;6(Suppl 1):26–28. Acupuncture and control were both found to be effective; significance was not specified.

Stable Bronchial Asthma

Biernacki W, Peake MD. Acupuncture in treatment of stable asthma. *Respir Med*. 1998;92(9):1143–1145. Acupuncture and control were both found to be effective per two of three measures; significance was not specified.

Christensen PA, Laursen LC, Taudorf E, Sorensen SC, Weeke B. Acupuncture and bronchial asthma. *Allergy*. 1984;39:379–385. Acupuncture was found to be significantly effective; effectiveness of control was not specified.

Mitchell P, Wells JE. Acupuncture for chronic asthma: a controlled trial with six months follow-up. *Am J Acupunct*. 1989;17(1):5–13. Acupuncture and control were both found to be significantly effective.

Takishima T, Mue S, Tamura G, Ishihara T, Watanabe K. The bronchodilating effect of acupuncture in patients with acute asthma. *Ann Allergy*. 1982;48:44–49. (Infectious type asthma, mixed type asthma, perennial asthma, paroxysmal type asthma.) Acupuncture was found to be significantly more effective than control.

Tandon MK, Soh PFT, Wood AT. Acupuncture for bronchial asthma? *Med J Aust*. 1991;154:409–412. Acupuncture was found to be significantly more effective than each control.

Moderate/Severe Stable Bronchial Asthma

Tandon MK, Soh PFT. Comparison of real and placebo acupuncture in histamine-induced asthma. *Chest*. 1989;96:102–105. No significant difference in effectiveness was found between acupuncture and control.

Tashkin DP, Kroening RJ, Bresler DE, Simmons M, Coulson AH, Kerschnar H. A controlled trial of real and simulated acupuncture in the management of chronic asthma. *J Allergy Clin Immunol*. 1985;76(6):855–864. No significant difference in effectiveness was found between acupuncture and control.

Chronic Obstructive Pulmonary Disease

Neumeister W, Kuhlemann H, Bauer T, Krause S, Schultze-Werninghaus G, Rasche K. Effect of acupuncture on quality of life, mouth occlusion pressures and lung function in COPD [In German]. *Med Klin*. 1999;94(1 Spec No):106–109. Acupuncture was found to be significantly more effective than control.

CARDIOVASCULAR CONDITIONS

Diastolic Hypertension

Williams T, Mueller K, Cornwall MK. Effect of acupuncture-point stimulation on diastolic blood pressure in hypertensive subjects: a preliminary study. *Phys Ther*. 1991;71(7): 523–529. Acupuncture was found to be significantly more effective than control in short term only.

Coronary Artery Disease with Variable Heart Rate

Shi X, Wang ZP, Liu KX. Effect of acupuncture on heart rate variability in coronary heart disease patients [In Chinese]. *Chung Kuo Chung Hsi I Chieh Ho Tsa Chih*. 1995;15(9): 536–538. Acupuncture was found to be significantly more effective than control.

GASTROINTESTINAL CONDITIONS

Nausea and Vomiting

Seasickness

Bertolucci LE, DiDario B. Efficacy of a portable acustimulation device in controlling seasickness. *Aviat Space Environ Med*. 1995;66(12): 1155–1158. Acupuncture was found to be significantly more effective than control.

Nausea and Vomiting Related to Pregnancy

Belluomini J, Litt RC, Lee KA, Katz M. Acupressure for nausea and vomiting of pregnancy: A randomized, blinded study. *Obstet Gynecol*. 1994;84(2):245–248. Acupuncture was found to be significantly more effective than control.

Nausea and Vomiting Associated with Nalbuphine Premedication

Dundee JW, Chestnutt WN, Ghaly RG, Lynas AGA. Traditional Chinese acupuncture: a potentially useful antiemetic? *Br Med J*. 1986; 293:583–584. Acupuncture was found to be significantly more effective than each control.

Dundee JW, Ghaly G. Local anesthesia blocks the anti-emetic effect of P6 acupuncture. *Clin Pharmacol Ther*. 1991;50(1):78–80. Acupuncture was found to be significantly more effective than control.

Dundee JW, Ghaly RG, McKinncy MS. P6 acupuncture anti-emesis comparison of invasive and non-invasive techniques. *Anesthesiology*. 1989;71(3A):A130. Acupuncture was found to be significantly more effective than each of three controls.

Nausea and Vomiting During Cesarean Section under Spinal Anesthesia

Stein DJ, Birnbach DJ, Danzer BI, Kuroda MM, Grunebaum A, Thys DM. Acupressure versus intravenous metoclopramide to prevent nausea and vomiting during spinal anesthesia for cesarean section. *Anesth Analg*. 1997;84(2): 342–345. Acupuncture and one control were both found to be significantly more effective than a second control.

Nausea and Vomiting after Surgery

Dundee JW, Ghaly RG. Does the timing of P6 acupuncture influence its efficacy as a postoperative anti-emetic? *Br J Anaesth*. 1989;63: 630P. Acupuncture was found to be significantly more effective than each control.

Fry ENS. Acupressure and postoperative vomiting. *Anaesthesia*. 1986;41:661–662. Acupuncture was found to be significantly more effective than control.

Weightman WM, Zacharias M, Herbison P. Traditional Chinese acupuncture as an antiemetic. *Br Med J*. 1987;295:1379–1380. No significant difference in effectiveness was found between acupuncture and control; relative effectiveness was not specified.

Nausea and Vomiting after Strabismus Surgery

Chu YC, Lin SM, Hsieh YC, et al. Effect of BL-10 (tianzhu), BL-11 (dazhu) and GB-34 (yanglinquan) acuplaster for prevention of vomiting after strabismus surgery in children. *Acta Anaesthesiol Sin.* 1998;36(1):11–16. Acupuncture was found to be significantly more effective than control.

Schlager A, Offer T, Baldissera I. Laser stimulation of acupuncture point P6 reduces postoperative vomiting in children undergoing strabismus surgery. *Br J Anaesth.* 1998;81(4): 529–532. Acupuncture was found to be significantly more effective than control.

Nausea and Vomiting after Tonsillectomy

Shenkman Z, Holzman RS, Kim C, et al. Acupressure-acupuncture antiemetic prophylaxis in children undergoing tonsillectomy. *Anesthesiology.* 1999;90(5):1311–1316. Acupuncture was found to be nonsignificantly more effective than control.

Nausea and Vomiting after Gynecologic Surgery

Alkaissi A, Stalnert M, Kalman S. Effect and placebo effect of acupressure (P6) on nausea and vomiting after outpatient gynaecological surgery. *Acta Anaesthesiol Scand.* 1999;43(3): 270–274. Acupuncture was found to be significantly more effective than control per first of two measures.

Allen DL, Kitching AJ, Nagle C. P6 acupressure and nausea and vomiting after gynaecological surgery. *Anaesth Intensive Care.* 1994;22(6): 691–693. No significant difference in effectiveness was found between acupuncture and control; relative effectiveness was not specified.

Nausea and Vomiting after Gynecologic Laparoscopy

al-Sadi M, Newman B, Julious SA. Acupuncture in the prevention of postoperative nausea and vomiting. *Anaesthesia.* 1997;52(7):658–661. Acupuncture was found to be significantly more effective than control.

Yang LC, Jawan B, Chen CN, Ho RT, Chang KA, Lee JH. Comparison of P6 acupoint injection with 50% glucose in water and intravenous

droperidol for prevention of vomiting after gynecological laparoscopy. *Acta Anaesthesiol Scand.* 1993;37:192–194. Acupuncture and first control were both found to be significantly more effective than a second control.

Nausea and Vomiting after Cesarean Section

Ho CM, Hseu SS, Tsai SK, Lee TY. Effect of P-6 acupressure on prevention of nausea and vomiting after epidural morphine for post-cesarean section pain relief. *Acta Anaesthesiol Scand.* 1996;40(3):372–375. Acupuncture was found to be significantly more effective than control.

Xerostomia

Blom M, Dawidson I, Angmar-Mansson B. The effect of acupuncture on salivary flow rates in patients with xerostomia. *Oral Surg Oral Med Oral Pathol.* 1992;73(3):293–298. Acupuncture was found to be significantly effective; effectiveness of control was not specified.

Xerostomia Induced by Radiation

Blom M, Dawidson I, Fernberg JO, Johnson G, Angmar-Mansson B. Acupuncture treatment of patients with radiation-induced xerostomia. *Eur J Cancer B Oral Oncol.* 1996;32B(3): 182–190. Acupuncture and control were both found to be significantly effective.

UROLOGIC CONDITIONS

Female Urethral Syndrome

Zheng H, Wang S, Shang J, et al. Study on acupuncture and moxibustion therapy for female urethral syndrome. *J Tradit Chin Med.* 1998; 18:122–127. Acupuncture was found to be significantly more effective than control.

Female Lower Urinary Tract Infection

Aune A, Alraek T, LiHua H, Baerheim A. Acupuncture in the prophylaxis of recurrent lower urinary tract infection in adult women. *Scand J Primary Health Care.* 1998;16(1):37–39.

Acupuncture was found to be significantly more effective than control in preventing recurrence.

Neurogenic Bladder after Spinal Cord Injury

Cheng PT, Wong MK, Chang PL. A therapeutic trial of acupuncture in neurogenic bladder of spinal cord injured patients: a preliminary report. *Spinal Cord*. 1998;36(7):476–480. Acupuncture was found to be significantly more effective than control.

RHEUMATOLOGIC CONDITIONS

Systemic Lupus Erythematosus

Feng SF, Fang L, Bao GQ, et al. Treatment of systemic lupus erythematosus by acupuncture. *Chin Med J*. 1985;98(3):171–176. Acupuncture was found to be significantly effective; effectiveness of control was not specified.

Progressive Systemic Sclerosis with Hand and Finger Coldness

Maeda M, Kachi H, Ichihashi N, Oyama Z, Kitajima Y. The effect of electrical acupuncture-stimulation therapy using thermography and plasma endothelin (ET-1) levels in patients with progressive systemic sclerosis (PSS). *J Dermatol Sci*. 1998;17(2):151–155. Acupuncture was found to be more effective than control; significance was not specified.

Primary Raynaud's Syndrome

Appiah R, Hiller S, Caspary L, Alexander K, Creutzig A. Treatment of primary Raynaud's syndrome with traditional Chinese acupuncture. *J Intern Med*. 1997;241(2):119–124. Acupuncture was found to be significantly more effective than control per several outcome measures.

Primary Sjögren's Syndrome

List T, Lundeberg T, Lundstrom I, Lindstrom F, Ravald N. The effect of acupuncture in the treatment of patients with primary Sjögren's syndrome. A controlled study. *Acta Odontol Scand*. 1998;56(2):95–99. Acupuncture was found to be nonsignificantly more effective than control.

REPRODUCTIVE DYSFUNCTIONS

Nonorganic Male Sexual Dysfunction

Aydin S, Ercan M, Caskurlu T, et al. Acupuncture and hypnotic suggestions in the treatment of non-organic male sexual dysfunction. *Scand J Urol Nephrol*. 1997;31(3):271–274. Acupuncture was found to be nonsignificantly more effective than each control.

Male Subfertility Due to Low Sperm Quality

Siterman S, Eltes F, Wolfson V, Zabludovsky N, Bartoov B. Effect of acupuncture on sperm parameters of males suffering from subfertility related to low sperm quality. *Arch Androl*. 1997;39(2):155–161. Acupuncture was found to be significantly more effective than control.

ENDOCRINOLOGIC CONDITIONS

Menopausal Dysfunction

Kraft K, Coulon S. Effect of a standardized acupuncture treatment on complaints, blood pressure and serum lipids of hypertensive, postmenopausal women: a randomized, controlled clinical study [In German]. *Forsch Komplementarmed*. 1999;6(2):74–79. Acupuncture was found to be significantly more effective than control per one of two measures.

OBSTETRIC CONDITIONS

Malposition of Fetus

Li Q, Wang L. Clinical observation on correcting malposition of fetus by electro-acupuncture. *J Tradit Chin Med*. 1996;16(4):260–262. Acupuncture was found to be significantly more effective than the first of two controls on the first of two measures.

Breech Presentation

Cardini F, Weixin H. Moxibustion for correction of breech presentation: a randomized controlled trial. *JAMA*. 1998;280(18):1580–1584. Acupuncture was found to be significantly more effective than control per two of three measures.

Prolonged Labor

Tempfer C, Zeisler H, Heinzl H, Hefler L, Husslein P, Kainz C. Influence of acupuncture on maternal serum levels of interleukin-I, prostaglandin F2alpha, and beta-endorphin: a matched pair study. *Obstet Gynecol*. 1998; 92(2):245–248. Acupuncture was found to be significantly more effective than control.

Zeisler H, Tempfer C, Mayerhofer K, Barrada M, Husslein P. Influence of acupuncture on duration of labor. *Gynecol Obstet Invest*. 1998; 46(1):22–25. Acupuncture was found to be significantly more effective than control in the first stage; no significant difference in effectiveness was found between acupuncture and control in the second stage.

NEUROLOGIC CONDITIONS

Insomnia

Montakab H. Acupuncture and insomnia [In German]. *Forsch Komplementarmed*. 1999; 6(Suppl 1):29–31. Acupuncture was found to be significantly more effective than control.

Tinnitus

Furugard S, Hedin PJ, Eggertz A, Laurent C. Acupuncture worth trying in severe tinnitus [In Swedish]. *Lakartidningen*. 1998;95(17): 1922–1928. Acupuncture was found to be significantly more effective than control over the shorter term; no significant difference was found over the longer term.

Nielsen OJ, Moller K, Jorgensen KE. The effect of traditional Chinese acupuncture on severe tinnitus. A double-blind, placebo-controlled clinical study with an open therapeutic surveillance [In Danish]. *Ugeskar Laeger*. 1999; 161(4):424–429. No significant difference was found in effectiveness between acupuncture and control; relative effectiveness was not specified.

Impaired Balance

Balance Disorders after Whiplash Injury

Fattori B, Borsari C, Vannucci G, et al. Acupuncture treatment for balance disorders following whiplash injury. *Acupunct Electrother Res*. 1996;21(3–4):207–217. Acupuncture was found to be significantly more effective than control per several clinical outcome measures.

Epilepsy

Chronic Intractable Epilepsy

Kloster R, Larsson PG, Lossius R, et al. The effect of acupuncture in chronic intractable epilepsy. *Seizure*. 1999;8(3):170–174. Acupuncture and control were both found to be nonsignificantly effective.

Dementia

Traumatic Cerebral Dementia

Zhang AR, Pan ZW, Lou F. Effect of acupuncturing houxi and shenmen in treating cerebral traumatic dementia [In Chinese]. *Chung Kuo Chung Hsi I Chieh Ho Tsa Chih*. 1995;15(9): 519–521. Acupuncture was found to be significantly more effective than control.

Peripheral Neuropathy

Peripheral Neuropathy Related to HIV Infection

Shlay JC, Chaloner K, Max MB, et al. Acupuncture and amitriptyline for pain due to HIV-related peripheral neuropathy: a randomized controlled trial. Terry Beirn Community Programs for Clinical Research on AIDS. *JAMA*. 1998;280(18):1590–1595. Acupuncture and control were both found to be effective; significance was not specified.

Stroke

Acute Cerebral Infarction

Si QM, Wu GC, Cao XD. Effects of electroacupuncture on acute cerebral infarction. *Acupunct Electrother Res*. 1998;23(2):117–124. Acupuncture was found to be significantly more effective than control.

Acute Focal Ischemic Stroke

Gosman-Hedstrom G, Claesson L, Klingenstierna U, et al. Effects of acupuncture treatment on daily life activities and quality of life: a controlled, prospective, and randomized study of acute stroke patients. *Stroke*. 1998;29(10): 2100–2108. No significant difference in effectiveness was found between acupuncture and control with three of four measures.

Subacute Stroke

Kjendahl A, Sallstrom S, Osten PE, Stanghelle JK, Borchgrevink CF. A one year follow-up study on the effects of acupuncture in the treatment of stroke patients in the subacute stage: a randomized, controlled study. *Clin Rehabil*. 1997;11(3):192–200. Acupuncture significantly was found to be more effective than control at one-year follow-up.

Hemiplegia

Hemiplegia Due to Stroke

Chen YM, Fang YA. 108 cases of hemiplegia caused by stroke: the relationship between CT scan results, clinical findings and the effect of acupuncture treatment. *Acupunct Electrother Res*. 1990;15:9–17. Acupuncture was found to be significantly more effective than control.

Guo ZX, Wang RS, Guo XC. Clinical observation on treatment of 40 cases of apoplexy hemi-plegia complicated shoulder-hand syndrome with electro-acupuncture [In Chinese]. *Chung Kuo Chung Hsi I Chieh Ho Tsa Chih*. 1995; 15(11):646–648. Acupuncture was found to be significantly more effective than control.

Wong AM, Su TY, Tang FT, Cheng PT, Liaw MY. Clinical trial of electrical acupuncture on hemiplegic stroke patients. *Am J Phys Med Rehabil*. 1999;78(2):117–122. Acupuncture was found to be significantly more effective than control.

PSYCHOLOGIC CONDITIONS

Depression

Luo H, Meng F, Jia Y, Zhao X. Clinical research on the therapeutic effect of the electro-acupuncture treatment in patients with depression. *Psychiatry Clin Neurosci*. 1998;52 Suppl:S338–S340. Acupuncture was found to be significantly more effective than control per two of three measures.

Roschke J, Wolf C, Kogel P, Wagner P, Bech S. Adjuvant whole body acupuncture in depression: a placebo-controlled study with standardized mianserin therapy [In German]. *Nervenarzt*. 1998;69(11):961–967. Acupuncture was found to be more effective than one of two controls; significance was not specified.

ADDICTIONS

Alcohol Addiction

Leung ASH. Acupuncture treatment of withdrawal symptoms. *Am J Acupunct*. 1977;5(1): 43–50. Acupuncture was found to be more effective than control regarding alcohol addiction; significance was not specified.

Sapir-Weise R, Berglund M, Frank A, Kristenson H. Acupuncture in alcoholism treatment: a randomized out-patient study. *Alcohol Alcohol*. 1999;34(4):629–635. No significant difference in effectiveness was found between acupuncture and control; relative effectiveness was not specified.

Worner TM, Zeller B, Schwarz H, Zwas F, Lyon D. Acupuncture fails to improve treatment outcome in alcoholics. *Drug Alcohol Dependence*. 1992;30:169–173. No significant difference in effectiveness was found between acupuncture and control; relative effectiveness was not specified.

Short-Term Withdrawal from Nicotine

Cottraux JA, Harf R, Boissel JP, Schbath J, Bouvard M, Gillet J. Smoking cessation with behavior therapy or acupuncture: a controlled study. *Behav Res Ther*. 1983;21(4):417–424. Acupuncture and control were both found to be significantly effective.

He D, Berg JE, Hostmark AT. Effects of acupuncture on smoking cessation or reduction for motivated smokers. *Prev Med*. 1997;26(2):208–214. Acupuncture was found to be significantly more effective than control.

Lamontagne Y, Annable L, Gagnon MA. Acupuncture for smokers: lack of long-term therapeutic effect in a controlled study. *CMA J*. 1980;122:787–790. Acupuncture and control were both found to be significantly effective.

Steiner RP, Hay DL, Davis AW. Acupuncture therapy for the treatment of tobacco smoking addiction. *Am J Chin Med*. 1982;10(1–4):107–121. Acupuncture and control were both found to be significantly effective.

White AR, Resch KL, Ernst E. Randomized trial of acupuncture for nicotine withdrawal symptoms. *Arch Intern Med*. 1998;158(20):2251–2255. No significant difference in effectiveness was found between acupuncture and control.

Long-Term Withdrawal from Nicotine

Clavel-Chapelon F, Paoletti C, Benhamou S. Smoking cessation rates 4 years after treatment by nicotine gum and acupuncture. *Prev Med*. 1997;26(1):25–28. No significant difference in effectiveness was found between acupuncture and controls.

Cottraux JA, Harf R, Boissel JP, Schbath J, Bouvard M, Gillet J. Smoking cessation with behavior therapy or acupuncture: a controlled study. *Behav Res Ther*. 1983;21(4):417–424. Acupuncture and control were both found to be significantly effective.

Cottraux J, Schbath J, Messy P, Mollard E, Juenet C, Collet L. Predictive value of MMPI scales on smoking cessation programs outcomes. *Acta Psychiatr Belg*. 1986;86:463–469. Acupuncture was found to be more effective than controls; significance was not specified.

Gillams J, Lewith GT, Machin D. Acupuncture and group therapy in stopping smoking. *The Practitioner*. 1984;228:341–344. Acupuncture was found to be nonsignificantly more effective than control.

MacHovec FJ, Man SC. Acupuncture and hypnosis compared: fifty-eight cases. *Am J Clin Hypnosis*. 1978;21(1):45–47. Acupuncture and control were both found to be significantly effective.

Parker LN, Mok MS. The use of acupuncture for smoking withdrawal. *Am J Acupunct*. 1977;5(4):363–366. Acupuncture was found to be nonsignificantly more effective than control.

Vandevenne A, Rempp M, Burghard G, Kuntzman Y, Jung F. Study of the specific contribution of acupuncture to tobacco detoxification [In French]. *Semaine Hopitaux Paris*. 1985;61:2155–2160. Acupuncture was found to be nonsignificantly more effective than control.

Waite NR, Clough JB. A single-blind, placebo-controlled trial of a simple acupuncture treatment in the cessation of smoking. *Br J Gen Pract*. 1998;48(433):1487–1490. Acupuncture was found to be significantly more effective than control.

Cocaine Addiction

Otto KC, Quinn C, Sung YF. Auricular acupuncture as an adjunctive treatment for cocaine addiction. A pilot study. *Am J Addict*. 1998;7(2):164–170. Acupuncture was found to be more effective than control per the first of two measures; significance was not specified.

Bullock ML, Kiresuk TJ, Pheley AM, Culliton PD, Lenz SK. Auricular acupuncture in the treatment of cocaine abuse. A study of efficacy and dosing. *J Subst Abuse Treat*. 1999; 16(1):31–38. No significant difference in effectiveness was found between acupuncture and each control; relative effectiveness was not specified.

MULTISYSTEM CONDITIONS

Electromagnetic Field Hypersensitivity

Arnetz BB, Berg M, Anderzen I, Lundeberg T, Haker E. A nonconventional approach to the treatment of "environmental illness." *J Occup Environ Med*. 1995;37(7):838–844. Acupuncture and control were both found to be significantly effective per several measures.

REFERENCES

Birch S, Hammerschlag R. *Acupuncture Efficacy: A Summary of Controlled Clinical Trials*. Tarrytown, NY: The National Academy of Acupuncture and Oriental Medicine; 1996:xii–xiii.

Hammerschlag R, Morris MM. Clinical trials comparing acupuncture with biomedical standard care: a criteria-based evaluation of research design and reporting. *Complement Ther Med*. 1997;5:133–140.

MEDLINE Database, National Library of Medicine, National Institutes of Health. Available at: http://www.ncbi.nlm.nih.gov. Accessed June 1, 2000.

ter Riet G, Kleijnen J, Knipschild P. Acupuncture and chronic pain: a criteria-based meta-analysis. *J Clin Epidemiol*. 1990a;43(11):1191–1199.

ter Riet G, Kleijnen J, Knipschild P. A meta-analysis of studies into the effect of acupuncture on addiction. *Brit J Gen Pract*. 1990b;40:379–382.

Vincent CA, Richardson PH. The evaluation of therapeutic acupuncture: concepts and methods. *Pain*. 1986;24: 1–13.

CHAPTER 53

Electroacupuncture: Mechanisms and Clinical Application

George A. Ulett, Songping Han, and Ji-sheng Han

INTRODUCTION

Traditional Chinese acupuncture is a 3,000-year-old folk therapy. It is based upon metaphysical concepts of "ch'i" (Qi), a supposed body energy that runs through hypothesized channels called meridians. On these meridians are 365 designated acupuncture points that can be used for stimulation via needles or moxibustion (lighted punks of *Artemis vulgaris*) to balance yin and yang by relieving blockages in the

George A. Ulett, MD, PhD, is Clinical Professor of Psychiatry at the University of Missouri School of Medicine, Missouri Institute of Mental Health, and author of more than 250 scientific publications. He is a clinical professor at St. Louis University, a former professor of psychiatry at Washington University School of Medicine, and former director of the Missouri Department of Mental Health. He has practiced, researched, and taught acupuncture for over 30 years.

Ji-sheng Han, MD, graduated from the Shanghai Medical College in 1953. Currently a Professor of Physiology in the Neuroscience Research Institute, Peking University, he is a member of the Chinese Academy of Sciences and president of the Chinese Association for the Study of Pain (CASP).

Songping Han, PhD, received his bachelor of medicine degree from Beijing Medical College in 1982 and his PhD in neuropharmacology from Saint Louis University School of Medicine in 1990. He is a faculty member of Saint Louis University School of Medicine. He is interested in both basic and clinical research of complementary and alternative medicine. As a researcher, he is also active in promoting acupuncture by helping doctors to have a better understanding of the neurochemical mechanisms of acupuncture therapy in order to further increase the therapeutic efficacy by using new technologies.

Source: Adapted by permission of Elsevier Science from Electroacupuncture, *Biological Psychiatry*, Vol. 44, p. 129–138, Copyright 1998 by the Society of Biological Psychiatry.

flow of Qi. Diagnosis is made by feeling 12 organ-specific pulses located on the wrists and with cosmological interpretations including a representation of five elements: wood, water, metal, earth, and fire.

One of us (Ulett) learned traditional Chinese acupuncture 30 years ago. It was found useful in treating patients with chronic pain, but the metaphysical explanations and the necessity for mystical rituals were troublesome. A few years later, in 1971, President Nixon visited China, and acupuncture became a household word in the United States. The American Medical Association was also troubled by metaphysical explanations and declared in the *St. Louis Post Dispatch* in 1974 that acupuncture was "quackery" (1974). This article discouraged U.S. medical schools from interest in this type of therapy. Some even called it "Oriental hypnosis."

Our laboratory in St. Louis, Mo., was then studying neurophysiological concomitants of hypnosis and received a grant from the National Institutes of Health (NIH) to compare these two treatments (Parwatikar et al, 1979; Ulett et al, 1979). We were able to report that acupuncture was not hypnosis (Ulett, 1983). We found that although acupuncture needles alone gave some pain relief, when electricity was added the modulation was 100% more effective.

Increasingly research publications gave strong evidence that acupuncture could be explained on a physiological rather than metaphysical basis (Pomeranz and Stux, 1979). In 1987 Professor Ji-sheng Han published a collection of research studies on acupuncture from his laboratory in Beijing Medical University covering a 25-year period (Han, 1987). In 1990 Han demonstrated the differential release of brain neuropeptides by different frequencies of stimulation (Han and Sun, 1990). This chapter reviews some of Dr. Ji-sheng Han's work in the past 25 years on the physiological mechanism of electroacupuncture-induced analgesia.

SUMMARY OF RESEARCH ESTABLISHING THE NEUROCHEMICAL BASIS OF ACUPUNCTURE ANALGESIA

Acupuncture Increased the Pain Threshold in Human Volunteers

The first paper demonstrating the analgesic effect of acupuncture using experimentally induced pain and quantitative methods to determine acupuncture-induced changes in pain threshold in medical student volunteers at Beijing Medical University was published in 1973 in the *Chinese Medical Journal* (Research Group, 1973). Pain was induced by modified potassium iontophoresis with gradually increasing anodal currents (0.1 to 0.3 mA/step) passing through the skin on the head, thorax, back, abdomen, and leg. The pain threshold was estimated by the current (mA) needed to produce pain. Measurements were taken every 10 minutes for 100 minutes after the insertion of the needle into the Hoku (LI-4) and Zusanli points (ST-36), which was manipulated (300 insertion/twistings per minute, manual acupuncture) for 50 minutes (N = 60). Data were expressed as average percent changes in these skin areas. Intramuscular injection of morphine (10 mg) was used as positive control, which produced an 80% to 90% increase in pain threshold ($p < .05$), suggesting that the method is valid.

Acupuncture at the Hoku point produced an increase in the pain threshold with a peak increase occurring 20 to 40 minutes after the needle insertion. The threshold returned to the preacupuncture level 45 minutes after the needles were removed, with a half-life of 16:21:9. This result confirmed the analgesic effect of acupuncture. There was no difference in the an-

algesic effect of acupuncture whether the needle was placed in the left or right hand. Furthermore, a greater increase in the pain threshold was produced when both the Hoku and Zusanli points were stimulated simultaneously with acupuncture as compared with the results when either one of these two points was stimulated alone (see Figure 53–1).

The analgesic effect was completely prevented by the injection of procaine into the Hoku point prior to needling. In addition, needling on the affected limbs of 12 hemiplegic and 13 paraplegic patients had no effect on the pain threshold on the unaffected side, indicating the involvement of sensory nerves. The gradual increase and return in the pain threshold suggest that acupuncture-induced analgesia is mediated by humoral factors.

Rats Developing Tolerance to Electroacupuncture Analgesia Also Tolerant to Morphine Analgesia

Several strategies were then employed to characterize the chemical nature of the factors responsible for acupuncture analgesia. An important piece of evidence suggesting the importance of endogenous opioid substances in mediating acupuncture analgesia was derived from cross-tolerance experiments (Han et al, 1981). Repeated electroacupuncture was applied to rats at the Zusanli and Sanyinjiao points for six sessions using 2 to 15 Hz, of 0.3 milliseconds duration, 30 minutes for each session with 30-minute intervals. The amplitude of the pulse was 1 V every 10 minutes, reaching 3 V as maximum. Repeated electroacupuncture resulted in tolerance (ie, a gradual decrease of acupuncture effect). In these rats, the analgesic effect of a challenging dose of morphine (6 mg/kg, IV) was also reduced correspondingly. The analgesic effect of both electroacupuncture and morphine returned to the control level at similar rates following a period of recovery (Y = 0.78X + 22.4, r = .996, $p < 0.1$). In addition, morphine tolerance developed in rats following chronic injection of morphine (5 to 50 mg/kg, three times/day

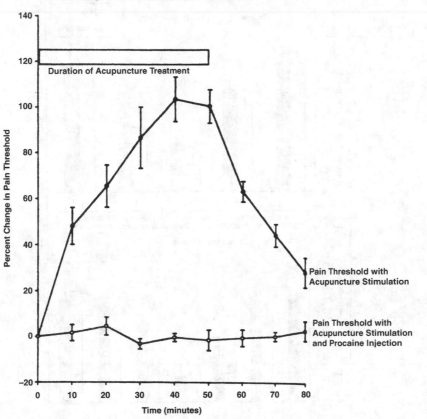

Figure 53–1 The effect of manual acupuncture on the pain threshold in human volunteers, applied at the Hoku point. *Source:* Adapted by permission of Elsevier Science from Electroacupuncture, *Biological Psychiatry*, Vol. 44, pp. 129–138, Copyright 1998 by the Society of Biological Psychiatry.

for 8 days). The effect of morphine returned to the control level 9 days after the cessation of morphine treatment. A similar attenuation of electroacupuncture analgesia was also observed in these rats ($Y = 0.74X + 28.4$, $r = .938$, $p < .01$). These findings suggest that electroacupuncture analgesia and morphine analgesia share the same or similar mechanisms (see Figure 53–2).

Acupuncture-Induced Analgesic Effect Can Be Transferred

Neurochemical factors responsible for acupuncture analgesia may be produced in, and re-leased from, the central nervous system (CNS). If this is true, the infusion of the cerebrospinal fluid (CSF) taken from an animal that has undergone acupuncture into a naive animal might produce a significant increase in the pain threshold in the recipient animal. This hypothesis was tested in a cross-perfusion/infusion experiment (Research Group, 1974). Finger acupuncture by pressing the Quenlun point (on top of the Achilles tendon) of the rabbit for 30 minutes produced a dramatic analgesic effect. This was determined by the changes in avoidance response latency during a noxious stimulation produced by radiant heat from an incandescent lamp (12 V, 50 W

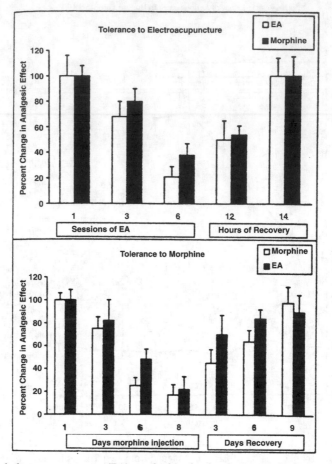

Figure 53–2 Repeated electroacupuncture (EA) resulted in the development of tolerance to EA and the cross-tolerance to morphine. *Source:* Adapted by permission of Elsevier Science from Electroacupuncture, *Biological Psychiatry*, Vol. 44, pp. 129–138, Copyright 1998 by the Society of Biological Psychiatry.

in 8.75-mm cine-projector). The lateral ventricle of the rabbit was perfused with artificial cerebral spinal fluid (CSF) at a rate of 10 to 15 µL/minute during acupuncture. The CSF from the donor rabbit (0.3 to 0.5 mL) was then infused into the lateral ventricle of a naive recipient rabbit. A rather marked nociceptive effect was observed in the recipient rabbit. Perfusion or infusion of the ventricle with control artificial CSF had no significant effect on avoidance response latency in donor or recipient rabbits. These results clearly

demonstrated that the acupuncture-induced analgesia is mediated by substances that are released from the central nervous system (CNS).

Microinjection of Opioid Receptor Antagonist (Naloxone) Attenuated the Analgesic Effects

To examine the biochemical and anatomical characteristics of the receptors responsible for acupuncture analgesia, an opioid receptor antagonist was introduced into selected brain regions by the microinjection technique in an attempt to prevent the acupuncture-induced analgesia (Zhou et al, 1981). Intravenous injection of morphine (4 mg/kg) or finger acupuncture (Kuenlun point, 10 minutes) produced a significant analgesic effect in rabbits, as shown by the increase of the avoidance response latency. Naloxone, an opioid receptor antagonist, was microinjected into the following nuclei: accumbens, amygdala, habenula, or periaqueductal gray (PAG), at a rate of 0.25μ L/minute for 20 minutes either unilaterally or bilaterally. Microinjection of naloxone into any one of these four nuclei significantly attenuated the analgesic effect induced by morphine or acupuncture. These results suggest that the analgesic effect of morphine and acupuncture is mediated by opioid receptors in these brain areas. Results obtained from experiments using chemical blockade, and from studies using lesion methods, further suggest that acupuncture analgesia and morphine analgesia may require a neural connection among those nuclei using endorphins as transmitters.

Microinjection of Antiserum against β-Endorphin into the Periaqueductal Gray (Brain Tissue) (PAG) Attenuated the Electroacupuncture Analgesic Effect

At least three kinds of endorphins and their receptors have been found in the CNS. Results from studies using naloxone indicate the involvement of opioid receptors but do not indicate which types of endorphins are involved. Specific antiserum raised against a certain type of endorphin can neutralize and prevent the action of that endorphin. Antiserum that recognizes (HO) or does not recognize (UA) rabbit-endorphin was injected bilaterally at a volume of 4 L into the rabbit PAG through chronically implanted cannulae (Xie et al, 1983). Changes in avoidance and response latency (ARL) were determined before and after electroacupuncture at the points Zusanli and Quenlun for 10 minutes or after the intravenous injection of morphine. The antinociceptive effect of electroacupunc-

ture, but not of morphine, was attenuated by HO antiserum. In contrast, neither saline nor UA affected the analgesic effect of electroacupuncture or morphine. These results suggest that morphine produces an analgesic effect by direct activation of opioid receptors in the PAG, whereas the effect of electroacupuncture is mediated by endorphins.

Enkephalins and Dynorphins Are Selectively Released into the CSF by Electroacupuncture

Different endorphins have different distribution patterns and biological functions in the CNS. It would have great clinical advantage if one could selectively stimulate the release of a certain type of endorphin without affecting others. The selectivity of acupuncture on endorphin release was examined using electroacupuncture of different frequencies (Fei et al, 1978). The spinal subarachnoid space of the rat was perfused with artificial CSF before and after electroacupuncture at the Zusanli and Sanyinjiao points using 2, 15, or 100 Hz. CSF was collected for measurement of methionin enkephalin, dynorphin A, or dynorphin B using radioimmunoassay. Methionin enkephalin and dynorphins were selectively released into the CSF by electroacupuncture of low and high frequencies, respectively. Similar results were also obtained from studies in humans (see Figure 53–3).

Electroacupuncture Produced Corresponding Increases in Pain Threshold and Endorphin Immunoreactivity

Electroacupuncture also increases the tissue content of endorphins (Chen et al, 1983). Rats were divided into three groups according to the degree of analgesia produced by electroacupuncture (15 Hz, 3 V for 30 minutes). The electroacupuncture-induced increase in tail flick latency was less than 20%, between 21% and 70%, and over 70% in these groups, respectively. The brain was removed after electroacupuncture for mea-

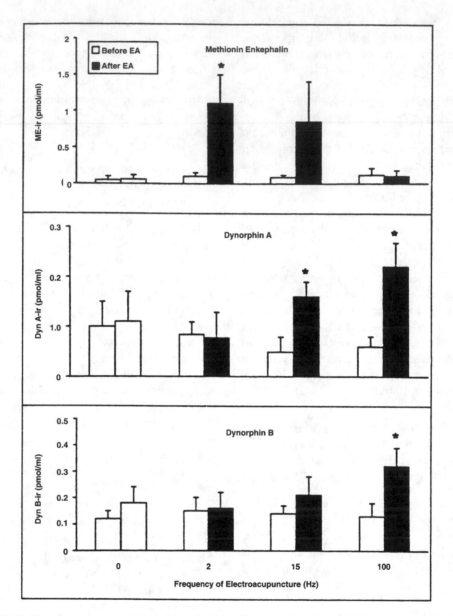

Figure 53–3 Electroacupuncture (EA) of low and high frequencies releases different types of endogenous opioids from the CNS. ME = methionin enkephalin; Dyn = dynorphin. *Source:* Adapted by permission of Elsevier Science from Electroacupuncture, *Biological Psychiatry*, Vol. 44, pp. 129–138, Copyright 1998 by the Society of Biological Psychiatry.

surement of cerebral-endorphin immunoreactivity (β-endorphin-ir) with radioimmunoassay. The results show no changes in β-endorphin-ir in rats with low analgesic effect and a dramatic increase in β-endorphin-ir in rats with high analgesic effect. There was a strong correlation between electroacupuncture-induced analgesia and β-endorphin-ir in brain tissue (see Figure 53–4).

CLINICAL APPLICATIONS OF NEUROELECTROACUPUNCTURE

The development of a scientific neuroelectroacupuncture has made it possible to consider a wide variety of clinical applications that have been demonstrated and now stand ready for replication and double-blind studies. These include the following.

Pain

Traditionally acupuncture has been widely used as a treatment for various types of acute and chronic pain. A 70% rate of success for pain elimination or modulation has been reported clinically in patients with low-back strain, arthritis, myofascial discomfort, migraine, and other painful disorders (Ulett, 1989; Ng et al, 1992; Thomas and Lundberg, 1994; Anderson et al, 1976).

Depression

The successful treatment of major depression has been demonstrated in China to require twice-daily, 30-minute periods of electrostimulation

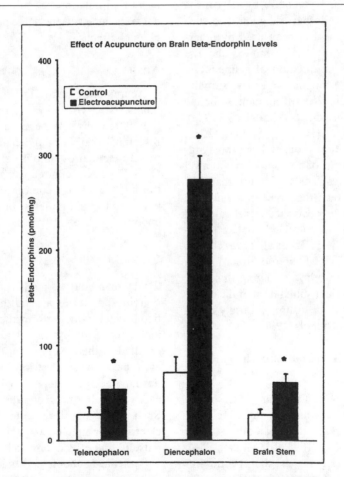

Figure 53–4 Acupuncture produces concomitant increases in pain threshold and brain beta-endorphin levels (* = *p* < .05 compared with control groups). *Source:* Adapted by permission of Elsevier Science from Electroacupuncture, *Biological Psychiatry*, Vol. 44, pp. 129–138, Copyright 1998, Elsevier Science.

(Han, 1986; Lou et al, 1990). Medical insurance reimbursement does not presently cover such treatments in U.S. hospitals. Our experience therefore has been limited to weekly office treatments for less severe depression. This less intense schedule, however, has permitted a decrease, and in some cases, an elimination of the need for antidepressant medication.

Addiction

Wen first demonstrated the use of ear acupuncture for addiction by placing a needle in the concha, an area innervated by the vagus nerve (Wen and Cheung, 1973). Wen stressed the necessity of electrical stimulation of the concha in his treatment for heroin addiction, and such electrical stimulation has been used by others (Katims et al, 1992). Han reported the use of transcutaneous stimulation of acupuncture points with a Han's acupoint and nerve stimulator (HANS) at identified frequencies for the treatment of heroin addicts (Han et al, 1994a). The alternating high- (100 Hz) and low- (2 Hz) frequency stimulation produced the most significant improvement on the opioid withdrawal syndrome. A clinical study on more than 500 heroin addicts shows that the treatment with HANS significantly decreased heart rate and palpitation and produced a euphorialike sensation and warm feeling (Wu et al, 1995). It also produced a significant hypnotic effect and an increase in body weight. Following this lead, we have used electrical stimulation of the dorsal interosseous muscle for treating a variety of addictions (Ulett and Nichols, 1996).

Cerebrovascular Accidents and Their Sequelae

Recent reports suggest that early intervention following a stroke may assist with earlier rehabilitation and decrease nursing home stay by 50% (Johansson et al, 1993; Magnusson et al, 1994). Studies by Han suggest that specific frequencies of stimulation may be effective for treatment of spinal spasticity (Han et al, 1994b). Although these preliminary reports appear prom-

ising, replication of these studies in the United States is needed.

Gastrointestinal Disorders

In traditional Chinese medicine, stimulation of the point Zusanli (tibialis anticus motor point) has long been advocated for the treatment of both diarrhea and constipation. Such normalization of colon function could theoretically be explained by impulses reaching the lumbar plexus. The effects of such stimulation have been reported both in animals and humans (Li et al, 1992; Jin et al, 1992). In the light of research emphasizing the importance of specific frequencies of stimulation, it could well be that different frequencies at the same point have different clinical effects.

Anxiety

Acupuncture has long been associated with homeostatic (yin and yang), regulation, or calming effect. This may be explained in light of the research report above indicating that electroacupuncture releases opioid neuropeptides in the CNS. We have reported using Pavlovian conditioning techniques combined with electroacupuncture to train patients for the self-release of endorphins (Ulett, 1996).

CONCLUSION

Our own studies, published reports from research laboratories around the world, and particularly the work performed in the Beijing Medical University by Han and his group, have resulted in the development of a new scientifically based neuroelectric acupuncture. A basis has now been developed for further physiological investigations and controlled clinical studies. Such increasing evidence for a scientific neuroelectric acupuncture will gain its acceptance as a useful and effective procedure to be taught in U.S. medical schools.

Acupuncture has a great potential of being used for various medical purposes. For example, we and others have shown that the doses of anesthetics and postoperational analgesics can be significantly reduced when a HANS is used during a surgical procedure (acupuncture-assisted analgesia). This can result in a reduced risk of complications associated with the operation and the duration of hospital stay. In another example, instead of using daily application of methadone or other potent or long-lasting opioid receptor agonists in the treatment of heroin addiction, HANS stimulates the suppressed endophinergic neurons in the CNS to attenuate the heroin withdrawal syndrome and to restore the function of these neurons. The important next step in acupuncture research is to have a better understanding of the neurochemical mechanism of acupuncture in order that the therapeutic effectiveness of acupuncture can be further increased.

REFERENCES

Anderson SA, Hansson G, Holmgren E, Renberg O. Evaluation of the pain suppressive effect of different frequencies of peripheral electrical stimulation in chronic pain conditions. *Acct Northup Scan.* 1976;47:149–159.

Chen QS, Xie GX, Han JS. Effect of electroacupuncture on the content of immunoreactive beta-endorphin in rats' brain regions. *Kexue Tonga.* 1983;28:312–319.

Fei H, Xie GX, Han JS. Differential release of metenkephalin and dynorphin in spinal cord by electroacupuncture of different frequencies. *Kexue Tongbo.* 1978; 31:1512–1515.

Han JS. Electroacupuncture: an alternative to antidepressants for treating affective diseases? *J Neurosci.* 1986; 29:79–92.

Han JS. *The Neurochemical Basis of Pain Relief by Acupuncture.* Beijing, China: Chinese Medical Science and Technology Press, 1987.

Han JS, Chen XH, Yuan Y, Yan SC. Transcutaneous electrical nerve stimulation for treatment of spinal spasticity. *Chin Med J.* 1994a;107:5–11.

Han JS, Li SJ, Tang J. Tolerance to electroacupuncture and its cross tolerance to morphine. *Neuropharmacology.* 1981;20:593–596.

Han JS, Sun SL. Differential release of enkephalin and dynorphin by low- and high-frequency electroacupuncture in the central nervous system. *Acupunct Sci Int.* 1990;1:19–27.

Han JS, Wu LZ, Cui CL. Heroin addicts treated with transcutaneous electrical nerve stimulation of identified frequencies. *Regul Pept.* 1994b;54:115–116.

Jin H, Zhou L, Lee K, Chang T, Chey W. The inhibition by electrical acupuncture on gastric acid secretion is mediated via endorphin and somatostatin in dogs. *Clin Res.* 1992;40:167A.

Johansson K, Lindgren I, Widner H, Wiklund I, Johansson BB. Can sensory stimulation improve the functional outcome in stroke patients? *Neurology.* 1993;43: 2189–2192.

Katims JJ, Ng L, Lowinson JH. Acupuncture and transcutaneous electrical nerve stimulation: afferent nerve stimulation (ANS) in the treatment of addiction. In: Lowinson J, ed. *Substance Abuse: A Comprehensive Textbook.* 2nd ed. Baltimore, MD: Williams and Wilkins; 1992:574–583.

Li Y, Tougas G, Chiverton S, Hunt R. The effect of acupuncture on gastrointestinal function and disorders. *Am J Gastroenterol.* 1992;87:1372–1381.

Lou HC, Shen YC, Zhou D, Jia KY. A comparative study of the treatment of depression by electro-acupuncture. *Acupunct Sci Int J.* 1990;1:20–26.

Magnusson M, Johansson K, Johansson B. Sensory stimulation with electroacupuncture promotes normalization of postural control after stoke. *Stroke J Cereb Circ.* 1994;25:1176–1180.

Ng L, Katims JJ, Lee M. Acupuncture: a neuromodulation technique for pain control. In: Aronoff G, ed. *Evaluation and Treatment of Chronic Pain.* 2nd ed. Baltimore: Williams & Wilkins; 1992:291–298.

Parwatikar S, Brown M, Stern J, Ulett G, Sletten I. Acupuncture, hypnosis and experimental pain: I. Study with volunteers. Acupuncture and electrotherapeutics. *Res Int J.* 1979;3:161–190.

Pomeranz B, Stux F, eds. *Scientific Basis of Acupuncture.* New York: Springer Verlag; 1979.

Research Group of Acupuncture Anesthesia, Peking Medical College. The effect of acupuncture on the human skin pain threshold. *Chin Med J.* 1973;3:151–157.

Research Group of Acupuncture Anesthesia, Peking Medical College. The role of neurotransmitters of brain in finger-acupuncture analgesia. *Scientia Sinica.* 1974;17: 112–130.

St. Louis Post Dispatch. August 4, 1974.

Thomas M, Lundberg T. Importance of modes of acupuncture in the treatment of chronic nociceptive low-back pain. *Acta Anaesthesiol Scand.* 1994;38:63–69.

Ulett G. Acupuncture is not hypnosis: physiological studies. *Am J Acupunct.* 1983;11:5–13.

Ulett G. Acupuncture. In: Tollsion C, Kriegel M, eds. *Interdisciplinary Rehabilitation of Low-Back Pain.* Baltimore: Williams & Wilkins; 1989:85–100.

Ulett G. Conditioned healing with electroacupuncture. *Alternative Ther.* 1996;2:56–60.

Ulett G, Nichols J. *The Endorphin Connection.* Gleve, Australia: Wild and Woolley; 1996.

Ulett G, Parwatikar S, Stern J, Brown M. Acupuncture, hypnosis and experimental pain: II. Study with patients. Acupuncture and electrotherapeutics. *Res Int J.* 1979; 3:191–201.

Wen H, Cheung S. Treatment of drug addiction by acupuncture and electrical stimulation. *Asian J Med.* 1973;9: 138–141.

Wu LZ, Cui CL, Hans JS. Han's acupoint nerve stimulator (HANS) for the treatment of opiate withdrawal syndrome. *Chin J Pain Med.* 1995;1:30–38.

Xie GX, Hans JS, Hollt V. Electroacupuncture analgesia blocked by microinjection of anti-beta-endorphin antiserum into periaqueductal gray of the rabbit. *Int J Neurosci.* 1983;18:287–292.

Zhou ZF, Du MY, Wu WY, Jiang Y, Han JS. Effect on intracerebral microinjection of naloxone on acupuncture- and morphine-analgesia in the rabbit. *Scientia Sinica.* 1981;24:1166–1178.

BIBLIOGRAPHY

Brown M, Ulett G, Stern J. Acupuncture loci and techniques for location. *Am J Chin Med.* 1974;2:67–74.

Gunn CC. Motor points and motor lines. *Am J Acupunct.* 1978;6:55–58.

Han JS. *The Neuro-Chemical Basis of Pain Relief by Acupuncture.* Vol. 2. China: Hubei Science and Technology Press, 1999.

Liu KY, Varela M, Oswald R. The correspondence between acupuncture points and motor points. *Am J Chin Med.* 1975;3:347–358.

Saletu B, Saletu M, Brown M, Stern J, Sletten I, Ulett G. Hypnosis and acupuncture analgesia: a neurophysiological reality? *Neuropsychobiology.* 1975;1:518–542.

Thomas M, Lundberg T. Importance of modes of acupuncture in the treatment of chronic nociceptive low-back pain. *Acta Anaesthesiol Scand.* 1994;38:63–69.

Ulett G. *Principles and Practice of Physiologic Acupuncture.* St. Louis, MO: Warren H. Green; 1982.

Ulett G. *Beyond Yin and Yang: How Acupuncture Really Works.* St. Louis, MO: Warren H. Green; 1992.

Ulett G, Han S. *Neuro-Electric Stimulation: The Scientific Acupuncture Alternative.* St. Louis, MO: Warren Green, 2001.

Wang J, Mao L, Hans JS. Antinociceptive effects induced by electroacupuncture and transcutaneous electrical nerve stimulation in the rat. *Int J Neurosci.* 1992a;65: 117–129.

Wang JQ, Mao L, Hans JS. Comparison of the antinociceptive effects induced by electroacupuncture and transcutaneous electrical nerve stimulation in the rat. *Int J Neurosci.* 1992b;65:117–129.

Wells E, Jackson R, Diaz R, Stanton V. Acupuncture as an adjunct to methadone treatment services. *Am J Addict.* 1995;4:198–214.

Wen H, Cheung S. Treatment of drug addiction by acupuncture and electrical stimulation. *Asian J Med.* 1973;9: 138–141.

Part XIII

Chiropractic

CHAPTER 54

The Discipline of Chiropractic

54.1 Utilization Data: Chiropractic Utilization and Cost-Effectiveness

Charles A. Simpson

INTRODUCTION

Some 50,000 chiropractic physicians compose the third largest healing profession in the United States. For the last 100 years, chiropractors have served patients with a unique array of services and a track record of effectiveness and positive clinical outcomes. The popularity of chiropractic care among patients has allowed robust development of what began as a humble and marginalized health care discipline.

The clinical niche that chiropractic occupies has become increasingly relevant to medical directors and administrators who are focused on quality, outcomes, patient satisfaction, and cost-effectiveness. Viewed initially as an attractive add-on to traditional services by providing a competitive advantage, chiropractic has attracted interest for its ability to reduce medical costs overall by providing effective and efficient health care interventions, particularly for musculoskeletal conditions.

For these reasons, particularly popularity and cost-effectiveness, chiropractic services are now included in the offerings of a substantial number of health plans across the country. The present extent of chiropractic integration into managed care plans exceeds that of any other alternative discipline (J. McAndrews, DC, American Chiropractic Association, oral communication, Sept. 1994). Recent surveys indicate inclusion in health plan coverage as high as 87% (Azevedo, 1994). As alternative therapies become integrated in mainstream environments, the experiences of chiropractic integration may provide a useful model for the transition of other complementary disciplines.

CHIROPRACTIC UTILIZATION

Consumer Interest in Chiropractic

The public is attracted by the benefits of chiropractic treatment. A Louis Harris poll (1994) found that more than one-third of the 1,253 adults surveyed had sought professional care

Charles A. Simpson, DC, has been a practicing chiropractor for over 20 years. He is founder and currently Chief Medical Director of Complementary Healthcare Plans (CHP) of Portland, Oregon. CHP provides integrated acupuncture, chiropractic, naturopathic medicine, and massage therapy services for health plans, health maintenance organizations, and preferred-provider organizations in Oregon and Washington state.

Courtesy of Charles A. Simpson, DC, Cornelius, Oregon

for back trouble during the preceding 5 years. Of those seeking care, 59% had seen chiropractors, 69% had seen medical doctors (MDs), 33% physical therapists, and 13% doctors of osteopathy (DOs). (Many saw more than one provider.) Of those who saw a chiropractor, 63% were very satisfied with their care; 50% to 56% of the respondents reported high satisfaction with other providers.

The Harris poll (Harris, 1994) also found that one-half of the general public views chiropractors as the most skilled specialists in manipulative procedures. Of those who visited any practitioner for back trouble, 59% saw chiropractors as most skilled in the care of back problems. In the general public, 70% consider it important to have chiropractic as a basic benefit in their health plans. To some degree, this is true because most chiropractors deal with a very specific scope of practice, focused primarily on musculoskeletal problems. Of the 27 million Americans who visit a chiropractor each year, approximately 85% seek treatment for back and neck pain, 10% for headaches or extremity pain, and 5% for other conditions (Hurwitz et al, 1998).

Even more dramatic differences in patient satisfaction have been found between chiropractic patients and those seeing practitioners from other disciplines (Cherkin and MacCornack, 1989). A survey of back pain patients in a Seattle area HMO found, "The percentage of chiropractor patients 'very satisfied' with the care they received was triple that for patients [of other practitioners] (66% compared with 22%)." Chiropractic patients were three times as likely to perceive their provider as confident and comfortable in dealing with low-back pain. A patient's perception of his or her chiropractor's confidence, experience, and competence in dealing with health problems is one of the paramount issues of "bedside manner" and, ultimately, patient satisfaction. Cherkin and MacCornack's (1989) survey found chiropractic care highly regarded because chiropractors were able to identify the problems for which patients were seen, knew how to treat them, and were able to pass some of that sense of confidence along to the patient.

Use of chiropractic and other complementary and alternative medicine (CAM) health care services in the United States is extensive and growing. It has been estimated that there were 425 million visits to nontraditional providers in 1990 (Eisenberg et al, 1993). It is estimated that in 1997, this utilization increased to 629 million visits, an increase of 47% (Eisenberg et al, 1998). Expenditures for CAM services were reported at about approximately $13.7 billion in 1990 and $21.2 billion in 1997.

Use of chiropractic services experienced similar increases. Spending for chiropractic services represents about 1% of all health care expenses, totaling nearly $9 billion in 1990 (Eisenberg et al, 1993). The total number of visits to chiropractors rose over 30% between 1990 and 1997. Although the utilization of these services is significant, experience with managing this care has been limited in most health systems. Utilization management strategies frequently employed by managed care organizations are traditional gatekeeper arrangements or strict limitations of the benefit. In these environments, appropriate referral and use of CAM care may be limited. Referral to chiropractors appears to be widely variable. As few as 3.3% (Druss and Rosenheck, 1999) and as many as 65% (National Market Measures, 1999) of mainstream practitioners report that they refer patients for chiropractic care (see Table 54.1–1). Surveys of chiropractors by the American Chiropractic Association show that less than 5% of new patients are referred by physicians inside or outside of managed care plans. Benefit design limitations, whether through caps on services, high copayments, preauthorization, or similar strategies, may contain cost but do little to ensure quality of care.

Treatment of Back Pain in Managed Care

The incidence of back pain is high in the general population. An estimated 80% of adults will have at least one episode of disabling low-back pain in their lifetime and many suffer chronic or recurring pain (Kelly and White, 1980). Back pain is one of the two most common reasons patients go to doctors, second only to the common cold (Cypress, 1983). For managed care organizations seeking to improve the delivery of appropriate health care, the development of medical management strategies for costly and prevalent conditions such as back pain will become increasingly important.

Back pain is also the second most common reason for absenteeism among workers in both industrial and nonindustrial employment (Rowe, 1969). It is estimated that among male workers alone, over 100 million workdays are lost every year due to back pain (Salkever, 1985). To an employer sponsor of health benefits, having a managed care plan with a comprehensive and coordinated response to the problem of disabling backache is a significant benefit. Not only can medical costs be contained, but the costs of lost productivity can be decreased as well.

The significant impact of back pain on public health was the impetus for the formulation of clinical practice guidelines recently published by the Agency for Health Care Policy and Research (Bigos et al, 1994). These guidelines were developed to assist provider and patient decisions about appropriate health care. A multi-disciplinary panel of clinicians and other experts reviewed the scientific literature and employed expert clinical opinion to define the current state of knowledge about back pain and its treatment. The panel recommended a series of palliative and treatment approaches. The initial intervention recommended was the use of nonprescription analgesics (such as acetaminophen, aspirin, and ibuprofen) to "provide sufficient pain relief for most patients with acute low-back symptoms." In the event of failure to improve, manipulation was recommended with the indication, "manual loading of the spine using short or long leverage methods is safe and effective for patients in the first month of acute low-back symptoms . . . ." Prescribed pharmaceuticals (nonsteroidal anti-inflammatory drugs [NSAIDs]) were recommended, but muscle relaxants and narcotic analgesics were not. Other commonly prescribed cures were found to have "no proven efficacy," and were not recommended. These included prolonged bed rest, traction, ultrasound, and transcutaneous electrical nerve stimulation (TENS).

A study by the RAND Corporation estimated that doctors of chiropractic (DCs) perform over 90% of the spinal manipulative procedures in the United States (Shekelle et al, 1991). While traditional medicine has been slow to accept and refer to chiropractors, the efficacy of manipulative treatments has been increasingly well documented in the past several years. In one study, a randomized comparison contrasted chiropractic management with hospital outpatient treatment of back pain patients (Meade et al, 1990). Outcomes were tracked by the Oswestry Disability Questionnaire and clinical tests of straight leg raising and lumbar flexion. Follow-up at intervals from 6 weeks to 2 years showed greater improvement in the chiropractor-treated group of patients. Although more hospital-treated patients received treatment during the second year (24% versus 17% of DC-treated patients), chiropractic patients maintained better improvement on outcomes scores and fewer absences from work.

Back pain has traditionally been viewed as a benign self-limiting condition. More recent investigation suggests that while this condition is not life-threatening, it is far more prevalent, recurrent, and persistent than previously thought. Direct medical costs in the United States are estimated at $25 billion a year (Frymoyer and Cats-Baril, 1991). The total cost to society, including medical and disability payments, is estimated at up to $50 billion annually (Nachemson, 1992). Many observers have reported short-term benefits of manipulative treatment for acute low-back pain. Additionally, there is information available that begins to suggest a long-term benefit from chiropractic treatment as well.

CHIROPRACTIC COST-EFFECTIVENESS

Concern for increased medical costs for a health plan often prevents consideration of add-on benefits such as mental health, vision

Table 54.1–1 Data on the Utilization of Chiropractic Based on Surveys of the Use of Alternative Therapies

Source	Universe Surveyed	Response	Parameter	Chiropractic
National Market Measures, 1999	Randomly selected managed care organizations (MCOs)	N = 114 of 449 MCOs	Of MCOs offering alternative therapies, percentage offering chiropractic	65.0%
Madigan Army Medical Center (Drivdahl and Miser, 1998)	Patients in a family practice	N = 177	Of patients using alternative medicine, percentage using chiropractic	64.0%
Kaiser Permanente, Division of Research (Gordon et al, 1998)	Kaiser physicians • Primary care clinicians • OB/Gyn clinicians Kaiser patients	N = 624 N = 157 N = 17,735	Percentage of clinicians who used or recommended chiropractic Used chiropractic past year Ever used chiropractic	33.6% 37.6% 8.5% 23.4%
Stanford Center for Research (Astin, 1998)	Demographically representative individuals randomly selected from a panel	N = 1,035	Of those using alternative medicine in previous year, percentage who used chiropractic	15.7%
Center for Alternative Medicine Research (Eisenberg et al, 1998)	Nationally representative random households; residents surveyed by telephone	N = 2,055 (1997 survey)	Prevalence and frequency of use of chiropractic among adult respondents	11.0%
Departments of Psychiatry and Public Health, Yale University (Druss and Rosenheck, 1998)	Participants in 1996 Medical Expenditure Panel Survey of noninstitutionalized civilians	N = 16,068 adults	From broader population in survey, statistics on visits to chiropractors in past year	3.3%

Source:
Astin J. Why patients use alternative medicine: Results of a national study. *JAMA.* 1998;279(19):1548–1553.
Drivdahl CE, Miser WF. The use of alternative health care by a family practice population. *J Am Board Fam Pract.* 1998 May–June; 11(3):193–199.
Druss B, Rosenheck R. Association between use of unconventional therapies and conventional medical services. *JAMA.* 1999;282(7):651–656.
Eisenberg D, Davis R, Ettner S, Appel S, Wilkey S, Van Rompay M, Kessler R. Trends in alternative medicine use in the United States, 1990–1997: Results of a follow-up national survey. *JAMA.* 1998;280(18):1569–1575.
Gordon N, Sobel D, Tarazona E. Use of and interest in alternative therapies among adult primary care clinicians and adult members in a large health maintenance organization. *WJM.* 1998;169(3):153–161.
National Market Measures. *The Landmark Report II.* Sacramento, CA: Landmark Healthcare; 1999.

care, or alternatives to traditional health care. In the case of chiropractic, many have argued that rather than increasing medical costs, it may reduce costs overall by reducing the intensity of services and by replacing more costly procedures.

Cost comparisons between medical and chiropractic treatment for back injuries frequently show an advantage for chiropractic care. A study of 3,062 Utah industrial injury cases compared MD and DC providers for the same ICD-9 codes *(International Classification of Diseases,* 9th ed) (Jarvis et al, 1991). Both time-loss and non–time-loss claims were considered. While a true cohort analysis was not possible given the available data, the study concluded that "chiropractic care is less costly than medical care in certain ICD-9 categories and no more costly than medical care in the remaining ICD-9 categories."

A study of Florida back injury cases examined 10,652 closed cases to compare chiropractic case management with mainstream medical care (Wolk, 1988). The results indicated that the cost of chiropractic treatment was significantly lower (58% less). Additionally, hospitalization rates were much lower for the chiropractic patients (20%, compared with hospitalization rates of 52% for medical patients). Although case mix and severity could not be considered, the difference in cost and the potential for cost savings are significant.

Data from earlier studies have been reinforced in an episode analysis by MEDSTAT, a database and information management company (Stano et al, 1992). There are findings that indicate that chiropractic patients have lower medical costs, largely as a result of lower inpatient utilization. The authors of this study recommend examination of the effects of substituting chiropractic for other forms of care, as well as the policy implications for managing health care. Economic analysis of chiropractic costs on health insurance coverage in Virginia considered the impact of chiropractic inclusion (Dean and Schmidt, 1992). Chiropractic costs compared favorably with other forms of treatment, but more importantly, had an offsetting impact, thereby reducing other medical costs. The provision of chiropractic benefits could be achieved with "minimal, even negligible, impacts on the costs of health insurance." Another study, commissioned initially by the province of Ontario, reviewed the scientific literature and the cost experience in the province (Manga and Angus, 1993). Chiropractic care was shown to be safe and clinically effective, as well as cost-effective. The study found potential for savings, and recommended "a shift from medical to chiropractic management of low-back pain."

In summary, there is increasing evidence that chiropractic care is appropriate and effective. A body of consistent data also suggests that chiropractic patients are well satisfied with their care. In addition, the research findings indicate that chiropractic is cost-effective. These positive findings, paired with high utilization by patients, identify chiropractic as an appropriate treatment for inclusion in integrative medicine programs.

REFERENCES

Azevedo D. Are we asking too much of the gatekeepers? *Med Econ.* April 1994;11:121–130.

Bigos S, Bowyer O, Braen G, et al. *Acute Low Back Pain in Adults: Clinical Practice Guidelines.* Rockville, MD: Agency for Healthcare Policy and Research, Public Health Survey; 1994. AHCPR Publication 95-0642.

Cherkin D, MacCornack, F. Patient evaluation of low back pain from family physicians and chiropractors. *West J Med.* 1989;328:246–252.

Cypress D. Characteristics of physician visits for back symptoms: a national perspective. *Am J Public Health.* 1983;73:389–395.

Dean D, Schmidt R. *A Comparison of the Costs of Chiropractors versus Alternative Medical Practitioners.* Richmond, VA: Virginia Chiropractic Association; 1992.

Druss B, Rosenheck R. Association between use of unconventional therapies and conventional medical services. *JAMA.* 1999;282(7):651–656.

Eisenberg D, Davis R, Ettner S, Appel S, Wilkey S, Van Rompay M, Kessler R. Trends in alternative medicine use in the United States, 1990–1997: Results of a follow-up national survey. *JAMA.* 1998;280(18):1569–1575.

Eisenberg DM, Kessler RC, Foster C, Norlock FE, Calkins DR, Delbanco TL. Unconventional medicine in the United States. *N Engl J Med.* 1993;328:246–252.

Frymoyer J, Cats-Baril W. An overview of the incidences and costs of low back pain. *Orthop Clin North Am.* 1991;22:263–271.

Harris L. *Americans' Perception of Chiropractors and Their Treatment for Back Problems.* New York: Louis Harris and Associates of New York; 1994.

Hurwitz E, Coulter I, Adams A, Genovese B, Shekelle P. Utilization of chiropractic services in the United States and Canada: 1985–1991. *Am J Pub Health.* 1998;88(5):771–776.

Jarvis K, Phillips RB, Morris EK. Cost per case comparison of back injury claims of chiropractic versus medical management for conditions with identical diagnostic codes. *J Occup Med.* 1991;33(8):847–852.

Kelly J, White A. Epidemiology and impact of low back pain. *Spine.* 1980;5:133–142.

Manga P, Angus D. *The Effectiveness and Cost-Effectiveness of Chiropractic Management of Low Back Pain.* Ottawa, Canada: Pran Manga and Associates; 1993.

Meade T, Dyer S, Browne W, Townsend J, Frank A. Low back pain of mechanical origin: Randomized comparison of chiropractic and hospital outpatient treatment. *BMJ.* 1990;300:1431–1437.

Nachemson A. Newest knowledge of low back pain: A critical look. *Clin Orthop.* 1992;279:8–20.

National Market Measures. *The Landmark Report II.* Sacramento, CA: Landmark Healthcare;1999.

Rowe M. Low back pain in industry: A position paper. *J Occup Med.* 1969;11:161–169.

Salkever D. *Morbidity Costs: National Estimates and Economic Determinate.* Rockville, MD: U.S. Department of Health and Human Services; 1985:1–13. DHHS Publication 86-3393.

Shekelle P, Adams A, Chassin M, et al. *The Appropriateness of Spinal Manipulation for Low Back Pain: Project Overview and Literature Review.* Santa Monica, CA: RAND Corp; 1991.

Stano M, Ehrhart J, Allenburg TJ. The growing role of chiropractic in health care delivery. *J Am Health Policy.* 1992;2(6):39–45.

Wolk S. *Chiropractic Versus Medical Care: A Cost-Analysis of Disability and Treatment for Back-Related Workers' Compensation Cases.* Arlington, VA: Foundation for Chiropractic Education and Research; 1988.

54.2 An Overview of the Profession of Chiropractic

David Chapman-Smith

DEFINITION AND LEGAL SCOPE OF PRACTICE

Chiropractic (from Greek, meaning treatment by hand) is a health profession concerned with the diagnosis, treatment, and prevention of disorders of the musculoskeletal system and the effects of these disorders on the nervous system and general health. Chiropractic practice emphasizes clinical interventions that support the natural ability of the body to heal itself (homeostasis) and includes:

- Manipulation and mobilization of spinal and other joints, also known as joint adjustment.

David Chapman-Smith, LLB, received his honors degree in law from Auckland University, New Zealand, and was a litigation partner there in the firm of Holmden Horrocks & Co. until his move to Toronto, where he now has his legal practice. He currently serves as Secretary-General for the World Federation of Chiropractic and General Counsel for the Ontario Chiropractic Association. A recognized author and spokesman for the profession, he is co-editor of national chiropractic clinical guidelines in the United States and Canada, has been editor of the newsletter *The Chiropractic Report* for the past 14 years, and is the author of the recently published book *The Chiropractic Profession.*

Source: Adapted with permission from D. Chapman-Smith, *The Chiropractic Profession,* © 2000, NCMIC Group Inc.

- Soft tissue techniques.
- Exercise and rehabilitative programs.
- Other supportive methods, such as the use of back supports and orthotics, interferential therapies, ultrasound, etc.
- Patient education on spinal health, posture, nutrition, and other lifestyle modifications.

The legally defined scope of practice of chiropractic is not the same in every country, state, or province, but always has these common features:

1. Primary contact or care—meaning patients can consult a chiropractor directly without any requirement of medical referral
2. The right and duty to perform a diagnosis, including the right to perform and/or order diagnostic skeletal X-rays and other imaging studies
3. The use of spinal manipulation and a range of other manual and physical therapeutics
4. No use of prescription drugs or surgery

The legal scope of practice may appear in one or more of three levels of legislation:

1. Statute
2. Regulations or rules under that statute enacted by government
3. In-practice standards issued by the chiropractic board or regulatory authority established under the statute

A summary of all U.S. state scope-of-practice laws and other licensure requirements can be obtained from an annual directory published by the Federation of Chiropractic Licensing Boards (FCLB), 901 54th Avenue, Suite 101, Greeley, CO 80634, Telephone: (970) 356-3500, e-mail: fclb@fclb.org, Web site: www.fclb.org.

EPIDEMIOLOGY AND TREATMENT

Various studies on the use of chiropractic services, including a recent large survey in the United States and Canada (Hurwitz et al, 1998),

report that approximately 95% of chiropractic patients seek care for neuromusculoskeletal pain or disorders. Approximately 65%, or two out of three patients, have low-back pain and/or leg pain. Approximately 10% have headache. See Table 54.2–1 for a summary of conditions treated in chiropractic practice. Nonmusculoskeletal conditions (5%) include circulatory, digestive, gynecological, and respiratory problems that may improve or resolve completely when a related spinal problem is corrected. A recent national survey in Sweden (Leboeuf-Yde et al, 1999) indicates that 23%, or about one in four, of patients receiving chiropractic treatment for musculoskeletal pain report significant nonmusculoskeletal benefits after chiropractic treatment, primarily with respect to digestive and respiratory problems.

Goals of Chiropractic Practice

Following from the above, the goals of chiropractic practice are to:

1. Meet the patient's immediate needs, often the relief of pain.
2. Address the cause of the symptoms by restoring normal ranges of movement and function to the joints, muscles, and other structures of the musculoskeletal or locomotor system.

Table 54.2–1 Breakdown of Patient Complaints Seen in Chiropractic Practice

Complaint	Percentage
Back pain	70%
Low-back pain	65%
Midback pain	5%
Other neuromusculoskeletal pain	25%
Head/neck pain	15%
Extremity pain	10%
Nonneuromusculoskeletal disorders	5%
Allergies, asthma, etc	

Source: Adapted with permission from D. Chapman-Smith, *The Chiropractic Profession,* © 2000, NCMIC Group Inc.

3. Thereby allow the nervous system to function without interference, better regulating the various body systems and general health.

Within their scope of practice, chiropractors employ a range of techniques of spinal adjustment as described in Exhibit 54.2–1.

SAFETY AND EFFECTIVENESS

There is now good research evidence of the safety and effectiveness of chiropractic treatment for the conditions most commonly seen in practice—acute and chronic back pain (Manga et al, 1993; Meade et al, 1990; van Tulder et al, 1997), neck pain (Hurwitz et al, 1996, Coulter et al 1996), and headache (Nilsson et al, 1997; Boline et al, 1995).

The only risk of significant harm is vertebral artery injury and stroke as the result of cervical manipulation, but that is a very remote risk at 1 to 2 incidents per 1 million treatments (Haldeman et al, 1999), a much lesser risk than the morbidity and mortality arising from medications and surgeries given to equivalent patients in medical practice (Coulter et al, 1996). The scientific literature on the safety and effectiveness of spinal manipulation and mobilization has been reviewed in studies by the RAND Corporation, which has reported that these procedures are appropriate for many forms of back pain (Shekelle et al, 1991), neck pain, and headache (Coulter et al, 1996). See Chapter 56 for more information on safety and effectiveness.

EDUCATION AND LICENSURE

Necessary Qualifications for the Right To Practice

Many countries and jurisdictions, including all U.S. states and Canadian provinces, have legislation regulating the practice of chiropractic. To practice, a chiropractor must have a license or registration with the licensing board with the following preconditions:

Exhibit 54.2–1 Classification System for Chiropractic Manipulative/Adjustive Techniques

Manual Articular Manipulative and Adjustive Procedures
- Specific contact thrust procedures
  1. High-velocity thrust
  2. High-velocity thrust with recoil
  3. Low-velocity thrust
- Nonspecific contact thrust procedures
- Manual force, mechanically assisted procedures
  1. Drop-table and terminal point adjustive thrust
  2. Flexion-distraction table adjustment
  3. Pelvic block adjusting
- Mechanical force, manually assisted procedures
  1. Fixed stylus, compression wave adjustment
  2. Moving stylus instrument adjustment

Manual Nonarticular Manipulative and Adjustive Procedures
- Manual reflex and muscle relaxation procedures
  1. Muscle energy techniques
  2. Neurologic reflex techniques
  3. Myofascial ischemic compression procedures
  4. Miscellaneous soft-tissue techniques
- Miscellaneous procedures
  1. Neural retraining techniques
  2. Conceptual approaches

Source: Reprinted from S. Haldeman et al., eds., *Quality Assurance and Practice Parameters, Guidelines for Chiropractic Quality Assurance,* © 1993, Aspen Publishers, Inc.

1. Graduation with a doctor of chiropractic degree from a duly accredited chiropractic college
2. Completion of national board examinations
3. Completion of state/provincial licensing board examinations
4. Satisfaction of various conditions common to licensed health professions, such

as being of sound character, holding malpractice insurance, and completing mandatory continuing education and/or practice review requirements.

Education

In North America, there is a minimum of 6 years full-time, university-level education, which includes 2 years of college credits in qualifying subjects and then a 4-year undergraduate program at chiropractic college. A typical program, with subjects and hours of study, is shown in Table 54.2–2. This training is followed by national and state/provincial licensing board examinations. Postgraduate specialties include chiropractic sciences, neurology, nutrition, orthopedics, radiology, rehabilitation, and sports chiropractic.

Although many chiropractic colleges are private institutions, they are not free to establish their own entrance requirements, curricula, faculty, staff, governance, facilities, research, or patient care. In these and other areas, uniform minimum requirements are established through an official accreditation system. In the United States, the accrediting agency for the chiropractic profession is the Council on Chiropractic Education (CCE). It is based in Scottsdale, Arizona, and has been recognized by the U.S. Department of Education since 1974. In Canada, the accrediting agency is the Canadian Council on Chiropractic Education (CCE Canada), which is formally affiliated with the CCE and has reciprocal standards. There are chiropractic colleges, and all have accredited status with the CCE. Additionally, 13 of them are accredited by non-chiropractic regional accrediting agencies such as the North Central Association of Schools and Colleges.

Licensure Examinations

A doctor of chiropractic seeking a license to practice must pass the following board exams:

- Part I—basic science in seven areas (general anatomy, spinal anatomy, physiology,

chemistry, pathology, microbiology, and public health)
- Part II—clinical science in six areas (general diagnosis, neuromusculoskeletal diagnosis, radiography, principles of chiropractic, chiropractic practice, and associated clinical sciences)
- Part III—clinical competency in nine areas (case history, physical examination, neuromusculoskeletal examination, X-ray examination, clinical laboratory and special studies examination, diagnosis/clinical impression, chiropractic techniques, supportive techniques, and case management)

Prior to 1965, at a time when chiropractic examining boards had fewer resources, chiropractors in most U.S. states took the same basic science board examinations as medical doctors. Accordingly, they were required to meet the same standard. Since that time, chiropractic examinations have become separate, while remaining at an equivalent standard with medicine.

The regulatory process for chiropractic practice has created two national organizations in the United States. The Federation of Chiropractic Licensing Boards (FCLB), established in 1933, seeks to unify standards and requirements of individual state boards and publishes their state licensure requirements annually. It is affiliated with and has appointed members on the National Board of Chiropractic Examiners (NBCE). The NBCE, established in 1963, administers the state and national board licensing examinations. It has developed examination systems that are now used nationally and internationally, including the three-part exam referred to above. At this writing, 46 states require or accept NBCE exams for licensure, and others have requirements similar to, or modeled on, the NBCE exams:

National Board of Chiropractic Examiners
901 54th Avenue
Greeley, CO 80634
Phone: (970) 356-9100
E-mail: nbce@nbce.org
Web site: www.NBCE.org/nbce

Table 54.2–2 Subjects Taught in a Typical Semester-Based Chiropractic Program, by Year and Number of Hours

Division	First Year (Hrs)	Second Year (Hrs)	Third Year (Hrs)	Fourth Year (Hrs)
Biological Sciences	Human Anatomy (180) Microscopic Anatomy (140) Neuroanatomy (72) Neuroscience I (32) Biochemistry (112) Physiology I (36)	Pathology (174) Lab Diagnosis I (40) Microbiology & Infectious Disease (100) Neuroscience II (87) Nutrition (58) Immunology (13)	Lab Diagnosis II (32) Toxicology (13)	Clinical Nutrition (26) Community Health (39)
Chiropractic Sciences	Chiropractic Principles I (56) Basic Body Mechanics (96) Chiropractic Skills I (100)	Chiropractic Principles II (58) Chiropractic Skills II (145) Spinal Mechanics (42)	Chiropractic Principles III (42) Clinical Biomechanics (100) Chiropractic Skills III (145) Auxiliary Chiropractic Therapy (58) Introduction to Jurisprudence & Practice Development (16)	Integrated Chiropractic Practice (95) Jurisprudence & Practice Development (46)
Clinical Sciences	Normal Radiographic Anatomy (16) Radiation Biophysics and Protection (44)	Intro. Diagnosis (87) Intro. Bone Pathology (48) Skeletal Radiology (39)	Orthopedics & Rheumatology (92) Neurodiagnosis (42) Differential Diagnosis (32) Diagnosis & Symptomatology (116) Radiological Technology (39) Arthritis & Trauma (48)	Clinical Psychology (46) Emergency Care (52) Child Care (20) Female Care (29) Geriatrics (20) Abdomen, Chest & Special Radiographic Procedures (40)
Clinical Education	Observer I (28)	Observer II (73)	Observer III (406)	Internship (752) Clerkships • Auxiliary Therapy (33) • Clinical Lab (21) Clinical X-ray • Technology (71) • Interpretation (69) • Observer IV (31)
Research			Applied Research & Biometrics (32)	Research Investigative Project
Totals	912	978	1,213	1,390

Total hours over four years: 4,493 plus research project.

Courtesy of the Canadian Memorial Chiropractic College, Toronto, Ontario, Canada (December 1, 2000).

JOINT MANIPULATION

Appropriate Course of Treatment

Reporting on the appropriateness of spinal manipulation for low-back pain, a 1991 RAND Corporation expert panel, which was composed of three chiropractors, two medical orthopedists, an internist, a family practitioner, a neurologist, and an osteopath, unanimously concluded, "An adequate trial of spinal manipulation is a course of 2 weeks for each of two different types of spinal manipulation (4 weeks total); after which, in the absence of documented improvement, spinal manipulation is no longer indicated" (Shekelle et al, 1991).

Typically, a patient is given manipulation three times weekly at first, then less frequently. This amounts to approximately 12 treatments over 4 weeks. This approach to frequency and duration of care has been endorsed in subsequent formal evidence-based chiropractic practice guidelines in the United States (Haldeman et al, 1993) and Canada (Henderson et al, 1994).

Some patients will only require one or a few treatments. If there is documented improvement after 4 weeks, but not complete relief of symptoms or restored function, the course of manipulations may continue. Typically, it will end within 8 weeks for uncomplicated conditions, within 16 weeks for other conditions unless there has been major trauma and/or complications. Some patients, because of lasting effects of trauma and/or the demands of their work and lifestyle, will require long-term supportive care. Others elect to have preventive or maintenance care.

Level of Expertise

Skilled spinal manipulation requires extended training and full-time practice. The prominent orthopedic surgeon and researcher William Kirkaldy-Willis, MD, editor of the text, *Managing Low-Back Pain* (1992), advises family physicians to refer patients who may benefit from manipulation to a chiropractor or other specialist. Alan Stoddard, DO, MD, a British osteopath and specialist in physical medicine, has stated:

The art of manipulation depends on the ability of the practitioner to combine the forces he uses such that the maximum leverage occurs precisely at the level of the restricted joint. Such skill takes a great deal of practice to perfect. Clearly those engaged in continuous practice are likely to be more skilled than those who manipulate only on rare occasions. The concert pianist practices his art daily to maintain a high standard. This applies equally to the art of manipulation (Stoddard, 1979).

INSURANCE COVERAGE AND REIMBURSEMENT

Since the degree to which there is government and private third-party payment for chiropractic services constantly changes according to time and jurisdiction, the following is a summary overview only.

Government Funding

Worldwide over the past 20 years, four government commissions have been asked to study and report on whether there should be government funding for chiropractic services. These commissions were convened in Australia (1986) (Thompson, 1986), New Zealand (1978) (Hasselberg, 1979), Sweden (1987) (Commission on Alternative Medicine, 1988), and Ontario, Canada (1993) (Manga et al, 1993)—all said yes. These recommendations have led to varying degrees of coverage in Australia (veterans only), Canada (partial funding for all patients in most provinces), and Sweden (partial funding for all patients in approximately one-third of the health regions). There is also government funding in:

- Denmark (nationally, for all patients)
- Israel (nationally through health maintenance organizations for all patients)
- Italy (only on medical referral in designated interdisciplinary clinics)

- Norway (nationally for all patients)
- Switzerland (Switzerland was the first country to establish government funding for chiropractic services)
- The United Kingdom (for patients receiving chiropractic services through National Health Service contracts)
- The United States (for seniors under Medicare, the military and in some cases for the disadvantaged under Medicaid)

Workers' Compensation and Automobile Insurance

These plans typically include coverage of chiropractic services on a similar basis to medical services in U.S. states, Canadian provinces, Australian states, and several European countries.

Employee Benefit Plans

Private insurance coverage under employee benefit plans has become available wherever the profession has become established (Jensen et al, 1997). In the United States, HMO coverage for chiropractic appears to be increasing, as reflected in the findings of the Landmark Report II (1999), which indicated that approximately 67% of managed care organizations surveyed offered chiropractic benefits. In conventional insurance plans, preferred provider organizations (PPOs), and point-of-service plans, more than 80% of employees have full or partial coverage for chiropractic services. Jensen et al (1997) reported that chiropractic coverage was provided by a range of insurers:

- Conventional insurance plans—84%
- Preferred provider organizations—83%
- Point-of-service plans—81%
- Managed care plans—44%

As mentioned, coverage in managed care plans expanded from 44% to 67% by 1999.

Chiropractic in Mauritius

Mauritius, an island country in the Indian Ocean, provides a colorful example. Dr. Rajinder Roy became the first chiropractor to establish a practice in Mauritius in 1994. Shortly thereafter, insurers began referring him back pain patients who were scheduled to be flown to South Africa for back surgery. Surgery was not needed in the first 20 consecutive cases and, as a result, many insurers now provide third-party funding for chiropractic services from him and others.

REFERENCES

Boline PD, Kassak K, Bronfort G, Nelson C, Anderson A. Spinal manipulation versus amitriptyline for the treatment of chronic tension-type headaches: A randomized clinical trial. *J Manipulative Physiol Ther* 1995;18:148–154.

Commission on Alternative Medicine, Social Departementete, Legitimization for Vissa Kiropraktorer, Stockholm, SOU (English Summary). 1987:12-13—16.

Coulter ID, Hurwitz EL, Adams AH, et al. The appropriateness of manipulation and mobilization of the cervical spine. Santa Monica, CA: RAND, 1996; Document No. MR-781-CR.

Haldeman S, Chapman-Smith D, Petersen D, eds. *Guidelines for Chiropractic Quality Assurance and Practice Parameters. Proceedings of the Mercy Center Consensus Conference*. Gaithersburg, Maryland: Aspen Publishers; 1993:179–184.

Haldeman S, Kohlbeck FJ, McGregor M. Risk factors and precipitating neck movements causing vertebrobasilar artery dissection after cervical trauma and spinal manipulation. *Spine*. 1999; 24(8):785–794.

Hasselberg PD. Chiropractic in New Zealand, Report of a Commission of Inquiry. Wellington, New Zealand: Government Printer; 1979.

Henderson D, Chapman-Smith D, Mior S, Vernon H, eds. *Clinical Guidelines for Chiropractic Practice in Canada*. Suppl. to JCCa. 1994;38(1).

Hurwitz EL, Aker PD, Adams AH, Meeker, WC, Shekelle P. Manipulation and mobilization of the cervical spine: A systematic review of the literature. *Spine*. 1996;21:1746–1760.

Hurwitz EL, Coulter I, Adams A, Genovese B, Shekelle P. Utilization of chiropractic services in the United States and Canada: 1985–1991. *Am J Pub Health*. 1998;88(5):771–776.

Jensen G, Morrisey M, Gaffney S, Liston DK. The new dominance of managed care: Insurance trends in the 1990s. *Health Affairs*. 1997;16:125–136.

Kirkaldy-Willis W, Burton C, eds. *Managing Low-Back Pain*, 3rd ed. New York: Churchill Livingston, 1992.

Leboeuf-Yde C, Axén I, Ahlefeldt G, Lidefelt P, Rosenbaum A, Thurnherr T. The types and frequencies of improved nonmusculoskeletal symptoms reported after chiropractic spinal manipulative therapy. *J Manipulative Physiol Ther*. 1999; 22(9):559–564.

Manga P, Angus D, Papadopoulos C, Swan W. *The Effectiveness and Cost-Effectiveness of Chiropractic Management of Low-Back Pain*. Ottawa, Ontario: Pran Manga and Associates, University of Ottawa, 1993;65–70.

Meade TW, Dyer S, Browne W, Townsend J, Frank AO. Low back pain of mechanical origin: Randomized comparison of chiropractic and hospital outpatient treatment. *Br Med J*. 1990;300:1431–1437.

National Market Measures. *The Landmark Report II*. Sacramento, CA: Landmark Healthcare; 1999.

Nilsson N, Christensen HW, Hartvigsen J. The effect of spinal manipulation in the treatment of cervicogenic headache. *J Manipulative Physiol Ther*. 1997;20(5):326–330.

Shekelle P, Adams A. The appropriateness of spinal manipulation for low-back pain: Indications and ratings by a multidisciplinary expert panel. Santa Monica, CA: RAND; 1991. Monograph No. R-4025/2-CCR/FCER.

Stoddard A. *The Back: Relief from Pain*. Canada: Prentice-Hall; 1979:17.

Thompson C. Second Report, Medicare Benefits Review Committee. Canberra, Australia: Commonwealth Government Printer, June 1986: Chapter 10 (Chiropractic).

van Tulder MW, Koes BW, Bouter LM. Conservative treatment of acute and chronic nonspecific low back pain: A systematic review of randomized controlled trials of the most common interventions. *Spine*. 1997 Sep 15;22(18):2128–2156.

54.3   Resources

David Chapman-Smith

PROFESSIONAL ASSOCIATIONS

The two largest national associations in the world are the American Chiropractic Association (ACA) and the Canadian Chiropractic Association (CCA). In the United States, there is a second national association named the International Chiropractors' Association (ICA). The ACA and ICA conduct an increasing number of joint educational, public education, and political action initiatives. Since health care laws and

rights and funding arrangements are mainly matters of state/provincial law rather than national law in the United States and Canada, chiropractors' first professional memberships are often with their state or provincial associations.

The organization representing state associations in the United States is the Congress of Chiropractic State Associations (COCSA). The organization representing national associations throughout the world is the World Federation of Chiropractic (WFC). This is a member of the Council of International Organizations of Medical Sciences (CIOMS) and is in official relations with the World Health Organization (WHO).

American Chiropractic Association (ACA)
1701 Clarendon Boulevard
Arlington, VA 22209
Phone: (703) 276-8800; fax: (703) 243-2593
E-mail: memberinfo@americhiro.org
Web site: www.amerchiro.org

Canadian Chiropractic Association (CCA)
1396 Eglinton Avenue West
Toronto, Ontario M6C 2E4, Canada
Phone: (416) 781-5656; fax: (416) 781-7344
E-mail: ccachiro@inforamp.net
Web site: www.ccachiro.org

International Chiropractors' Association (ICA)
1110 Glebe Road, Suite 1000
Arlington, VA 22201
Phone: (703) 528-5000; fax: (703) 528-5023
E-mail: chiro@erols.com
Web site: www.chiropractic.org

Congress of Chiropractic State Associations (COCSA)
PO Box 2054
Lexington, SC 29071-2054
Phone: (803) 356-6809; fax: (803) 356-6226
E-mail: jjordan@chirolink.com

World Federation of Chiropractic
3080 Yonge Street, Suite 5065
Toronto, Ontario M4N 3N1, Canada
Phone: (416) 484-9978; fax: (416) 484-9665
E-mail: info@wfc.org
Web site: www.wfc.org

PROFESSIONAL LIABILITY INSURANCE

Chiropractors may obtain their professional liability/malpractice insurance from many private companies. The National Chiropractic Mutual Insurance Company (NCMIC Insurance) was established by the profession and is by far the largest carrier for chiropractors in the United States.

NCMIC Insurance
1452 29th Street, Suite 200
West Des Moines, IA 50266-1307
Phone: (515) 222-1736; fax: (515) 222-2951
Web site: www.ncmic.com

RESEARCH ORGANIZATIONS

Leading research organizations are the Foundation for Chiropractic Education and Research (FCER), which funds research and awards for postgraduate education from private funding, and the Consortial Center for Chiropractic Research (CCCR), which has significant funding support from the U.S. government through the National Center for Complementary and Alternative Medicine, National Institutes of Health, and the Bureau of Health Professions, Health Resources and Services Administration.

Foundation for Chiropractic Education and Research (FCER)
PO Box 4689
704 East 4th Street
Des Moines, IA 50306-4689
Phone: (515) 282-7118; fax (515) 282-3347
E-mail: fcernow@aol.com

Consortial Center for Chiropractic Research
c/o Palmer College of Chiropractic
1000 Brady Street
Davenport, IA 52803
Phone: (319) 884-5162; fax: (319) 884-5227

SOURCES OF FURTHER INFORMATION

For more comprehensive summary information on chiropractic see the recent books:
The Chiropractic Profession: Its Education, Practice, Research and Future Directions (Chapman-Smith, NCMIC Group Inc., West Des Moines, Iowa, 2000; Telephone: 1-877-291-7312)
Chiropractic in the United States: Training, Practice and Research (ed. Cherkin and Mootz, AHCPR Publication No. 98-N002, Public Health

Service, U.S. Department of Health and Human Services, 1997). Listed below are a selection of chiropractic clinical texts and peer-reviewed journals.

Clinical Texts

Haldeman S, ed. *Principles and Practice of Chiropractic*. Stamford, CT: Appleton and Lange; 1992.

Bergmann T, Peterson D, Lawrence D, ed. *Chiropractic Technique*. St. Louis: Mosby Yearbook Inc.; 1998.

Liebenson C, ed. *Rehabilitation of the Spine: A Practitioner's Manual*. Baltimore: Williams & Wilkins; 1996.

Stude DE, ed. *Spinal Rehabilitation*. Stamford, CT: Appleton and Lange; 1999.

Murphy DR, ed. *Conservative Management of Cervical Spine Syndromes*. New York: McGraw-Hill; 1999.

Foreman SM, Croft CA, eds. *Whiplash Injuries: The Cervical Acceleration/Deceleration Syndrome*. Baltimore: Williams & Wilkins; 1988.

Vernon H, ed. *Upper Cervical Syndrome: Chiropractic Diagnosis and Treatment*. Baltimore: Williams & Wilkins; 1998.

Curl DD, ed. *Chiropractic Approach to Head Pain*. Baltimore: Williams & Wilkins; 1994.

Hammer WI, ed. *Functional Soft-Tissue Examination and Treatment of Manual Methods,* 2nd ed. Gaithersburg, MD: Aspen Publishers; 1999.

Hyde TE, Gengenbach M, eds. *Conservative Management of Sports Injuries*. Baltimore: Williams & Wilkins; 1997.

Anrig C, Plaugher G, eds. *Pediatric Chiropractic*. Baltimore: Williams & Wilkins; 1997.

Cramer GD, Darby SA, eds. *Basic and Clinical Anatomy of the Spine: Spinal Cord and ANS*. St. Louis: Mosby Yearbook; 1995.

Yochum TR, Rowe LJ, eds. *Essentials of Skeletal Radiology*. Baltimore: Williams & Wilkins; 1996.

Marchiori DM, ed. *Clinical Imaging: With Skeletal Chest and Abdomen Patterned Differentials*. St. Louis: Mosby; 1999.

Souza TA, ed. *Differential Diagnosis for the Chiropractor: Protocols and Algorithms*, 2nd ed. Gaithersburg, MD: Aspen Publishers, 2001.

Newsletter

The Chiropractic Report
Chiropractic Report Inc.
Toronto
Phone: (416) 484-9601
Web: www.chiropracticreport.com.

Peer-Reviewed Journals

Chiropractic Technique
Lippincott Williams & Wilkins (for the National College of Chiropractic)
Baltimore, MD
Phone: (410) 528-8555

Journal of Manipulative and Physiological Therapeutics
Mosby (for the National College of Chiropractic)
St. Louis, MO
Phone: (314) 453-4351

Journal of the Neuromusculoskeletal System
Data Trace (for the American Chiropractic Association)
Baltimore, MD
Phone: (410) 494-4994

Topics in Clinical Chiropractic
Aspen Publishers, Inc
Gaithersburg, MD 20878
Phone: (301) 417-7500

CHAPTER 55

Cost Comparison of Chiropractic and Medical Treatment: A Literature Review

Richard A. Branson

INTRODUCTION: PREVALENCE AND COST

Spinal disorders of musculoskeletal origin are a major health and economic problem in Western industrialized societies. Ten to 23% of family physician patients present with musculoskeletal problems (Hoffman, 1997; Kahl, 1987). In 1990, 9.4% of the U.S. population saw a health care provider for low-back pain (Waddell, 1996). Each year there are an estimated 15 million office visits for mechanical low-back pain, placing it fifth among symptomatic reasons for all physician visits (Hart et al, 1995). Low-back problems are the seventh leading reason for all U.S. hospitalizations. The lifetime prevalence of low-back pain and neck pain has been reported at 62% and 71%, respectively (Makela et al, 1991; McKinnon et al, 1997). The 6-month prevalence of low-back pain and headaches has been reported at 41% and 26%, respectively (Korff et al, 1988).

The estimated cost of back disorders in 1994 was $38 to $50 billion, with over $6.5 billion spent on physician services alone (Frymoyer and Durett, 1997). Furthermore, disability-related costs in 1994 were estimated to be nearly $14

billion (Frymoyer and Durett, 1997). One of the most significant reasons to explore cost-effectiveness associated with low-back pain interventions relates to the magnitude of the indirect long-term costs associated with occupational back injuries. Less than 10% of industrial back problems become chronic, yet they account for 80% of the total costs (Frymoyer and Durett, 1997). Despite the greater resources expended and better understanding of spinal disorders, the prevalence and attendant costs appear to be increasing.

Traditional medical treatment of common uncomplicated spinal conditions lacks evidence for both treatment and cost-effectiveness (Koes et al, 1991; Manga et al, 1994; Rodriquez et al, 1992). A recent systematic review of 190 randomized clinical trials of common interventions for the treatment of acute and chronic low-back pain found strong evidence supporting effectiveness of only 5 of 14 conservative treatments (van Tulder et al, 1997). Wahlgren and coworkers (1997) found two-thirds of patients with low-back pain who received 1 month of care from a primary care physician still progressed to a chronic state, experiencing pain at 6 and 12 months after the initial onset of pain. Twenty percent of patients with low-back pain in the United States who see an orthopedic or neurosurgeon will have a spinal operation within 1 year (Cheadle et al, 1994). The issue of chronic disability from musculoskeletal disorders is profound. Injured workers who do not return to work within the first 3 to 6 months following an injury have less than a 20% chance of ever returning to productive employment (Cheadle et al, 1994).

Richard A. Branson, DC, is a 1991 graduate of Western States Chiropractic College. He has served in private practice and at Northwestern College of Chiropractic in Minnesota as a radiology instructor, staff clinician, and assistant professor of research. He is currently Director of Chiropractic for the Institute of Athletic Medicine, an outpatient rehabilitation service of Fairview Health Systems, and also serves as the Chief Chiropractic Consultant for Blue Cross Blue Shield of Minnesota. He maintains an active interest in chiropractic research.

Chiropractic has received increasing attention in recent years both by consumers and the health care industry. Approximately 4.8 million people a year consult a chiropractor for low-back pain (Waddell, 1996). Chiropractors are the second most commonly used health professional for low-back pain care (Shekelle et al, 1992). In 1994, $2.65 billion was spent on chiropractic services (Frymoyer and Durett, 1997). A 1995 survey revealed that 56% of medical doctors have referred patients to a chiropractor (McKinnon et al, 1997). Ninety percent of spinal manipulation for low-back pain, neck pain, and headaches is performed by chiropractors (Shekelle, 1994).

Fourteen systematic reviews of randomized clinical trials on spinal manipulation therapy for back and neck pain have been published since 1984 (van Tulder et al, 1997; Shekelle et al, 1992; Brunarski, 1984; Ottenbacher and Difablo, 1985; Koes et al, 1991; Assendelft et al, 1992; Anderson et al, 1992; Assendelft et al, 1996a; Aker et al, 1996; Coulter et al, 1996; Hurwitz et al, 1996; Bronfort, 1997; Shekelle and Coulter, 1997). These reviews evaluate the methodological quality of the clinical trials. Ten of the 14 reviews concluded that spinal manipulative therapy was a beneficial form of treatment (see Table 55–1).

SAFETY AND RISKS

The safety of any therapeutic intervention is an important factor in cost-effectiveness. If two interventions for a given condition have equal costs yet one has a greater risk of complications, the treatment with a lower risk may have greater value. Estimates of serious complications from spinal manipulation have been extensively reported in the literature (Frisoni and Anzola, 1991; Gatterman, 1990; Klougart et al, 1996; Rivett and Milburn, 1996; Schellhas et al, 1980). The best estimates of risk are derived from a comprehensive review of the literature by Assendelft et al (1996b). They estimated vertebrobasilar accidents to be 1 per 20,000 and possibly as few as 1 per 1 million manipu-

lations and cauda equina syndrome, the most serious complication of lumbar spinal manipulation, to be less than 1 per 1 million manipulations. No randomized clinical trial or case-control study evaluating spinal manipulation has reported complications from spinal manipulation (Manga et al, 1994). Terrett (1995) reviewed cases of serious complications from spinal manipulation and found 40 cases of medical misrepresentation or inaccurate reporting by medical and medicolegal authors. Terrett suggests that these complications are less frequent than the literature reports. Furthermore, a recent publication (Dabbs and Lauretti, 1995) reported that cervical manipulation for neck pain is several hundred times safer than the use of prescription and over-the-counter nonsteroidal anti-inflammatory drugs.

COST-EFFECTIVENESS

Determining cost-effective and effective treatment of spine-related disorders is an important means to help consumers obtain the greatest health benefit from a given investment in treatment in today's health care market. Cost-effectiveness comparisons can help determine the most efficient method to allocate limited health care resources among interventions and choose between two or more competing treatments for the same illness (Clark, 1996). Simply put, the goal is to maximize health outcomes and minimize costs.

The purpose of this study was to review and summarize the literature after 1980 that evaluated retrospective and prospective studies comparing costs of medical and chiropractic care. There are three reasons why this review was limited to publications after 1980 (Assendelft et al, 1993). First, more current treatment and compensation costs are based on better documentation. Second, diagnosis and treatment opinions change with time, and such change affects cost of care. Finally, recent dramatic changes have occurred in health care affecting chiropractic and its position in delivery of care to patients with neuromusculoskeletal conditions.

Table 55–1 Systematic Reviews of Spinal Manipulation and Mobilization of the Spine

Author, Year	Condition Reviewed	Number of Trials	Conclusions
Brunarski, 1984	Musculoskeletal conditions	15	Limited empirical evidence supporting SMT.
Ottenbacher and Difabio, 1985	Musculoskeletal conditions	9	Limited empirical evidence supporting SMT. Serious flaws in the methodology.
Koes et al, 1991	Back and NP	35	Efficacy of SMT not convincingly demonstrated. Serious flaws in the methodology.
Assendelft et al, 1992	LBP treated by DC	5	Efficacy of SMT not convincingly demonstrated. Serious flaws in the methodology.
Shekelle et al, 1992	LBP	25	SMT is of short-term benefit in some patients, particularly those with uncomplicated LBP.
Anderson et al, 1992	LBP	23	SMT was consistently more effective than a number of comparative therapies.
Assendelft et al, 1996	LBP treated by DC	8	Efficacy of SMT not convincingly demonstrated.
Gross et al, 1996	Acute and chronic NP	5	SMT in combination with other treatments provides short-term relief of NP.
Coulter et al, 1996	NP and HA	11	SMT provides short-term effects for subacute and chronic HA.
Hurwitz et al, 1996	NP and HA	14	SMT provides short-term benefits for NP and HA.
Koes et al, 1996	Back and NP	38	Efficacy of SMT not convincingly demonstrated.
van Tulder et al, 1997	Acute and chronic LBP	25	SMT is an effective treatment of acute and chronic LBP
Bronfort, 1997	LBP, NP, HA, and nonmusculoskeletal conditions	58	SMT appears to have a short-term effect on acute LBP, chronic LBP, NP, and muscle tension HA.
Shekelle and Coulter, 1997	NP and HA	9	SMT is an appropriate therapy for selected patients with neck pain and headache.

SMT = spinal manipulative therapy; LBP = low-back pain; NP = neck pain; HA = headaches; DC = doctor of chiropractic.
Source: Reprinted from R.A. Branson, Cost Comparison of Chiropractic and Medical Treatment of Common Musculoskeletal Disorders: A Review of the Literature after 1980, *Topics in Clinical Chiropractic*, Vol. 6, No. 2, pp. 57–68, © 1999, Aspen Publishers, Inc.

Method

A literature search was made using MEDLINE database literature from 1976 through November 1998 and the CHIROLARS database literature from 1980 through November 1998. The search employed medical subject headings with free-text words. The key words used were "cost-effectiveness, cost-benefit analysis, cost analysis, workmen's compensation, osteopathy, medical care," and "chiropractic." A hand search of related books and other published literature was also performed. A study was included if it compared medical and chiropractic costs, if it was published after 1980, and if it was published in English. Any abstracts or unpublished studies were excluded.

Results

The MEDLINE and CHIROLARS search identified 683 studies. Twenty-two of these studies fulfilled the inclusion criteria. A hand search of books and bibliographies of identified studies revealed an additional two studies. The 24 studies that fulfilled the inclusion criteria are summarized in Tables 55–2 and 55–3.

Nineteen of the 24 studies were retrospective, and 5 were prospective. Ten of the 24 were workers' compensation studies. Nine of the 24 studies contained data from private insurance sources. Seven of the 9 studies with data from private insurance sources were from the same database and analyzed by the same author. Total cost comparison revealed that 15 of the 19 retrospective studies were in favor of chiropractic and 4 of the 19 were in favor of medical care. Three of the 5 prospective studies were in favor of medical care, and 2 out of 5 found no difference between chiropractic and medical treatment. Sixteen of 24 studies described patients with only low-back or thoracic problems. Eight of 24 studies had a broader focus of conditions, such as neck pain and other musculoskeletal injuries. Twelve of the 24 studies were published after 1994.

Discussion

Sixteen of the 24 studies reported lower mean total costs associated with chiropractic treatment. Other authors have reported that older cost-effectiveness literature had more favorable cost outcomes for chiropractic treatment. They found more modern (post-1980) studies had mixed results and favored medical treatment more frequently. This author's review of post-1980 studies does not concur with these findings. One possible explanation for this difference is that there are more published studies on cost-effectiveness of medical and chiropractic care since

the pre-1994 publication date of those studies. As stated earlier, 12 of the 24 studies were published after 1994. That is a 48% increase in the literature on this subject in a 4-year period. This alone testifies to the recent increase in interest of cost-effectiveness of chiropractic care.

Ten of the 24 studies used data from before 1990. Five of these had lower average total chiropractic costs, and 5 had lower average total medical costs (Dean and Schmidt, 1992; Nyiendo and Lamm, 1991; Greenwood, 1985; Shekelle et al, 1995; Wolk, 1988). Most studies reported a higher number of treatment visits with chiropractors, yet the average total costs were more often lower. When average total costs were higher, it was reportedly from higher chiropractic radiograph utilization (Carey et al, 1995), and greater severity and chronicity of chiropractic patients (Nyiendo and Lamm, 1991).

Benefits of Cost-Effectiveness Studies

The literature indicates there are many benefits to performing cost-effectiveness comparisons (Detsky and Naglie, 1990; Drummond et al, 1997; Conrad and Deyo, 1994). It can help providers and consumers make economic decisions about health care. It can also assist third-party payers, hospitals, health maintenance organizations, and those involved in policy making focus on appropriate utilizations of limited health care dollars.

Limitations of Cost-Effectiveness Studies

Cost-effectiveness research also has its limitations. Most of the studies reviewed were retrospective and used insurance databases that were developed for administrative purposes and not for research. This often does not allow accurate comparisons of patient characteristics such as severity and chronicity. The need to differentiate between chronic and acute conditions is very important for organizations such as health maintenance organizations and for the development of treatment guidelines.

Only three studies controlled for patient severity (Smith and Stano, 1997; Stano and Smith,

Table 55–2 Retrospective Studies Comparing Costs of Chiropractic and Medical Care

Author, Year	Condition	Source and Year of Data	Population	Chiropractic Claims	Medical Claims	Patient Characteristics Similar between Groups
Jarvis et al, 1997	9 common low-back injuries	Utah Workmen's Compensation; 1989 claims data	Total (injury) / Total (strain) / Total (nonsurgical) / Patient compensation	1989 Claims N=277 $665 $876 $703 $83	1989 Claims N=715 $877 $3,836 $1,282 $366	Gender composition similar
	9 common low-back injuries	1986 claims data	Total (injury) / Total (strain) / Total (nonsurgical) / Patient compensation	1986 Claims N = 365 $710 $716 $628 $73	1986 Claims N=844 $1,753 $1,485 $679 $1,077	Gender composition similar
Smith and Stano, 1997	9 common low-back injuries	National private fee-for-service insurance; 2 years of insurance claims (7/88–6/90)	Same provider / 1st episode / 2nd episode / 3rd episode / Total all treatment	N=97 $282 $439 $318 $1,038	N=101 $919 $983 $1,166 $3,068	Severity similar, DC patients had more chronic cases
Stano and Smith, 1996	9 common low-back injuries	National private fee-for-service insurance; 2 years of insurance claims (7/88–6/90)	Total / Outpatient costs	N=1,575 $518 $447	N=4,608 $1,020 $598	Insurance type, age, gender, region and time between episodes
Stano, 1995	Update of Stano and Smith, 1993	National private fee-for-service insurance; (claims—7/88–6/90)	Total / Outpatient costs	N=2,408 $493 $425	N=4,391 $1,000 $554	Severity, insurance type, age, gender, region
Stano, 1994	Common low-back conditions	National private fee-for-service insurance; (claims—7/88–6/90)	Total / Outpatient costs	N=2,664 $5,577 $3,326	N=7,918 $6,910 $3,438	Insurance type, age, gender, region, work status
Stano, 1993	Common low-back conditions	National private fee-for-service insurance; (claims—7/88–6/90)	Average total cost of care	N=2,668 $573	N=5,212 $1,112	No

continues

Table 55–2 continued

continues

Author, Year	Condition	Source and Year of Data	Population	Chiropractic Claims	Medical Claims	Patient Characteristics Similar between Groups
Stano, 1993	493 ICD-9 codes: musculoskeletal	National private fee-for-service insurance; (claims—7/88–6/90)	Total Inpatient Outpatient	N=92,585 $3,799 $1,380 $2,419	N=303,056 $4,937 $2,385 $2,550	
Stano, 1993	493 ICD-9 codes: musculoskeletal	National private fee-for-service insurance; 2 years of insurance (claims—7/88–6/90)	Total Inpatient Outpatient	N=10,088 $3,840 $1,770 $2,069	N=32,127 $5,168 $2,249 $2,522	Insurance type, age, gender, region, and work status
Tuchin and Bonello, 1995	Back injuries	Australian Workers' Comp.; 1 year (7/91–6/92); random sample	Total	N=20 cases randomly selected $300	N=20 cases randomly selected $647	Age, gender, injury location, type, and mechanism; worksite
Mosely et al, 1996	Back and neck pain	Louisiana HMO; 1 year (claims—10/94–10/95)	Total Imaging	N=121 $539 $30	N=1,838 $774 $94	Age, gender, surgical patients; patient satisfaction
Erball, 1992	Mechanical lower-back pain	Australian Workers' Compensation, 1 year (claims—4/90–3/91)	Total Provider costs Drugs, tests, etc* Patient compensation	N=998 $963 $369 $202 $392	N=993 $2,308 $209 $528 $1,569	Groups similar in gender composition but MD groups had older patients, more blue-collar workers
Dean and Schmidt, 1992	11 spinal conditions	National Medical Care Utilization and Expenditure Survey, 1980	Average total payments	N=384 $114	N=333 $85	No
Jarvis et al, 1991	Back injury claims	Utah Workers' Compensation Fund, 1986	Total Patient compensation	N=837 $526 $68	N=769 $684 $668	Chiropractic group was older, had greater number of diagnoses

Table 55–2 continued

Author, Year	Condition	Source and Year of Data	Population	Chiropractic Claims	Medical Claims	Patient Characteristics Similar between Groups
Jarvis, 1989	Back injury claims	Utah Workers' Compensation Fund, 1986	Total (no surgery) Total (includes surgery) Provider costs	N=400 $775 $775 $166	N=459 $966 $1,665 $846	
Nyiendo and Lamm, 1991	Back injury claims	State Accident Insurance Fund of Oregon (6/85–12/85)	Total Patient compensation	N=121 $2,047 $1,217	N=102 $1,275 $1,271	
Johnson et al, 1989	Back injury claims	Iowa State Workers' Compensation records, 1984	Patient compensation	N=266 DC $263 DO $1,565	N=102 $617	No
Wolk, 1988	Back injury claims	Florida State Workers' Compensation records (7/85–6/86)	Without surgery Total With surgery Total	DC N=444 $1,204 DO N=181 $945 DC N=558 $1,204 DO N=411 $1,002	MD N=814 $2,213 MD N=1,100 $2,352	No
Greenwood, 1985	Back and neck injury claims	West Virginia Compensation Fund, 1980–1981	Average provider cost Patient compensation	N=200 $1,274 $1,887	N=187 $544 $1,100	Surgical cases excluded
Bergemann and Cichoke, 1980	Back injury claims	Oregon Workers' Compensation Board, 1974–1975	Total office visit cost Patient compensation	N=113 $181 $276	N=114 $327 $650	Age; chiropractic group had more males

Source: Reprinted from R.A. Branson, Cost Comparison of Chiropractic and Medical Treatment of Common Musculoskeletal Disorders: A Review of the Literature after 1980, *Topics in Clinical Chiropractic,* Vol. 6, No. 2, pp. 57–68, © 1999, Aspen Publishers, Inc.

Table 55–3 Prospective Studies Comparing Costs of Chiropractic and Medical Care

Author, Year	Condition	Source and Year of Data	Parameters	Chiropractic/ Osteopathic	General Practitioners	Surgeons	Similarity of Populations
Carey et al, 1995	Acute low-back pain	North Carolina estimated charges for care (6/92–3/93)	Total (injury)	DC N=606 $681	MD N=644 $509 HMO N=202 $365	Orthopedist surgeon (OR) N=181 $809	No
Shekelle et al, 1995	Low-back pain	Secondary analysis from the 1982 U.S. Census RAND health insurance experiment	Total Outpatient Inpatient Provider costs	DC N=462 $281 $281 $0 $264	GP N=263 $199 $210 $2,000 $247	OR N=85 $531 $281 $2,500 $180	No
			Total Outpatient Inpatient Provider costs	DO N=72 $338 $280 $4,000 $238	Internist N=60 $332 $218 $1,400 $180	Orthopedist N=129 $348 $239 $2,000 $212	
Skargren et al, 1998	Low-back and neck pain	Swedish medical costs, converted into 1995 American currency	Total w/ surgery Total, no surgery Surgery costs	DC N=219 $2,928 $2,739 $189	PTN=192 $2,954 $2,248 $706		Age, gender, exercise level, smokers, work satisf, previous episodes, expectations, location and duration of pain, function
Skargren et al, 1997	Low-back and neck pain	Follow-up of study on Swedish medical costs, 1997 Total costs—12 months of care	Total with surgery Total, no surgery Surgery costs	DC N=179 $4,051 $3,492 $382	PTN=144 $4,010 $2,943 $994		Same as above
Cherkin et al, 1998	Low-back pain	(11/93–9/95) DC treatment in solo practice; PT treatment in HMO; patient education (booklet) in HMO	Two years of treatment Total costs per subject	DC N=122 $429	PTN=133 $437	Patient education N=66 $153	Age, gender, employment, smokers, general health, mental health, previous episodes, duration of pain, function, medication use

Source: Reprinted from R.A. Branson, Cost Comparison of Chiropractic and Medical Treatment of Common Musculoskeletal Disorders: A Review of the Literature after 1980, *Topics in Clinical Chiropractic,* Vol. 6, No. 2, pp. 57–68, © 1999, Aspen Publishers, Inc.

1996; Skargren et al, 1997), and four controlled for patient chronicity (Dabbs and Lauretti, 1995; Stano and Smith, 1996; Nyiendo and Lamm, 1991; Skargren et al, 1997). Standardization of patient diagnosis within and between providers cannot be controlled in retrospective studies. Prospective studies do have better control of the conditions surrounding the study, yet they also are subject to methodological criticisms (Conrad and Deyo, 1994; Manga and Angus, 1998).

Two studies compared average charges by each provider (Dean and Schmidt, 1992; Carey et al, 1995). Both of these studies concluded that medical care was more cost-effective than chiropractic care. Payments received are often less than billable charges primarily because discounting is usually larger for chiropractors than for medical doctors (Manga and Angus, 1998).

Another limitation of these studies is the absence of information of direct costs of care. None of the 24 studies measured all direct costs of care for an episode. Direct costs include expenditures of all visits to the provider, prescription and nonprescription drugs or supplements, laboratory costs, diagnostic imaging, referrals to specialists, and hospital costs. Furthermore, evaluation of indirect costs such as workdays lost by the patient and possibly a caregiver such as a family member, friend, or neighbor to assist in various domestic duties should be included in a complete cost-effectiveness evaluation.

The idea of bias must be considered in a cost-effectiveness analysis. Studies that have been funded by an entity with a vested interest should identify the funding source. Another important issue is whether the results can be generalized to other populations. For example, workers' compensation studies may not be generalized to other patient populations. Caution should be taken when generalizing any results in other settings.

Other Reviews of the Literature on Cost-Effectiveness

Six studies have been published since 1985 that review the literature on the cost-effective-

ness of chiropractic and medical care. Two limited their review to workers' compensation studies (Assendelft and Boulter, 1993; Johnson et al, 1985), one included a review of specialists' and generalists' care (Solomon et al, 1997), two reported on treatment effectiveness and cost-effectiveness for the Canadian government (Manga and Angus, 1998; Manga et al, 1993), and one focused on the treatment of low-back pain and its economic implications in the Virginia state health care system (Schifrin, 1992).

Johnson and colleagues (1985) reviewed 17 workers' compensation studies dated 1940 to 1981 comparing medical and chiropractic care. They found that 14 of the 17 studies had lower total costs when patients were treated by chiropractors.

Assendelft and Boulter (1993) reviewed the literature for all workers' compensation studies that compared medical and chiropractic treatment from 1940 to 1990. Six studies after 1980 and 11 studies prior to 1980 were included in their review. They concluded that most of the studies were of poor methodological quality and "chiropractic cost-effectiveness is not yet convincingly proven."

A recent study by Solomon et al (1997) reviewed and methodologically critiqued the literature on cost, outcomes, and patient satisfaction of rheumatic and musculoskeletal conditions. They compared outcomes of care from generalists and specialists. They investigated five different conditions: low-back pain, work-related injuries, osteoarthritis, acute arthritis (crystal and septic arthritis), and rheumatoid arthritis. They reviewed seven studies on low-back pain and one on work-related injuries that compared chiropractic and medical costs of care. They concluded that generalists' care of low-back pain is equally effective and less expensive yet it is less satisfying to patients than chiropractic care. A 1993 publication by the Ontario Chiropractic Association reviewed the literature on the treatment effectiveness and cost-effectiveness in chiropractic. The authors summarized the original lengthy paper in a more recent publication (Manga et al, 1994). They concluded that the current body of evidence supports the effectiveness and cost-effectiveness of chiropractic treatment for low-back pain. A recent update of this work reached the same conclusion (Manga and Angus, 1998).

Schifrin (1992) reviewed 22 cost-effectiveness studies on low-back pain for the American Chiropractic Association. Four post-1980 studies, 14 pre-1980 studies, and 2 British studies were reviewed. He concluded that chiropractic provides "important and therapeutic benefits at economical costs."

Other Studies of Interest

Cost-effectiveness studies have been published comparing traditional medical treatments for low-back pain (Hill and Hardy, 1996; Shvartzman et al, 1992). They concluded that conservative and multidisciplinary care is equally or more cost-effective than surgery or orthopedic outpatient care.

Meade et al (1990) published a randomized clinical trial comparing medical and chiropractic treatment of low-back pain. They found that chiropractic treatment was more effective than hospital outpatient care for patients with chronic and severe low-back pain of this type. The authors commented on the potential economic implications of their results. They determined that the average cost of chiropractic treatment was less than hospital outpatient treatment. They concluded that savings of approximately $40 million would have been possible if patients with no contraindications to spinal manipulation had been referred for chiropractic care instead of hospital outpatient treatment. A 3-year follow-up confirmed their initial findings that chiropractic care provided more benefit and longer term satisfaction than hospital outpatient care (Meade et al, 1995).

Recently, a randomized prospective trial compared cost-effectiveness of chiropractic treatment to physical therapy and patient education (Cherkin et al, 1998). It found the use of an educational booklet to be the most cost-effective method of care for low-back pain. There are several limitations in this study similar to other cost analysis publications. These include different settings for chiropractic and physical therapy services, lack of medication cost analysis, and incorrect crossover in the control population.

CONCLUSION

In general, it appears that chiropractic intervention is more cost-effective when compared with traditional medical intervention. One other conclusion that can be drawn from these data is the need for well-designed prospective randomized clinical trials on chiropractic and medical treatment incorporating the economic analysis of common musculoskeletal disorders. The lack of prospective cost-effectiveness literature is not limited to musculoskeletal disorders. A recent review evaluating randomized clinical trials found only 121 of 50,000 published trials (0.2%) included economic analysis (Adams et al, 1992).

The importance of containing the rising health care costs is undisputed. Finding the most cost-effective treatment for common musculoskeletal conditions should be a high priority in a market in which health care costs are increasing and health care dollars are declining.

A recent survey of 18 insurance companies that offer some form of reimbursement for complementary therapies reported that all covered chiropractic services (Pelletier et al, 1997). This survey also reported important factors influencing coverage of complementary and alternative therapies. The top three factors given by most of the insurers were consumer interest, proof of clinical efficacy, and state-mandated coverage. Currently all 50 states license chiropractors, and 41 of the 50 states mandate insurance coverage for chiropractic services (Pelletier et al, 1997). Nearly 5 million people each year see a chiropractor for low-back pain.

Nine of 14 systematic reviews of spinal manipulation endorse its efficacy. In reviews published after 1980, 16 studies reported lower total costs for chiropractic treatment. A number of economists and researchers have concluded that wider incorporation of chiropractic benefits in health plans could produce significant economic benefit (Manga et al, 1994; Manga, 1995; Manga and Angus, 1998; Meade et al, 1995; Schifrin, 1992). The economic impact may be more meaningful in some Canadian provinces and U.S. states where financial incentives currently exist for patients to use medical rather than chiropractic care.

The economic trends evident in the literature since 1980 favor chiropractic. However, most of the research on cost-effectiveness is limited because of its largely actuarial and retrospective nature. Capturing actual reimbursement charges prospectively has only been done in two studies (Skargen et al, 1998; Cherkin et al, 1998). Unfortunately, the data are not readily generalizable because of the populations studied and the nature of the delivery systems.

Higher quality research will be needed to better understand cost-effectiveness of chiropractic methods and the extent to which chiropractic care impacts both direct and indirect costs associated with chronic disability. Given the limited state of cost-effectiveness data for all interventions, chiropractic consistently shows benefit of a magnitude that should favorably affect coverage policy. Available cost data on chiropractic help to bolster arguments for its inclusion in care delivery and coverage.

REFERENCES

Adams ME, McCall NT, Gray DT, Orza MJ, Chalmers TC. Economic analysis in randomized control trials. *Med Care.* 1992;30:231–243.

Aker P, Gross AR, Goldsmith CH, Pelseo P. Conservative management of mechanical neck pain: systematic overview and meta-analysis. *BMJ.* 1996;313:1291–1296.

Anderson R, Meeker WC, Wirick BE, Mootz RD, Kirk DH, Adams A. A meta-analysis of clinical trials of spinal manipulation. *J Manipulative Physiol Ther.* 1992;15:487–494.

Assendelft WJJ, Boulter LM. Does the goose really lay golden eggs? A methodological review of workmen's compensation studies. *J Manipulative Physiol Ther.* 1993;16:162–168.

Assendelft WJJ, Boulter LM, Knipschild PG. Complications of spinal manipulation. A comprehensive review of the literature. *J Fam Pract.* 1996a;42:475–480.

Assendelft WJJ, Koes BW, van der Heijden GJMG, Boulter LM. The efficacy of chiropractic manipulation for back pain: blinded review of relevant randomized clinical trials. *J Manipulative Physiol Ther.* 1992;15:487–494.

Assendelft WJJ, Koes BW, van der Heijden GJMC, Boulter LM. The effectiveness of chiropractic treatment of low back pain: an update and attempt at statistical pooling. *J Manipulative Physiol Ther.* 1996b;19:499–507.

Bergemann BW, Cichoke AJ. Cost effectiveness of medical vs. chiropractic treatment of low-back injuries. *J Manipulative Physiol Ther.* 1980;3:143–147.

Bronfort G. *Efficacy of Manual Therapies of the Spine* [thesis]. Amsterdam, The Netherlands: Thesis Publishers Amsterdam; 1997.

Brunarski DJ. Clinical trials of spinal manipulation: a critical appraisal and review of the literature. *J Manipulative Physiol Ther.* 1984;7:243–249.

Carey PG, Garrett J, Jackman A, et al. The outcomes and costs of care for acute low back pain among patients seen by primary care practitioners, chiropractors, and orthopedic surgeons. *N Engl J Med.* 1995;333:913–917.

Cheadle A, Franklin C, Wolfhagen C, et al. Factors influencing the duration of work-related disability: a population based study of Washington state workers' compensation. *Am J Public Health.* 1994;84(2):190–196.

Cherkin DC, Deyo RA, Battie M, Street J, Barlow W. A comparison of physical therapy, chiropractic manipulation and provision of an educational booklet for the treatment of patients with low back pain. *N Engl J Med.* 1998;339:1021–1029.

Clark RE. Understanding cost-effectiveness. *Spine.* 1996;21:646–650.

Conrad DA, Deyo RA. Economic decision analysis in the diagnosis and treatment of low back pain. A methodological primer. *Spine.* 1994;19(suppl):2101–2106.

Coulter ID, Hurwitz EL, Adams AH, et al. *The Appropriateness of Manipulation and Mobilization of the Cervical Spine.* Santa Monica, CA: RAND; 1996.

Dabbs V, Lauretti WJ. A risk assessment of cervical manipulation vs. NSAIDs for the treatment of neck pain. *J Manipulative Physiol Ther.* 1995;18:530–536.

Dean DH, Schmidt RM. *A Comparison of the Costs of Chiropractors Versus Alternative Medical Practitioners.* Richmond, VA: Virginia Chiropractic Association; 1992.

Detsky AS, Naglie G. A clinician's guide to cost-effectiveness analysis. *Ann Intern Med.* 1990;113:147–154.

Drummond MF, Richardson S, O'Brien BJ, Levine M, Heyland D. Users' guide to the medical literature XIII. How to use an article on economic analysis of clinical practice. *JAMA.* 1997;277:1552–1557.

Erball PS. Mechanical low-back pain: a comparison of medical and chiropractic management within the Victorian work care scheme. *Chiro J Aust.* 1992;22:47–53.

Frisoni GB, Anzola GP. Vertebrobasilar ischemia after neck motion. *Stroke.* 1991;22:1452–1460.

Frymoyer JW, Durett CL. *The Economics of Spinal Disorders.* 2nd ed. Philadelphia: Lippincott-Raven; 1997.

Gatterman MI. Complications of and contraindications to spinal manipulative therapy. In: Gatterman MI, ed. *Chiropractic Management of Spine-Related Disorders.* Baltimore: Williams & Wilkins; 1990.

Greenwood JG. Work-related back and neck injury cases in West Virginia. The issues in chiropractic treatment of low-back injuries. *Orthop Rev.* 1985;14:51–63.

Hart LG, Deyo RA, Cherkin DC. Physician office visits for low back pain. Frequency, clinical evaluation, and treatment patterns from a U.S. national study. *Spine.* 1995;20:11–19.

Hill PA, Hardy PA. The cost-effectiveness of a multidisciplinary pain management program in a district general hospital. *Pain Clinic.* 1996;9:181–188.

Hoffman D. Musculoskeletal problems are common in family practice. *Am Fam Physician.* 1997;54(8):2524.

Hurwitz EL, Aker PD, Adams AH, Meeker WC, Shekelle PG. Manipulation and mobilization of the cervical spine. A systematic review of the literature. *Spine.* 1996; 21:1746–1760.

Jarvis KB. Cost per case analysis of Utah industrial back injury claims. Chiropractic management versus medical management for diagnostically equivalent conditions. *DC Tracts.* 1989;1:67–79.

Jarvis KB, Phillips RB, Danielson C. Managed care preapproval and its effect on the cost of Utah worker compensation claims. *J Manipulative Physiol Ther.* 1997; 20:372–376.

Jarvis KB, Phillips RE, Morris EK. Cost per case comparison of back injury claims of chiropractic versus medical management for conditions with identical diagnostic codes. *J Occup Med.* 1991;33:847–852.

Johnson MR, Ferguson AC, Swank LL. Treatment and cost of back or neck injury – a literature review. *Res Forum.* Spring 1985:68–78.

Johnson MR, Schultz MK, Ferguson AC. A comparison of chiropractic, medical, and osteopathic care for work-related sprains and strains. *J Manipulative Physiol Ther.* 1989;12:335–344.

Kahl IF. Musculoskeletal problems in the family practice setting: guidelines for curriculum design. *J Rheumatol.* 1987;14(4):811–814.

Klougart N, Leboeuf-Yde C. Rasmussen LR. Safety in chiropractic practice, part 1: the occurrence of cerebrovascular accidents after manipulation to the neck in Denmark from 1978–1988. *J Manipulative Physiol Ther.* 1996;19:371–377.

Koes BW, Assendelft WJJ, van der Heijden GJMG, Boulter LM. Spinal manipulation for low back pain. An updated systematic review of randomized clinical trials. *Spine.* 1996;21:2860–2873.

Koes BW, Assendelft WJJ, van der Heijden, GJMC, Boulter LM, Knipschild PG. Spinal manipulation and mobilization for back and neck pain: a blinded review. *BMJ.* 1991;303:1298–1303.

Koes BW, Boulter LM, Beckerman H. van der Heijden GJMG, Knilschild PG. Physiotherapy exercises and back pain: a blended review. *BMJ.* 1991;302:1572–1576.

Korff MV, Dworkin SF, Resche LL, Kruger A. An epidemiologic comparison of pain complaints. *Pain.* 1988; 32:173–183.

Makela M, Hellovaara M, Sievers K, et al. Prevalence, determinants, and consequences of chronic neck pain in Finland. *Am J Epidemiol.* 1991;134:1356–1367.

Manga P. Letter to the editor. *Spine.* 1995;20:2170–2173.

Manga P, Angus D. *Enhanced Chiropractic Coverage under OHIP as a Means of Reducing Health Care Costs, Attaining Better Health Outcomes, and Achieving Equitable Access to Health Services.* Ontario, Canada: University of Ottawa; 1998.

Manga P, Angus D, Papdopoulos C, et al. *The Effectiveness and Cost-Effectiveness of Chiropractic Management of Low Back Pain.* Richmond Hill, Ontario, Canada: Kenilworth Publishing; 1993.

Manga P, Angus D, Swan WR. Findings and recommendations from an independent review of chiropractic management of low back pain. *J Neuromusculoskel Syst.* 1994;2:1–8.

McKinnon ME, Vickers MR, Ruddock VM, Townsend J, Meade TW. Community studies of health service implications of low back pain. *Spine.* 1997;21:2161–2166.

Meade TW, Dyer S, Browne W, Frank AO. Randomized comparison of chiropractic and hospital outpatient management for low back pain: results from extended follow up. *BMJ.* 1995; 311:349–350.

Meade TW, Dyer S, Browne W, Townsend J, Frank AO. Low back pain of mechanical origin: randomized comparison of chiropractic and hospital outpatient treatment. *BMJ.* 1990;300:1431–1437.

Mosely CD, Cohen IG, Arnold RM. Cost-effectiveness of chiropractic care in a managed care setting. *Am J Managed Care.* 1996;2:280–282.

Nyiendo J, Lamm L. Disabling low back Oregon workers' compensation claims. Part III: diagnostic and treatment procedures and associated costs. *J Manipulative Physiol Ther.* 1991;14:287–297.

Ottenbacher K, Difablo RP. Efficacy of spinal manipulation/mobilization therapy: a meta-analysis. *Spine.* 1985; 10:833–837.

Pelletier KR, Marie A, Krasner M, Haskell W. Current trends in the integration and reimbursement of complementary and alternative medicine by managed care, insurance carriers, and hospital providers. *Am J Health Promotion.* 1997;12:112–123.

Rivett DA, Milburn P. A prospective study of complications of cervical spine manipulation. *J Manipulative Physiol Ther.* 1996;4:166–170.

Rodriquez AA, Bilkey WJ, Agre JC. Therapeutic exercises in chronic neck and back pain. *Arch Phys Med Rehabil.* 1992;73:870–875.

Schellhas KP, Latchaw RE, Wendling LR, Gold LHA. Vertebrobasilar injuries following cervical manipulation. *JAMA.* 1980;244:1450–1453.

Schifrin LG. *Mandated Health Insurance Coverage for Chiropractic Treatment: An Economic Arrangement with Implications for the Commonwealth of Virginia.* Richmond, VA: Foundation of Chiropractic Education and Research; 1992.

Shekelle PG. Spinal manipulation. *Spine.* 1994;19:858–861.

Shekelle PG, Adams AH, Chassin MR, Hurwitz EL, Brook RH. Spinal manipulation for low-back pain. *Ann Intern Med.* 1992;117:590–598.

Shekelle PG, Coulter I. Cervical spine manipulation. Summary report of a systematic review of the literature and a multidisciplinary panel. *J Spinal Disord.* 1997; 10:223–228.

Shekelle PG, Markovich M, Louie R. Comparing the costs between provider types of episodes of back pain care. *Spine.* 1995;20:221–227.

Shvartzman L, Weingarten E, Sherry H, Levin S, Persaud A. Cost-effectiveness analysis of extended conservative therapy versus surgical intervention in the management of herniated lumbar intervertebral disc. *Spine.* 1992;17: 176–182.

Skargren E, Carlsson PG, Oberg B. One-year follow-up comparison of the cost and effectiveness of chiropractic and physiotherapy as primary management for back pain. *Spine.* 1998;23:1875–1884.

Skargren EI, Oberg BE, Carlsson PG, Gade M. Cost and effectiveness analysis of chiropractic and physiotherapy treatment for low back and neck pain. Six-month follow-up. *Spine.* 1997;22:2167–2177.

Smith M, Stano M. Cost and recurrences of chiropractic and medical episodes of low-back care. *J Manipulative Physiol Ther.* 1997;20:5–12.

Solomon DH, Bates DW, Panush RS, Katz JN. Costs, outcomes, and patient satisfaction by provider type for patients with rheumatic and musculoskeletal conditions: a critical review of the literature and proposed methodologic standards. *Ann Intern Med.* 1997;127:52–60.

Stano M. A comparison of health care costs for chiropractic and medical patients. *J Manipulative Physiol Ther.* 1993; 16:291–299.

Stano M. An overview of the ACA cost of care analysis project. *J Chiro.* 1993;30:41–45.

Stano M. The economic role of chiropractic: an episode analysis of relative insurance costs for low back care. *J Neuromusculoskel Syst.* 1993;1:64–68.

Stano M. Further analysis of health care costs for chiropractic and medical patients. *J Manipulative Physiol Ther.* 1994;17:442–446.

Stano M. The economic role of chiropractic: further analysis of relative insurance costs for low back care. *J Neuromusculoskel Syst.* 1995;3:139–144.

Stano M, Smith M. Chiropractic and medical costs of low back care. *Med Care.* 1996;34:191–204.

Terrett AGJ. Misuse of the literature by medical authors in discussing spinal manipulative therapy injury. *J Manipulative Physiol Ther.* 1995;18:203–210.

Tuchin PJ, Bonello R. Preliminary findings of analysis of chiropractic utilization and cost in the workers compensation system of New South Wales, Australia. *J Manipulative Physiol Ther.* 1995;18:503–511.

van Tulder MW, Koes MW, Boulter LM. Conservative treatment of acute and chronic nonspecific back pain. A systematic review of randomized controlled trials of the most common interventions. *Spine.* 1997;22: 2128–2156.

Waddell G. Keynote address for primary care forum. *Spine.* 1996;21:2820–2825.

Wahlgren DR, Atkinson JH, Epping-Jordan JE, et al. One-year follow-up of first onset low back pain. *Pain.* 1997; 73:213–221.

Wolk S. *Chiropractic Versus Medical Care: A Cost Analysis of Disability and Treatment for Back-Related Workers' Compensation Cases.* Richmond, VA: Foundation of Chiropractic Education and Research; 1988.

CHAPTER 56

Effectiveness and Safety of Spinal Manipulation for Low-Back Pain, Neck and Head Pain

William C. Meeker

The purpose of this review is to describe the effectiveness and safety of spinal manipulation for several common musculoskeletal pain complaints. The primary focus will be on studies that have evaluated outcomes of care using randomized clinical trial designs. However, where necessary in discussions of safety, observational study designs must also be examined.

SPINAL MANIPULATION

Spinal manipulation has a broad operational definition with many technical distinctions. It is practiced by several professions including osteopathic and medical physicians, physical therapists, and others, but chiropractors deliver 94% of manipulative procedures in practice in the United States (Shekelle, 1994). In general, manipulation denotes the application of physical forces to bodily tissues, most often joints and muscles. Forces are usually delivered by hand, but there are exceptions (Haldeman, 1992; Haldeman et al, 1992). The application of manipulative forces can vary considerably in terms of amplitude, velocity, direction, duration, and

William C. Meeker, DC, MPH, is the Director of Research for the Palmer Center for Chiropractic Research in Davenport, Iowa, and the Principal Investigator of the Consortial Center for Chiropractic Research, one of 13 research centers established by the National Center for Complementary and Alternative Medicine (NCCAM). Dr. Meeker has served the American Public Health Association on the Governing Council for 4 years and was recently appointed to the Advisory Council of the NCCAM. He is also the editor of the *Journal of the Neuromusculoskeletal System.*

frequency, and there are various schools of thought as to the most effective forms. For example, high-velocity, low-amplitude maneuvers are known as "adjustments" in chiropractic, while low-velocity, variable-amplitude maneuvers are often termed "mobilization." The interested reader can refer to excellent textbooks on manipulation for additional technical detail (eg, Bergmann et al, 1993).

The hypothesized biological effects of manipulation can be categorized as either mechanical or neurological or both, and detailed discussions of putative explanatory mechanisms exist in the literature (Gatterman, 1995). The most frequently studied outcomes of manipulation have been symptom reduction (usually pain) and improvement in physical functioning, primarily because most experimental clinical research to date has focused on painful back, neck, and head complaints. These outcomes are appropriate and important to patients.

SPINAL MANIPULATION AND LOW-BACK PAIN

There now exist at least 39 randomized clinical trials comparing manipulation to some other form of treatment for various forms of low-back pain, and many more observational studies. Twenty-six of the randomized trials favored manipulation, while 13 did not find an advantage to manipulation. However, in no case was the comparison treatment found to be more effective than manipulation, a consistent finding. To more precisely summarize the extant trials, low-back pain is divided below into acute and chronic (including "subacute") categories. The pain is generally deemed subacute or chronic if it has existed for more than 6 weeks.

There are 12 trials that evaluated patients with acute low-back pain, usually of less than 6 weeks' duration (Table 56–1). Manipulation was delivered as the sole treatment, or sometimes in combination with other treatments. The comparison treatments were mostly physical therapy modalities such as exercise, back school, shortwave diathermy, infrared heat, electrical stimulation, and massage, but nonsteroidal anti-inflammatory drugs (NSAIDs) and analgesics were also compared. Six of the trials reported in favor of manipulation; three reported no statistically significant differences between the com-

parison groups, and three trials found statistically significant differences in a subgroup of the study sample only. Outcomes of interest included rate of recovery, pain reduction, and improvement in physical functioning.

Eight trials focused only on patients with chronic/subacute low-back pain (Table 56–2). Manipulation was again delivered solely or in combination with other treatments. Comparisons were to physical therapy, diathermy, back education, Transcutaneous Electrical Nerve Stimulation (TENS), corsets, bed rest, analgesics, massage, and sham manipulation. Five of these reported results favoring manipulation while two reported no additional benefit from manipulation. One study did not draw a statistical conclusion. Again, the outcomes of interest focused

---

Table 56–1 Trials Comparing Spinal Manipulation with Other Conservative Treatments in Acute Low-Back Pain

Author and Year	Comparison Treatment	N = Total Sample Size	Finding on Spinal Manipulation
Bergquist-Ullman and Larsson, 1977	Back school	97	Positive
Delitto et al, 1992	Flexion exercises	24	Positive
Farrell and Twomey, 1982	Shortwave diathermy and exercises	48	Positive
Godfrey et al, 1984	Massage and electrical stimulation	81	Equivocal
Hadler et al, 1987	Spinal mobilization	54	Positive Subgroup only
Helliwell and Cunliffe, 1987	Analgesics	14	Equivocal
MacDonald and Bell, 1990	Exercises and advice on posture	95	Positive Subgroup only
Mathews et al, 1987	Infrared heat	291	Positive Subgroup only
Nwuga, 1982	Shortwave diathermy and exercises	51	Positive
Rasmussen, 1979	Shortwave diathermy	24	Positive
Sanders et al, 1990	No treatment control	12	Positive
Waterworth and Hunter, 1985	Shortwave diathermy and exercises; NSAIDs	108	Equivocal

Table 56–2 Trials Comparing Spinal Manipulation with Other Conservative Treatments in Chronic or Subacute Low-Back Pain

Author and Year	Comparison Treatment	N = Total Sample Size	Finding on Spinal Manipulation
Arkuszewski, 1986	Bed rest, analgesics, and massage	100	Positive
Evans et al, 1978	Analgesics	32	Positive
Gibson et al, 1985	Shortwave diathermy	75	Equivocal
Herzog et al, 1991	Back school	29	No conclusion
Koes et al, 1992	Physiotherapy, usual care by a general practitioner	192	Positive
Pope et al, 1994	Massage, corset, TENS	164	Equivocal stimulation
Triano et al, 1995		209	Positive
Waagen et al, 1986	Massage and sham manipulation	19	Positive

on pain reduction, and recovery and improvement in physical functioning.

Fifteen trials included mixed patient populations of acute, subacute, and chronic low-back pain (Table 56–3). Of these, nine reported results favoring manipulation and one reported a favorable result in a subgroup. The rest of the studies did not find a statistically significant difference in favor of manipulation.

It should be noted that 11 trials (4 of these are not included in previous Tables 56–1, 56–2, and 56–3) included some form of placebo therapy comparison (see Table 56–4). Most often this was detuned diathermy or a sham manipulation of some type. The results appear to rule out the probability that the effect of manipulation is due to nonspecific mechanisms. In 7 of 11, manipulation was more effective; 1 study had a subgroup that showed more benefit; and in 3 studies, manipulation was equal to the placebo.

Systematic Reviews of Trials of Spinal Manipulation for Low-Back Pain

The historical association of spinal manipulation with chiropractic probably explains the interesting finding that there are more reviews of original research data in the scientific literature on manipulation than there are randomized trials. The reviews were systematically described in the *Journal of the American Medical Association* (Assendelft et al, 1995). Fifty-one reviews were found, of which 34 concluded that the evidence favored spinal manipulation for low-back pain, while 17 were neutral. All the reviews were coded for quality and characteristics of good scholarship. Nine of the 10 highest quality reviews favored manipulation. Other factors related to a conclusion in favor of manipulation were the inclusion of a clinician trained in manipulation on the study team and a more comprehensive literature review. Further discussion of some of the individual reviews can yield additional information on the efficacy and effectiveness of spinal manipulation.

In 1992, two quantitative metanalyses of spinal manipulation appeared in the refereed literature. Shekelle and colleagues (1992) at RAND found 25 controlled trials and were able to combine the results of 9 into one quantitative point estimate of effect size. They found that the difference in probability of recovery from

Table 56–3 Trials Comparing Spinal Manipulation with Other Conservative Treatments in Mixed Populations with Low-Back Pain

Author and Year	Comparison Treatment	N = Total Sample Size	Finding on Spinal Manipulation
Blomberg et al, 1994	Optimized activation conventional treatment	101	Positive
Bronfort, 1989	Medical treatment (eg, medication)	19	No conclusion
Cherkin et al, 1998	Physical therapy and educational booklet	321	Positive
Coxhead et al, 1981	Exercises, corset, or traction	292	Positive
Doran and Newell, 1975	Physiotherapy, analgesics, corset	452	Equivocal
Hoehler et al, 1981	Massage	95	Positive
Kinalski et al, 1989	Physiotherapy	111	Positive
Meade et al, 1990	Physiotherapy	741	Positive
Postacchini et al, 1988	Physiotherapy, drug therapy, bed rest, back school	325	Positive Subgroup only
Rupert et al, 1985	Drugs and bed rest, home care instructions	Sample size not reported	Positive
Siehl et al, 1971	Conservative treatment, surgery	47	Positive
Skargren et al, 1998	Physical therapists	323	Equivocal (at 1 year)
Skargren et al, 1997	Physical therapists	323	Equivocal (at 6 months)
Wreje et al, 1992	Massage	39	Positive
Zylbergold and Piper, 1981	Heat and exercises	18	Equivocal

uncomplicated acute low-back pain at 3 weeks is 0.17 with manipulation. Since the recovery rate without manipulation in these trials approximated 50%, the increase to 67% indicated an improvement of 34%. The authors concluded that manipulation hastened recovery for acute low-back pain, and that for chronic back pain, the results were insufficient to draw a conclusion. They also concluded that the general quality of the studies was low and that long-term benefits (beyond 3 months) were not well studied.

Anderson and colleagues (1992) conducted a quantitative metanalysis in which they statisti-cally pooled the results of 23 randomized clinical trials of manipulation for low-back pain. Their analysis, which used a different statistical technique and the examination of a larger number of outcome variables at a variety of time points, indicated that manipulation was favored at approximately the same strength as the metanalysis conducted by Shekelle et al (1992). The average outcome, expressed as a Cohens D-index, suggested that the average patient receiving manipulation experienced a better outcome than 54% to 85% of the patients receiving the comparison treatments, depending on the specific outcome variable and when it was assessed.

Table 56–4 Trials Comparing Manipulation with Placebo Therapy

Author and Year	Comparison Treatment	N = Total Sample Size	Finding on Spinal Manipulation
Bergquist-Ullman and Larsson, 1977	Shortwave diathermy at lowest intensity	147	Positive
Gibson et al, 1985	Detuned shortwave diathermy	75	Equivocal
Glover et al, 1974	Detuned shortwave diathermy	84	Equivocal
Koes et al, 1992	Detuned shortwave diathermy and detuned ultrasound	129	Positive
Ongley et al, 1987	Nonforceful manipulation	81	Positive
Postacchini et al, 1988	Antiedema gel	160	Positive Subgroup only
Rupert et al, 1985	Sham manipulation, massage	Sample size not reported	Positive
Sanders et al, 1990	Sham manipulation	12	Positive
Sims-Williams et al, 1979	Microwave at lowest setting	94	Equivocal
Sims-Williams et al, 1978	Microwave at lowest setting	94	Positive
Triano et al, 1995	High-velocity, low-force mimic	209	Positive

Another systematic qualitative review of spinal manipulation for low-back pain was conducted by Koes et al (1996). This paper reviewed 36 randomized trials and scored them for methodological quality. While 8 of the top 10 highest quality studies favored manipulation, the authors were conservative in their conclusions, stating that spinal manipulation had not been proven in consistently sound studies. They also concluded that the evidence for chronic back pain was perhaps more compelling than for acute back pain due to the publication of several studies since 1992. They called for additional research to explain the heterogeneity of findings. In a discussion published with the paper, Meeker (1996) pointed out that in the overall context of clinical trial research on back pain, no other treatment has received more scientific attention than spinal manipulation.

Finally, the clinical trial data on manipulation have been sufficient to cause at least two government-sponsored groups of policy experts—in the United States (Bigos et al, 1994) and the United Kingdom (Royal Commission of General Practitioners, 1996)—to come to the con-sensus that spinal manipulation should be recommended as a treatment for back pain. The U.S. Agency for Health Care Policy and Research, based on the research evidence, rated spinal manipulation at the highest level (Grade B) of any treatment option for low-back pain. Only nonsteroidal anti-inflammatory drugs received the same rating, while all other treatments for back pain received lower ratings and poorer recommendations. In summary, evidence exists to support the efficacy and effectiveness of spinal manipulation for low-back pain, especially within the first 3 months. Although favorable long-term outcomes have been reported (eg, Meade et al, 1995), these data are insufficient to draw definite conclusions.

SPINAL MANIPULATION AND NECK PAIN

Several years ago, a study conducted by RAND identified 67 studies that dealt with the outcomes of spinal manipulation of the cervical spine (Hurwitz et al, 1996). Fourteen of the studies were randomized trials that were then systematically reviewed for quality and results. Overall, while the quality of the randomized trials on neck pain ranged widely, with some problems identified in design, execution, and statistical analysis, they were judged to have similar quality to those already discussed on low-back pain. As with the studies on low-back pain, none of the studies indicated that the comparison treatment was more effective than manipulation. However, not all of the studies found a statistically significant difference in favor of manipulation, even when the results showed trends in that direction.

At this time, at least 20 randomized controlled trials of cervical manipulation have been conducted in patients with neck pain or forms of headache. Eleven of the trials dealt with acute, subacute, or chronic neck pain (see Table 56–5); and 9 addressed headache (Table 56–6).

Three trials assessed manipulation for acute neck pain (Table 56–5). In all cases, manipulation was combined with some other modality. Comparison treatments were various combinations of analgesics, cervical collars, exercise, rest, and postural advice. The results tended to favor the group that received manipulation in one study (Nordemar and Thorner, 1981) and statistically significant differences favoring manipulation were seen in two studies (McKinney, 1989; Mealy et al, 1986).

Eight trials assessed manipulation for subacute and chronic neck pain (Sloop et al, 1982; Lowe et al, 1983; Brodin, 1985; Vernon et al, 1990; Cassidy et al, 1992; Koes et al, 1993; Skargren et al, 1997; Jordan et al, 1998). Generally, results favored manipulation over the comparison treatments, but only two demonstrated statistically significant results (Brodin, 1982; Vernon et al, 1990). Three of the trials (Howe et al, 1983; Koes et al, 1992; Sloop, 1982) had data suitable for pooling in a small quantitative meta-analysis (Hurwitz et al, 1996). The effect size point estimate was 0.42, favoring spinal manipu-

Table 56–5 Randomized Trials of Spinal Manipulation for Neck Pain

Author and Year	Comparison Treatment	N = Total Sample Size	Finding on Spinal Manipulation
Brodin, 1985	Salicylates, modalities, advice	73	Positive
Cassidy et al, 1992	Mobilization	100	Equivocal
Howe et al, 1983	Azapropazone	52	Equivocal
Jordan et al, 1998	Intensive training, physiotherapy	119	Equivocal
Koes et al, 1993	Exercise, modalities, general practitioner care, detuned diathermy	64	Equivocal
McKinney, 1989	Analgesics, collar, rest	61	Positive
Mealy et al, 1986	Analgesics, collar, advice, exercise	170	Positive
Nordemar and Thorner, 1981	Analgesics, cervical collar	30	Equivocal
Skargren et al, 1997	Physical therapist	323	Equivocal
Sloop et al, 1982	Diazepam	39	Equivocal
Vernon et al, 1990	Mild mobilization	9	Positive

Table 56–6 Randomized Clinical Trials of Spinal Manipulation and Headache

Author and Year	Comparison Treatment	N = Total Sample Size	Finding on Spinal Manipulation
Boline et al, 1995	Amitriptyline	126	Positive
Bove and Nilsson, 1998	Laser and soft tissue treatment	75	Equivocal
Jensen et al, 1990	Cold packs	19	Positive
Hoyt et al, 1979	Palpation, rest	22	Positive
Carlsson et al, 1990	Acupuncture	52	Positive
Parker et al, 1978	Manipulation, mobilization by MD, physical therapist	85	Positive/equivocal
Nelson et al, 1998	Amitriptyline, combination of spinal manipulation therapy and amitriptyline	218	Positive
Nilsson et al, 1997	Low-level laser therapy with deep friction massage	53	Positive
Nilsson, 1995	Deep massage, laser therapy	38	Equivocal

lation. Translation of this result to a 100-mm visual analog pain scale yielded a difference of 12.6 mm (95% confidence interval, –0.15- 25.5). The results indicated a high probability (90%) that manipulation conferred an advantage of about 13% on a visual analog pain scale, a difference that would be clinically important to most patients.

In a separate effort (Aker et al, 1996), a team of investigators reviewed trials that evaluated conservative management of neck pain, including spinal manipulation. They analyzed the same nine studies mentioned above, and conducted a more comprehensive statistical metanalysis of five of them. The pooled effect size was –0.6 (95% confidence interval –0.9- –0.4) in favor of manipulation, equivalent to an improvement of 16.2 points on a 100-point visual analog pain scale. The results were robust in several different scenarios, for example, dropping out the worst quality study. They concluded that manipulation had more evidence to support its effectiveness than many other common treatments for neck pain.

A study that has become a scientific landmark on whiplash-associated disorders also took up the task of reviewing the voluminous literature on neck pain and its treatment (Cassidy et al, 1995). As in other similar government-sponsored efforts, a systematic approach was taken, with final group consensus reached on specific recommendations. The interested reader is recommended to the full text to appreciate the scientific context that exists on the topic of musculoskeletal pain disorders. The conclusions of the blue-ribbon panel were disappointing; its findings were that there is a dearth of high-quality research on the topic overall. However, spinal manipulation and mobilization were singled out as procedures that had evidence to support them. The consensus recommendation was that a short regimen of spinal manipulation and mobilization can be used for whiplash-associated disorders.

In summary, randomized clinical trials on acute and chronic neck pain, combined with metanalyses, support the effectiveness of spinal manipulation in clinical practice.

SPINAL MANIPULATION AND HEADACHE

There have been at least nine randomized clinical trials (Table 56–6) that assessed the effectiveness of spinal manipulation for headache, five of them reviewed by Hurwitz et al (1996). Two of the trials focused on migraine (Parker et al, 1978; Nelson et al, 1998), while the rest assessed muscle tension or cervicogenic headache. The best-rated study on muscle tension headache (Boline et al, 1995) compared manipulation performed by a chiropractor to low-dose amitriptyline over a 6-week course. Four weeks after concluding treatment, patients who received manipulation maintained their improvement from baseline while patients on amitriptyline did not. Statistically significant differences were found with respect to mean headache intensity, frequency, medication use, and functional status. Three other trials also found significant differences in favor of manipulation. However, a much-publicized study in the *Journal of the American Medical Association* did not find that manipulation was better than a control treatment for chronic muscle tension headache (Bove and Nilsson, 1998).

In the two randomized trials on migraine headache (Parker et al, 1978; Nelson et al, 1998), the group receiving chiropractic manipulation in one study suffered statistically less pain intensity when compared with manipulation and mobilization performed by a physical therapist or medical physician, but there were no statistically significant differences on frequency or duration of headache. The other study found that spinal manipulation seemed to be as effective or better than amitriptyline alone, and interestingly, better than the combination of manipulation and amitriptyline.

Two trials by the same investigators (Nilsson et al, 1995, 1997) examined the effects of manipulation on cervicogenic headache. In the first, patients under manipulation improved to a greater degree than the comparison group on all outcome variables, but statistical significance was not reached. The authors concluded that

methodological problems, including the small sample, precluded strong conclusions. In the second trial, spinal manipulation was found to have a clear advantage over the comparison treatment of low-level laser and friction massage.

In summary, the clinical trial data supporting the effectiveness of spinal manipulation for headache appear promising for some headache subgroups, but insufficient to draw strong conclusions because of mixed results. Additional research needs to be done, particularly on patients with clear diagnoses.

SAFETY OF SPINAL MANIPULATION

Contraindications to spinal manipulation are well described in chiropractic textbooks (eg, Bergmann et al, 1993) and are an important part of explicitly developed chiropractic practice guidelines (Haldeman et al, 1992). Most are logical extensions of known physiology and anatomy. Nonetheless, there are very few systematic prospective studies of complications arising from spinal manipulation. Thus information with regard to the potential harm from spinal manipulation must be derived from case reports, case series, and two cohort studies (Senstad et al, 1997; Klougart et al, 1996). Senstad focused on common, nonserious reactions to treatment with spinal manipulation, while Klougart and colleagues examined serious complications. The following paragraphs in this section focus on serious complications.

The issue is further clouded by a lack of knowledge about the denominator that is needed to calculate a risk rate. The actual number and type of patients and the number of manipulations they received during a given period of time are relatively unknown. Furthermore, the rarity of serious incidents and the poor documentation that is often found in case reports make cause-and-effect relationships difficult to determine.

Hurwitz et al (1996) extensively discussed the benefits and risks of spinal manipulation of the cervical spine. They found 118 case reports of complications allegedly arising from this procedure in the English language literature. Most were cerebrovascular accidents. Twenty-one patients died, and 52 survived with serious impairments, usually of a neurological nature. The authors attempted to calculate the risk of cervical spinal manipulation by extrapolating a denominator from a community-based study of the use of chiropractic services (Shekelle and Brook, 1991), and by assuming that the published cases represent only one-tenth of the actual incidence. The risk for a complication was estimated to be 1 per 1 million manipulations. Under the same assumptions, the rate of serious complications was estimated to be 6 per 10 million manipulations, and the rate of death from cervical spine manipulation 3 per 10 million manipulations.

Complications from lumbar spinal manipulation are extremely rare, on the order of one case per 100 million manipulations (Shekelle et al, 1992). The most serious complication is cauda equina syndrome. One review (Haldeman and Rubinstein, 1992) found 13 cases that have occurred between 1911 and 1992. An additional 16 cases were found, but they were related to manipulation under anesthesia, a procedure rarely performed by chiropractors.

The most recent comprehensive review (Assendelft et al, 1996) included case reports in all other languages. They retrieved 295 cases of complications from all types of spinal manipulation and provided a detailed analysis. They noted that no complications have been reported in any of the randomized clinical trials of spinal manipulation to date.

Since the reviews mentioned above, there has been one retrospective cohort study that examined the incidence of cerebrovascular accidents after manipulation of the cervical spine (Klougart et al, 1996), in which the number of patients and treatments was fairly well known. A cerebrovascular accident is the most serious complication of manipulation. Conducted in Denmark, the review covered the period 1978–1988 and the experience of 99% of the practicing chiropractors in the country. Five cases of cerebrovas-cular accidents were identified—approximately 1 case occurring in every 1 million cervical manipulations. Of these five incidents, one resulted in a fatality—approximately 1 case in 5 million.

The context for such risk rates should be kept in mind. For example, the risk of a serious complication from NSAIDs is 3.2 per 1,000 over age 65 (approximately 3,200 per million); and 0.39 per 1,000 *under* age 65 (390 per million). Serious complications in this case are defined as gastrointestinal events that include bleeding, perforation, or other adverse event resulting in hospitalization or death (Hurwitz et al, 1996).

There are numerous additional discussions of the risks of spinal manipulation (eg, see Haldeman, 1992) and the interested reader is referred to them for additional insight. Most authors have agreed, that while the true risks for manipulation are somewhat unknown, they are apparently rare. In skilled hands, for the proper indications, spinal manipulation is a safe procedure.

CONCLUSION

In over 50 randomized trials, spinal manipulation has been tested against a wide variety of comparison treatments with generally favorable results for quality-of-life outcomes important to patients. In at least certain kinds of patients, manipulation appears to be effective for those with acute, subacute, and chronic low-back pain, especially for short-term outcomes. Results for neck pain are weaker, but still substantial enough to consider manipulation as a viable treatment option when compared to other relatively untested consecutive treatments for the spine. Results for headache in general are mixed; however, patients with cervicogenic, muscle tension, and migraine headache may benefit. The risk of morbidity associated with lumbar manipulation is exceedingly small. The risk from cervical manipulation is slightly higher for greater harm, but also very rare. In skilled hands, for the proper indications, spinal manipulation is remarkably safe and generally effective for these forms of common musculoskeletal complaints.

REFERENCES

Aker P, Gross AR, Goldsmith CH, Peloso P. Conservative management of mechanical neck pain: Systematic overview and meta-analysis. *BMJ.* 1996;313:1291–1296.

Anderson R, Meeker WC, Wirick BE, Mootz RD, Kirk DH, Adams A. A meta-analysis of clinical trials of spinal manipulation. *J Manipulative Physiol Ther.* 1992;15(3):181–194.

Arkuszewski Z. The efficacy of manual treatment in low back pain: A clinical trial. *Manual Med.* 1986;2:68–71.

Assendelft WJJ, Bouter LM, Knipschild PG. Complications of spinal manipulation. A comprehensive review of the literature. *J Fam Pract.* 1996;42:475–480.

Assendelft WJJ, Koes BW, Knipschild PG, Bouter LM. The relationship between methodological quality and conclusions in reviews of spinal manipulation. *JAMA* 1995;274:1942–1948.

Bergmann TF, Peterson DH, Lawrence DJ. *Chiropractic Technique: Principles and Procedures.* New York: Churchill Livingston; 1993.

Bergquist-Ullman M, Larsson U. Acute low back pain in industry. A controlled prospective study with special reference to therapy and confounding factors. *Acta Orthop Scand* 1977;170(Suppl):11–117.

Bigos S, Bowyer O, Braen G, et al. *Acute Low Back Problems in Adults.* Clinical Practice Guideline No. 14. Rockville, MD: Agency for Health Care Policy and Research; 1994. AHCPR Publication 95-0642.

Blomberg S, Hallin G, Grann K, Berg K, Sennerby U. Manual therapy with steroid injections in low-back pain. *Spine.* 1994;19:569–577.

Boline PD, Kassak K, Bronfort G, Nelson C, Anderson A. Spinal manipulation versus amitriptyline for the treatment of chronic tension-type headaches: A randomized clinical trial. *J Manipulative Physiol Ther.* 1995;18:148–154.

Bove G, Nilsson N. Spinal manipulation in the treatment of episodic tension-type headache: A randomized controlled trial. *JAMA.* 1998;280(18):1576–1579.

Brodin H. Cervical pain and mobilization. *Manuelle Med.* 1982;20:90–94.

Bronfort G. Chiropractic versus general medical treatment of low-back pain: A small-scale controlled clinical trial. *Am J Chiro Med.* 1989;2:145–150.

Carlsson J, Fahlcrantz A, Augustinsson L. Muscle tenderness in tension headache treated with acupuncture or physiotherapy. *Cephalalgia.* 1990;10:131–141.

Cassidy JD, Duranceau J, Liang MH, Salmi LR, Skovron ML, Spitzer WO. Scientific monograph of the Quebec task force on whiplash-associated disorders. *Spine.* 1995;20(8S):1S–74S.

Cassidy JD, Lopes AA, Yong-Hing K. The immediate effect of manipulation versus mobilization on pain and range of motion in the cervical spine: A randomized controlled trial (see author correction). *J Manip Physiol Ther.* 1992;15:570–575.

Cherkin DC, Deyo RA, Battie M, Street J, Barlow W. A comparison of physical therapy, chiropractic manipulation, and provision of an educational booklet for the treatment of patients with low back pain. *N Engl J Med.* 1998;339(15):1021–1029.

Coxhead CE, Meade TM, Inskip H, North WRS, Troup JDG. Multicentre trial of physiotherapy in the management of sciatic symptoms. *Lancet.* 1981;1:1065–1068.

Delitto A, Cibulka MT, Erhard RE, Bowling RW, Tenhula JA. Evidence for use of an extension-mobilization category in acute low-back syndrome. A prescriptive validation pilot study. *Phys Ther.* 1992;73:216–223.

Doran DM, Newell DJ. Manipulation in treatment of low back pain. A multicentre study. *BMJ.* 1975;2:161–164.

Eisenberg DM, Kessler RC, Foster C, Norlock FE, Calkins DR, Delbanco TL. Unconventional medicine in the United States: Prevalence, costs, and patterns of use. *N Eng J Med.* 1993;328:246–252.

Evans DP, Burke MS, Lloyd KN, Roberts EE, Roberts GM. Lumbar spinal manipulation on trial. *Rheumatol Rehab.* 1978;17:46–53.

Farrell JP, Twomey LT. Acute low back pain. Comparison of two conservative treatment approaches. *Med J Aust.* 1982;1:160–164.

Gatterman MI, ed. *Foundations of Chiropractic. Subluxation.* St Louis: Mosby-Year Book, Inc; 1995.

Gibson T, Harkness J, Blackgrave P, Grahame R, Woo P, Hills R. Controlled comparison of short-wave diathermy treatment with osteopathic treatment in non-specific low back pain. *Lancet.* 1985;1:1258–1261.

Glover JR, Morris JG, Khosla T. Back pain: a randomized trial of rotational manipulation to the trunk. *Br J Ind Med.* 1974;31:59–64.

Godfrey CM, Morgan PP, Schatzker J. A randomized trial of manipulation for low back pain in a medical setting. *Spine.* 1984;9:301–304.

Hadler NM, Curtis P, Gillings DB, Stinnett S. A benefit of spinal manipulation as adjunctive therapy for acute low-back pain: A stratified controlled trial. *Spine.* 1987;12:702–706.

Haldeman S, ed. *Principles and Practice of Chiropractic.* Norwalk, CT: Appleton and Lange; 1992.

Haldeman S, Chapman-Smith D, Petersen D, eds. *Guidelines for Chiropractic Quality Assurance and Practice Parameters.* Gaithersburg, MD: Aspen Publishers, Inc; 1992.

Haldeman S, Rubinstein SM. Cauda equina syndrome in patients undergoing manipulation of the lumbar spine. *Spine.* 1992;17:1469–1473.

Helliwell PS, Cunliffe G. Manipulation in low-back pain. *Physician.* April 1987;187–188.

Herzog W, Conway PJ, Willcox BJ. Effects of different treatment modalities on gait symmetry and clinical measures for sacroiliac joint patients. *J Manipulative Physiol Ther.* 1991;14:104–109.

Hoehler FK, Tobis JS, Buerger AA. Spinal manipulation for low back pain. *JAMA.* 1981;245:1835–1838.

Howe DH, Newcombe RG, Wade MT. Manipulation of the cervical spine. A pilot study. *J R Coll Gen Pract.* 1983;33:574–579.

Hoyt WH, Shaffer F, Bard DA, Benesler JS, Blankenhorn GD. Osteopathic manipulation in the treatment of muscle-contraction headache. *J Am Osteopath Assoc.* 1979;78:322–325.

Hurwitz EL, Aker PD, Adams AH, Meeker, WC, Shekelle P. Manipulation and mobilization of the cervical spine. A systematic review of the literature. *Spine.* 1996;21:1746–1760.

Jensen OK, Nielsen FF, Vosmar L. An open study comparing manual therapy with the use of cold packs in the treatment of post-traumatic headache. *Cephalalgia.* 1990;10:241–250.

Jordan A, Bendix T, Nielsen H, Hansen FR, Host D, Winkel A. Intensive training, physiotherapy, or manipulation for patients with chronic neck pain. A prospective, single-blinded, randomized clinical trial. *Spine.* 1998;23(3):311–308.

Kinalski R, Kuwik W, Pietrzak L. The comparison of the results of manual therapy versus physiotherapy methods used in treatment of patients with low back syndromes. *Manual Med.* 1989;4:44–46.

Klougart N, LeBoeuf-Yde C, Rasmussen LR. Safety in chiropractic practice. Part I. The occurrence of cerebrovascular accidents following cervical spine adjustment in Denmark during 1978–1988. *J Manipulative Physiol Ther.* 1996;19:371–377.

Koes BW, Assendelft AJJ, van der Heijden GJMG, Bouter LM. Spinal manipulation for low back pain. An updated systematic review of randomized clinical trials. *Spine.* 1996;21:2860–2873.

Koes BW, Bouter LM, Mameren HV, et al. A randomized clinical trial of manual therapy and physiotherapy for persistent back and neck complaints: Subgroup analysis and relationship between outcome measures. *J Manipulative Physiol Ther.* 1993;16(4):211–219.

Koes BW, Bouter LM, Van Mameren H, et al. The effectiveness of manual therapy, physiotherapy, and treatment by the general practitioner for nonspecific back and neck complaints: A randomized clinical trial. *Spine.* 1992;17(1):28–35.

MacDonald RS, Bell CMJ. An open controlled assessment of osteopathic manipulation in nonspecific low back pain. *Spine.* 1990;15:364–370.

Mathews JA, Mills SB, Jenkins VM, et al. Back pain and sciatica: Controlled trials of manipulation, traction, sclerosant and epidural injections. *Br J Rheumatol.* 1987;26:416–423.

McKinney LA. Early mobilisation and outcome in acute sprains of the neck. *BMJ.* 1989;299:1006–1008.

Meade TW, Dyer S, Browne W, Frank AO. Randomised comparison of chiropractic and outpatient management for low back pain: Results from extended follow up. *BMJ.* 1995;311:349–351.

Meade TW, Dyer S, Browne W, Townsend J, Frank AO. Low back pain of mechanical origin: Randomized comparison of chiropractic and hospital outpatient treatment. *BMJ.* 1990;300:1431–1437.

Mealy K, Brennan H, Fenelon GC. Early mobilisation and outcome in acute sprains of the neck. *BMJ (Clin Res Ed).* 1986;292:656–657.

Meeker W. Point of view. *Spine.* 1996;21:2873.

Nelson CF, Bronfort G, Evans R, Boline P, Goldsmith C, Anderson AV. The efficacy of spinal manipulation, amitriptyline and the combination of both therapies for the prophylaxis of migraine headache. *J Manipulative Physiol Ther.* 1998;21(8):511–519.

Nilsson N. A randomized controlled trial of the effect of spinal manipulation in the treatment of cervicogenic headache. *J Manipulative Physiol Ther.* 1995;18:435–440.

Nilsson N, Christensen HW, Hartvigsen J. The effect of spinal manipulation in the treatment of cervicogenic headache. *J Manipulative Physiol Ther.* 1997;20(5):326–330.

Nordemar R, Thorner C. Treatment of acute cervical pain: A comparative group study. *Pain.* 1981;10:93–101.

Nwuga VCB. Relative therapeutic efficacy of vertebral manipulation and conventional treatment in back pain management. *Am J Phys Med.* 1982;2:143–146.

Ongley MJ, Dorman TA, Klein RG, Eek BC, Hubert LJ. A new approach to the treatment of low back pain. *Lancet.* 1987;2:143–146.

Parker GB, Tupling H, Pryor DS. A controlled trial of cervical manipulation for migraine. *Aust NZ J Med.* 1978;8:589–593.

Pope MH, Phillips RB, Haugh LD, Hsieh CJ, MacDonald L, Haldeman S. A prospective randomized three-week trial of spinal manipulation, transcutaneous muscle stimulation, massage and corset in the treatment of subacute low back pain. *Spine.* 1994;19:2571–2577.

Postacchini F, Facchini M, Palieri P. Efficacy of various forms of conservative treatment in low back pain. A comparative study. *Neuro-Orthopedics.* 1988;6:28–35.

Rasmussen GG. Manipulation in treatment of low back pain. A randomized clinical trial. *Manuelle Med.* 1979;1:8–10.

Royal Commission of General Practitioners. *Clinical Guidelines for the Management of Acute Low Back Pain.* London: HMSO; September 1996.

Rupert RL, Wagnon R, Thompson P, Ezzeldin MT. Chiropractic adjustments: Results of a controlled clinical trial in Egypt. *ICA Int Rev Chiro.* Winter 1985;58–60.

Sanders GE, Reinert O, Tepe R, Maloney P. Chiropractic adjustive manipulation on subjects with acute low back pain: Visual analog pain scores and plasma β-endorphin levels. *J Manipulative Physiol Ther.* 1990;13:391–395.

Senstad O, Lebouef-Yde C, Borchgrevink C. Frequency and characteristics of side effects of spinal manipulative therapy. *Spine.* 1997;22:435–441.

Shekelle PG. *The Use and Costs of Chiropractic Care in the Health Insurance Experiment.* Santa Monica, CA: RAND; 1994.

Shekelle PG, Adams AH, Chassin MR, Hurwitz EL, Brook RH. Spinal manipulation for low-back pain. *Ann Intern Med.* 1992;117:590–598.

Shekelle PG, Brook RH. A community-based study of the use of chiropractic services. *Am J Public Health.* 1991;81(4):439–442.

Siehl D, Olson DR, Ross HE, Rockwood EE. Manipulation of the lumbar spine with the patient under general anesthesia: An evaluation by EMG and clinical neurologic examination of its use for lumbar nerve root compression. *J Am Osteopath Assoc.* 1971;70:433–441.

Sims-Williams H, Jayson M, Young SM, Baddeley H. Controlled trial of mobilization and manipulation for patients with low back pain in general practice. *BMJ.* 1978;2:1338–1340.

Sims-Williams H, Jayson MIV, Young SMS, Baddeley H, Collins E. Controlled trial of mobilization and manipulation for low back pain: Hospital patients. *BMJ.* 1979;2:1318–1320.

Skargren EI, Carlsson PG, Oberg BE. One-year follow-up comparison of the cost and effectiveness of chiropractic and physiotherapy as primary management for back pain. Subgroup analysis, recurrence, and additional health care utilization. *Spine.* 1998;23(17):1875–1883.

Skargren EI, Oberg BE, Carlsson PG, Gade M. Cost and effectiveness analysis of chiropractic and physiotherapy treatment for low back and neck pain. Six-month follow-up. *Spine.* 1997;22(18):2167–2177.

Sloop PR, Smith DS, Goldenberg EVA, Dore C. Manipulation for chronic neck pain. A double-blind controlled study. *Spine.* 1982;7:532–535.

Triano JJ, McGregor M, Hondras MA, Brennan PC. Manipulative therapy versus education programs in chronic low back pain. *Spine.* 1995;20:948–955.

Vernon HT, Peter A, Burns S, Viljakaanen S, Short L. Pressure pain threshold evaluation of the effect of spinal manipulation in the treatment of chronic neck pain: A pilot study. *J Manipulative Physiol Ther.* 1990;13:13–16.

Waagen GN, Haldeman S, Cook G, Lopez D, DeBoer KF. Short-term trial of chiropractic adjustments for the relief of chronic low-back pain. *Manual Med.* 1986;2:63–67.

Waterworth RF, Hunter IA. An open study of diflunisal, conservative and manipulative therapy in the management of low back pain. *NZ Med J.* 1985;98:372–375.

Wreje U, Nordgren B, Aberg H. Treatment of pelvic joint dysfunction in primary care: A controlled study. *Scand J Primary Health Care.* 1992;10:310–315.

Zylbergold RS, Piper MC. Lumbar disc disease: Comparative analysis of physical therapy treatments. *Arch Phys Med Rehabil.* 1981;62:176–179.

CHAPTER 57

Overcoming Barriers to the Integration of Chiropractic

J. Michael Menke

INTRODUCTION

Low-back pain is the third most common acute condition seen by primary care providers (Bigos et al, 1994). This condition and its sequela tend to generate high utilization of outpatient medical services. These conditions are typically chronic, involving recurring symptoms for which there is little intervention except medication and exercise.

The treatment of back pain is an area of health care in which chiropractic could make a major contribution. In the search for new ways to manage chronic and debilitating illness, there is a need to maximize patient services and control health care costs. According to numerous controlled clinical trials and metanalyses, spinal manipulation is one of the most effective treatments for low-back pain. Chiropractors provide 94% of all spinal manipulation services in the United States (Shekelle, 1994). In a metanalysis of research on chiropractic cost-effectiveness, chiropractic was found to accrue lower costs in

J. Michael Menke, MA, DC, has a background in research, clinical practice, and consulting. As a statistician and research methodologist, he has participated in 10 randomized controlled clinical trials in chiropractic and for 16 years has served as an adjunct faculty member at Palmer College of Chiropractic-West. As a practitioner and director of a busy full-time private practice, for 12 years he provided chiropractic services, co-managing cases with spinal orthopedists, internists, and physiatrists at Stanford University Medical Center and three large medical groups. In 1999, he initiated Palmer's program for interdisciplinary internships, rounds, and rotations in mainstream medical settings and has been involved in integrative curriculum design with two university medical schools.

16 of 24 studies (Branson, 1999; see Chapter 55).

Chiropractic Utilization

Eisenberg and colleagues (1998) found that chiropractic services are provided more frequently than other forms of alternative care (more than 969 visits per 1,000 as compared with 574 visits to massage therapists). Other recent studies have found that chiropractic treatment is provided by managed care organizations with twice the frequency of any other complementary therapy (67% offered chiropractic; the other most frequently provided service was acupuncture, covered by 31% of insurers) (National Market Measures, 1999).

Research over two decades has consistently identified high patient satisfaction with chiropractic treatment (see Chapter 53). More than 100 controlled clinical trials have found it efficacious (see Chapter 56). Economically, chiropractic is currently one of the most viable, cost-effective forms of complementary and alternative medicine (CAM) service provision, when applied to common musculoskeletal problems (see Chapter 55). In addition, chiropractic offers major potential in the treatment of serious spine disorders in the context of highly successful multidisciplinary programs such as the Texas Back Institute in Plano, Texas (see Chapter 38). However, despite this promising potential, there are certain health care environments in which chiropractic is not yet considered as a treatment option. It is valuable to identify factors that tend to impede the full expression of chiropractic in a health system. This chapter addresses these issues.

BARRIERS TO CHIROPRACTIC

Perceptions of the Research

Currently, there is a perception that there is little or no research on chiropractic. In reality, literally thousands of studies have been published on spinal manipulation, the treatment of choice in chiropractic practice. Of these, approximately 110 are of high enough research quality to provide useful clinical and health policy information. In terms of the quality issue, in the clinical trials on back pain, chiropractic research has received quality scores comparable to evaluations of conventional therapies. Additional informative and critical chiropractic appraisals and research are cited in the MEDLINE databases of the National Institutes of Health (NIH) in more than 2,000 journal articles on chiropractic.

It is also noteworthy that this research is predominantly published in peer-reviewed medical journals, such as the *Journal of the American Medical Association*, the *New England Journal of Medicine*, the *British Medical Journal*, and *Spine*. Of the current literature, approximately 70% is published in medical journals and 30% in chiropractic journals. Principal investigators on the majority of these studies are physicians and medical researchers. The legitimate nature of this research is an important aspect of its credibility.

Data on Safety

Chiropractic safety has been well established through research, and the safety record of chiropractic is exceptional. What is known in quantitative terms about the safety of chiropractic? Researchers have reported serious complications to occur at a rate of approximately 1 in 1 million manipulations (Klougart et al, 1996; Hurwitz et al, 1996). Extensive metanalysis by the RAND Corporation also places the incidence of fatalities due to chiropractic treatment conservatively at less than approximately 1 in 3 million treatments (Shekelle, 1994). Reported safety rates are reflected in the Table 57–1.

Comparison with other forms of treatment for the same condition provides an additional frame of reference. For example, with respect to side effects and complications, chiropractic has been found to be far safer than the use of nonsteroidal, anti-inflammatory medications and cortisone therapies (see Chapter 56).

Table 57–1 Complication Rates Associated with Chiropractic Treatment

Complication	Frequency
Stroke (caused by vertebrobasilar accident)[1]	1 in 1,000,000
Major impairment[2]	1 in 1,000,000
Death[3]	Less than 3 in 10,000,000
Low-back (lumbar) nerve damage[4]	Approximately 1 in 100,000,000

Courtesy of J. Michael Menke, San Jose, California.

REFERENCES

1. Klougart N, LeBoeuf Y de C, Rasmussen LR. Safety in chiropractic practice. Part I. The occurrence of cerebrovascular accidents following cervical spine adjustment in Denmark during 1978–1988. *J Manipulative Physiol Ther.* 1996;19:371–377.
2. Hurwitz EL, Aker PD, Adams AH, Meeker WC, Shekelle PG. Manipulation and mobilization of the cervical spine: A systematic review of the literature. *Spine.* 1996;21:1746–1760.
3. Shekelle PG, Brook RH. A community-based study of the use of chiropractic services. *Am J Public Health.* 1991;81:439–442.
4. Shekelle PG, Adams AH, Chassin MR, Hurwitz EL, Brook RH. Spinal manipulation for low-back pain. *Ann Intern Med.* 1992;117:590–598.

Scope of Practice

Issues regarding scope of practice may surface when chiropractic is considered for inclusion in a mainstream medical environment. There may be the concern that chiropractors treat beyond their scope of practice. There is also the fear that they may not detect more serious underlying pathology and delay critical referral to appropriate medical care. The profession has matured to recognize the value of medical care in cases that are beyond the benefits of chiropractic treatment. The complementary chiropractic approach—chiropractic as a part of the health care system—is being taught more frequently in the chiropractic college curriculum as part of differential diagnosis, pathology classes, and chiropractic treatment classes.

Some physicians have concerns that chiropractors might co-opt patients, in the capacity of primary care providers. Physicians do not want to work in a competitive environment but may be willing to work in a collaborative and complementary mode, mutually referring and co-managing patient conditions as appropriate.

COMPLEMENTARY AND ALTERNATIVE CHIROPRACTIC

On the Web site of the National Center for Complementary and Alternative Medicine, the distinction is made between complementary treatment and alternative therapies. The distinction may sound like hair-splitting, given that the two concepts are commonly used interchangeably to describe therapies not typically taught in medical education. In England and Europe, however, there has been an emphasis on the inclusion of nonmedical therapies in conventional treatment, which are therefore described as complementary. In the United States, nonmedical treatments are often considered outside medicine or alternative. This distinction is relevant to chiropractic, which encompasses two general styles of practice within the discipline.

Complementary chiropractic practitioners can be distinguished by their willingness to work in conjunction with physicians and other practitioners. This requires a different emphasis on patient care and a different scope and style of practice. Complementary chiropractors tend to specialize in treating musculoskeletal conditions. In contrast, alternative providers typically treat a wider variety of conditions, with particular emphasis on correcting subluxation lesions of the spine. In the alternative chiropractic approach, subluxation detection and treatment are fundamental to the course of treatment. This in itself becomes a barrier to integration since the subluxation concept is not accepted by conventional medicine. This style of practice is sometimes associated with the overuse of radiographs and extended treatment plans.

It should be noted that the alternative chiropractic approach continues to help thousands of patients each year. Many patients like this approach and continue to use it. However, given that the primary focus of treatment is subluxation, which cannot be reliably detected, it is difficult to define treatment endpoints and therefore to define success. For insurers and consumers who want facts and figures, this approach does not provide the kind of data that allows the tracking of treatment effectiveness.

The key questions to ask a chiropractor to determine if his or her practice style is alternative or complementary include:

1. When do you release a patient from care?
2. How do you know the treatment plan has been completed?

An alternative approach is reflected in the response, "The patient is never released from care because patients need maintenance care in order to preserve good health." Another indicator of alternative practice is overreliance on radiographs to assess patient condition. This is an approach that measures subtle rejuxtapositions of adjacent vertebrae over an extensive course of treatment.

On the other hand, complementary chiropractic protocol tends to be more empirically defined. It involves monitoring patients' symptoms periodically throughout the course of treatment and at the endpoint. This is symptom-based care; the patient is discharged when the symptoms are resolved or maximum benefit has been achieved and referral to a specialist is necessary. Complementary practitioners tend to use outcome measures to assess patient status, including the level of pain, functionality, ability to perform activities of daily living, and quality of life as evidence of response to treatment. The following aspects of practice style are characteristic of complementary chiropractic.

Complementary Practice

Style

A chiropractor providing treatment in a complementary approach:

- refers the patient to an appropriate specialist when there is no response to treatment.
- encourages patient independence and self-care.
- provides treatment based on empirical evidence gathered through assessment and response to treatment.

Competency

A chiropractor providing treatment in a complementary approach:

- uses differential diagnosis to rule out underlying pathology.
- is knowledgeable regarding other medical disciplines.
- consults with other health care providers regarding treatment.
- is aware of the protocol for making professional referrals.

Scope of Practice and Practice Guidelines

A chiropractor providing treatment in a complementary approach:

- limits intervention primarily to musculoskeletal pain and dysfunction.

- bases assessment on physical examination and standard diagnosis using ICD-9 or ICD-10 codes (International Classification of Diseases, ninth revision).
- reserves radiographs and other forms of diagnostic imaging for high-risk cases.
- uses common medical nomenclature.

Interventions are provided on a finite treatment plan with these guidelines:

- All conditions should respond within six to eight visits.
- If there is 50% to 75% improvement at the end of treatment period, the chiropractor continues to treat patient for another six to eight visits and then reevaluates.
- If patient reaches maximum benefit sooner or fails to progress, the chiropractor discharges or refers patient out as appropriate.

The profile of the complementary chiropractor is one who uses radiographs judiciously and treats conservatively with the goal of promoting maximal benefit. There is a commitment to cost-containment and effectiveness. The practitioner also educates patients thoroughly in prevention and self-care. This is a genuine value-added service in an integrated environment, particularly for those patients with chronic conditions such as pain.

THE IMPORTANCE OF CREDENTIALING

In the development of integrative medical services, credentialing chiropractic provides at least three important functions. One is to distinguish complementary from alternative practitioners. Another is to identify those candidates most likely to adapt well to mainstream medical environments and participation on the multidisciplinary team. It is also a means of determining excellence in practitioners. The steps in credentialing most relevant to these issues include:

- *Creating the comprehensive provider application.* The credentialing organization can include questions regarding practice style in the dimensions discussed above, including defining the treatment plan as well as determining the endpoint of treatment, the use of radiographs, and the type of techniques used in practice.

- *Evaluating the practitioner's curriculum vitae.* This may also suggest his or her practice philosophy. If the practitioner has given seminars, the topic will usually reflect the style of practice. Practitioners who have work experience in mainstream health care environments, either as a chiropractor or as an allied health care professional, are candidates who may adapt well to an integrative environment.
- *Conducting a peer review of the practitioner's application and all related documents.*
- *Determining the practitioner's capabilities for data reporting and profiling.* Complementary practitioners will be more likely to participate in data reporting. They may be more proficient in charting and record keeping.
- *Conducting an interview (frequently during the on-site visit).*
- *Reviewing the provider's office, records, and operations on site.* A site visit provides an opportunity to review treatment plans and their rationale. Key considerations are whether the treatment plan reflects appropriate use of radiographs and whether subjective and objective measures are used to monitor treatment.

CHIROPRACTIC EDUCATION

Coursework at Chiropractic Institutions

Many of the concerns regarding chiropractic practice can be addressed through a better understanding of chiropractic education. At this point in time, chiropractic education is extensive and rigorous. Medical education and chiropractic education both require 4 years of study, with chiropractic education requiring 4,822 class hours, comparable to medical education's 4,667 hours.

For the most part, textbooks, course requirements, and objectives are equivalent for the same courses in chiropractic and medical education. However, chiropractic does not currently offer a postgraduate residency, whereas medical education has a residency requirement.

Graduation from an accredited college of chiropractic is required of any and all chiropractors who are licensed in any of the 50 United States; Washington, DC; and territories. Chiropractic education emphasizes courses in anatomy, biomechanics, and therapeutic techniques, whereas medical education emphasizes pathology, microbiology, and pharmacology. Chiropractic educational institutions must undergo a rigorous review process biannually, which is conducted by the Council on Chiropractic Education of the U.S. Department of Health and Human Services. The accreditation process evaluates the credentials of the faculty, the inclusion of ongoing research, and the overall quality of chiropractic education.

Chiropractic education includes coursework that thoroughly reviews all the systems of the body and trains practitioners in the basic techniques of physical examination, such as listening to the heart, taking blood pressure readings, and providing cranial nerve examination to detect signs of potential stroke. (See Table 57–2.) There are additional courses in pathology focused on the detection and evaluation of clinical symptoms and referral to the appropriate provider in cases of suspected underlying pathology, such as cancers. Typically the primary care physician is the point of referral in these cases.

Schools of chiropractic provide coursework in differential diagnosis that train practitioners to identify conditions that are more appropriately treated by medical doctors and should be referred out. Coursework in differential diagnosis is comparable to that of medical schools. These classes involve the same curriculum design, have the same number of credit hours, and use the same textbooks as those of medical schools.

Woven throughout the curriculum is content on the musculoskeletal system, including bones,

Table 57–2 Chiropractic Coursework

Course Area	Credit Hours
Adjustive technique and analysis	555
Clinical practice, differential diagnosis	410
Diagnostic imaging	305
Chiropractic principles	245
Orthopedics	135
Biochemistry	150
Microbiology	120
Physical therapy techniques	120
Nutrition	90
Public health	70
Biomechanics	65
Gynecology, obstetrics	65
Professional practice	65
Psychology	55
Research	50
Geriatrics, pediatrics	45
First aid	45
Dermatology (and skin pathologies)	30
Otolaryngology	25
Other coursework including pathology	177

Source: Reprinted from *Chiropractic in the United States: Training, Practice and Research*, D.C. Cherkin and R.D. Mootz, eds., ACHPR Publication No. 98-N002, Rockville, MD: Agency for Health Care Policy and Research: 1997.

joints, muscles, ligaments, tendons, bursa anatomy, and related physiology. There is a heavy emphasis on neurology, neuroanatomy, and neurophysiology, which supports the treatment focus on the musculoskeletal system.

Goals of Chiropractic Education

- *To treat within the scope of practice.* While scope of practice is defined legally by each state, the treatment approach is conveyed through the college curriculum. Scope of practice is reviewed in depth in the coursework on professional practice and ethics.
- *To train sufficiently in differential diagnosis so that practitioners will not overlook more serious conditions, thereby delaying treatment.* Chiropractic education entails coursework in serious pathologies and how they may manifest clinically, for the purpose of identifying and referring out such conditions. Course content includes gastrointestinal conditions, the genitourinary systems, cardiovascular function, neurophysiology, and pathology.
- *To train in clinical safety.* Students are taught to identify and rule out patients who are not good candidates for manipulation due to a variety of physical conditions such as hypertension, suspected fracture, underlying pathology, torn ligaments, or other effects of trauma. Ruling out these conditions reflects the proper use of diagnostic imaging, such as radiographs. Proper manipulation technique is taught under supervision by highly experienced clinical instructors who train students in the safest techniques for providing chiropractic adjustments. Skills are tested at the end of each course, and again before allowing entry into the clinic. By the time students graduate, they have received thorough training in the techniques of performing adjustments safely. In fact, malpractice premiums are lowest for new graduates probably because they are trained to err on the side of caution.

CHIROPRACTIC AND PHYSICAL THERAPY

Although chiropractic is currently experiencing high utilization in managed care networks, the integration of chiropractic into hospitals, spine centers, and university medical centers is occurring at a slower rate. One of the major barriers to the integration of chiropractic in these environments has been the confusion of chiropractic with physical therapy in the minds of policy makers and the general public.

In conversations with medical and managed care directors about the inclusion of chiropractic, the response to these issues has often been, "We have no need for chiropractors—we already have physical therapists." The fundamental question then is, "Does chiropractic spinal manipulation for low-back pain offer any additional benefit over physical therapy that would suggest a rationale for inclusion?"

At first, this author wondered if physical therapists and chiropractors were vying for the same types of patients. When attending lectures given by physical therapists, the author has been impressed with their approach to problems and found them to be thorough and careful. It was only after interviewing chiropractors who worked with physical therapists, physiatrists, orthopedists, and neurosurgeons that an analysis evolved that drew distinctions between the two disciplines, although clearly there is some overlap (see Table 57–3).

Chiropractic focuses primarily on conditions of the spine. In terms of musculoskeletal conditions, physical therapy has a record of particular effectiveness in joint rehabilitation of shoulders, hips, and knees, and in postsurgical rehabilitation. Physical therapy is also utilized in rehabilitation for patients with a wide range of physical trauma, including stroke and burns.

The primary therapy provided in chiropractic treatment is spinal manipulation. In fact, chiropractors perform approximately 94% of all the spinal manipulation procedures in the United States. In contrast, physical therapists use a broad range of therapeutic techniques that include exercise, body mechanics, ergonomics, manual therapy, patient education, and self-care.

In chiropractic, manipulation of the spinal joints is almost always a component of treatment. This is where essentially all chiropractic benefit occurs. The effectiveness of this approach has been borne out in a large body of research in the peer-reviewed journals. A thorough review of treatment for back pain by the Agency for Health Care Policy and Research (AHCPR) involved an analysis of more than 10, 000 studies (Bigos et al, 1994). This metanalysis found spinal manipulation to be one of three treatments efficacious in the treatment of low-back pain. The other two were anti-inflammatory medications and bed rest of not more than 4 days' duration.

Physical therapy includes a form of spinal manipulation similar to that used by chiropractors, but physical therapists perform less than 5% of the spinal manipulation in the United States (Bigos et al, 1994). Physical therapists also provide other forms of less vigorous mobilizations and gentler movements of the spinal joints. Physical therapy has a record of extensive benefit for a wide range of conditions, whereas chiropractic treatment is focused primarily on interventions that address the health and function of the spine. Ultimately, the strengths of physical therapy and chiropractic could be blended nicely in a form of complementary treatment for musculoskeletal conditions. Chiropractic has established itself as a reliable intervention for low-back pain of a simple mechanical origin. But ultimately, patients must also learn how to take care of themselves to prevent problems in the future and to avoid overutilization and overdependence on health care. Physical therapists and chiropractors are both highly competent at patient education, exercise, and rehabilitation.

CONCLUSION

The safety and popularity of chiropractic and its effectiveness for certain conditions make it a viable candidate for greater inclusion in health care. Medical and managed care directors may find it useful to include a chiropractor on the multidisciplinary team—one who is compatible in a medical environment. The complementary chiropractor must have the ability to triage serious medical conditions, thereby differentiating acute situations from chronic aches and pains. For chiropractic to become an integrated discipline on the health care team, appropriate referral protocol is also an essential component of practice. With the professions working shoulder to shoulder, new protocols and critical pathways will evolve.

New benchmarks of excellence will provide the context for the systematic and relevant measurement of outcomes in response to singular and combination treatments. Then perhaps the

Table 57–3 Practice Style

Physical Therapists	*Complementary Chiropractors*
• Evaluate the condition and define treatment plan. • May also determine the condition (over half the states allow patients to attend physical therapy without a physician referral).	• Determine the condition and define treatment plan. • Are trained in differential diagnosis.
• Have wide range in education and competencies. —nonspinal musculoskeletal conditions —postsurgical rehabilitation —sports injuries • Are trained in treatment of spinal conditions.	• Focus primarily on treatment of spinal conditions since that is the focus of therapeutic intervention. • May treat joint problems in shoulders, knees, or hips, but typically those related to spinal dysfunction.
• Use wide range of techniques including exercise, body mechanics, ergonomics, manual therapy, patient education, and self-responsibility.	• Perform spinal manipulation (94% of all U.S. procedures). Almost all patients receive spinal manipulation, if indicated. • Refer outpatients not appropriate for manipulation.
• Employ adjunctive therapies including spinal manipulation, but only for certain indications. • Selects from broad range of adjunctive therapies, as appropriate.	• Employ adjunctive therapies including nutrition and exercise. • Use physiotherapy modalities to support spinal manipulation, such as light, heat, water, ice or cold packs, electrical stimulation, and ultrasound, massage, office- or home-based traction.
• See wider variety of patients, such as burn or stroke victims, and others with serious conditions that result from major trauma to the body.	• See patients with spinal problems; they tend to have less serious conditions and some ambulatory capacity.
• Use various approaches to manipulation, in the context of mobilization. • Use manipulation as required by the situation.	• Use spinal manipulation as mainstay of chiropractic practice; procedure involves high-velocity, low-amplitude (short thrust).
• Has regional approach to soft tissue, focusing on muscles and ligaments with skeletal structure as supportive.	• Focus on skeletal juxtaposition—joints and lack of mobility and how that affects the soft tissue.
• Focus primarily on musculoskeletal system and related soft tissue.	• Include role of nerve supply to the region in diagnosis and treatment.
• In rehabilitation, emphasize active patient participation.	• Require patient to be passive during the treatment and active participation is required only for posttreatment rehabilitation.

Courtesy of J. Michael Menke, MA, DC, with data from D. Saunders, Saunders Group.

safest and best that each profession has to offer will become apparent. From this foundation, care can be provided for patients challenged by chronic pain and other conditions that create cost overruns and dependency on the health care system.

REFERENCES

Bigos S, Bowyer O, Braen G, et al. *Acute Low Back Problems in Adults*. Clinical Practice Guideline No. 14. Rockville, MD: Agency for Health Care Policy and Research; 1994. AHCPR publication 95-0642.

Branson RA. Cost comparison of chiropractic and medical treatment of common musculoskeletal disorders: A review of the literature after 1980. *Top Clin Chiro*. 1999;6(2):l57–168.

Eisenberg D, et al. Trends in alternative medicine use in the United States, 1990–1997: results of a follow-up national study. *JAMA*.1998:280:1569–1575.

Hurwitz EL, Aker PD, Adams AH, Meeker WC, Shekelle P. Manipulation and mobilization of the cervical spine. A systematic review of the literature. *Spine*. 1996;21:1746–1760.

Klougart N, LeBoeuf-Y de C, Rasmussen LR. Safety in chiropractic practice. Part I. The occurrence of cerebrovascular accidents following cervical spine adjustment in Denmark during 1978–1988. *J Manipulative Physiol Ther*.1996:19:371–377.

National Market Measures. *The Landmark Report II*. Sacramento, CA: Landmark Healthcare; 1999.

Shekelle PG. *The Use and Costs of Chiropractic Care in the Health Insurance Experiment*. Santa Monica, CA: RAND, 1994.

Massage

CHAPTER 58

The Developing Discipline of Therapeutic Massage

58.1   Utilization Data: Massage Therapy in the United States

American Massage Therapy Association

Americans are turning to therapeutic massage to obtain relief from injuries and certain chronic and acute conditions, to help them deal with the stresses of daily life, and to maintain good health. In a 1998 national survey of consumers by Opinion Research Corporation (ORC), 52% of the 1,007 adults surveyed said they think of massage as therapeutic (ORC, 1998).

The American Massage Therapy Association (AMTA) is a professional organization of more than 44,000 members in 30 countries. The association also helps consumers and medical professionals find qualified, professional massage therapists nationwide, through its *Find A Massage Therapist* national locator service. The free national locator service is available via AMTA's Web site at www.amtamassage.org and toll-free at (888) 843-2682 ((888) THE-AMTA).

Source: This chapter was derived from materials copyrighted by the American Massage Therapy Association® and is published with its permission.

Medical professionals are developing a greater understanding of the efficacy and benefits of massage and are more commonly integrating the services of massage therapists into patient care. According to a national survey conducted by the State University of New York at Syracuse (Grant et al, 1995), 54% of primary care physicians and family practitioners said they would encourage their patients to pursue therapeutic massage as a treatment. Of those, 34% said they are willing to refer the patient to a massage therapist. Some health insurance companies, realizing the cost savings of massage, may cover sessions with a massage therapist when they are a prescribed aspect of treatment. In the 1999 consumer survey by ORC, of the 17% of adults who said they had discussed massage with their doctors, 69% reported that the conversation regarding massage was favorable (ORC, 1999).

PATTERNS OF UTILIZATION

- Consumers spend between $4 and $6 billion annually on visits to massage therapists—approximately 27% of the $21.2 billion spent on complementary health care in 1997 (Eisenberg et al, 1998).
- Consumers visit massage therapists 114 million times each year—approximately 18% of the 629 million annual visits to alternative health care providers (Eisenberg et al, 1998).
- A total of 22% of the adult U.S. population reports having massages in the past 5 years, 13% in the past 12 months (ORC, 1998). Those who seek massage therapy from a trained professional average seven visits per year (InterActive Solutions, 1998).

DEMOGRAPHICS OF USE

- Massage is sought out by large numbers of people in all age brackets (ORC, 1999):

  18–24   24%
  25–34   29%
  35–44   27%
  45–54   31%
  55–64   35%
  Over 65 16%
- In 1998, massage use ranged from 12% to 30% (ORC, 1998).

  - In 1999, massage use in different age cohorts ranged from 16% to 35%, and was most popular among those well educated (35%) and the affluent—people earning $50,000 or more (34%) (ORC, 1999).
  - More women than men used massage therapy (18% compared with 11%) (ORC, 1999).
  - Residents of the West were twice as likely as those of the South to have had a massage in the past 12 months (23% compared to 12%) (ORC, 1999).

USE IN CLINICAL ENVIRONMENTS

- Fifty-four percent of primary care physicians and family practitioners say they would encourage their patients to pursue massage therapy as a complement to medical treatment (Grant et al, 1995).
- Doctors are prescribing massage to help patients manage stress and pain.
- Massage is an important component of physical therapy, sports medicine, and some nursing practices.
- HMO members using complementary and alternative medicine services rate their satisfaction with HMO-defined acupuncture, naturopathic, and massage benefits as high (Weeks, 1998).
- Of the types of alternative care commonly available, people say they would be most likely to use massage therapy (80%), vitamin therapy (80%), herbal therapy (75%), and chiropractic (73%) (InterActive Solutions, 1998).

CONDITIONS THAT MAY BE HELPED BY THERAPEUTIC MASSAGE

An increasing number of research studies show massage reduces heart rate, lowers blood pressure, increases blood circulation and lymph flow, relaxes muscles, improves range of motion, and increases endorphins (enhancing medical treatment). Although therapeutic massage does not increase muscle strength, it can stimulate weak, inactive muscles and, thus, partially compensate for the lack of exercise and inactivity resulting from illness or injury. It also can hasten and lead to a more complete recovery from exercise or injury. People with the following conditions have reported that therapeutic massage has lessened or relieved many of their symptoms:

- arthritis, asthma, headache, circulatory problems, digestive disorders, insomnia, immune function, and stress
- musculoskeletal conditions, including acute and chronic pain, carpal tunnel syndrome, myofascial pain, sports injuries, reduced range of motion, and temporomandibular joint dysfunction (TMJ)

Contraindications include certain forms of cancer, some cardiac problems, infectious diseases, phlebitis, and some skin conditions.

WORK SITE UTILIZATION

• The Touch Research Institutes (TRI) at the University of Miami has documented the positive effects of massage therapy on job performance and stress reduction. The research indicates that a basic 15-minute chair massage, provided twice weekly, results in decreased job stress and significant increase in productivity (Field et al, 1996).
• A growing number of businesses and organizations offer massage in the workplace, including the U.S. Department of Justice, Boeing, Reebok, and a number of Fortune 500 companies, to address musculoskeletal problems, stress, and conditions related to ergonomic stress (Lippin, 1996).

AVAILABILITY OF PRACTITIONERS

• The number of massage therapists is between 150,000 and 190,000, including students (AMTA, 1999).
• AMTA membership has increased three-fold in the 1990s to over 42,000 members (AMTA, 1999).

REFERENCES

American Massage Therapy Association. Market analysis exhibit. Evanston, IL: American Massage Therapy Association; January 1999.

Caravan Opinion Research Corporation International. Public attitudes towards massage study. Princeton, NJ: Opinion Research Corporation International; 1998; 1999.

Eisenberg DM, Davis RB, Ettner SL, et al. Trends in alternative medicine use in the United States, 1990–1997. *JAMA*. 1998;280(18):1569–1575.

Field T, Ironson G, Scafidi F, et al. Massage therapy reduces anxiety and enhances EEG pattern of alertness and math computations. *Int J Neurosci*. 1996;86:197–205.

Grant W, Kamps C, Blumberg D, Hendricks S, Dewan M. The physician and unconventional medicine. *Alternative Ther Health Med*. 1995;1:31–35.

InterActive Solutions. *The Landmark Report on Public Perceptions of Alternative Care*. Sacramento, CA: Landmark Healthcare; 1998.

Lippin RA. Alternative medicine moves into the workplace. *Alternative Ther Health Med*. 1996;2(1):47–51.

Weeks J. First retrospective member survey on HMOs. *St. Anthony's Alternative Med Integration Coverage*. 1998;2(8):1.

58.2   Therapeutic Massage: An Overview of the Discipline

Linda Chrisman

INTRODUCTION

Massage therapy encompasses a wide variety of therapeutic techniques. All include the hands-on manipulation of muscles and soft tissues to prevent and alleviate discomfort, pain, muscle spasm, and stress. Massage can enhance the functioning of all major aspects of physiology—the circulatory, lymphatic, muscular, skeletal, and nervous systems. It also appears to systemically improve the rate at which the body recovers from injury and illness (American Massage Therapy Association [AMTA], 2000).

There are more than 150 variations of massage, bodywork, and somatic therapy techniques (Associated Bodywork and Massage Professionals [ABMP], 2000). Therapeutic massage typically consists of a blend of Swedish massage, neuromuscular massage, and acupressure techniques (Field, 1999). Massage therapists are frequently trained in several different modalities and incorporate these methods, as needed, into their practices. Some techniques emphasize muscle or soft tissue manipulation. Others focus on a nurturing form of touch to relieve suffering. Bodywork may also involve gentle movements that are facilitated by the therapist or are learned by the client as part of a self-care program. In the mind-body methods, massage therapists are trained to facilitate an awareness of the role that emotions play in relation to chronic tension

---

Linda Chrisman, MA, CMT, is an educator, writer, and practitioner with over 20 years of experience in the field of somatic bodywork. A graduate of Stanford University and the California Institute of Integral Studies, she has been certified in a number of disciplines, including Trager therapy and therapeutic massage. Ms. Chrisman practices and teaches in the San Francisco Bay area, where she specializes in Rosen Method bodywork and Continuum Movement, and provides consulting services in the field of integrative medicine.

or pain. Clinical experience suggests that massage is beneficial to a broad range of patients, unless they have a fracture, are recovering from surgery, or have some other type of special needs (AMTA, 2000).

HISTORY

Massage has been used worldwide for thousands of years to promote health and healing. References to massage are found in the Bible, the Vedas of India, and Chinese medical texts more than 4,000 years old (Greene, 2000). In the West, massage was advocated as early as 400 B.C. by Hippocrates. Modern Western massage is credited primarily to Peter Ling, a nineteenth-century Swedish athlete. His approach, which became known as Swedish massage, continues to be one of the most commonly used massage techniques in the Western world.

The first massage therapy clinics in the United States were opened after the Civil War by two Swedish physicians. Between 1880 and 1910, "a considerable number of American physicians used massage in their practices." (Greene, 2000) With the introduction of new medical technologies in the early 1900s, the time-intensive practice of massage was delegated to nurses and assistants. In the 1930s and 1940s, these practitioners also became less interested in massage therapy and increasingly emphasized the use of more technologic forms of treatment. However, massage therapy was still routinely practiced in hospitals throughout the United States until the 1950s (Field, 1999).

MEDICAL BENEFITS

Massage facilitates general physiological responses that enhance health and wellness and promote the healing process, through mechanisms such as improved circulation and the clearing of metabolic wastes. It also provides specific benefits for particular conditions. In addition, massage retains the human factor in the increasingly technologically oriented practice of medicine. Therapeutic massage can be a valuable, cost-effective primary or adjunctive therapy that is compatible with many other medical approaches to treatment (Greene, 2000).

Physiologic Mechanisms

Therapeutic massage has been found to complement certain forms of medical treatment (unless contraindicated) through a number of physiological mechanisms (AMTA, 2000):

- Enhanced immune function, as measured by an increase in natural killer cells (Ironson et al, 1996)
- Increased circulation of blood and movement of lymph fluids (Hollis, 1987)
- Elevated production of endorphins, which act as natural painkillers (AMTA, 2000)
- Decreased stress and improved relaxation as measured by urinary cortisol, norepinephrine, and epinephrine levels (Field et al, 1996)
- Decrease in depression associated with shifts from right frontal EEG activation to left frontal EEG activation (Jones, Field, and Davalos, in press).

Therapeutic Applications

Massage has clinical applications as an adjunctive therapy for a wide range of general conditions, which include:

- Use in the intensive care unit for stress and pain management (Dunn, Sleep, and Collett, 1995)
- Moderation of pain from cancer (Weinrich and Weinrich, 1990)
- Prevention of perineal trauma in childbirth (Labrecque, Marcoux, Pinault et al, 1994)
- Improvement in mother-infant bonding (White-Traut and Nelson, 1988)

- Promotion of faster healing for strained muscles and sprained ligaments (AMTA, 2000)
- Reduction of pain, swelling, and muscle spasms, as well as tension and stiffness (AMTA, 2000)
- Provision of greater joint flexibility and range of motion (AMTA, 2000)
- Enhancement of overall wellness (Field, 1999).

Research and clinical studies indicate improvement in a surprisingly diverse range of conditions and diagnoses, including:

- Anxiety (Sunshine, Field, Schanberg et al, 1996; Field et al, 1992; Field et al, 1996)
- Arthritis: osteoarthritis and rheumatoid arthritis (Greene, 2000)
- Asthma, bronchitis, sinusitis (Field, Henteleff et al, 1998)
- Autism (Greene, 2000)
- Bulemia in adolescents (Field et al, 1998)
- Burn patients (Field, Peck et al, 1998)
- Carpal tunnel syndrome (Greene, 2000)
- Chronic fatigue syndrome (Field, Sunshine et al, 1997)
- Circulatory problems (lymphedema) (Hollis, 1987)
- Depression (Field, 1999)
- Diabetes (Field, Hernandez-Reif, La Greca et al, 1997)
- Digestive disorders: spastic colon, constipation, diarrhea, and nausea (Greene, 2000)
- Fibromyalgia (Sunshine, Field, and Schanberg et al, 1996)
- Headache (Greene, 2000)
- Hypertension (Greene, 2000)
- Insomnia (Greene, 2000)
- Myofascial pain (Hollis, 1987)
- Pain, including chronic pain (Field, Hernandez-Reif, Taylor et al, 1997; Pope, Philips, and Haugh et al, 1994)
- Pregnancy (Field, Hernandez-Reif, Taylor et al, 1997)
- Premature birth: infant massage (Field et al, 1986)
- Premenstrual syndrome (Greene, 2000)

- Restricted range of motion (AMTA, 2000)
- Soft tissue rehabilitation in spinal cord injury patients (Mowen, 2000)
- Sports injuries (Greene, 2000)
- Strained muscles, ligaments (Hollis, 1987)
- Stress (Field, Ironson, Pickens et al, 1996)
- Temporomandibular joint (TMJ) dysfunction (Greene, 2000).

Contraindications

Massage therapists warn of contraindications for massage (Hollis, 1987); however, there is little research that identifies specific contraindications (Field, 1999). It is important to note that, although a rigorous approach such as Swedish massage might be contraindicated for some conditions, a gentle style of touch, such as the Rosen method or acupressure, could be beneficial for the same conditions (Saputo, 2000).

Major contraindications include:

- Advanced heart disease (Greene, 2000)
- Conditions prone to hemorrhage (Greene, 2000)
- High fever (Field, 1999)
- Infectious or contagious skin conditions (Field, 1999)
- Kidney failure (Greene, 2000)
- Low platelet count, because vigorous massage may cause bruising (Field, 1999)
- Tumors and infected lymph nodes (Field, 1999)
- Varicose veins or phlebitis. The concern is that massage might dislodge a blood clot and result in pulmonary embolism. This issue has not been examined through systematic research or case reports (Field, 1999).
- Open wounds or lesions, new scar tissue, and burn areas. Massage is not recommended for fragile healing tissue. However, massage of burn areas with cocoa butter can alleviate itching (Field, 1999). Massage therapy has also been used to reduce anxiety and indirectly reduce pain before and during the painful procedure of debridement (Field, Peck et al, 1998). In addition,

massage that focuses on the tissue that remains intact has been found to ameliorate the general perception of pain (McKinnon, 2000).

RESEARCH

The MEDLINE database of the National Library of Medicine currently includes approximately 5,000 citations on massage. This reflects the major expansion in massage research over the past 20 years. Studies have also been conducted in Europe that have not yet been translated into English (Greene, 2000). Two sources of research on massage in the United States are the Touch Research Institutes (TRI) at the University of Miami School of Medicine and the National Center for Complementary and Alternative Medicine (NCCAM) at the National Institutes of Health (NIH).

Touch Research Institute (TRI)
1400 NW 10th Avenue, Suite 610
Miami, FL 33136
Phone: (305) 243-6781
Web site: http://www.miami.edu/touch-research

TRI has conducted more than 55 studies (published or in review) that evaluate the effects of massage therapy in clinical situations ranging from posttraumatic stress to migraine headache. The Institute works in conjunction with other major universities, including Duke, Harvard, Princeton, and the University of Maryland. An example of the work of TRI is evident in its seminal research on the importance of touch in the development of premature infants. (See Chapter 59 for summaries of their selected clinical findings and a bibliography of published studies.)

National Center for Complementary and Alternative Medicine (NCCAM) at the NIH
NCCAM Clearinghouse
PO Box 8218
Silver Spring, MD 20907-8218
Toll-free phone: (888) 644-6226
Web site: <http://www.nccam.nih.gov>

NCCAM has funded several studies on the benefits of massage, and more research is in progress.

NIH-funded studies on therapeutic massage produced findings on both physiologic mechanisms and clinical outcomes:

- Cortisol levels and blood pressure dropped more quickly in postabdominal surgery patients undergoing massage therapy, compared with controls.
- Cancer patients who received massage therapy while undergoing bone marrow transplant were much less anxious and fatigued.
- HIV-exposed infants who underwent massage therapy fared better than those who did not, in terms of improved weight gain, neonatal performance, and decreased stress behaviors.
- Medical and nursing students under stress who received massage therapy demonstrated increased immune response greater than that of controls, as measured by immunoglobulin levels.

At the time of this writing, the NIH is funding 13 research projects that involve a massage component, including studies that focus on various aspects of back pain, immune function, prostatitis, infant health, and depression in pregnant women.

MEDLINE Database of the National Library of Medicine

The MEDLINE database of the National Library of Medicine is accessed via the PubMed home page. Citations from the peer-reviewed literature can be accessed using the terms *massage* and *therapeutic massage* at http://www.ncbi.nlm.nih.gov.

LICENSING AND TRAINING

Massage therapy is a developing profession. Massage standards, training, and licensure vary greatly from region to region, and there is currently a minimum of professional standardization. However, the positive outcomes experienced in the profession are a testimony to the safety and effectiveness of the discipline. The safety of this practice is reflected in the exceptionally low malpractice rates, which typically range from approximately $200 to $250 per year (McKinnon, 2000; ABMP, 2000; AMTA, 2000).

Licensing

Standards for massage therapists, like those of most other health care professionals, are determined at the state level. Massage is licensed in 29 states and in Washington, DC. In other states, there are no educational requirements, in which case, standards are determined by the city or local municipality. National organizations are not currently in agreement on this issue; some recommend licensure as a minimum requirement, whereas others do not (Field, 1999). When developing credentialing guidelines in a particular region, check with state and city government to obtain the regulations relevant to that jurisdiction (McKinnon, 2000).

Certification

The National Certification Examination is considered a voluntary examination in most states. The National Certification Board for Therapeutic Massage and Bodywork (NCBTMB) administers this examination and certifies massage therapists who successfully pass the exam and maintain their status through continuing education. Due to the variety of diverse approaches within the profession, the exam is limited as a means for evaluating massage therapists. The examination is most relevant to practitioners of classic Swedish massage, rather than to providers of bodywork or somatic education.

Another issue associated with standards development is the determination of requisite classroom education. For potential practitioners with a high school education, 500 hours may be considered a minimum. On the other hand, for professionals trained in another area of health care, such as nursing, 100 classroom hours can provide sufficient training for the development of a highly competent practitioner, because of the additional skills and experience that they bring to the work (McKinnon, 2000).

Accredited Training

Accreditation for schools of massage training is a rigorous process in some states and can involve months of effort to provide the required documentation. However, despite governmental regulatory efforts to assure adequate training, there are currently no consistent national educational standards that define what should be taught and by whom. For example, in some training institutes, experienced massage therapists teach anatomy. In others, anatomy is taught by professionals with a background in nursing, medicine, or chiropractic, who typically provide more in-depth training. These issues are particularly complex for health care organizations

entering the field that desire benchmarks with which to assess the educational background of candidates (McKinnon, 2000).

Standards

These issues are also particularly complex for health care organizations considering the hiring or credentialing of massage therapists. A strategy for defining standards is to develop standards that reflect the level of expertise in the service area. This can be done by contacting the national massage associations, obtaining lists of the insured practitioners in the area, and sending out requests for résumés. Reviewing the credentials of the applicant pool will provide a sense of the range of training and experience available. This enables the organization to set a standard that is high enough to assure quality service provision but does not overly restrict the pool of applicants (which can occur in a rural area, for example) (McKinnon, 2000).

REFERENCES

Associated Bodywork and Massage Professionals (ABMP); Web site http://www.abmp.com; accessed June 2000.

American Massage Therapy Association (AMTA); Web site http://www.amta.com. Accessed June 2000.

Dunn C, Sleep J, Collett D. Sensing an improvement: an experiential study to evaluate the use of aromatherapy, massage, and periods of rest in the intensive care unit. *J Adv Nurs*. 1995;21:34–40.

Field T. Massage therapy. In: *Essentials of Complementary and Alternative Medicine*. Jonas W, Levin J, eds. Baltimore: Lippincott Williams & Wilkins. 1999; 383–391.

Field T, Henteleff T, Hernandez-Reif M, et al. Children with asthma have improved pulmonary function after massage therapy. *J Pediatr*. 1998;132:854–858.

Field T, Hernandez-Reif M, La Greca A, et al. Glucose levels decreased after giving massage therapy to children with diabetes mellitus. *Spectrum*. 1997;10:23–25.

Field T, Hernandez-Reif M, Taylor S, et al. Labor pain is reduced by massage therapy. *J Psychosom Obstet Gynecol*. 1997;18:286–291.

Field T, Ironson G, Pickens J, et al. Massage therapy reduces anxiety and enhances EEG pattern of alertness and math computations. *Int J Neurosci*. 1996;86:197–205.

Field T, Peck M, Krugman S, et al. Massage therapy effects on burn patients. *J Burn Care Rehabil*. 1998;19:241–244.

Field T, Schanberg S, Cafidi F, et al. Tactile/kinesthetic stimulation effects on preterm neonates. *Pediatrics*. 1986;77:654–658.

Field T, Schanberg S, Kuhn C, et al. Bulimic adolescents benefit from massage therapy. *Adolescence*. 1998;33(131); 555–563.

Field T, Sunshine W, Hernandez-Reif M, et al. Chronic fatigue syndrome: massage therapy effects on depression and somatic symptoms in chronic fatigue syndrome. *J Chronic Fat Syndrome*. 1997;3:43–51.

Greene E. Massage therapy. In: *Clinician's Complete Reference to Complementary and Alternative Medicine*, Novey D, ed. St. Louis: Mosby; 2000:338–348.

Hollis N. *Massage for Therapists*. Oxford, England: Blackwell Publishers; 1987.

Ironson G, Field T, Scafidi F, et al. Massage therapy is associated with enhancement of the immune system's cytotoxic capacity. *Int J Neurosci*. 1996;84:205–218.

Jones N, Field T, Davalos M. Massage attenuates right frontal EEG asymmetry in one-month-old infants of depressed mothers. *Infant Behav Dev*. In press.

Labrecque M, Marcoux S, Pinault JJ, et al. Prevention of perinatal trauma by perineal massage during pregnancy: a pilot study. *Birth*. 1994;21:20–25.

McKinnon J. McKinnon Institute. Oral communication, May 2000.

Mowen K. Spinal cord injuries and soft tissue rehabilitation. *Massage Bodywork*. Feb/March 2000;36–44.

Pope MH, Philips RB, Haugh LD, et al. A prospective randomized three-week trial of spinal manipulation, transcutaneous muscle stimulation, massage and corset in the treatment of subacute low back pain. *Spine*. 1994;19:2571–2577.

Saputo L. Oral communication, July 2000.

Sunshine W, Field T, Schanberg S, et al. Massage therapy and transcutaneous electrical stimulation effects on fibromyalgia. *J Clin Rheumatol*. 1996;2:18–22.

Weinrich SP, Weinrich MC. The effect of massage on pain in cancer patients. *Appl Nurs Res*. 1990;3:140–145.

White-Traut RC, Nelson MN. Maternally administered tactile, auditory, visual, and vestibular stimulation: relationship to later interactions between mothers and premature infants. *Res Nurs Health*. 1988;11:31–39.

58.3   Resources in the Discipline of Massage Therapy

Linda Chrisman

NATIONAL ASSOCIATIONS

There are currently two primary national associations and numerous others that focus on specific techniques or populations within the field of massage. The two national associations are ABMP and AMTA. During the past decade, membership has doubled for the major professional bodywork organizations. These associations can assist health care organizations in locating trained, qualified massage therapists.

Associated Bodywork and Massage Professionals (ABMP)

1271 Sugarbush Drive
Evergreen, CO 80439-7347
Toll-free phone: (800) 458-2267
Fax: (303) 674-0859
Email: expectmore@abmp.com
MassageFinder, a referral service at no cost, a toll-free phone: (800) 458-2267

ABMP is a professional membership association founded in 1987 to provide massage, bodywork, and somatic therapy practitioners with professional services, information, and regulatory advocacy. Its current membership totals over 31,000. Members must meet educational requirements and adhere to a published code of ethics. Benefits include:

- Assistance in locating products, equipment, and services, including a directory of resources and a resource guide to professional training for practitioners
- Information and publications on marketing and operating a business successfully
- Comprehensive liability insurance and other member benefits
- Member certification
- Member referrals available to the public and to prospective employers at no cost

American Massage Therapy Association (AMTA)

820 Davis Street, Suite 100
Evanston, IL 60201-4444
Phone: (847) 864-0123
Fax: (847) 864-1178
Email: info@inet.amtamassage.org
Web site: http://www.amtamassage.org
Find a Massage Therapist[SM] provides referrals at (847) 864-0123 or at the Web site (click on *Find a Massage Therapist*)

AMTA has more than 42,000 members in over 20 countries. The association sets practice standards and ethics for the professional and has certification programs for sports massage therapists. Requirements for membership include:

- Graduation from a training program accredited or approved by the Commission on Massage Training Accreditation (COMTA), which requires at least 500 hours of classroom instruction
- An appropriate current city, state, or provincial license, or
- Certification by the NCTMB

International Massage Association and National Association of Massage Therapy

3000 Connecticut Avenue NW, Suite 102
Washington, DC 20008
Phone: (202) 387-6555
Fax: (800) 776-NAMT.

ASSOCIATIONS WITHIN THE FIELD OF MASSAGE AND BODYWORK

Craniosacral Therapy

The Upledger Institute
11211 Prosperity Farms Road, Suite D-325
Palm Beach Gardens, FL 33410-3487
Phone: (800) 233-5880

Geriatric Massage

Day-Break Geriatric Massage Project
Phone: (317) 722-9896

Infant Massage

International Association of Infant Massage
1891 Goodyear Avenue, Suite 622
Ventura, CA 93003
Phone: (800) 248-5432

Rolfing®

Guild for Structural Integration
PO Box 1559
Boulder, CO 80306-1559
Phone: (303) 447-0122 or (800) 447-0150

Rosen Method

Rosen Method, The Berkeley Center
825 Bancroft Way
Berkeley, CA 94710

Phone: (510) 845-6606
The Rosen Method Professional Association (practitioner referrals)
Phone: (800) 893-2622

Shiatsu

American Oriental Bodywork Therapy Association
1010 Haddonfield Berlin Road
Kirkwood Voorhees, NJ 08043
Phone: (856) 782-1616

Trager Psychophysical Integration

The Trager Institute
21 Locust Avenue
Mill Valley, CA 94941
Phone: (415) 388-2688
Web site: http://www.trager.com

BOOKS

Overviews

Claire T. *Bodywork.* New York: William Morrow; 1995.
Knaster M. *Discovering the Body's Wisdom.* New York: Bantam Books; 1996.
Montague A. *Touching: the Human Significance of Skin.* 3rd ed. New York: Harper & Row; 1986.

Texts

Beck MF. *Milady's Theory and Practice of Therapeutic Massage.* 3rd ed. Albany, NY: Milady Publishing; 1999.
Burch S. *Recognizing Health and Illness: Pathology for Massage Therapists.* Lawrence, KS: Health Positive Publications; 1997.
Chaitow LJ. *Soft Tissue Manipulation.* Wellingborough: Thornsons; 1988.
Field T. *Touch.* Cambridge, MA: Harvard University Press; 1997.
Fritz S. *Mosby's Fundamentals of Therapeutic Massage.* 2nd ed. St. Louis: Mosby-Year Book; 1999.
Hollis M, Jones E, Watt J, Wamner J. *Massage for Therapists.* 2nd ed. Oxford, England: Blackwell Scientific Publications;, 1998.

Loving JE. *Massage Therapy: Theory and Practice*. Stamford, CT: Appleton & Lange; 1998.

Lowe W. *Fundamental Assessment in Massage Therapy*. 3rd ed. Bend, OR: Orthopedic Massage Education and Research Institute; 1997.

Manheim CJ. *The Myofascial Release Manual*. 2nd ed. Thorofare, NJ: Slack; 1994.

Tappan F, Benjamin P. *Tappan's Handbook of Healing Massage Techniques*. 3rd ed. Englewood Cliffs, NJ: Prentice Hall; 1998.

Werner R, Benjamin B. *A Massage Therapist's Guide to Pathology*. Baltimore: Lippincott Williams & Wilkins; 1998.

Mind-Body Practices

Johnson DH, ed. *Bone, Breath, and Gesture: Practices of Embodiment*. Berkeley, CA: North Atlantic Books; 1995. Interviews and chapters from the innovators and practitioners of mind-body massage and bodywork.

Keleman S. *Emotional Anatomy: The Structure of Experience*. Berkeley, CA: Center Press; 1985. The seminal text on the expression of mind and emotions in the body.

Periodicals

Massage and Bodywork Quarterly, from American Bodywork and Massage Professionals
Phone: (303) 674-8478
See also the preceding entry for ABMP.

Massage Therapy Journal, from American Massage Therapy Association
Phone: (847) 864-0123; also see the preceding entry for AMTA.

Touchpoints, from Touch Research Institute, Department of Pediatrics (D-820)
University of Miami School of Medicine
PO Box 016820
Miami, FL 33101
The quarterly publication of the Touch Research Institute, which reviews its current research and that of other research institutions; annual subscription for $10
Phone: (305) 243-6781

58.4   Perspective: The Applications of Massage in Mind-Body Medicine

Len Saputo

In modern culture, psychotherapy is almost the norm. Despite the fact that many people apply therapy to their lives diligently and even achieve a deeper understanding of their psycho-

Len Saputo, MD, is founder and President of the Health Medicine Forum, a nonprofit public educational foundation that has linked more than 2,500 practitioners. The Forum's Web site address is <http://www.healthmedicine.com>. He is also president of <AlternativeHealth.com>, a Web site that provides cybercast presentations on complementary therapies.

Courtesy of Len Saputo, MD, Walnut Creek, California.

logical issues, they often remain "stuck in their heads," unable to change unhealthy behavior patterns significantly.

This dilemma is relevant not only to the individuals who suffer these conditions, but also to the health care systems that fund their treatment. We must find a better way to relieve emotional pain and suffering and must do this cost-effectively.

The major underlying premise of "mind/body medicine" is that mind and body are inseparably connected. They each represent a perspective of the whole person and provide a window through which we can gain important information. By considering the body and mind in tandem, we create a golden opportunity to learn how they influence one another and how they collectively affect our health.

THE MIND-BODY DYNAMIC

Whenever we experience an event, we simultaneously respond both physically and emotionally. Our body posture and breathing mechanics are affected in a measurable way by every emotional response we have. Put simply, we develop "holding patterns" that persist long after the conscious mind has forgotten the original experience—they reflect the physical (somatic) manifestations of persisting emotional residues.

One of the types of treatment that appears to be the most effective in releasing these "stored-in-the-body" experiences is bodywork—certain forms of massage and breathwork. An experienced bodywork practitioner can detect the client's holding patterns and carefully guide him/her through the remembering process. By releasing tense areas through massage or trigger-point therapy and breathing exercises, long-forgotten experiences often surge into conscious awareness.

This style of body-mind medicine releases tensions and can help to bring about a greater sense of physical well-being. It also assists the client in dealing with the impact of physical (somatic) and emotional residues, which can be re-experienced in the present, at a time later in life when the individual is better equipped to deal with their impact.

The "felt" meaning of earlier emotional traumas may be re-lived during bodywork sessions. Getting "out of one's head" and into an experiential state can provide the opportunity to face emotional issues that could not be dealt with when they originally occurred. This type of bodywork reconnects the individual with his or her fundamental nature and core personality in a way that is very therapeutic and growth enhancing.

Bodywork is not in itself psychotherapy. There are numerous disciplines within the fields of bodywork that train practitioners in both counseling and massage. These include the "somatic therapies," such as Rosen Method bodywork and Rolfing®. Another useful approach is for a bodyworker and a psychologist to work together. However, there is an ever-growing trend in modern health care to integrate both approaches into a single therapy. Psychologists are beginning to incorporate massage into the scope of their practices, and bodyworkers are being trained to bring psychology into their practices.

For patients who feel stuck with their psychological and/or physical health issues, this integrative style of therapy can provide a simple and powerful adjunct to standard medical treatment. The proper application of mind-body strategies as early in the disease process as possible minimizes both human suffering and health care expenditures over the long term.

58.5   Case Study: The Role of Massage in Trauma Care

Judith McKinnon and Robyn Scherr

In February 2000, the McKinnon Institute had the honor of providing trauma support for Alaska Airlines employees following the crash of Flight 261. With short notice, a team of professional McKinnon massage therapists was able to recruit and organize the needed personnel to provide emergency therapeutic services to employees.

The role of our team in the trauma support was informed by the training we had received from two professional massage instructors on the Institute staff. Mark Bitzer had provided posttrauma massage for rescue workers responding to the Oklahoma City bombing. Maureen Manley had traveled several times to Croatia, teaching massage and dance in the aftermath of the first round of major civil conflict in the former Yugoslavian republic.

The lessons they learned through these intense interventions and the team's experience with the Alaska Airlines crash have provided insight into the issues massage therapists may face when entering a trauma environment. These experiences provide the basis for future strategies in the provision of massage therapy in crisis situations.

Judith McKinnon is Director of the McKinnon Institute of Professional Massage in Oakland, California, which she founded in 1973. She has served as a gubernatorial appointee to the Physical Therapy Examining Committee, and she successfully drafted and lobbied for legislation on behalf of over 2,000 vocational schools in California.

Robyn Scherr is a freelance writer who worked for 10 years as a graphic designer and technical writer before becoming a massage therapist. She holds certifications in four massage disciplines, and the work of her private practice includes a focus on working with trauma.

Source: Adapted with permission from J. McKinnon, Touching Grief When Disaster Strikes, *Massage & Bodywork*, Vol. 15, No. 2, pp. 102–106, © 2000, Massage & Bodywork Magazine.

THE VALUE OF MASSAGE THERAPY IN TRAUMA SITUATIONS

After the Oklahoma City bombing, massage therapists worked in a volunteer capacity to provide massages to exhausted rescue workers and numbed survivors (Bitzer, 2000). Health care professionals have reported benefit when massage has been made available in crisis situations, such as the San Francisco earthquake of 1986. Volunteer professionals also provided services to traumatized communities following Hurricane Andrew. The literature indicates that children who experienced the trauma of the hurricane were especially responsive to the provision of professional massage services (Field et al, 1996). As educators and clinicians in the field of massage therapy, our perception is that touch may be one of the most immediate needs for many people in moments of trauma. The sense of touch tends to be a grounding experience. Massage is also valuable because it can prepare people to receive the benefits of counseling or psychotherapy. In the context of trauma, the availability of professional massage allows psychological needs to be addressed with an immediate, practical, and effective approach.

The Client and the Team

We must also remember that there are many avenues of healing and that no one approach or combination will work for every client all of the time. When presented with particularly jarring, traumatic, or overwhelming circumstances, our usual modes of coping may not be what we most need. In a crisis situation, we may not recognize what we require to heal.

For this reason, experience suggests that it is best, whenever possible, to provide a variety of modalities at trauma sites. The provision of multiple types of expertise is both practical and effective in such situations. Psychotherapists, clergy, massage therapists, and others have complementary skills in dealing with people experiencing and recovering from trauma. It is when working together within our scopes of practice that we are able to do the greatest good.

Specifics of Working with Trauma Clients

People who have been exposed to a disaster or significant trauma frequently experience great distress. How individuals handle their stress, however, may vary significantly. Some may be quite composed; others are visibly shaken and fragile. Their initial presentation is an invaluable indicator in deciding whether and how to work with a particular client. It is by no means the only one. Particularly in trauma situations, the client's emotions may shift quickly during a session, and a massage practitioner must keep a close eye on client reactions. If the client appears to be overwhelmed, becoming emotionally withdrawn, or has unusual responses to the intervention, it is completely appropriate to stop the session and explore the best avenues to address the client's needs in the moment. As massage therapists, we must recognize that we are not rescue workers, psychotherapists, or religious counselors. Sometimes, the greatest good we can do for our clients is to help them find what they need at that particular time or the most appropriate redress to their immediate needs.

Informed Consent and Personal Boundaries

Following the Alaska Airlines crash, staff from the McKinnon Institute provided massage services at two airline facilities to a range of employees, from mechanics to supervisors, in all stages of grief. Many had worked their entire scheduled off-duty time since the crash. Some of the airline staff had been on duty in Seattle, Anchorage, or Portland, and were then flown to the Bay Area to provide support and to pick up the extra workload. They were all physically exhausted and emotionally strained, and had hours or days to go before they would have the time to relax and reflect on the past week's events.

For many of our clients, this was their first massage. This brought up the issue of informed consent. It is always essential that a client give consent, because touch involves fundamental personal boundaries. In this charged atmosphere, working with people who had not experienced therapeutic touch, we were especially thorough in our explanations and inquired frequently about clients' comfort levels.

Individualizing the Treatment

We worked with members of the airline staff to provide the support they needed so they felt alert, contained, and able to perform their jobs without being overwhelmed. For some, that meant vigorous and superficial sports massage, for others, slow, deep-tissue release or subtle energy work.

Teamwork in the Trauma Environment

Working in teams was invaluable. Not only were we able to see more clients than a practitioner working alone, but we were also able to support each other. This helped us to maintain our professional boundaries, so we were better able to assist our clients. Maintaining our professional, compassionate distance allowed us to observe our clients more accurately and to treat them appropriately and effectively. Working in teams also allowed us to take breaks. It was tempting to work straight through our shifts, but we all realized that we were much more valuable to our clients when we took the time we needed to nourish and refresh ourselves.

Criteria for Working in Trauma Situations

When working in trauma situations, professional massage therapists ideally:

- Identify the support systems that are in place in order to coordinate with other professionals on site, as appropriate.

- Obtain informed consent for any modality they practice. For massage therapists, it is important to remember that clients may not be familiar with the terms and practices of the therapy and may need more careful explanations.
- Remember that client needs and emotions can shift quickly in a trauma situation. The provider must be prepared for sudden changes that might require a different approach.
- Proceed slowly and provide clear transitions. Clients in trauma situations have experienced abrupt changes in their lives. It is best to allow them to become accustomed to touch.
- Stay grounded and maintain good boundaries. Massage providers may encounter many strong emotions in a highly charged atmosphere and will be able to do their best work if they maintain their center.

It has become apparent in the last decade that therapeutic massage has much to offer health care. The work of the Touch Research Institutes on posttraumatic stress in children indicates the relevance of massage to the needs of individuals who have experienced trauma (Field et al, 1996). Our experience with the Alaska Airlines disaster affirms this benefit. Therapeutic massage also has meaningful applications for the trauma of hospital workers (Field, Quintino, Henteleff et al, 1997), combat exposure, fire fighting, and law enforcement. Other populations for whom this approach is relevant include victims of physical and sexual abuse (Field et al, 1997), and battered women and children. Research and clinical experience indicate that, for many types of problems and conditions, touch is the missing link in the healing process. It is apparent that massage has a major contribution to make in the health of our society and in health care delivery.

REFERENCES

Bitzer M. McKinnon Institute of Professional Massage. Oral communication, May 2000.

Field T, Quintino O, Henteleff T, Wells-Keife L, Delvecchio-Feinberg G. Job stress reduction therapies. *Altern Ther Health Med*. 1997;3:54–56.

Field T, Seligman S, Scafidy F, Schanberg S. Alleviating post traumatic stress in children following hurricane Andrew. *J Appl Dev Psychol*. 1996;17:37–50.

58.6   Definitions: Massage and Bodywork

Vickie S. Ina and Linda Chrisman

Within the professional massage therapy community, the distinction is made between massage, bodywork, energy therapies, and movement therapies. This list of definitions, although not exhaustive, includes techniques that may not traditionally be thought of as massage. However, all of these disciplines have value as adjunctive and primary therapies. They reflect the broad range of mind-body approaches that utilize the therapeutic benefits of touch and movement.

BASIC TECHNIQUES

Swedish Massage—The most common form of massage, which focuses on relaxing muscles

Source: Portions of this chapter have been adapted from Vickie Ina, Emeryville, California.

and easing aches and pains for increased freedom of movement and better posture.

Esalen Massage—A more relaxed form of massage, emphasizing long-flowing strokes for deep relaxation, nurturance, and sensate awareness.

Sports Massage—A technique similar to Swedish and deep-tissue massage, adapted to address the effects of athletic performance on the body. The goals include warmup, improved range of motion and muscle flexibility, increased circulation, increased nutrients and oxygen to the tissue, and enhanced elimination of metabolic byproducts. Sports massage also therapeutically addresses muscle cramping, tears, bruising, aches, spasms, pain, and edema.

ACUPRESSURE AND PRESSURE-POINT THERAPIES

Acupressure—A technique that involves the surface stimulation of acupressure points digitally, manually, or with tools held in the hand. Acupressure massage is used to promote the flow of Qi or chi (pronounced chee) through the meridian system. Other related therapies include Jin Shin Do® and Jin Shin Jyutsu®.

Reflexology—Variation of pressure-point therapy applied to external reflex points that are believed to correspond to various areas of the body. Points on the feet, hands, or ears are massaged to bring about general healing.

Shiatsu—A Japanese technique whose name literally means "finger-pressure treatment," which restores energy to the body. There are several styles of this approach, including Zen Shiatsu, Oha Shiatsu, and Amma Therapy, a Korean variation.

Touch for Health—A combination of acupressure touch, applied kinesiology, and massage.

Trigger-Point or Myotherapy—This method involves specific finger or thumb pressure on release points in the muscles and connective tissue to relieve pain and referred pain patterns, hypersensitivity and muscle spasms, stiffness or loss of movement, and inflammation. Applica-

tions of trigger-point therapy include treatment of sports injuries and chronic back pain.

Tuina (Tui Na Tsang)—Focuses specifically on visceral massage for various digestive disorders.

DEEP-TISSUE TECHNIQUES

Deep-Tissue Massage—Releases the chronic patterns of tension in the body through slow strokes and deep finger pressure on contracted areas, either following or massaging across the grain of muscles, tendons, and fascia, with primary focus on the deeper layers of muscle tissue. Rolfing® is perhaps the best-known method of deep-tissue massage.

Aston-Patterning—A somatic education method, including deep-tissue bodywork, that analyzes patterns of movement to identify areas of ease and discomfort in order to teach people how to live more optimally in their bodies.

Hakomi Integrative Somatics—A mind-body education method that combines movement, body awareness, and touch to address physical and emotional trauma.

Hellerwork—A form of deep-tissue bodywork that also includes movement education and guided verbal dialogue. Hellerwork was developed from Rolfing.®

Lomi Method—A form of bodywork that includes deep-tissue massage, as well as Gestalt therapy, mindfulness meditation techniques, and breath work.

Myofascial Release—The use of deep-tissue massage in which long-stretching strokes are used to facilitate the release of chronic muscular tensions in the fascia that may be restricting posture, movement, and circulation.

Neuromuscular Therapy—A method to balance the nervous and musculoskeletal systems and relieve pain and dysfunction. Trigger-point massage and myotherapy are related forms.

Rolfing® (Structural Integration)—A form of deep-tissue work and movement education for reordering the body so as to bring its major segments—head, shoulder, thorax, pelvis, and legs—into a finer alignment with gravity.

ENERGY THERAPIES

Energy Therapies—Certain forms of healing in traditional cultures focus on the vital energy or life force of the body, including electric, magnetic, and electromagnetic fields. Acupressure, like acupuncture, is believed to affect the flow of energy along electromagnetic pathways called *meridians*. Other forms of energy therapy, such as therapeutic touch, do not use physical touch but are intended to affect the energy field around the body.

Polarity Therapy—A system of bodywork that integrates the holding of pressure points and gentle stretching to balance the energy systems of the body.

Reiki—A simple laying-on-of-hands technique to balance the energy systems of the body.

Therapeutic Touch—A method developed by nurses and derived from the laying-on of hands, which does not involve direct contact with the body. This technique is also known as the Krieger-Kunz Method of Therapeutic Touch.

MASSAGE FOR SPECIFIC POPULATIONS

Geriatric Massage—A gentle form of massage therapy adapted to the specific physiologic needs of older (and in some cases, frailer) people.

Infant Massage—Gentle techniques intended to promote bonding between parent and infant and to accustom a young child to the positive aspects of touch. Research indicates that massage is essential to proper human development (see Chapter 59).

On-Site Massage—Back and neck massage performed with the client seated in a specially designed massage chair, fully clothed. This type of massage can be provided at the work site or other public environments.

Pre- and Postnatal Massage—Gentle techniques for pregnant mothers and newborns.

MIND-BODY TECHNIQUES (SOMATIC THERAPIES)

Somatic Therapy is a generic term that includes touch and movement therapies. Thomas Hanna originated the phrase to distinguish Hanna somatics and other mind-body approaches from massage.

Alexander Technique®—A method in which new patterns of movement and posture are taught through coaching, verbal cues, and touch. The goal is to develop and maintain a more effective alignment of the head, neck, and back to improve overall physical and emotional functions.

Body-Mind Centering—A method that includes touch, movement, guided imagery, developmental repatterning, and dialogue to release restrictive habits of movement. This technique has been shown to be effective in the rehabilitation of injuries and neuromuscular disorders.

Continuum Movement—A method that involves sound, breath, and subtle movement to disrupt habitual movement patterns and facilitate new movement possibilities. This therapy is particularly effective in rehabilitation from spinal cord injury and a variety of other neuromuscular conditions.

Feldenkrais Method®—A method of gentle touch that involves movement reeducation to improve posture and flexibility and alleviate muscular tension and pain. Feldenkrais has proved to be effective for a wide variety of conditions.

Hanna Somatics®—A method that involves slow-motion movement to improve muscular control and enable the client to better locate, sense, and gain control of muscles in various areas of the body.

Somatic Experiencing—A noninvasive somatic education method that includes touch, imagery, movement, and dialogue to access and integrate deeply held emotional or physical trauma.

Rosen Method®—This approach uses gentle touch and verbal exchange between practitioner and client to draw the client's attention to areas in which tension is held chronically. This can facilitate the release of muscular tension and, in some cases, suppressed emotions.

Trager®—A technique that utilizes rhythmic rocking movements to relax the body and the mind.

Zero Balancing—A method for aligning body structure and energy.

MOVEMENT THERAPIES

Pilates (Physical-Mind Method)—A series of nonimpact exercises designed by Joseph Pilates to develop strength, flexibility, balance, and inner awareness.

Qigong (Chi gung)—Forms of ancient Chinese practice that incorporate breath, slow movement, visualization, and meditation to stimulate health and healing.

T'ai Chi—A type of Qigong based on Taoist principles of health that involves a series of slow, relaxed, fluid movements.

Yoga—Movement and postures achieved through gradual stretching and breath practice that promote stamina, circulation, flexibility, and healing, developed in the Indian culture more than two millennia ago.

SPECIFIC THERAPEUTIC TECHNIQUES

Craniosacral Therapy—A therapy that involves gentle, noninvasive touch by the practitioner to enhance functioning of the cerebrospinal system by identifying and releasing critical points of restriction. In adults, the therapy often focuses on the relationship of the skull to the spine. In infants, therapy may also focus on the subtle relationship of the cranial plates and the effects of birth trauma.

Manual Lymph Drainage—A gentle, whole-body massage to stimulate lymphatic flow and decrease edema.

Ortho-bionomy™—A gentle technique that guides the body into comfortable positions that encourage the spontaneous release of muscular tension.

BIBLIOGRAPHY

American Massage Therapy Association (AMTA); Web site http://www.AMTAmassage.com. Accessed May 2000.

Kaptchuk T. *The Web that Has No Weaver: Understanding Chinese Medicine*. New York: Congdon and Weed; 1992.

Knaster M. *Discovering the Body's Wisdom*. New York: Bantam Books; 1996.

Murray M, Pizzorno J. *Encyclopedia of Natural Medicine, Revised*. Sacramento, CA: Prima Publishing; 1997.

CHAPTER 59

Research on the Benefits of Therapeutic Massage

59.1 Research on the Effectiveness of Massage
Tiffany M. Field
59.2 Bibliography: Research by the Touch Research Institutes
Tiffany M. Field

59.1   Research on the Effectiveness of Massage

Tiffany M. Field

INTRODUCTION

The Touch Research Institutes (TRI) at the University of Miami School of Medicine is the first center in the world devoted entirely to the scientific study of touch and its application in the fields of science and medicine. Since 1982, TRI's team of researchers, representing Harvard, Princeton, Duke, McGill, and the University of Maryland, has explored the connection between touch therapy and the effective treatment of disease. Their work continues to demonstrate that touch therapy has significant beneficial effects on human well-being. Specifically, massage has been shown to encourage a wide range of healing benefits, by reducing stress hormones, encouraging weight gain in premature infants, alleviating depression, decreasing pain, and enhancing the immune response.

CURRENT STUDIES

Pediatric Pain Management

The crippling effects of pain are associated with diseases such as cancer and juvenile rheumatoid arthritis. However, relatively little research has been conducted on pediatric pain management. Traditionally, treatment relies on the use of medications that alter the body's biochemistry, but pediatricians are understandably reluctant to prescribe potentially addictive drugs to children. As a result, children with juvenile arthritis are given anti-inflammatory drugs to reduce pain. Massage is now being evaluated as an alternative therapy because of its capacity to

Tiffany M. Field is Director of the Touch Research Institutes (TRI) at the University of Miami School of Medicine. She is recipient of the American Psychological Association Boyd McAndless Distinguished Young Scientist Award and has received a Research Scientist Award from the National Institute of Mental Health for her research career. Dr. Field is the author of *Infancy* (Harvard University Press, 1990), *Touch Therapy* (Churchill Livingston, 2000), and numerous other books, as well as more than 350 journal articles. She has also served as the editor of a series of volumes on high-risk infants and another series on stress and coping.

Courtesy of Tiffany Field, Miami, Florida.

increase serotonin levels with the potential to mediate pain. Researchers are evaluating the use of massage to offset the need for addictive pain medications (Field et al, 1997).

Treatment for Newborns

Child abuse, neglect, and drug exposure during pregnancy continue to proliferate and are related to behavioral problems, depression, anxiety, and poor interpersonal relationships among children. TRI has recruited retired volunteers to massage premature, drug-exposed, and failure-to-thrive newborns. The results suggest that it may be as beneficial to touch as to be touched. The volunteers showed a significant decrease in depression, increased feelings of self-worth, improved sleep patterns, and fewer doctor visits, while the children were more responsive following the treatment program (Field et al, 1998).

Treatment for HIV Patients

HIV-positive men were evaluated to determine the effects of massage therapy on the immune system. After 45 minutes of massage therapy, 5 days a week for a month, their anxiety and stress levels were decreased. Of even greater significance were the findings of enhanced immune response. Participants' natural killer cell counts increased, providing increased protection against opportunistic infections such as pneumonia (Ironson et al, 1996).

Alertness and Anxiety

Massage therapy has been found to reduce anxiety. In a study involving cognitive processing, researchers observed enhanced EEG patterns of alertness and improved math computation (Field et al, 1996a). Twenty-six adults were given chair massage and 24 control group adults were asked to relax in the massage chair for 15 minutes, two times a week for 5 weeks. On the first and last days of the study, they were monitored with an EEG before, during, and after

the sessions. Before and after the sessions, participants completed questionnaires regarding life events and job stress, completed the POMS Chronic Depression Scales, and performed math computations. In addition, they were evaluated for biochemical markers of stress by testing saliva samples for cortisol levels. Statistical analyses revealed the following:

- Frontal delta power increased for both groups, suggesting relaxation.
- The massage group showed decreased frontal alpha and beta power (suggesting enhanced alertness) while the control group showed increased alpha and beta power.
- The massage group showed increased speed and accuracy on math computations while the control group did not change.
- Anxiety levels were lower following the massage, but not following the control sessions; however, mood state was less depressed following both the massage and control sessions.
- On the first day only, salivary cortisol levels were lower following the massage, but not following the control sessions.
- At the end of the 5-week period, depression scores were lower for both groups, but job stress scores were lower only for the massage group.

Asthma

Children with asthma were found to have improved pulmonary functions after massage therapy (Field et al, 1998a). Thirty-two children with asthma (sixteen 4- to 8-year-olds and sixteen 9- to 16-year-olds) were randomly assigned to receive either massage therapy or relaxation therapy. The children's parents were taught to provide one therapy or the other for 20 minutes before bedtime each night for 30 days. The younger children who received massage therapy showed an immediate decrease in behavior anxiety and cortisol levels after massage. Also, their attitude toward asthma and their peak air flow and other pulmonary functions improved over the course of the study. The older children who received massage therapy reported lower anxiety after the massage. Their attitude toward asthma also improved over the study, but only one measure of pulmonary function improved (forced respiratory flow from 25% to 75%). The reason for the smaller therapeutic benefit in the older children is unknown; however, it appears that daily massage improves airway caliber and control of asthma.

Bulimic Adolescents Benefit from Massage Therapy

Twenty-four female adolescent bulimic inpatients were randomly assigned to a massage therapy or a standard treatment (control) group (Field et al, 1998c). Results indicated that the massaged patients showed immediate reductions in anxiety and depression (both self-report and behavior observation). In addition, by the last day of the therapy, they had lower depression scores, lower cortisol levels (reflecting decreased stress), higher dopamine levels, and showed improvement on several other psychological and behavioral measures. These findings suggest that massage therapy is effective as an adjunct treatment for bulimia.

Burn Injuries Improved with Massage Therapy

Twenty-eight adult patients with burns were randomly assigned before debridement to either a massage therapy group or a standard treatment control group (Field et al, 1998b). In the massage group, levels of anxiety and cortisol decreased, and behavior ratings, activity, vocalizations, and anxiety improved after the massage therapy sessions on the first and last days of treatment. Longer-term effects were also significantly better for the massage therapy group, including decreases in depression and anger, and decreased pain on the McGill Pain Questionnaire, the Present Pain Intensity scale, and a Visual Analogue Scale. Although the underlying mechanisms are not known, these data suggest

that debridement sessions were less painful after the massage therapy sessions due to a reduction in anxiety, and that the clinical course was probably enhanced as the result of a reduction in pain, anger, and depression.

Massage Stimulates Growth in Preterm Infants

Forty preterm infants (average gestational age = 30 weeks; mean birth weight = 1,176 g; mean duration intensive care = 14 days) were assigned to treatment and control groups once they were considered medically stable. Assignments were based on a random stratification of gestational age, birthweight, intensive care duration, and study entrance weight. The treatment infants (N = 20) received tactile/kinesthetic stimulation for three 15-minute periods per day for a 10-day period. Sleep/wake behavior was monitored and Brazelton assessments were performed at the beginning and at the end of the treatment period. The treated infants averaged 21% greater weight gain per day (34 g versus 28 g) and were discharged 5 days earlier. No significant differences were demonstrated in sleep/wake states and activity levels between the groups. The treated infants' performance was superior on the habituation cluster items of the Brazelton scale. The treatment infants were also more active during the stimulation sessions than during the non-stimulation observation sessions (particularly during the tactile components of the sessions) (Scafidi et al, 1990).

Massage Therapy for Infants and Children with Medical Conditions

Studies were reviewed regarding the effects of massage therapy on infants with a variety of conditions including premature birth, cocaine exposure, HIV infection, and parenting by depressed mothers (Field, 1994). Additional childhood conditions reviewed included abuse (sexual and physical), asthma, autism, burns, cancer, developmental delays, dermatitis (psoriasis), diabetes, eating disorders (bulimia), juvenile rheumatoid arthritis, posttraumatic stress disorder, and psychiatric problems. Generally, massage therapy resulted in lower anxiety, decreases in stress hormones, and improved clinical course. Studies that trained parents, grandparents, and volunteers to provide the massage found that the therapy enhanced the wellness of the caregiver and provided cost-effective treatment for the children.

Migraine Headaches Can Be Reduced by Massage Therapy

Twenty-six adults with migraine headaches were randomly assigned to a wait-list control group or to a massage therapy group, who received two 30-minute massages per week for five consecutive weeks (Hernandez-Reif et al, 1998a). The massage therapy subjects reported fewer distress symptoms, less pain, more headache-free days, fewer sleep disturbances, and increased serotonin levels.

Multiple Sclerosis Patients Benefit from Massage Therapy

Twenty-four adults with multiple sclerosis were randomly assigned to a standard medical treatment control group or a massage therapy group that received 45-minute massages twice a week for 5 weeks (Hernandez-Reif et al, 1998b). The massage group had lower and less depressed mood immediately following the massage sessions and, by the end of the study, they had improved self-esteem, better body image, less negative image of disease progression, and enhanced social functional status.

Preschool Children's Sleep and Wake Behavior

In this study, preschool children received 20-minute massages twice a week for 5 weeks (Field et al, 1996b). They were evaluated after the massage sessions on the first and last days of the study. The behavior of the children who received massage was compared with children in the wait-list (the control) group. The massaged children had better behavior ratings on general state of well-being, vocalization, activity, and cooperation. Their behavior had also improved by the end of the study, according to ratings by their teachers. At the end of the 5-week period, parents rated their children as having less aversion to touch and more extraverted behaviors.

Nicotine Cravings Are Reduced by Hand or Ear Massage

Attempts at smoking cessation have been correlated with severe withdrawal symptoms, including intense cigarette cravings, anxiety, and depressed mood (Hernandez-Reif et al, 1999). Twenty adult smokers (mean age = 32.6 years) were randomly assigned to a self-massage treatment or a control group. The treatment group was taught to conduct a hand or ear self-massage during three periods of cravings each day for 1 month. Self-reports revealed lower anxiety scores, improved mood, and fewer withdrawal symptoms. In addition, by the last week of the study, the self-massage group smoked fewer cigarettes per day than participants in the control group. The present findings suggest that self-massage may be an effective addition to smoking cessation programs to alleviate smoking-related anxiety, reduce cravings and withdrawal symptoms, improve mood, and reduce smoking.

CONCLUSION

Studies conducted at TRI have documented the impressive benefits of massage therapy:

- Premature infants who receive early massage therapy continue to do better at 6 to 8 months follow-up.
- HIV-positive patients experience immune enhancement and increases in natural killer cell function.
- Individuals with chronic pain may require less medication due to the release of serotonin, a pain-alleviating substance.

As the scientific community continues to investigate alternatives to conventional therapies, ongoing research regarding touch therapies becomes even more vital. This research has shown clearly that touch therapy can play an important role in treating diverse medical conditions.

REFERENCES

Field T. Massage therapy for infants and children. *J Dev Behav Pediatr.* 1994;16:105–111.

Field T, Henteleff T, Hernandez-Reif M, et al. Children with asthma have improved pulmonary functions after massage. *J Pediatr.* 1998a;152:854–858.

Field T, Ironson G, Scafidi F, et al. Massage therapy reduces anxiety and enhances EEG pattern of alertness and math computations. *Int J Neurosci.* 1996a;86:197–205.

Field T, Kilmer T, Hernandez-Reif M, Burman I. Preschool children's sleep and wake behavior: effects of massage therapy. *Early Child Dev Care.* 1996b;120:39–40.

Field T, Peck M, Krugman S, Tuchel T, Schanberg S, Kuhn C, Burman I. Burn injuries benefit from massage therapy. *J Burn Rehabil.* 1998b;19:241–244.

Field T, Schanberg S, Kuhn C, et al. Bulimic adolescents benefit from massage therapy. *Adolescence.* 1998c;131:555–563.

Hernandez-Reif M, Dieter J, Field T, Swerdlow B, Diego M. Migraine headaches are reduced by massage therapy. *Int J Neurosci.* 1998a;96:1–11.

Hernandez-Reif M, Field T, Field T, Theakston H. Multiple sclerosis patients benefit from massage therapy. *J Bodywork Movement Ther.* 1998b;2(3):168–174.

Hernandez-Reif M, Field T, Hart S. Smoking cravings are reduced by self-massage. *Prev Med.* 1999;28:28–32.

Ironson G, Field T, Scafidi F, et al. Massage therapy is associated with enhancement of the immune system's cytotoxic capacity. *Int J Neurosci.* 1996;84:205–218.

Scafidi F, Field TM, Schanberg S. Massage stimulates growth in preterm infants: a replication. *Infant Behav Dev.* 1990;13:167–188.

59.2   Bibliography: Research by the Touch Research Institutes

Tiffany M. Field

PUBLISHED RESEARCH

Effects of Touch on Infants and Preterm Neonates

Cigales M, Field T, Lundy B, Cuadra A, Hart S. Massage enhances recovery from habituation in normal infants. *Infant Behav Dev.* 1997;20:29–34.

Field T, Grizzle N, Scafidi F, Abrams S, Richardson S. Massage therapy for infants of depressed mothers. *Infant Behav Dev.* 1996;19:109–114.

Field T, Hernandez-Reif M, Quintino O, Schanberg S, Kuhn C. Elder retired volunteers benefit from giving massage therapy to infants. *J. Appl Gerontol.* 1998;17:229–239.

Field T, Malphurs J, Carraway K, Pelaez-Nogueras M. Carrying position influences infant behavior. *Early Child Dev Care.* 1996;121:49–54.

Field T, Scafidi F, Schanberg S. Massage of preterm newborns to improve growth and development. *Pediatr Nurs.* 1987;13:385–387.

Field T, Schanberg S, Bauer C, Tucci K, Roberts J, Morrow C, Kuhn CM. Massage stimulates growth in preterm infants: a replication. *Infant Behav Dev.* 1990;13:167–188.

Field T, Schanberg S, Scafidi F, et al. Tactile/kinesthetic stimulation effects on preterm neonates. *Pediatrics.* 1986;77:654–658.

Pauk J, Kuhn C, Field T, Schanberg S. Positive effects of tactile versus kinesthetic or vestibular stimulation on neuroendocrine and ODC activity in maternally deprived rat pups. *Life Sci.* 1986;39:2081–2087.

Pelaez-Nogueras M, Gewirtz JL, Field T, et al. Infant preference for touch stimulation in face-to-face interactions. *J Appl Dev Psychol.* 1996;17:199–213.

Prodromidis M, Field T, Arendt R, Singer L, Yando R, Bendell D. Mothers touching newborns: a comparison of rooming-in versus minimal contact. *Birth.* 1995;22:196–200.

Scafidi F, Field T. HIV-exposed newborns show inferior orienting and abnormal reflexes on the Brazelton Scale. *J Pediatr Psychol.* 1997;22:105–112.

Scafidi F, Field T, Schanberg S, Bauer C, Vega-Lahr N, Garcia R. Effects of tactile/kinesthetic stimulation on the clinical course and sleep/wake behavior of preterm neonates. *Infant Behav Dev.* 1986;9:91–105.

Scafidi F, Field T, Wheeden A, et al. Cocaine-exposed preterm neonates show behavioral and hormonal differences. *Pediatrics.* 1996;97:851–855.

Touch in Pregnancy and Labor

Field T, Hernandez-Reif M, Hart S, Theakston H. Pregnant women benefit from massage therapy. *J Psychosom Obstet Gynecol.* 1999;20:31-38.

Field T, Hernandez-Reif M, Taylor S, Quintino O, Burman I. Labor pain is reduced by massage therapy. *J Psychosom Obstet Gynecol.* 1997;18:286–291.

Touch in Postpartum Depression

Field T, Grizzle N, Scafidi F, Schanberg S. Massage and relaxation therapies' effects on depressed adolescent mothers. *Adolescence.* 1996;31(124):903–911.

Lundy BL, Field T, Cuadra A, Nearing G, Cigales M, Hashimoto M. Mothers with depressive symptoms touching newborns. *Early Dev Parenting.* 1996;5:124–130.

Malphurs J, Raag T, Field T, Pickens J, Pelaez-Nogueras M. Touch by intrusive and withdrawn mothers with depressive symptoms. *Early Dev Parenting.* 1996;5:111–115.

Pelaez-Nogueras M, Field T, Hossain Z, Pickens L. Depressed mothers' touching increases infants positive affect and attention in still-face interactions. *Child Dev.* 1996;67:1780–1792.

The Needs of Children and Adolescents

Field T, Harding J, Soliday B, Lasko D, Gonzalez N, Valdeon C. Touching in infant, toddler and preschool nurseries. *Early Child Dev Care.* 1996;126:101–110.

Field T, Henteleff T, Hernandez-Reif M. Children with asthma have improved pulmonary functions after massage therapy. *J Pediatr.* 1998;132:854–858.

Field T, Hernandez-Reif M, LaGreca A, Shaw K, Schanberg S, Kuhn C. Massage therapy lowers blood glucose levels in children with diabetes mellitus. *Diabetes Spectrum.* 1997;10:237–239.

Field T, Hernandez-Reif M, Seligman S, et al. Juvenile rheumatoid arthritis: benefits from massage therapy. *J Pediatr Psychol.* 1997;22:607–617.

Field T, Kilmer T, Hernandez-Reif M, Burman I. Preschool children's sleep and wake behavior improve after massage therapy. *Early Child Dev Care.* 1997;120:39–44.

Field T, Lasko D, Mundy P, Henteleff T, Talpins S, Dowling M. Autistic children's attentiveness and responsivity improve after massage therapy. *J Autism Dev Disord.* 1997;27:333–338.

Field T, Morrow C, Valdeon C, Larson S, Kuhn C, Schanberg S. Massage therapy reduces anxiety in child and adolescent patients. *J Am Acad Child Adolesc Psychiatry.* 1992;31:125–130.

Field T, Quintino O, Hernandez-Reif M, Koslovsky G. Attention deficit hyperactivity disorder adolescents benefit from massage therapy. *Adolescence.* 1998;33:103–108.

Field T, Seligman S, Scafidy F, Schanberg S. Alleviating posttraumatic stress in children following Hurricane Andrew. *J Appl Dev Psychol.* 1996;17:37–50.

Field T, Shanberg S, Kuhn C, et al. Bulimic adolescents benefit from massage therapy. *Adolescence.* 1997;33:131.

Hernandez-Reif M, Field T, Krasnegor J, Martinez E. Cystic fibrosis symptoms are reduced with massage therapy intervention. *J Pediatr Psychol.* 1999;24:183–189.

Schachner L, Field T, Hernandez-Reif M, Duarte A, Krasnegor J. Atopic dermatitis symptoms decrease on children following massage therapy. *Pediatr Dermatol.* 1998;15:390–395.

The Effects of Touch on Specific Conditions

Field T. American adolescents touch each other less and are more aggressive toward their peers as compared with French adolescents. *Adolescence.* 1999;34:753–758.

Field T. Preschoolers in America are touched less and are more aggressive than preschoolers in France. *Early Child Dev Care.* 1999;151:11–17.

Field T, Hernandez-Reif M. Sleep problems in infants decrease following massage therapy. *Early Child Dev Care.* In press.

Field T, Hernandez-Reif M, Hart S, et al. Sexual abuse effects are lessened by massage therapy. *J Bodywork Movement Ther.* 1997;1:65–69.

Field T, Ironson G, Scafidi F, et al. Massage therapy reduces anxiety and enhances EEG pattern of alertness and math computations. *Int J Neurosci.* 1996;86:197–205.

Field T, Peck M, Krugman S, et al. Burn injured benefit from massage therapy. *J Burn Care Rehabil.* 1997;19:241–244.

Field T, Quintino O, Henteleff T, Wells-Keife L, Delvecchio-Feinberg G. Job stress reduction therapies. *Alternative Ther Health Med.* 1997;3:54–56.

Field T, Sunshine W, Hernandez-Reif M, et al. Chronic fatigue syndrome: massage therapy effects on depression and somatic symptoms in chronic fatigue syndrome. *J Chronic Fatigue Syndrome.* 1997;3:43–51.

Hart S, Field T, Hernandez-Reif M, Lundy B. Preschoolers' cognitive performance improves following massage. *Early Child Dev Care.* 1998;143:59–64.

Hernandez-Reif M, Field T, Dieter J, Swerdlow B, Diego M. Migraine headaches are reduced by massage therapy. *Int J Neurosci.* 1998;96:1–11.

Hernandez-Reif M, Field T, Hart S. Smoking cravings are reduced by self massage. *Prev Med.* 1999;28:28–32.

Hernandez-Reif M, Field T, Theakston H. Multiple sclerosis patients benefit from massage therapy. *J Bodywork Movement Ther.* 1998;2:168–174.

Ironson G, Field T, Scafidi F, et al. Massage therapy is associated with enhancement of the immune system's cytotoxic capacity. *Int J Neurosci.* 1996;84:205–218.

Jones NA, Field T. Right frontal EEG asymmetry is attenuated by massage and music therapy. *Adolescence.* 1999;34:529–534.

Sunshine W, Field T, Schanberg S, et al. Massage therapy and transcutaneous electrical stimulation effects on fibromyalgia. *J Clin Rheumatol.* 1996;2:18–22.

PART XV

Clinical Nutrition

CHAPTER 60

The Field of Clinical Nutrition

60.1 Utilization and Effectiveness Data: Nutritional Supplements and Clinical Nutrition

Nancy Faass

The use of clinical nutrition in the United States is increasing and is reflected in the greater utilization of vitamin supplements.

- A study performed at Cornell University estimated sales for dietary supplements in the United States for 1997 at approximately $11.8 billion with a projected growth rate of 10% to 14% (Nesheim, 1999).
- Data from the Food and Drug Administration collected in 1995 indicate that more than 55% of adults surveyed used some type of dietary supplement (Yetley and Park, 1995).
- Another survey conducted in 2000 at the Centers for Disease Control and Prevention (CDC) found that approximately 40% of the 11,000 respondents surveyed had taken vitamins in the past month (Balluz et al, 2000).

Data from the U.S. nutrition industry indicate 1999 sales for natural products to be $28.2 bil-

As nutritional science has developed, so have its clinical applications. Clinical nutrition was initially limited to treating general malnutrition and specific nutritional deficiency states. In the past two decades, the field has gradually broadened to include the treatment of subclinical deficiencies and dependencies as well as the provision of nutrients as pharmacological agents. Scientific justification for an expanded definition of clinical nutrition has been considerably strengthened since that time. Laboratory tests can provide evidence of inadequate nutrition despite the lack of clinical findings of classical nutritional deficiency syndromes. Even in the absence of laboratory validation of nutritional deficiencies, numerous studies utilizing rigorous scientific designs have demonstrated impressive benefits from nutritional supplementation. It is now well established, for example, that nutritional factors are of major importance in the pathogenesis of both atherosclerosis and cancer and many other diseases

Melvyn Werbach, MD, 1996

Nancy Faass, MSW, MPH, is a writer and editor in San Francisco who provides book and project development.

Note: The author wishes to thank *Nutrition Business Journal* of San Diego and *Natural Foods Merchandiser* of Boulder, Colorado, for data and information, and Paul Saunders, ND, for reviewing portions of the manuscript.

lion. This amount encompasses money spent on dietary supplements such as vitamins and minerals, herbal/botanical products, sports nutrition, meal supplements, and specialty products, as well as natural and organic food and personal care products. A five-year summary of the nutrition industry reflects continuous growth in most all sectors (see Tables 60.1–1 and 60.1–2).

These products are marketed through a wide range of channels. The largest sector is the natural products retailers whose sales represent approximately 50% of the market (Traynor, 2000, p.1).

Growth in the sale of natural products in major sectors in 1999 included:

- natural products retailers—49%
- mass market outlets—28%
- multilevel marketers—16%
- Internet—0.5%
- mail order—4%
- direct sale by practitioners—4%

Table 60.1–1 U.S. Nutrition Industry 1994–1999, Products

Products	1994*	1995*	1996*	1997**	1998**	1999**
Vitamins	$3.9 B	$4.3 B	$4.7 B	$5.3 B	$5.6 B	$5.8 B
Herbs/Botanicals	2.0 B	2.5 B	3.0 B	3.5 B	4.0 B	4.1 B
Sports Nutrition	900 M	990 M	1.1 B	720 M	760 M	790 M
Mineral Supplements	690 M	800 M	890 M	1.1 B	1.1 B	1.3 B
Meal Supplements	450 M	560 M	590 M	1.7 B	1.8 B	2.0 B
Specialty/Other Products	670 M	750 M	920 M	980 M	1.2 B	1.5 B
Total Supplements	8.6 B	9.8 B	11.2 B	13.3 B	14.5 B	15.4 B

Source: Adapted with permission from the *Nutrition Business Journal*, San Diego, California, © 1999.

*Source: Nutrition Business International, LLC. Unpublished data; written communication, J. Martens, 8/00; (c) 1999.

**Source: Nutrition Business Journal. Annual Industry Overview 2000;V(7/8).4. Note that industry figures for 1997 and 1998 were recalculated at that time.

Table 60.1–2 U.S. Nutrition Industry 1994–1999, Channels. Figures include the above products and also natural/organic food, functional foods, and natural personal care products.

Sales Channels	1994*	1995*	1996*	1997**	1998**	1999**
Retail-Health Food Stores	8.0 B	9.1 B	10.3 B	11.6 B	12.5 B	13.5 B
Retail-Mass Market	3.8 B	4.4 B	5.2 B	19.9 B	22.0 B	23.9 B
Mail Order	650 M	740 M	810 M	970 M	1.0 B	1.0 B
Multilevel Marketing	3.5 B	3.8 B	4.0 B	4.5 B	4.8 B	4.9 B
Practitioner	360 M	500 M	640 M	810 M	870 M	1.0 B
Internet				20 M	60 M	170 M
Totals***	16.4 B	18.6 B	21.0 B	37.8 B	41.6 B	44.5 B

Source: Adapted with permission from the *Nutrition Business Journal*, San Diego, California, © 1999.

*Source: Nutrition Business International, LLC. Unpublished data; written communication, J. Martens, 8/00; (c) 1999.

**Source: Nutrition Business Journal. Annual Industry Overview 2000;V(7/8).4. Note that industry figures for 1997 and 1998 were recalculated at that time.

***Totals on sales channels reflect entire nutrition industry, which includes natural/organic food, functional foods, and natural personal care products.

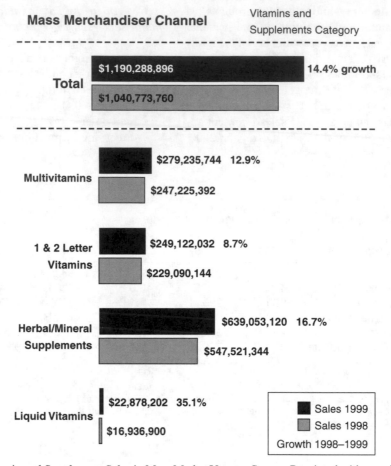

Figure 60.1–1 Vitamin and Supplement Sales in Mass Market Venues. *Source:* Reprinted with permission from *Natural Foods Merchandiser*, June 2000, p. 35, © 2000, New Hope Communications.

The rapid growth of this industry is occurring in most sectors and channels. One of the fastest growing channels for the sale of nutritional supplements is mass market outlets, which experienced sales growth in vitamin and supplement sales of 44% in 1998 and 14.4% in 1999 (see Figure 60.1–1).

RESEARCH ON SUPPLEMENT USE

The National Health and Nutrition Examination Survey

A retrospective evaluation of massive U.S. federal data looked at the use of dietary sup-

plements in the United States. The Third National Health and Nutrition Examination Survey, 1988–1994 (NHANES III) (1998) is a nationally representative survey of the civilian, noninstitutionalized U.S. population, 2 months of age or over. Participants were surveyed regarding their use of vitamin and/or mineral supplements in the past month and other dietary supplements as well. The survey found that approximately 40% of the population interviewed took dietary supplements during the month prior to the interview. Higher levels of education, income, and self-reported health status were all positively related to supplement use. During that period, 67% of supplement users took only one supplement, the majority of them taking a combination vitamin/mineral product (46%). The demographic pattern of usage during that period was:

- females (44%)
- males (35%)
- non-Hispanic Whites (43%)
- non-Hispanic Blacks (30%)
- Mexican Americans (29%).

CDC Study: Americans' Use of Vitamins

In order to determine how common vitamin and mineral supplementation is in the United States, researchers from the Centers for Disease Control (CDC) reevaluated the national use of supplements as reported in NHANES III (Balluz et al, 2000). More than 11,000 respondents reported taking at least one vitamin or mineral supplement within the previous 30 days—a number judged to be equivalent to 40% of the U.S. population. The most common vitamins taken include vitamin C (ascorbic acid), vitamin B_1 (thiamin), vitamin B_2, vitamin B_3 (niacin), vitamin B_6 (pyroxidine), vitamin B_{12} (cobalamin), folate (folic acid), vitamin E, vitamin A, and vitamin D. The Division of Environmental Hazards and Health Effects at the CDC in Atlanta, Ga., noted that at least 300 nonvitamin and nonmineral products were also reportedly taken. More women (57%) than men (43%) took supplements. In the past few years, folic acid supplements have been encouraged among women of childbearing age to reduce the likelihood of their bearing children with neural tube defects. This study found that women were more likely to take these supplements than men were, particularly women of childbearing age (20 to 49 years). The researchers note that Americans spend up to $1.7 billion each year on vitamins and minerals.

British Cohort Study of Supplement Use by Women

Research data from a British study focused on the use of dietary supplements by women (Kirk et al, 1999). The study reviewed patterns of diet and lifestyle for 13,822 subjects from the U.K. Women's Cohort Study (8,409 who used supplements and 5,413 who did not). Essentially, supplement users tended to eat a better diet; had higher intakes of all nutrients, except for fat and vitamin B_{12}; tended to be vegetarian; consumed more fruit and vegetables; were more physically active; and had a lower alcohol intake. Supplement use was less likely in respondents with a body mass index above 25 and those who reported smoking regularly. The study concluded that supplement use is associated with a healthier lifestyle and an adequate nutrition intake.

DATA ON COST AND EFFECTIVENESS OF NUTRITION

Supplemental Calcium for the Prevention of Hip Fracture*

The cost-effectiveness of daily calcium supplementation for the prevention of primary osteoporotic hip fractures was assessed using raw data (Bendich et al, 1999) from clinical trials and the National Health and Nutrition Examination Survey (NHANES, 1998). The metanalysis was based on the published relative risk estimates from three double-blind, placebo-controlled clinical trials (Chapuy et al, 1992; Reid et al, 1995; Dawson-Hughes et al, 1997) and the analysis of NHANES data on the daily intake of calcium supplements by adults in the United States. These data were then used to estimate the preventable proportion of hip fractures. The National Hospital Discharge Survey (1995) database provided the number and demographic characteristics of patients discharged with a primary diagnosis of hip fracture.

The 1990 itemized costs of hip fractures, as estimated by the U.S. Office of Technology As-

---

*Source: Adapted by permission of Excerpta Medica, Inc. from A. Bendich et al., Supplemental calcium for the prevention of hip fracture: Potential health-economic benefits, *Clinical Therapeutics,* Vol. 21, No. 6, pp. 1058, Copyright 1999 by Excerpta Medica, Inc.

sessment, were inflated to 1995 dollars using the medical care component of the Consumer Price Index. Using these inflated itemized costs, researchers then estimated the weighted average expenditures, reflecting both the types of services associated with specific hospital discharge destinations and the demographic characteristics of discharged patients. The cost of supplements containing 1,200 mg/day of elemental calcium for the mean duration (34 months) of the three clinical trials was calculated on the basis of 1998 unit-price and market-share data for six representative products.

For 1995, the data indicate that 290,327 patients aged 50 years or older were discharged from U.S. hospitals with a primary diagnosis of hip fracture, at an estimated direct cost of $5.6 billion. Based on the risk reductions seen in three clinical trials, it is estimated that almost half of the hip fractures are avoidable among individuals 50 years or older through the preventive use of calcium supplementation. Nationwide, there are an estimated 134,764 hip fractures and $2.6 billion in direct medical costs that could have been avoided if individuals aged 50 years or older consumed approximately 1,200 mg of supplemental calcium per day. Additional savings could be expected because this intervention is also associated with significant reductions in the risk for all nonvertebral fractures.

Comparing the cost of calcium with the expected medical savings from hip fractures avoided, it is cost-effective to preventively provide 34 months of calcium supplementation to all women aged 75 years or older. If, as the published studies suggest, shorter periods of supplementation result in an equivalent reduction in the risk of hip fractures, calcium supplementation becomes cost-effective for all adults aged 65 years or older. The data support the value of encouraging older adults to increase their intake of dietary calcium and to consider taking a daily calcium supplement. Even small increases in the usage rate of supplementation are predicted to reduce the morbidity and mortality associated with hip fracture at an advanced age and yield significant savings.

Medical Nutrition Therapy: Estimated Costs and Savings*

Longitudinal data from Group Health Cooperative of Puget Sound (Seattle, Wash.) were analyzed to assess the effects of medical nutrition therapy on members aged 55 years and older (Sheils et al, 1999). The subjects were health plan members who had diabetes (N = 12,308), cardiovascular disease (N = 10,895), or renal disease (N = 3,328), including Medicare beneficiaries enrolled in the plan's Medicare risk contract program and who had coverage for medical nutrition therapy services.

A retrospective analysis evaluated the differences in health care utilization levels of members who received medical nutrition therapy and those who did not, including those with diabetes, cardiovascular disease, and renal disease. Utilization was tracked per quarter for hospital discharges, physician visits, and other outpatient visits. Medical nutrition therapy was defined as services that assessed the nutrition status of a client, followed by provision of nutrition therapy, ranging from diet modification to the administration of enteral or parenteral nutrition. Although in general, Medicare does not reimburse for this type of therapy, Medicare Part B will reimburse for medically necessary nutrition care when ordered by a physician and delivered under a physician's supervision.

There is evidence in the medical literature that medical nutrition therapy can reduce morbidity and improve health outcomes for patients with diabetes and various types of cardiovascular disease. Fishbein (1985) concluded that poor diabetes control (including poor diet compliance) accounts for 44% to 54% of hospital admissions for this condition. Conversely, nutritional interventions have been documented to provide both health benefit and cost savings:

---

*Source: J.F. Sheils, R. Rubin and D.C. Stapleton, Medical Nutrition Therapy: Estimated Costs and Savings, Copyright The American Dietetic Association. Adapted by permission from *Journal of the American Dietetic Association*, Vol. 99, No. 4, pp. 428–435, © 1999.

- In weight reduction, including medical nutrition therapy for obese men and women, it has been associated with savings on prescription drug costs (Collins and Anderson, 1995).
- Coronary heart disease has been shown in a number of randomized control trials to respond to medical nutrition interventions, with a drop in mortality (Appel et al, 1997; Kannel, 1986). In one study, a 47% reduction in the incidence of coronary heart disease was observed for the intervention group studied over a 5-year (Hjermann et al, 1986).
- Studies also indicate that diet therapy can substantially lower patient blood pressure and effect reductions in the amount of medication needed in the treatment of hypertension. As a result, the cost of treatment was decreased, and the potential for side effects was reduced (Langford et al, 1985; Kaplan, 1983). In this study, differences in health care utilization were tracked and analyzed using multivariate regression models. Analysis of the data indicated a reduction in the utilization of health care services by patients receiving medical nutrition therapy.

This analysis showed that medical nutrition therapy was associated with:

- A reduction in use of hospital services
  —9.5% for patients with diabetes
  —8.6% for patients with cardiovascular disease
- A reduction in use of physician services
  —23.5% for patients with diabetes
  —16.9% for patients with cardiovascular disease
- No statistically significant impact for patients with renal disease.

Instituting such a program would potentially result in savings after the third year of the program. After an initial period of implementation, coverage for medical nutrition therapy could yield a net reduction in health services utilization and costs for at least some populations. In the case of persons aged 55 years and older, the savings in utilization of hospital and other services will actually exceed the cost of providing the medical nutrition benefit. These results suggest that coverage of this therapy has the potential to pay for itself by reducing the utilization of services.

LARGE STUDIES ON DIET

The Relationship between Nutritional Intake and Health

Enhanced Longevity. The positive effects of diet were the focus of a review that looked at the diet and health of more than 42,000 women in the Breast Cancer Detection Demonstration Project, with follow-up after five years. Participants were initially scored for their intake of fruits, vegetables, whole grains, low-fat dairy, and lean meats and poultry and then their general health status was tracked. Risk of fatal disease was reduced by 30% among the 20,000 women who followed this diet most closely (Kant et al, 2000).

Protective Effects of Fruits and Vegetables. Another study of interest looked at protective effects of green and yellow vegetables among more than 38,000 atomic bomb survivors in Japan. Consuming green-yellow vegetables two to four times a week was found to cut the risk of bladder cancer by almost 40%. A diet that included fruit cut risk as much as 40% to 50%. Chicken in the diet was associated with decreased risk to some degree. The consumption of the other dietary items, including meat and green tea, was not found to be related to risk. "The findings add to evidence that high consumption of vegetables and fruit are protective against bladder cancer" (Nagano et al, 2000).

Increased Risk Associated with Consumption of Red Meat. Eating red meat appears to cause an increase in the incidence of cancer. Recent research in Milan, Italy, evaluated the effects of diet in more than 10,000 hospital cases of cancer, compared with the health histories of approximately 8,000 other hospital patients who were cancer-free. Red meat consumption (seven or more times a week) was estimated to increase the risk of cancer by 50% or more for stomach, rectal, pancreatic, and bladder cancers. For colon cancer, the risk was almost doubled (risk ratio 1:9). For breast cancer, risk increased by approximately 20% and for ovarian cancer, by about 30%. No major differences were found due to age or gender (Tavani et al, 2000).

The Role of Carbohydrates in Weight Gain and in Heart Disease. A team of Harvard researchers tracked the effect of carbohydrates in the diet on weight gain and heart disease over a 10-year period, monitoring the diet and health of over 75,000 women, 38 to 63 years of age. The participants had no prior history of heart disease, stroke, or diabetes. The risk of heart disease was found to be "directly associated" with a diet high in carbohydrate content. Rather than categorizing foods as simple and complex carbohydrates, researchers rated carbohydrates on the Glycemic Index. Carbohydrates high on the Index tend to trigger greater release of insulin. Foods low on the Glycemic Index are metabolized more slowly and tend to be insulin-sparing. Over the course of the study, 761 cases of heart disease developed. Consumption of a diet high in carbohydrates was found to double the risk of heart attack in the top 40% of participants, with even greater risk among the top 20%. Researchers reported associations between high glycemic load, obesity, insulin resistance, and coronary heart disease (Liu et al, 2000).

Major Risk Factors Associated with Heart Disease. The Framingham Study was initiated in 1948 using a prospective epidemiological approach in order to investigate what was then an epidemic of coronary disease in the United States. Insights were provided into the prevalence, incidence, clinical spectrum, predisposing factors, and major risk factors for coronary disease, stroke, peripheral artery disease, and heart failure. The research served to dispel clinical misconceptions regarding hypertension, dyslipidemia, atrial fibrillation, and glucose intolerance. Diabetes was shown to operate more strongly in women, eliminating their advantage over men. Suboptimal values (and their relationship to cardiovascular disease) were established for a range of biochemical and physiological factors, including blood lipids, blood pressure, body weight, glucose, and fibrinogen. Seminal understandings regarding cholesterol and cholesterol fractions were established through this longitudinal study:

- Serum total cholesterol was shown to derive its atherogenic potential from its LDL component and also to reflect cholesterol being removed in the HDL fraction.
- The total HDL-cholesterol ratio was demonstrated to be the most efficient lipid profile for predicting coronary disease.
- High triglycerides associated with reduced HDL, indicating insulin resistance and small dense LDL, were shown to be associated with excess coronary disease.

All the risk factors tended to cluster, and this was shown to be promoted by insulin induced by weight gain. Multivariate risk profiles were produced in order to facilitate risk stratification of candidates for coronary disease, stroke, peripheral artery disease, and heart failure. The Framingham Study is now engaged in quantifying the independent contributions of homocysteine, Lp(a), insulin resistance, small dense LDL, C reactive protein, clotting factors, and genetic determinants of cardiovascular disease. It is now possible to estimate the lifetime risk of all the atherosclerotic cardiovascular disease outcomes (Kannel, 2000)

CONCLUSION

The availability of data from extended longitudinal studies and large populations provides the basis for a new level of sophistication in the science of nutrition. These data make possible more precise and targeted intervention in the prevention and treatment of chronic and degenerative disease. Paired with lifesyle intervention programs, they expand the range of interventions in the field of clinical nutrition.

REFERENCES

Appel LJ, Moore TJ, Obrzanek E, et al. A clinical trial of the effects of dietary patterns on blood pressure. *N Engl J Med.* 1997;336:1117–1124.

Balluz LS, Kieszak SM, Philen RM, Milimare J. Vitamin and mineral supplement use in the United States: Results from the third National Health and Nutrition Examination Survey. *Arch Fam Med.* 2000;9(3):258–262.

Bendich A, Leader S, Muhuri P. Supplemental calcium for the prevention of hip fracture: Potential health-economic benefits. *Clin Ther.* 1999;21(6):1058–1072.

Chapuy M, Arlot M, Duboeuf F, et al. Vitamin D_3 and calcium to prevent hip fractures in elderly women. *N Engl J Med.* 1992;327:1637–1642.

Collins RW, Anderson JW. Medication cost savings associated with weight loss for obese non-insulin-dependent diabetic men and women. *Prev Med.* 1995;24:369–374.

Dawson-Hughes B, Harris S, Krall E, Dallal G. Effect of calcium and vitamin D supplementation on bone density in men and women 65 years of age or older. *N Engl J Med.* 1997;337:670–676.

Fishbein HA. Precipitants of hospitalization in insulin-dependent diabetes mellitus (IDDM): A statewide perspective. *Diabetes Care.* 1985:8(Suppl 1):61–64.

Hjermann I, Holme I, Leren P. Oslo study diet and anti-smoking trial: Results after 102 months. *Am J Med.* 1986:80(2A):7–11.

Kannel WB. The Framingham Study: Its 50-year legacy and future promise. *J Atheroscler Thrombosis.* 2000;6(2): 60–66.

Kannel WB. Nutritional contributors to cardiovascular disease in the elderly. *J Am Geriatr Soc.* 1986:34(1): 27–36.

Kant AK, Schatzkin A, Graubard BI, Schairer C. A prospective study of diet quality and mortality in women. *JAMA.* 2000;283(16):2109–2115.

Kaplan NM. Non-drug treatment of hypertension. *Ann Intern Med.* 1983:102:359–373.

Kirk SF, Cade JE, Barrett JH, Conner M. Diet and lifestyle characteristics associated with dietary supplement use in women. *Public Health Nutr.* 1999:2(1):69–73.

Langford HG, Blaufox MD, Oberman A, et al. Dietary therapy slows the return of hypertension after stopping prolonged medication. *JAMA.* 1985:253:657–664.

Liu S, Willett WC, Stamfer MJ, et al. A prospective study of dietary glycemic load, carbohydrate intake, and risk of coronary heart disease in women. *Am J Clin Nutr.* 2000;71(6):1455–1461.

Nagano J, Kono S, Preston DL, et al. Bladder-cancer incidence in relation to vegetable and fruit consumption: A prospective study of atomic-bomb survivors. *Int J Cancer.* 2000;86(1):132–138.

National Health and Nutrition Examination Survey 1988–1994. Public use data. Hyattsville, MD: U.S. Department of Health and Human Services; 1998.

National Hospital Discharge Survey. Public use data. Hyattsville, MD: U.S. Department of Health and Human Services, 1995.

Nesheim MC. What is the research base for the use of dietary supplements? *Public Hlth Nutr.* 1999;2(1):35–38.

Reid I, Ames R, Evans M, et al. Long-term effects of calcium supplementation on bone loss and fractures in postmenopausal women: A randomized controlled trial. *Am J. Med.* 1995:98:331–335.

Sheils JF, Rubin R, Stapleton DC. The estimated cost and savings of medical nutrition therapy: The Medicare population. *J Am Diet Assoc.* 1999;99(4):428–435.

Tavani A, La Vecchia C, Gallus S, et al. Red meat intake and cancer risk: A study in Italy. *Int J Cancer.* 2000;86(3):425–428.

Traynor M. Natural products market tops $28 billion. *Natural Foods Merchandiser.* 2000;XXI(6):1, 21.

Werbach M. *Nutritional Influences on Illness: A Sourcebook of Clinical Research*, 2nd ed. Tarzana, CA: Third Line Press; 1996.

Yetley EA, Park YK. Diet and heart disease: Health claims. *J Nutr.* 1995;5(3 Suppl):679S–685S.

60.2   Resources in Clinical Nutrition

Nancy Faass

The field of clinical nutrition encompasses an enormous amount of information. For example, in MEDLINE there are more than 20,000 entries just under the single term "ascorbic acid." One strategy to become familiar with this field is to begin with an overview such as is found in the *Textbook of Nutritional Medicine* by Melvyn Werbach, MD. Once a foundational understanding of clinical nutrition has been established, knowledge can be kept current through a monthly audiotape such as *Functional Medicine Updates* by Jeffrey Bland, PhD. The following publications provide a foundation and ongoing updates in clinical nutrition, based on the peer-reviewed medical literature.

BOOKS

Reviews of the Clinical Research

The Work of Melvyn Werbach, MD

Melvyn Werbach, MD, compiles and summarizes the peer-reviewed clinical research on nutrition, organizing the clinical data by both disease category and nutrient or botanical. Each volume includes hundreds of abstracts and a complete bibliography. His publications include:

Werbach MR. *Foundations of Nutritional Medicine. A Sourcebook of Clinical Research*, 2nd ed. Tarzana, CA: Third Line Press, Inc; 1996.

Werbach MR. *Nutritional Influences on Illness: A Sourcebook of Clinical Research*, 2nd ed. Tarzana, CA: Third Line Press, Inc; 1996.

Werbach MR. *Nutritional Influences on Mental Illness: A Sourcebook of Clinical Research*, 2nd ed. Tarzana, CA: Third Line Press, Inc; 1999.

Werbach MR, Moss J. *Textbook of Nutritional Medicine*. Tarzana, CA: Third Line Press, Inc; 1999.

Werbach MR, Murray MT. *Botanical Influences on Illness: A Sourcebook of Clinical Research*. 2nd ed. Tarzana, CA: Third Line Press, Inc; 2000.

A CD-ROM is also available for keyword searching, which includes both *Nutritional Influences on Illness* (2nd ed., 1996) and *Nutritional Influences on Mental Illness* (1999). All the above books are published by and available from:

Third Line Press
4751 Viviana Drive
Tarzana, CA 91356
Phone: (818) 996-0076; fax: (818) 774-1575
Web site: http://www.third-line.com

Advanced Clinical Nutrition

The Work of Jeffrey Bland, PhD, and Colleagues

Yearly syllabuses are available from the annual conferences of HealthComm International, Inc. These conferences have each focused on a particular aspect of health, nutrition, the disease process, and the restoration of function, particularly at the biochemical and cellular level. HealthComm provides conferences, one-day regional workshops, texts, and audiotaped information. The information is thoroughly referenced from the peer-review literature.

Introductory texts include:

Bland JS, Costarella L, Levin B, et al. *Clinical Nutrition: A Functional Approach*. Gig Harbor, WA: The Institute for Functional Medicine; 1999.

Bland JS. *Fundamentals of Functional Medicine*. Gig Harbor, WA: The Institute for Functional Medicine; 1997.

Bland JS. *Genetic Nutritioneering*. Los Angeles: Keats Publishing; 1999.

More advanced text produced from the conferences include:

Bland JS. *Disorders of Intercellular Mediators and Messengers: Their Relationship to Functional Illness;* Gig Harbor, WA: The Institute for Functional Medicine; 1999.

Bland JS. *Improving Genetic Expression in the Prevention of the Diseases of Aging*; Gig Harbor, WA: The Institute for Functional Medicine; 1998.

Bland JS. *Improving Intercellular Communication in Managing Chronic Illness*; Gig Harbor, WA: The Institute for Functional Medicine; 1999.

Bland JS. *Nutritional Improvement of Health Outcomes: The Inflammatory Disorders*. Gig Harbor, WA: The Institute for Functional Medicine; 1997.

The syllabuses can be ordered from:

HealthComm International, Inc.
PO Box 1729
Gig Harbor, WA 98335
Phone: (800) 843-9660; fax: (253) 851-9749
Web site: http://www.healthcomm.com

A BREADTH OF RESOURCES IN CLINICAL NUTRITION

Crayhon R. *Robert Crayhon's Nutrition Made Simple*. New York: Evans and Company, Inc.; 1996.

This book, other texts, and seminar information can be obtained from:

Designs for Health Institute, Inc.
5345 Arapahoe Avenue
Boulder, CO 80303
Phone: (800) 847-8302 or (303) 415-0229; fax: (303) 415-0154

Integrative Medicine. *Access*. Newton, MA: Integrative Medicine; 2000.

This updatable looseleaf binder, published by Integrative Medicine, provides cross-referenced entries on herbs and nutrients with summaries of the research, including the analysis of botanicals from the German Commission E monographs.

This information, and other types of information resources on nutrition and botanical medicine, are provided through

Integrative Medicine
1029 Chestnut
Newton, MA 02464
Phone: (617) 720-4080

Murray MT. *Encyclopedia of Nutritional Supplements*. Rocklin, CA: Prima Publishing, 1996.

Murray MT, Pizzorno JE. *Encyclopedia of Natural Medicine*, revised 2nd ed. Rocklin, CA: Prima Publishing; 1997.

PDR Physicians' Desk Reference for Nonprescription Drugs and Dietary Supplements. Montvale, NJ: Medical Economics Data; 2000.

This resource can be ordered from:

Medical Economics Data
5 Paragon
Montvale, NJ 07645
Phone: (800) 922-0937 or (201) 358-7500

Pizzorno J, Murray M, eds. *Textbook of Natural Medicine*. New York: Churchill Livingston; 1999. This is a comprehensive, definitive text on naturopathic medicine.

Shils M, Olson J, Shike M, Ross AC, eds. *Modern Nutrition in Health and Disease*. 9th ed. Baltimore: Williams & Wilkins; 1998. This is an outstanding basic reference on nutrition in two volumes.

VIDEO AND AUDIOTAPES AND SERIES PUBLICATIONS

Integrated Medicine Videotapes by Dr. Leo Galland. A six-hour educational workshop on the principles and practices of integrated and nutritional medicine. Topics include 1) the mediators, antecedents, and triggers of illness; 2) nutritional influences on cell function and the effects of antioxidant nutrients; and 3) intestinal toxicity, dysbiosis, and leaky gut syndrome focusing on the causes, consequences, diagnosis, and treatment.

To order, call Nutrition Workshop, Inc. at 212-717-5170 or 772-3077; fax: (212) 794-0170.

Clinical Pearls News. This monthly health letter on nutrition and integrative medicine summarizes 75 to 100 peer-reviewed articles per issue. Summaries are drawn from more than 1,000 journals reviewed on a monthly basis. Key articles are accompanied by clinical commentary and author contact information. Interviews and case histories are also included. Contact:
ITServices at (916) 483-1085
E-mail: office@clinicalpearls.com
Web site: www.clinicalpearls.com

Current Contents Clinical Medicine and *Current Contents Life Sciences.* These monthly reviews of the clinical and scientific literature are available on print and diskette and may be obtained from:
The Institute for Scientific Information
350 Market Street
Philadelphia, PA 19104
Phone: (800) 523-1850, fax: (215) 386-2915

Functional Medicine Update. This is a monthly audiotape series—90 minute reviews on cassette, covering approximately 30 peer-reviewed articles in nutrition and complementary medicine. The tapes include interviews, clinical case studies, and summary cards.

Subscriptions are available through:
HealthComm International Inc.
PO Box 1729
Gig Harbor, WA 98335
Phone: (800) 843-9660, Fax: (253) 851-9749

WEB SITES AND DATABASES

Cochrane Collaboration. This international consortium seeks to meet the growing need for evidence-based documentation in medicine, including the field of complementary medicine. The Cochrane Collaboration is involved in the creation and maintenance of an international registry of completed and ongoing randomized controlled clinical trials and the development of guidelines and software to systematize and facilitate the preparation and updating of these systematic reviews.
Cochrane Complementary Medicine Field
Trial Registry Coordinator
Complementary Medicine Program
University of Maryland School of Medicine
2200 Kernan Drive
Baltimore, MD 21207-6697
Phone: (410) 448-6997; fax: (410) 448-6875

The Clinical Pearls Database. This database on CD-ROM reviews the research literature on nutrition. It contains more than 20,000 fully-referenced article summaries incorporating a decade of research. Also included are case studies, researched clinical protocols, and over 300 interviews with academic clinicians and researchers. All topics on the disk have extensive bibliographies. The CD-ROM or a subscription to the database on the Clinical Pearls Web site can be obtained from:
ITServices
3301 Alta Arden #2
Sacramento, CA 94525
Phone: (916) 483-1085, fax: (916) 483-1431
E-mail: office@clinicalpearls.com

Healthnotes Online. Healthnotes develops database content based on the peer-reviewed literature on treatment protocols utilizing vitamins and minerals; herbs; homeopathic remedies; diets and therapies; as well as drug-nutrient interactions. The information is appropriate for professional and public use.

Healthnotes
1505 SE Gideon, Suite 200
Portland, OR 97202
Phone (800) 659-6330 or (503) 234-4092
Web site: www.healthnotes.com

MEDLINE. MEDLINE on the Internet is a user-friendly system which tracks more than 6,000 medical journals from the U.S. and international literature. Go to <www.nlm.nih.gov>, click on Pub Med, and enter the key word you want to search. To find topics in nutrition, it is important to use the specific scientific or chemical term. For example, journal articles on vitamin C are listed under "ascorbic acid." Go to the location on the site called MeSH headings, enter the commonly used name, and the system will usually provide the terms used in MEDLINE.

FEDERAL INFORMATION RESOURCES AND WEB SITES

Telephone Resources

FDA Food Information Line
(888) SAFEFOOD—24 hours a day

USDA Meat and Poultry Hotline
(800) 535-4555; TTY (800) 256-7072

Web Sites

Centers for Disease Control and Prevention
http://www.cdc.gov

Food and Drug Administration (FDA)
http://www.fda.gov
FDA Food Safety Web site
http://www.cfsan.fda.gov

National Institutes of Health, Office of Dietary Supplements
http://dietary-supplements.info.nih.gov

U.S. Department of Agriculture (USDA)
Food Safety Web site
http://www.fsis.usda.gov

CHAPTER 61

Clinical Nutrition: A Functional Perspective

Jeffrey Bland

Have you ever wished that a blueprint or map existed to better integrate nutrition into clinical practice? One of the useful strategies developed in this area over the past decade is functional medicine. A functional approach involves paradigms for reevaluating the role of nutrition from a functional perspective.

THE FUNCTIONAL PERSPECTIVE

Perspective is extremely important because it is the key factor that differentiates among healing systems. The underlying perspective is the lens through which a clinician looks to understand the patient and to guide the course of action or treatment. A physician strongly oriented to a pharmacological approach may view the patient in terms of which medication is needed. A psychotherapist may ask which form of counseling or behavioral intervention is warranted. A nutritionist will ask which nutrient or

dietary therapy will be of greatest benefit. In each case, the underlying perspective informs the healing practice.

For functional medicine, this underlying perspective also involves a focus on process, dynamics, and purpose. The initial focus is not only on an endpoint or pathological state, but also on the dynamic processes that underlie and precede it. Acknowledging the existence of pathology as well as a need to understand it, functional medicine seeks a path of therapy that will engage, alter, and rebalance these underlying events. Diagnostic categories are recognized and utilized, but the practitioner also investigates the dietary, nutritional, lifestyle, environmental, structural, and psychosocial factors that interact to produce a change in the patient's state of well-being.

BIOCHEMICAL INDIVIDUALITY IN NUTRITION

The highly acclaimed biochemist Roger Williams, PhD (1998), suggested that each individual is unique. This uniqueness encompasses voluntary activities, such as decision making, personality development, emotional response, and involuntary activities such as the metabolism of nutrients, cellular processing of information, and communication among the body's organ systems. Individual uniqueness is the essential focus of the concept of biochemical individuality, which is central to every aspect of the practice of functional medicine, from assessment and diagnosis to the broad spectrum of treatment modalities such as clinical nutrition.

As traditionally practiced, medicine and nutrition have given consideration to the concept of individuality in the identification and treat-

Jeffrey Bland, PhD, has been actively involved in nutrition-related research for 20 years, and has served as Director of the Bellevue-Redmond Medical Laboratory, Professor of chemistry at the University of Puget Sound, and Senior Research Scientist at the Linus Pauling Institute of Science and Medicine. Dr. Bland was the founder and Chief Executive Officer of HealthComm International, Inc. Dr. Bland is currently President of Metagenics, Inc., a leading research and development company in the field of functional medicine. He is the author of many works on nutrition, including *Your Health Under Siege*; *Medical Applications of Clinical Nutrition*; *The 20-Day Rejuvenation Diet Program*, and *Genetic Nutritioneering* with NTC (1999). Dr. Bland has pioneered the concept that genetic expression—the way heredity is expressed in people's lives and health—can be altered through nutrition and lifestyle.

Courtesy of Jeffrey Bland, PhD, Gig Harbor, Washington.

ment of conditions such as phenylketonuria or maple sugar urine disease (Michals et al, 1996). Although medicine has long recognized that specific metabolic aberrations alter the afflicted individual's nutrition and health needs, it has taken the view that these defects are so rare as to be somewhat inconsequential (Zeman, 1991). Over the past decade, researchers in the field of functional medicine have come to appreciate the profound differences in biochemistry and physiological function that exist between apparently normal people. Through this focus, they have come to realize that all individuals have unique metabolic patterns that affect their nutrition and health needs. In comparing two individuals whose blood levels of B vitamins are nearly identical, for example, one might have five times as low a level of B vitamins in his or her *cells* as the other.

Individuals also respond uniquely to environmental toxins, food additives, and prescription medications. What is actually going on in any individual at any given moment illustrates one of the core principles of functional medicine: biochemical individuality. Children are taught that all snowflakes are a little different—no two are exactly alike. As adults, most of us have been bombarded with discussion about DNA and DNA typing. In a general sense, people appreciate individuality as a kind of uniqueness.

However, there are many aspects of life and events that most people don't believe are much affected by this component called individuality. As clinical scientists, many seem to have decided that individuality affects voluntary activities reflected in personality, but not everyday bodily processes and involuntary physiological functions. For example, it is common to say, "He's an odd one" or "She's her own person." Clinicians are much less likely to say, "She's got a unique knee jerk reflex in her patellar tendon" or "He has a unique way of opening and closing his lower esophageal sphincter." These constant, everyday, involuntary bodily processes are simply not widely recognized candidates for uniqueness, except in circumstances of illness or rare hereditary events.

A functional perspective views both voluntary and involuntary processes as highly variable. Individual factors that extend to a person's biochemical life may vary just as much as his or her psychological life. Biochemical individuality means that one person's way of digesting food is different from everyone else's way of digesting food; "the food that nourishes you is not the same food that nourishes me."

The following examples illustrate how biochemically diverse everyone is. Joosten and colleagues (1993) published the results from a study on the levels of vitamins B_{12} and B_6 and folic acid in 64 healthy older adults (mean age 76 years). The authors found that of these 64 subjects, 94% had perfectly normal blood levels of vitamins B_6 and B_{12} and folate. Yet despite apparently normal blood levels, over 63% of the participants had elevated serum metabolites, indicating deficiency of these vitamins *within* the cells. Even more striking was the individual variability in the serum metabolite levels. Subjects showing normal serum levels of vitamin B_6, vitamin B_{12} and folate differed as much as 500% (10 micromoles/L versus 50 micromoles/L) in their homocysteine levels. In the case of methylmalonic acid, some cases differed by 1,000% (100 nanomoles/L versus 1,000 nanomoles/L). This study clearly demonstrated how metabolically different healthy individuals can be, given strikingly similar and normal snapshot glances at vitamin status.

The B-complex vitamins are by no means the only examples of how different people can be biochemically. Vitamin E requirements have been reported to show, at minimum, a fivefold difference for normal, healthy adults, and an even greater individual variability when dietary intake of polyunsaturated fatty acids was substantially different (VERIS, 1993). In the case of vitamin C, plasma ascorbate levels in healthy adults regularly vary by 25% to 30%. However, according to recent findings published by researchers at the National Institutes of Health (NIH), actual cellular requirements for vitamin C in healthy adults may differ by a much greater degree (Levine et al, 1993; Washko et al, 1993).

Case Study:
The Treatment of Migraine Headache

A biomedical approach to migraine headache, for example, is to recognize the symptom pattern, rule out vascular and intracranial pathology, and determine the presence of hypertension or renal disease. Treatment centers on drugs like sumatriptan, propranolol, or ergotamine. Biofeedback is sometimes recommended.

The functional medicine practitioner asks, "What dietary, nutritional, genetic, environmental, lifestyle, psychosocial, or spiritual factors might be interacting in this patient's life?" and "What is the possible range of functional change that underlies this expression of symptoms?" A wide array of patient-centered solutions to migraine headache is the result. For example, remediation of migraine has been reported using oral magnesium therapy (M.A. Schmidt, CNC, CCN, unpublished data, written communication, 1996); supplementing with essential fatty acids (S. Baker, MD, oral communication, 1996); removing food, chemical, and inhalant triggers and employing sublingual neutralization therapy (P. Bolin, oral communication, 1996). Acupuncture, homeopathy, and the botanical feverfew (*Tanacetum parthenium*) have also shown success in migraine. None of these approaches alone is successful for all migraine sufferers, however. Consequently, a patient-centered approach that recognizes statistical tendencies and diagnostic categories, but is not constrained by them, is desirable.

The NIH researchers pointed out that previous attempts to set vitamin C guidelines have focused on urinary excretion of ascorbate and assumed that excess excretion corresponds to oversaturation of the body pools until the body stores become filled and excesses are excreted. However, for many nutrients (including magnesium, potassium, and sodium), urinary excretion does not indicate saturation. For other nutrients, such as glucose, excretion actually reflects pathology.

In essence, the first and foremost guiding principle of a functional approach—the principle of biochemical individuality—tells people that they are as different at the level of everyday involuntary biochemical processes as they are psychologically.

BALANCE PROMOTION AND HOMEODYNAMICS

The principle of balance promotion is based upon a second fundamental principle in functional nutrition—the concept of homeodynamics. Homeodynamics is a corollary of the familiar concept of homeostasis, developed by Claude Bernard (1865), a scientist and colleague of Pasteur. What Bernard proposed when he published his ideas in 1865 was the concept of a "milieu interieur," an interior environment, in which stability served as the "primary condition for freedom and independence of existence." Bernard viewed the preservation of constancy in this interior environment as the foremost goal of the organism and a goal toward which all vital mechanisms in the body were oriented.

A present-day medical dictionary defines homeostasis as "a tendency to stability in the normal body states (the internal environment) of the organism. It is achieved by a system of control mechanisms activated by compensating regulatory systems" (Dorland, 2000). Homeostatic systems are defined as control systems—a collection of interconnected components that function to keep a physical or chemical parameter of the internal environment relatively constant. For example, a high level of carbon dioxide in extracellular fluid triggers increased pulmonary ventilation, which in turn causes a decrease in carbon dioxide concentration.

Perhaps the best example of a homeostatic control system would be the body's thermoregulatory system. This system is designed to maintain our body temperature within about 3 degrees Fahrenheit (from 97 to 100). Most people experience convulsions at body temperatures of 106°F and cannot survive temperatures much greater than 109°F. At the other end of the spectrum, natural, self-protective heat-producing mechanisms occur with increasing exposure to cold, including vasoconstriction, increased thyroxine production, increased metabolic rate, and shivering. The thermoregulatory system maintains a relatively narrow temperature range throughout healthy life. Only with the loss of vitality (for example, in the loss of health that can accompany aging) does this thermoregulatory function become less physically and neurally sensitive. Body temperature is characterized by a relative homeostasis, a relative tendency toward constant, unchanging, fixed parameters. Of course, the same argument could be applied to the subtle control of blood pH between 7.35 and 7.45.

Within this relative constancy, there is another dynamic set of constantly changing conditions that are equally astonishing and more closely tied to biochemical individuality. In functional medicine, this alternative set of conditions is referred to as homeodynamics—collections of interconnected components that function not to keep a physical or chemical parameter of the internal environment relatively constant, but to maintain biochemical individuality. In other words, in the same way that homeostasis describes a set of regulatory factors that serve to keep all of the involuntary biochemical processes relatively the same, homeodynamics is used in a functional approach to describe another set of regulatory factors relevant to the unique involuntary biochemical processes.

Returning to the question of the body's thermoregulation, it is true that temperatures above the 110°F range will kill everyone. Temperatures in the low 90s will leave everyone shivering and blue. However, what is equally true is that thermoregulation is highly variable and falls into many unique patterns. Each person has a unique circadian rhythm for body temperature, and this rhythm changes from season to season as well as throughout the life cycle. Men respond differently than women to thermal stimulation. Thermoregulatory response to cold also varies across cultures.

Even chronic disease risk and obesity correlate with core body temperature. Persons with relatively low core temperatures experience a higher incidence of obesity by age 36, which can be predicted from the first week of neonatal life. Strong individuality is seen across thermoregulatory parameters, including intensity and onset of sweating or shivering, adjustment in metabolic rate, and temperature differential across tissue types. From a functional perspective, thermoregulation is hardly a fixed, one-size-fits-all physiological process. Understanding homeodynamic events is key to understanding thermoregulation at the individual biochemical level.

When using the term "dysfunction," clinicians and researchers should think not only about the loss of processes universally operating in human beings, but also about the loss of processes that are unique to the single individual in which the dysfunction occurs. This can only be understood within that individual's unique life context.

A homeodynamic understanding of nutrition forces people to think in terms of nutrient synergy, antagonism, and balance. The evolution of our clinical thinking about calcium and bone nicely illustrates this point. Historically, when nutrition researchers observed resorption of bone calcium, they perceived absolute quantitative calcium deficiency and recommended calcium carbonate supplements. However, "calcium deficiency" is not an isolated deficiency, but a problem of balance with both nutritional and nonnutritional parameters. Bone remineralization cannot be achieved with supplemental calcium carbonate alone. Other nutrients, such as magnesium, manganese, zinc, copper, boron, and phosphorus, are equally important in the bone matrix and formation of hydroxyapatite. These other nutrients must be present in certain ratios.

Clinicians now approach restoration of bone health through functional nutrition differently than they used to. It is also based on the knowledge that nutritional therapy is part of a broader picture that includes lifestyle medicine or "natural hygiene." The muscles around the bone have to move and people have to move them voluntarily, so they need to engage in physical activity for bones to mineralize. In space, when astronauts are in a zero gravity environment, minerals leach from their bones because load-bearing movement is difficult without gravity. Similarly, the bones of people who are bedridden lose minerals because those individuals are not upright and engaging in load-bearing activity that enables their bones to mineralize properly. An important objective of functional nutrition is the achievement and maintenance of an ever-changing balance in the individual, even though that target is difficult to hit.

NUTRIENT INTERACTIONS AND NUTRIENT RATIOS

Restoring balance to underlying metabolic patterns is a process that places a premium on the understanding of nutrient interactions. Nutrients do not travel alone through the body. They are accompanied by other nutrients and nonnutrient factors that play a critical role in the journey. An objective of nutritional therapy is to make sure this companionship takes place. Certain forms of minerals in an inorganic delivery form require adequate secretion of hydrochloric acid by the stomach for proper absorption. Many nutrients must attach to organic acids or amino acids for proper absorption. The companion presence of many different molecules has a dramatic effect on nutrient absorption. The presence of flavonoids along with vitamin C, for example, alters and enhances vitamin C absorption. Nutrients work synergistically. These companion relationships are critical points of emphasis in nutritional therapy.

The therapeutic steps used to treat Wilson's disease are a simple example of the importance of nutrient ratios. In this progressive disorder, which involves cirrhosis of the liver and de-

generation of brain tissue, zinc therapy lowers excessively high levels of copper in the blood (Chandra, 1994). This therapy recognizes the natural balance (and antagonism) that can occur in the body between copper and zinc.

PATTERN RECOGNITION

A next step in the evolution of functional assessment is the focus on human physiology as a dynamic process, involving the interrelationship of multiple systems. Functional assessment of only one pathway or one series of pathways may yield useful information, but it is still limited by being able to look only through this small window of metabolism. A more comprehensive level to which functional assessment will evolve will include multiple analytes whose story will become clear using sophisticated methods of pattern recognition.

Pattern recognition has been a part of assessment for centuries. For example, traditional Chinese medicine is concerned not with the mechanisms but with "patterns of disharmony." The clinician is trained to recognize the signature of the pattern and place it within a specific diagnostic category. In homeopathic medicine, pattern recognition is essentially what has given rise to the extensive *materia medica*. In psychotherapy, the events and stories of a patient's life are sifted through in an attempt to understand the patterns that produce disharmony. From this broader perspective, the pattern takes on primary importance because it is the pattern that leads to treatment decisions.

These considerations are examples of a functional approach to evaluation and treatment that is still evolving and in an early stage of development. The goal of functional practitioners is to recognize and understand as much as possible related to the dynamics that underlie health and disease.

REFERENCES

Bernard C. *An Introduction to the Study of Experimental Medicine.* Greene HC, trans. New York: Macmillan Co; 1865.

Chandra RK. Zinc and immunity. *Nutrition.* 1994;10: 79–80.

Dorland WAN. Dorland's Illustrated Medical Dictionary, 29th ed. San Mateo, CA: W.B. Saunders Co; 2000.

Joosten E, Van Den Berg A, Riezler R, et al. Metabolic evidence that deficiencies of vitamin B_{12} (cobalamin), folate, and vitamin B_6 occur commonly in older people. *Am J Clin Nutr.* 1993;58:468–476.

Levine M, Cantilena CC, Dhariwal KR. In situ kinetics and ascorbic acid requirements. *World Review of Nutrition and Dietetics.* 1993;72:114–127.

Michals K, Acosta PB, Austin V, et al. Nutrition and reproductive outcome in maternal phenylketonuria. *Eur J Pediatr.* 1996;155 (Suppl 1):S165–168.

The Vitamin E Research and Information Service (VERIS). *Review on Vitamin E.* LaGrange, IL: VERIS; 1993 Jan.

Washko PW, Wang Y, Levine M. Ascorbic acid recycling in human neutrophils. *J Biol Chem.* 1993;268: 15531–15535.

Williams RJ. *Biochemical Individuality: the Basis for the Genetotropic Concept.* Chicago: Keats/NTC Contemporary Publishing; 1998.

Zeman F. *Clinical Nutrition and Dietetics.* 2nd ed. New York: Macmillan Publishing; 1991; 624.

SUGGESTED READING

Costa M, Canale D, Fillicori M, et al. L-carnitine in idiopathic asthenozoospermia: a multi-center study. *Andrologia.* 1994;26:155–159.

Food and Nutrition Board, National Research Council, National Academy of Sciences. *Recommended Dietary Allowances.* 10th ed. Washington, DC: National Academy Press; 1989.

Frohlich J. Lipoproteins and homocysteine as risk factors for atherosclerosis assessment and treatment. *Can J Cardiol.* May 1995;11(suppl C):18–23.

Herbert V. The 1986 Herman Award Lecture. Nutritional science as a continuing unfolding story. *Am J Clin Nutr.* 1987;46(3):387–402.

Herbert V. Vitamin B-12; plant sources, requirements, and assays. *Am J Clin Nutr.* 1988;48(suppl 3):852–858.

Hoffman DR, Birch EE, Birch DG, et al. Effects of supplementation with omega-3 longchain polyunsaturated acids on retinal and cortical development in premature infants. *Am J Clin Nutr.* 1993;57(suppl):807S–845S.

Kramer R, Palmieri F. Metabolite carriers on mitochondria. In: Ernster L, ed. *Molecular Mechanisms in Bioenergetics.* Amsterdam: Elsevier Science Publishers; 1992.

Lonsdale D. *A Nutritionist's Guide to the Clinical Use of Vitamin B_1.* Tacoma, WA: Life Sciences Press; 1987.

Scheppach W, Sommer H, Kirchner T, et al. Effect of butyrate enemas on the colonic mucosa in distal ulcerative colitis. *Gastroenterology.* 1992;103:51–56.

Shuster MM. Biofeedback control of gastrointestinal motility. In: Masmajian JV, ed. *Biofeedback—Principles and Practice for Clinicians.* New York: Williams & Wilkins; 1979.

PART XVI

Herbal Therapy

CHAPTER 62

Trends in Botanical Therapy

62.1 Utilization Data: Botanical/Herbal and Homeopathic Products

Nancy Faass

TRENDS IN THE USE OF BOTANICALS

Interest in botanicals continues in a general upward trend among consumers, physicians, health systems, and health plans. Studies show the following increases in utilization:

- Eisenberg et al (1993) found herbal use in the U.S population to be 3%.
- Landmark Healthcare's *Report I* (InterActive Solutions, 1998) estimated approximate utilization in the U.S. to be 17%.
- In 1998, Stanford University/American Specialty Health research (2000) indicated herb use as high as 33%.
- Berman et al (1998) found primary care providers who would recommend herbs to be 33%.

However, in the natural products industry, data on consumer sales suggest that in 1999,

botanical sales began to plateau (*Nutrition Business Journal*, 1999, 2000) as reflected in Table 62.1–1. In mass merchandiser venues, data derived from bar code scanning indicate sales declined by 2.6%.

The international herbal industry has been estimated at more than $10 billion (Manitoba Agriculture and Food, 2000) and as high as $62 billion (Reuters, 2000). The largest markets for herbal medicines, both in terms of manufacturing and consumption, are in Europe, followed by Asia and Japan. The Asian market represents approximately half of the sales levels achieved in Europe (Manitoba Agriculture and Food, 2000). In Europe alone, projected sales in 1996 were estimated at $7 billion, with the following pattern of utilization (Blumenthal, 1998):

• Germany	$3.5 B
• France	1.8 B
• Italy	700 M
• United Kingdom	400 M
• Spain	300 M
• The Netherlands	100 M
• All others	130 M
• Total	$7.0 Billion

Nancy Faass, MSW, MPH, is a writer and editor in San Francisco who provides book and project development in integrative medicine and the social sciences.

Table 62.1–1 U.S. Botanical Sales Channels

Sales Channels	1995 ($)	1997 ($)	1998 ($)	1999 ($)
Natural Food Chains/Health Food Stores	900 M	1.2 B	1.4 B	1.4 B
Mass Market: (supermarket, drugstores, etc.)	260 M	560 M	780 M	760 M
Multilevel Marketing Firms	940 M	1.0 B	1.0 B	1.2 B
Mail Order Firms	220 M	320 M	360 M	340 M
Practitioners/Herbalists/Chinese Medicine	150 M	270 M	340 M	330 M
Specialty Asian Herb Shops	60 M	90 M	110 M	n.a.
Internet				40 M
Total Botanical Sales	2.5 B	3.5 B	4.0 B	4.1 B
Total Supplement Sales	$9.8 B	$12.6 B	$13.9 B	$15.4 B

Source: Reprinted with permission from the *Nutrition Business Journal*, San Diego, California, © 1999.

- WHO projections indicate that, worldwide, 80% of the population are dependent on plant medication (Farnsworth et al, 1985).

In the United States, health systems, hospitals, and health plans are responding to generally positive trends in consumer and physician interest:

- Developers of integrative medicine centers are creating botanical dispensaries to support prescriptions by practitioners (see Chapters 34–37).
- Dispensaries may also be viewed as profit centers or additional offerings in system pharmacies (see Chapter 7).
- CAM-interested health plans, such as Blue Cross of California and Oxford Health Plans, are beginning to offer members botanical products through catalogs at discounted rates.
- Some plans include botanicals as a part of benefit design.
- Specialty health plans such as Landmark Healthcare, Alternare, Alignis, and American Specialty Health Plans view botanicals as a part of the CAM services that they are offering plans and employers.
- The general trend over the past decade has been primarily one of growth.

Sales of certain specific herbs also increased significantly, as indicated by industry data (see Table 62.1–2). U.S. utilization mirrors some of the utilization patterns in Europe. In Germany in 1995, the most frequently prescribed botanical was *Gingko biloba* (with sales of $284 million) followed by horsechestnut, hawthorn, yeast, St. John's wort, myrtle, stinging nettle, echinacea, saw palmetto, and mild thistle (Schwabe/Pfaffrath, 1995).

THE MARKET FOR HOMEOPATHIC REMEDIES*

Sales of homeopathic remedies in the United States grew at a rate of 10% to 15% annually in 1997 and 1998, according to industry estimates. The lowest growth rates apply to direct-to-practitioner sales—once the largest source of sales. The largest market, with 40% to 45% of all homeopathics sales, has been the health food store, where growth is in the teens. The mass market has experienced higher growth and has begun to approach sales levels experienced in health food stores.

With the exception of Boiron, homeopathics manufacturers are privately held, thereby making

Source: Reprinted with permission from the *Nutrition Business Journal*, San Diego, California, © 1999.

Table 62.1–2 U.S. Botanical Sales—Most Frequently Purchased

Botanical	1995 ($)	1997 ($)	1998 ($)
Echinacea/Goldenseal	170 M	270 M	300 M
Garlic	150 M	210 M	230 M
Ginseng	190 M	240 M	250 M
Ginkgo biloba	170 M	250 M	310 M
St. John's wort	10 M	210 M	290 M
Saw palmetto	40 M	100 M	120 M
Combination formulas	900 M	1.2 B	1.4 B
Other herbs	840 M	1.2 B	1.2 B
Total	2.5 B	3.5 B	4.0 B

Source: Reprinted with permission from the *Nutrition Business Journal*, San Diego, California, © 1999.

firm estimates of the U.S. market for homeo-pathics manufacturers elusive. The market for homeopathic products was conservatively estimated to be:

- International market in 1997—$880 million
- U.S. market in 1997—over $120 million
- U.S. market from retail sales—$100 million
- Overall growth in U.S. market at 20%.

It has been estimated that more than 70 companies are marketing homeopathic remedies in the United States. The American Association for Homeopathic Pharmacists (AAHP) indicates that original manufacturers number only about 18 in the United States, although there are many more marketers and distributors. The AAHP (the manufacturers' trade association) and others believe the market is probably closer to $200 to $250 million, with growth of 10% to 15%. Health food store sales were estimated at approximately $125 million, rising to $250 million when mass market brands were included. Add to this practitioner sales, multilevel marketing, and catalog/Internet sales, and the market for homeopathic products increases to at least $300 million.

REFERENCES

American Specialty Health (ASH) and Stanford University. National consumer trends in complementary and alternative medicine. San Diego: ASH; 6/2000.

Annual industry overview 1999. *NBJ.* 1999;IV(6):3.

Annual industry overview 2000. *NBJ.* 2000;V(7/8):4.

Berman BM, Singh BB, Hartnol SM, et al. Primary care physicians and complementary-alternative medicine: training, attitudes, and practice patterns. *J Am Board Fam Pract.* 1998;11:272–281.

Blumenthal M, ed. *The Complete German Commission E Monographs: therapeutic Guide to Herbal Medicine.* Austin, TX: American Botanical Council and Boston: Integrative Medicine Communications, 1998.

Eisenberg DM, Kessler RC, Foster C, et al. Unconventional medicine in the United States. *N Engl J Med.* 1993; 328(4):246–252.

Farnsworth N, et al. Medicinal plants in therapy. *Bull World Health Org.* 1985;63:965–981.

InterActive Solutions. *Landmark Report I on Public Perceptions of Alternative Care.* Sacramento: Landmark Healthcare; 1998.

Manitoba Agriculture and Food, Web site at http://www.gov.mb.ca/agriculture/financial/agribus/ccg02s01.html. Accessed 8/00.

Reuters News Service. India begins to set traditional medicine house in order. Reuters News Service. 2000, July 13.

Schwabe/Pfaffrath. Arzneiverordnungs report (Drug Prescribing Report). Berlin: Phytopharm Consulting. 1995.

62.2   Herbal Medicine: A Modern Perspective

Michael T. Murray

The term "herb" by definition refers to a plant used for medicinal purposes. Are herbs effective medicinal agents or is their use merely a reflection of folklore, outdated theories, and myth? To some, herbs are thought of as ineffective medicines used prior to the advent of more effective synthetic drugs. To others, herbs are simply sources of compounds to isolate and then market as drugs. However, to a rapidly growing audience of patients and practitioners, herbs and crude plant extracts are effective medicines to be respected and appreciated.

For much of the world, herbal medicines are the only therapeutic agents available. In 1985, the World Health Organization estimated that perhaps 80% of the world population relied on herbs for primary health care needs (Farnsworth et al, 1985). This widespread use of herbal medicines is not restricted to developing countries; it has been estimated that 30% to 40% of all medical doctors in France and Germany rely on herbal preparations as their primary medication (Wagner interview, 1988). In the United Kingdom, the market for herbal and homeopathic remedies and aromatherapy oils increased by 41% between 1992 and 1996 (Ernst, 2000). In Germany, an herbal remedy (St. John's wort) is now the most frequently prescribed intervention for depression. In the United States, the sales

Michael T. Murray, ND, is one of the leading researchers and lecturers in the field of natural medicine. He is author of more than 24 books, including *The Healing Power of Herbs*, *The Encyclopedia of Nutritional Supplements* (1996), and co-author of *The Encyclopedia of Natural Medicine* with Joseph Pizzorno, ND. They are also co-editors of *The Textbook of Natural Medicine* (1999), a two-volume professional reference.

of St. John's wort rose by 2800% between 1997 and 1998 (Brevoort, 1998).

THE REBIRTH OF HERBAL MEDICINE

Throughout the world, but especially in Europe and Asia, a tremendous renaissance in the use and appreciation of herbal medicine has taken place. In Germany, estimates show that over $4 billion is spent on herbal products each year. In Japan, the figure is thought to be even higher. Botanical products are a major business in the United States as well, with an estimated annual sales figure of $3.98 billion for 1998, up from $1.3 billion in 1992, and climbing (American Botanical Council, unpublished data, 1998; Annual Industry Overview, 1999). However, it is interesting to note that while annual sales of ginseng products in the United States in 1992 were roughly $10 million (over 3 million pounds), roughly $100 million worth of American ginseng was exported (Deveny, 1992; Market Report, 1992). By 1998, the American market for ginseng had expanded to $250 million (Principe, 1989; Annual Industry Overview, 1999).

The rebirth of herbal medicine, especially in developed countries, is based largely on the renewed interest of scientific researchers. Their efforts have yielded an explosion of scientific information concerning plants, plant extracts, and constituents and their application as medical agents. It is ironic that this renewal comes not from traditional herbalists, but from renewed scientific investigation into the use of plant medicines.

THE ROLE OF HERBS IN MEDICINE

For the past two decades, about 25% of all prescription drugs in the United States have contained active constituents obtained from plants.

Digoxin, codeine, colchicine, morphine, vincristine, and yohimbine are some popular examples. Many over-the-counter preparations are composed of plant compounds as well. It is estimated that more than $11 billion worth of plant-based medicines are purchased each year in the United States alone, and $43 million worldwide (Fuchs, 1999).

Because a plant cannot be patented, very little research has been done in this century on whole plants or crude plant extracts as medicinal agents, per se, by large American pharmaceutical firms. Instead, pharmaceutical firms screen plants for biological activity and then isolate the so-called active constituents (compounds). (In fact, pharmacognosy, the study of natural drugs and their constituents, plays a major role in current drug development.) If the compound is powerful enough, the drug company will begin the formidable process to procure Food and Drug Administration (FDA) approval—formidable because in the United States FDA approval of a plant-based drug typically takes 10 to 18 years at a total cost of at least $230 million.

In contrast, European policies have made it economically feasible for companies to research and develop herbs as medicines. In Germany, herbal products can be marketed as medicines if they have been proved to be safe and effective (Keller, 1991). Actually, the legal requirements for herbal medicines are identical to those for all other drugs. Whether the herbal product is available by prescription or over the counter is based on its application and safety of use. Herbal products sold in pharmacies are reimbursed by insurance if they are prescribed by a physician.

The proof required by a manufacturer in Germany to illustrate safety and effectiveness for an herbal product is far less than the proof required by the FDA for drugs in the United States. In Germany, Commission E of the Federal Health Authority (comparable to the FDA) has developed a series of 200 monographs on herbal products. These reports, like the monographs produced in the United States by the FDA on over-the-counter medications, set standards for

safety and efficiency (Kleijnen and Knipschild, 1993). An herbal product is viewed as safe and effective when a manufacturer meets the quality requirements of the Commission's standards or produces additional evidence of safety and effectiveness, which can include data from the existing literature and anecdotal information from practicing physicians, as well as limited clinical studies.

The best single illustration of the difference in the regulatory issues on herbal products in the United States compared to Germany concerns *Ginkgo biloba*. In Germany, as well as France, extracts of *Ginkgo biloba* leaves are registered for the treatment of cerebral and peripheral vascular insufficiency (Kleijnen and Knipschild, 1993). Ginkgo products are available by prescription and over-the-counter purchase. Ginkgo extracts are among the three most widely prescribed drugs in both Germany and France, with a combined annual sales figure of more than $500 million. In contrast, in the United States, extracts, which are identical to those approved in Germany and France, are available as food supplements.

In the United States, no medicinal claims are allowed for most herbal products because the FDA requires the same standard of absolute proof that is required for new synthetic drugs. The FDA has rejected the idea of establishing an independent expert advisory panel for the development of standards similar to those of Germany's Commission E. Currently, herbal products continue to be sold as food supplements, and manufacturers are prohibited from making any diagnosis-relevant therapeutic claims for their products.

STATE OF THE RESEARCH

In the past 20 years, researchers have produced a tremendous amount of information concerning plants, crude plant extracts, and nutritional substances as medicinal agents. This can be reviewed in the MEDLINE database on the Internet (http://www.ncbi.nlm.nih.gov) or in medical libraries in yearly reference guides, *Chemical Abstracts*. In both MEDLINE and *Chemical Abstracts*, the information is usually indexed under the biochemical term or under the name of the active chemical constituents. Herbal reference books available in most book stores typically summarize the primary active chemical constituents of each herb.

Compare this to the lack of information that existed just 30 years ago, when it was impossible for the scientific establishment to determine the mechanisms by which most herbs promote their healing effects. Take aspirin, for example. The main mechanism for action responsible for aspirin's anti-inflammatory effect was not fully understood until the early 1970s, and its mechanism of action for pain relief is still being evaluated.

Since the mechanism of therapeutic action of herbs was not fully isolated and understood, many effective plant medicines were erroneously labeled as possessing no pharmacological activity. Today, however, researchers equipped with more sophisticated technology are rediscovering the wonder of plants as medicinal agents. Much of their increased understanding is, ironically, a result of synthetic drug research.

For example, one of the latest classes of widely used medications is the calcium channel-blocking drugs. These drugs block the entry of calcium into smooth muscle cells, thereby inhibiting contraction and promoting muscular relaxation. Calcium channel-blocking drugs are currently being used in the treatment of high blood pressure, angina, asthma, and other conditions associated with smooth muscle contraction. In many ways, the synthesis and understanding of these drugs symbolize the level of sophistication of the modern science of pharmacology. After these drugs were isolated and their mechanisms of action better understood, it was discovered that many herbs contain components that possess calcium channel-blocking activity. In most cases, the historical use of these herbs as medicine corresponded to their activity as muscle relaxants.

Many herbs possess pharmacological actions that are not consistent with modern pharmacological understanding. Numerous botanicals appear to impact homeostatic control mechanisms to aid normalization of many of the body's processes; when there is a hyperstate, the herb exerts a lowering effect to decrease or downregulate that function. And when there is a hypostate, it has a heightening or upregulating effect. This action is baffling to pharmacologists, but not to experienced herbalists, who have used terms such as "alterative," "amphiteric," "adaptogenic," or "tonic" to describe these effects.

THE ADVANTAGES OF HERBAL MEDICINES

The materia medica recorded in ancient China, Babylon, Egypt, India, Greece, and other parts of the world strongly suggest that herbal medicine was highly respected in ancient times (Griggs, 1981). In the context of modern medicine, what advantages do herbal medicines possess over synthetic drugs? Generally, herbal preparations tend to be less toxic than their synthetic counterparts and offer less risk of side effects. (Obviously, there are exceptions to this rule.) In addition, the mechanism of action is often to correct the underlying cause of ill health. In contrast, a synthetic drug is often designed to alleviate the symptom or effect, but may not address the underlying cause. It has also been demonstrated with many botanicals that the entire plant or crude extract is more effective than isolated constituents.

HERBAL MEDICINE AND THE PHARMACEUTICAL INDUSTRY

Since a plant cannot be patented, very little research has been done in the twentieth century on plants as medicinal agents, per se, by the large American pharmaceutical firms. Instead, plants were screened for biological activity and then the active constituents were isolated. Researchers have been dismayed by the fact that in many instances the isolated constituent was less active biologically than the crude herb. Since the crude herb provided no economic reward to the American pharmaceutical firm, the crude herb or extract never reached the marketplace. In contrast, European policies on herbal medicines made it economically feasible for companies to research and develop crude phytopharmaceuticals.

Another problem for herbal medicine in the United States has been the lack of standardization. The herb that best exemplifies this dilemma is digitalis. One batch of crude digitalis might have an extremely low level of active constituents, making the crude herb ineffective, while the next batch might be unusually high in active constituents, resulting in toxicity or even death when the standard amount is used. The lack of standardization made it easier for U.S. pharmaceutical firms to rationalize their economic need to isolate, purify, and chemically modify the active constituents of digitalis so that they could market these compounds as drugs. The problem with using the pure active constituent is that the safe dosage range is smaller. Digitalis toxicity and death have increased dramatically as a result of purification. Toxicity was less of a factor when using the crude herb because overconsumption of potentially toxic doses resulted in vomiting or diarrhea, thus avoiding the heart disturbance and death that occur now with pure digitalis cardiac glycoside drugs.

Fortunately, several European and Asian pharmaceutical firms began specializing in phytopharmaceuticals in the early part of the twentieth century. These companies have played a prominent role in researching, developing, and promoting herbal medicines.

Research is demonstrating that crude extracts often have greater therapeutic benefit than the isolated "active" constituent. This has been known for quite some time in other parts of the world, but in the United States isolated plant drugs are still thought of as having the greatest therapeutic effect. This myth is gradually eroding as our knowledge of herbal medicines increases. If current standardization techniques had been available earlier in the 20th century, it is possible that the majority of our current prescription drugs would be crude herbal extracts instead of isolated and modified active constituents.

HERBAL PREPARATION

Commercial herbal preparations are available in several different forms: bulk herbs, teas, tinctures, fluid extracts, and tablets or capsules. It is important for anyone who routinely uses or recommends herbs to understand the difference between these forms, as well as the methods of expressing strengths of herbal products. One of the major developments in the herb industry involves improvements in extraction and concentration processes.

Herbal Extracts

An extract is a concentrated form of the herb obtained by mixing the crude herb with an appropriate solvent (such as alcohol and/or water). When an herbal tea bag steeps in hot water, it is actually a type of herbal extract known as an infusion. The water serves as a solvent in removing some of the medicinal properties from the herb. Teas often are better sources of bioavailable compounds than the powdered herb, but they are relatively weak in action compared to tinctures, fluid extracts, and solid extracts. Herbal practitioners often use these latter forms for medicinal effects.

Tinctures are typically made by using an alcohol and water mixture as the solvent. The herb is soaked in the solvent for a specified amount of time, depending on the herb. This soaking lasts usually from several hours to a day, but some herbs may be soaked for much longer periods of time. The solution is then pressed out, yielding the tincture.

Fluid extracts are more concentrated than tinctures. Although they are most often made from hydroalcoholic mixtures, other solvents may be used (vinegar, glycerin, propylene glycol, etc). Commercial fluid extracts are usually made by distilling off some of the alcohol, typically by using methods that do not require elevated temperatures, such as vacuum distillation and countercurrent filtration.

A solid extract is produced by further concentration of the extract, using the mechanisms described above for fluid extracts as well as other techniques such as thin-layer evaporation. The solvent is completely removed, leaving a viscous extract (soft solid extract) or a dry solid extract, depending on the plant, plant portion, or solvent used and on whether a drying process was used. The dry solid extract, if not already in powdered form, can be ground into course granules or a fine powder. A solid extract can also be diluted with alcohol and water to form a fluid extract or tincture.

Analytical Methods

Improvements in analytical methods have led to definite improvements in harvesting schedules, cultivation techniques, storage, activity, stability of active compounds, and product purity. All of these gains have resulted in tremendous improvements in the quality of herbal preparations now available.

For example, optimal activity and quality collection should be done at a time when the active ingredient is present in the greatest amount. Improvements in analysis have led to more precise harvesting of many herbs.

Methods currently utilized in evaluating herbs and their extracts include the following:

- organoleptic
- microscopic
- physical
- chemical/physical
- biological

Organoleptic simply means "the impression of the organs." *Organoleptic analysis* involves the application of sight, odor, taste, touch, and occasionally even sound, to identify the plant. The initial sight of a plant or extract may be so specific that it is sufficient for identification. If this is not enough, perhaps the plant or extract has characteristic odor or taste. Organoleptic analysis represents the simplest, yet the most human, form of analysis.

Microscopic evaluation is indispensable in the initial identification of herbs, as well as in identifying small fragments of crude or powdered herbs, adulterants (eg, insects, animal feces, mold, and other fungi), and characteristic tissue features of the plant. Every plant possesses a characteristic tissue structure, which can be demonstrated through the study of tissue arrangement, cell walls, and configuration when samples are properly stained and mounted.

Physical methods are often used in crude plant evaluation to determine the solubility, specific gravity, melting point, water content, degree of fiber elasticity, and other physical characteristics.

Chemical/physical methods are also used to determine the percentage of active principles, alkaloids, flavonoids, enzymes, vitamins, essential oils, fats, carbohydrates, protein, ash, acid-insoluble ash, or crude fiber present.

The analytical process requires more precise assays to determine quality. Sophisticated techniques, such as high-pressure liquid chromatography and nuclear magnetic resonance, are often used to separate molecules. The readings from these machines provide a chemical fingerprint as to the nature of chemicals contained in the plant or extract. These techniques are invaluable in the effort to identify herbs, as well as to standardize extracts. The plant or extract can then be evaluated by various biological methods, mostly animal tests, to determine pharmacological activity, potency, and toxicity.

Techniques Used in the Production of Herbal Products

The range of sophistication in the processing of herbs is tremendous—from crude herb to highly concentrated standardized extracts. Nonetheless, there are some common stages (Bombardelli, 1991).

Collection and Harvesting

Wild-crafted. When plants are collected from their natural habitat, they are said to be wild-crafted. When they are grown, utilizing commercial farming techniques, they are said to be cultivated. When an herb is wild-crafted, there is a much greater chance that the wrong herb will be picked, a situation that could lead to serious consequences. The use of analytical methods can be employed to guarantee that the plant collected is the one desired.

Harvesting. The mode of harvesting varies greatly, from hand labor to the use of sophisticated equipment, but the mode is not as important as the time: a plant should be harvested when the part of the plant being used contains the highest possible level of active compounds. This is ensured by the use of analytical techniques.

Drying. After harvesting, most herbs have a moisture content of 60% to 80% and cannot be stored without drying. Otherwise, important compounds would break down or microorganisms would contaminate the material. Commercially, most plants are dried within a temperature range of 100°F to 140°F. With proper drying, the herb's moisture content will be reduced to less than 14%.

Garbling. Garbling refers to the separation of the portion of the plant to be used from other parts of the plant, dirt, and other extraneous matter. This step is often done during collection. Although there are machines that perform garbling, it is usually performed by hand.

Grinding or mincing. This process involves mechanically breaking down either leaves, roots, seeds, or other parts of a plant into very small units ranging from larger, coarse fragments to fine powder. The most widely used machine is the hammer mill. Other types of grinders include knife mills and teeth mills.

Extraction

The process of extraction is used in making tinctures, fluid extracts, and solid extracts. In this context, extraction refers to the separation by physical or chemical means of the desired material from a plant with the aid of a solvent. The U.S. health food industry often uses alcohol and water mixtures as botanical solvents; occasionally extractions involve the use of oil-based (lipophilic) solvents or hypercritical carbon dioxide.

The simplest process consists of soaking the herb in the alcohol/water solution for a period of time, followed by filtering. Typically, this process will yield a lower quality extract at a higher price because the solvent, usually alcohol, cannot be reused. It is, in essence, sold to the customer. Since tinctures are 1:5 concentrates, this means 80% of the bottle's content is alcohol and water and only 20% herbal material. Tinctures are typically not as cost-effective or as stable as solid extracts.

Strengths of Extracts. The potencies or strengths of herbal extracts are generally expressed in two ways. If they contain known active principles, their strengths are commonly expressed in terms of the content of these active principles. Otherwise, the strength is expressed in terms of their concentration. For example, tinctures are typically made at a 1:5 concentration. This means one part herb (in grams) is soaked in five parts liquid (in milliliters of volume). This means that there is five times the amount of solvent (alcohol or water) in a tincture as there is herbal material.

A 4:1 concentration means that one part of the extract is equivalent to, or derived from, four parts crude herb. This is the typical concentration of a solid extract. One gram of a 4:1 extract is concentrated from 4 g of crude herb.

Typically, 1 g of a 4:1 solid extract is equivalent to 4 mL of a fluid extract (one-seventh of an ounce) and 40 mL of a tincture (almost 1.5 oz). Some solid extracts are concentrated as much as 100:1, meaning it would take nearly 100 g of crude herb, or 100 mL of a fluid extract (approximately 3.5 oz), or 1,000 mL of a tincture (almost 1 qt) to provide an equal amount of herbal material in 1 g of a 100:1 extract.

Larger manufacturers utilize more elaborate techniques to ensure that an herb is fully extracted and that the solvent is reused. For example, countercurrent extraction is often used. In this process, the herb enters into a column of a large percolator composed of several columns. The material to be extracted is pumped at a given temperature and rate of speed through the different columns, where it mixes continuously with solvent. The extract-rich solvent then passes into another column, while fresh solvent once again comes into contact with herbal material as it is passed into a new chamber. In this process, complete extraction of health-promoting compounds can be achieved. The extract-rich solvent is then concentrated through one of a variety of techniques.

Concentration

After extraction of the herb, the resulting solutions can be concentrated into fluid extracts or solid extracts. In large manufacturing operations, the techniques and machines used (such as thin-layer evaporators) ensure that the extracted plant components are not damaged. These machines work by evaporating the solvent, thus isolating the plant compounds. The solvent vapors pass into a condenser, in which they recondense to liquid form and can be used again. The result is separation of the extracted materials from the solvent, so that the final product is a pure extract, and the solvent can be used again and again.

Drying of Extracts

Although a number of liquid-form extracts on the market can still be found (tinctures, fluid extracts, and soft extracts), a solid form is preferable. The primary reason is the greater chemical stability and reduced cost of the solid form (the alcohol in liquid-form extracts is often more expensive than the herb). In addition, tinctures, fluid extracts, and soft extracts are easily con-

taminated by bacteria and other microorganisms. Liquid forms of extracts also promote chemical reactions that break down the herbal compounds. Consequently, a number of drying techniques are employed, including freeze-drying and spray-drying (atomization). The result is a dried, powdered extract that can then be put into capsules or tablets.

Excipients

An excipient is an inert substance added to a prescription to give it a certain form or consistency. The same excipients used in the manufacture of drug preparations and vitamin and mineral supplements are often used in the production of tablets and capsules containing herbs or herbal extracts. Many manufacturers will provide a list of excipients contained in their products.

Quality Control in Herbal Products

Quality control refers to processes involved in maintaining the quality or validity of a product. Regardless of the form of herbal preparation, some degree of quality control should exist. Currently, no organization or government body certifies the labeling of herbal preparations.

Without quality control, one cannot be sure that the herb contained in the bottle is the same as that stated on the label. Chemical analysis of over 35 different commercial preparations of feverfew (*Tanacetum parthenium*) and taheebo (*Taebuia avellanedae*) for active components (parthenolide and lapachol, respectively) found a wide variation in the amounts of parthenolide in commercial preparations (Heptinstall et al, 1992). The majority of products contained no parthenolide or only traces. Analysis of 12 commercial sources of taheebo could identify lapachol (in trace amounts) in only one product (Awang, 1988).

Determining Quality

In the past, the quality of the extract produced was often difficult to determine, as many of the active principles of the herbs were unknown. However, recent advances in extraction processes, coupled with improved analytical methods, have reduced this problem of quality control (Bonati, 1991a; Bonati, 1991b; Karlsen, 1991). Expressing the strength of an extract by the concentration method does not accurately measure potency because there may be great variation among manufacturing techniques and raw materials. By using a high-quality herb (an herb high in active compounds), it is possible to create a more potent dried herb, tincture, or fluid extract compared to the solid extract that was made from a lower quality herb. Standardization is the solution to the problem.

Standardization

The term "standardized extract" (or "guaranteed potency extract") refers to an extract guaranteed to contain a standardized level of active compounds. Stating the content of active compounds rather than the concentration ratio allows for more accurate dosages to be made.

The best way to express the quality of an herb is in terms of its active components. Regardless of the form, the herb should be analyzed to ensure that it contains these components at an acceptable standardized level. More accurate dosages can then be given. This form of standardization is generally accepted in Europe and is beginning to be used in the United States as well.

This form of standardization (ie, stating the content of active constituents versus drug concentration ratio) allows the dosage to be based on active constituents (Bonati, 1991b). In Europe, *Vaccinium myrtillus*, *Silybum marianum*, and *Centella asiatica* extract dosage levels are based on their active constituent levels rather than drug ratio or total extract weight, for example, 40 mg of anthocyanosides for *Vaccinium myrtillus*, 70 mg of silymarin for *Silybum marianum*, and 30 mg of triterpenic acids for *Centella asiatica*. This type of dosage recommendation provides the greatest degree of consistency and assurance of quality.

Although referred to in terms of active constituents, it must be kept in mind that these are still crude extracts and not isolated constituents. For example, an *Uva ursi* extract standardized for its arbutin content, say 10%, still contains all of these synergistic factors that enhance the function of the active ingredient (arbutin). Another example of problems that can result from a lack of quality control is evident in a review of *Panax ginseng*.

Quality Control with Panax ginseng

Panax ginseng contains at least 13 different steroid-like compounds, collectively known as ginsenosides. These compounds are believed to be the most important active constituents of *Panax ginseng*. The usual concentration of ginsenosides in mature ginseng roots is between 1% and 3%. Ginsenoside Rg1 is present in significant concentrations in *Panax ginseng*. In contrast, American ginseng *(Panax quinquefolium)* contains primarily ginsenoside Rb1 and very little, if any, Rg1. This difference is extremely important, because, in general, Rb1 possesses a sedative effect, whereas Rg1 possesses a stimulatory effect.

Independent research and published studies have clearly documented a tremendous variation in the ginsenoside content of commercial preparations (Liberti and Marderosian, 1978; Soldati and Sticher, 1980). In fact, the majority of products on the market contain only trace amounts of ginsenosides, and many formulations contain no ginseng at all. The lack of quality control has led to several problems, ranging from toxic reactions to absence of medicinal effect.

Future Directions in Quality Control

Companies supplying standardized extracts currently offer the greatest degree of quality control, and hence these products typically provide the highest quality. Most standardized extracts are currently made in Europe under strict guidelines set forth by individual members of the European Economic Council (EEC) as well as those proposed by the EEC (Bonati, 1991a;

Bonati, 1991b; Karlsen, 1991). Included are guidelines for acceptable levels of impurities such as bacterial counts, pesticides, residual solvents, heavy metals, and product stability.

The production of standardized extracts serves as a model for quality control processes for all forms of herbal preparations. In general, it is believed that if the active components of a particular herb are known, the herbal product should be analyzed to ensure that it contains these components at an acceptable/standardized level. More accurate dosages can then be prescribed. Products should also be subjected to bacteriological counts. Currently, in many countries, numerous standardized extracts fulfill the requirements for marketing as drugs. These extracts have typically gone through the following major quality control steps:

- selection of suitable plant material
- botanical investigation, using organoleptic and microscopic techniques
- chemical analysis, using appropriate laboratory equipment
- screening for biological activity
- analysis of active fractions of crude extracts
- isolation of active principles
- determination of chemical structure of active principles
- comparison with compounds of similar structure
- analytical method developed for formulation
- detailed pharmacological evaluation
- studies performed to determine activity and toxicity of formulation
- studies on absorption, distribution, and elimination of herbal compounds
- clinical trials performed to determine activity in humans
- registration by national drug authorities

THE FUTURE OF HERBAL MEDICINE

Herbal medicine will certainly play a major role in future medicine. As more knowledge and understanding are gained about health and disease, medicine is adopting therapies that are more natural and less toxic. Lifestyle modification, stress reduction, exercise, meditation, dietary changes, and many other traditional naturopathic therapies are becoming much more valued in the mainstream. This illustrates the paradigm shift that is occurring, as these therapies gain acceptance as effective clinical options.

With the continuing advancement in science and technology, there has been a great improvement in the quality of the herbal medicines available. New developments in cultivation techniques, coupled with improvements in quality control and standardization of potency, will continue to increase the effectiveness of herbal medicines. The improvements in extraction and concentration processes also represent a major development in herbal medicine. Standardized extracts that state the level of active compounds provide the greatest benefit, owing primarily to more accurate dosages.

Improvements in plant cultivation techniques and the quality of herbal extracts (quality control and standardization) have led to the development of some very effective plant medicines. It is apparent that many of the "wonder drugs" of the future will be derived from plants or plant cell cultures and from cell cultures producing compounds naturally occurring in the human body (interferon, interleukin 2, various hormones, etc). Several herbal medicines described here may in fact already fulfill the role of wonder drug, for example, *Ginkgo biloba*, *Silybum marianum*, and *Panax ginseng*.

Many of the previous shortcomings of herbal medicine have been overcome (eg, the lack of scientific support, standardization, and quality control). The future of herbal medicine depends on several factors: continued research into herbal medicine, adoption by manufacturers of recognized standards of quality, continued existence of the naturopathic medical schools, and increased public awareness of the tremendous therapeutic value of herbs. Herbal medicine will undoubtedly play a major role in the medicine of the twenty-first century.

REFERENCES

Annual Industry Overview. *Nutr Bus J.* 1999;IV(6):1–5.

Awang DVC. Commercial taheebo lacks active ingredient. *Can Pharmacol J.* 1988;121:323–326.

Bombardelli E. Technologies for the processing of medicinal plants. In: Wijeskera ROB, ed. *The Medicinal Plant Industry.* Boca Raton, FL: CRC Press; 1991:96–98.

Bonati A. Formation of plant extracts into dosage forms. In: Wijeskera ROB, ed. *The Medicinal Plant Industry.* Boca Raton, FL: CRC Press; 1991a:107–114.

Bonati A. How and why should we standardize phytopharmical drugs for clinical validation? *J Ethnopharmacol.* 1991b;32:195–197.

Brevoort P. The booming U.S. botanical market: A new overview. *HerbalGram.* 1998;44:33–48.

Deveny K. Garlic and ginseng supplements become potent drugstore sellers. *The Wall Street Journal* 10/1/92, pp. B1, B5.

Ernst E. Prevalence of use of complementary/alternative medicine: A systmatic review. *Bull World Health Org.* 2000:78(2):252–257.

Farnsworth N, Akrtrlr O, Bingel AS, Soejarto DD, Guo Z. Medicinal plants in therapy. *Bull World Health Org.* 1985:63;965–981.

Griggs, B. *Green Pharmacy. A History of Herbal Medicine.* London: Robert Hale; 1981.

Heptinstall S, Awang DV, Dawson BA, Kindack D, Knight DW, Mag J. Parthenolide content and bioactivity of feverfew (*Tanacetum parthenium* (L.) Schultz-Bip.). Estimation of commercial and authenticated feverfew products. *J Pharm Pharmacol.* 1992:44;391–395.

Interview with Prof. H. Wagner. *HerbalGram.* 1988;19:16–17.

Karlsen J. Quality control and instrumental analysis of plant extracts. In: Wijeskera ROB, ed. *The Medicinal Plant Industry.* Boca Raton, FL: CRC Press; 1991:99–106.

Keller K. Legal requirements for the use of phytopharmaceutical drugs in the Federal Republic of Germany. *J. Ethnopharmacol.* 1991;32:225–229.

Kleijnen J, Knipschild P. Drug profiles—*Ginkgo biloba. Lancet.* 1993;340:1136–1139.

Liberti LE, Marderosian AD. Evaluation of commercial ginseng products. *J Pharmacol Sci.* 1978;67:1487–1489.

Market Report. *HerbalGram.* 1992;26:40.

Principe PP. The economic significance of plants and their constituents as drugs. *Econ Med Plant Res.* 1989;3:1–17.

Soldati F, Sticher O. HPLC separation and quantitative determination of ginsenosides from *Panax ginseng, Panax quinquefolium* and from ginseng drug preparations. *Planta Med.* 1980;39(4):348–357.

62.3   Credentialing Herbal Suppliers

Leah Kliger

The market for herbal/botanical supplements is booming. In two landmark studies, David Eisenberg, MD, and his colleagues (Eisenberg et al, 1993; Eisenberg, 1998) indicated about 12.5% of adults in the United States used some form of herbal remedy in the previous year. Researchers reported that consumers who used herbs spent an average of $75 per year on herbal products.

The *Nutrition Business Journal* estimates that from 1995 to 1997 (Nutrition Business Journal, 1999), the market for herbs grew at a rate of 43%. The growth in the following year was projected at 13%. In a context of high market demand and relatively low supply, the use of botanical products is predicted to continue to grow.

Patients and physicians, nurses, pharmacists, naturopathic doctors, acupuncturists, and other practitioners have a need for criteria by which

A frequent speaker on herbal medicine, Leah Kliger is Director of Integrative Medicine, Evergreen Healthcare, Kirkland, Washington, and is a health consultant who works with hospitals, physicians, and other health care practitioners to foster the development of integrative medicine.

Source: Adapted with permission from *Creating an Herbal Apothecary: An Implementation Guide for Hospitals, Physicians, and Other Health Care Practitioners,* by Leah Kliger, © 2000. Health Care Communications, P.O. Box 594, Rye, NY. (P) 914-967-6741.

to evaluate product quality; the potential for good or harm; and interactions with other herbal remedies, nutritional supplements, or pharmaceuticals.

Creating an herbal formulary may appear to be a daunting task. There are literally hundreds of thousands of medicinal plants in the world, numerous philosophies about healing with herbs, and thousands of herbal manufacturers and suppliers.

The quality of products varies widely, depending on conditions during harvesting and manufacturing. Chemical assays have been conducted by medicinal chemists to evaluate the potency of commercial botanical products, to determine whether the herb and the active ingredients stated on the label are contained within the product, and to determine whether they are of the potency indicated. In a particular analysis of *echinacea,* of ten different products evaluated, only one contained the exact amount indicated on the label of the herb *(USA Today,* 1997). An assay of St. John's wort the following year found even greater variability *(Los Angeles Times,* 1998).

In the evaluation of herbal products, questions to be considered include:

- Which herbal remedies should be stocked?
- Which are safe and effective?
- Which herbal traditions and practices must be taken into account?
- What types of preparations are most suitable for the therapeutic purposes? Tinctures? Capsules? Bulk herbs? Standardized products? Organic products?
- Which manufacturers and suppliers should be utilized as the source of the botanical products? On what basis will they be selected?
- How large or small should the formulary be? Should 50 remedies be stocked? 100? 700?
- Should herbs be stocked on the basis of popularity or is there value in stocking more obscure herbs with known benefit?
- Which are the primary medical conditions most often seen by practitioners?

- Which herbs have undergone the most scrutiny and research or clinical trials?
- Should the formulary include only brand names or those recommended by particular physicians? Should multilevel marketing products be considered?

EVALUATING SUPPLIES

What are the most important considerations when evaluating and selecting suppliers for the herbs to be stocked in an organization's formulary? This section offers suggestions for making those selections based on a credentialing process.

Develop a credentialing checklist to include the following questions:

Growing

- Are the supplier and its seed source reputable?
- What level of pesticides or herbicides is used?
- Are organic herbal products available and is there limited use of synthetic fertilizers?
- Is a soil analysis available? Is there evidence of heavy metals or other contaminants?
- What type of confirmation test is used to identify the plant and the proper plant parts?

Harvesting

- Is the plant processed within minutes of harvesting? Quick processing often means capture of volatile oils, and the plant's active constituents can be maximized.
- Has the proper part of the plant (ie, leaf, flower, or root) been selected to optimize scent, flavor, and medicinal properties?
- Are the herbs harvested at the right season (some believe time of day is also important)?

Processing/Manufacturing

- Are the raw materials purchased from a known and reputable source?
- What is the country of origin?

- Does the manufacturer follow stringent guidelines such as those of the American Herbal Products Association?
- Have harsh solvents/cleaning agents been used on the equipment, thereby creating the possibility of toxic residue on the herbs?
- Is the plant material quickly dried, thereby minimizing the opportunity for yeast, mold, or bacterial growth?
- Are guidelines in place for the handling of the botanical? Are the guidelines comparable to those for handling food-grade products?
- Is the manufacturing plant spotlessly clean?
- Are independent assays completed, are they performed in-house, and if not, who completes the evaluations?
- Is there any fumigation or irradiation of plant materials?
- Is there complete label disclosure?
- Are all ingredients listed on the label, including any solvents?
- Were any additives used, such as starch, wheat, corn, artificial flavors, colors, or binders?
- If additives were used, are they indicated on the label?
- Is there standardization of the active ingredient? Why or why not and how was the level of standardization determined?
- What is the in-house quality assurance program of the manufacturer?
- Are expiration dates noted on the label?
- Are there systems in place to track lot, batch, and shipping?

Formulating/Blending

- Are the amounts of botanicals in the formula based on published research?
- Who does the formulating and what are his or her credentials and training?
- What types of preparations are available (eg, bulk, teas, powder, tincture, extract, tablets, or encapsulations)?
- Does the manufacturer standardize the formula? Why or why not?

Clinical Research

- Are there any research affiliations with academic medical centers and/or pharmaceutical companies?
- Are researchers conducting clinical trials?
- At what level is the research funded?

Labeling

- Do the labels follow FDA guidelines?
- Are potentially harmful or adverse interactions listed on the box, the label, or on inserts?

Company Information and References

- How long has the company been in business?
- What kinds of references will it provide?

Health care professionals should send the checklist to a list of potential suppliers culled from a variety of sources such as the National Nutritional Foods Association (NNFA). The NNFA is the nation's largest natural products trade organization, which registers each product or member company and conducts random independent product evaluations. Obtaining good manufacturing practices (GMP) certification offered by the NNFA helps to ensure the safety, quality, purity, and label integrity of nutritional supplements and herbal remedies. Health care professionals may also wish to also decide to send this checklist to a select group of manufacturers who wholesale their products directly to practitioners such as medical doctors, naturopathic doctors, acupuncturists, chiropractors, and pharmacists.

Next Steps

- Ask for a written response to the credentialing checklist and analyze the responses for completeness.
- Winnow the list to no more than five to eight brands.
- Consider making one or more on-site visits to those on your short list of potential sup-

pliers in order to tour the manufacturing plant, talk to the owners, and discuss policies and procedures with the suppliers' quality assessment and research departments.

- Select one herbal remedy, eg, echinacea, from a potential supplier and have it assayed by a private laboratory.

- Negotiate favorable contract terms and price.
- Select and notify the supplier.
- Determine an ongoing supplier evaluation process.

REFERENCES

Eisenberg D, Davis R, Ettner S, et al. Trends in alternative medicine use in the United States, 1990–1997: results of a follow-up national survey. *JAMA.* 1998;280(18):1548–1552.

Eisenberg DM, Kessler RC, Foster C, et al. Unconventional medicine in the United States. *N Engl J Med.* 1993;328:246–252.

Industry Overview. *Nutr Bus J.* 1999; IV(6):3.

Los Angeles Times. August 31, 1998.

USA Today. November 25, 1997.

62.4   Selected References for Researching Herbal Medicines

Allison R. McCutcheon

MONOGRAPHS AND TEXTS

American Herbal Pharmacopoeia (AHP). *American Herbal Pharmacopoeia and Therapeutic Compendium.* Quality control, analytical and therapeutic monographs (astragalus, hawthorn berry, hawthorn leaf, schizandra berry, St. John's wort, valerian, willow bark). Santa Cruz, CA: American Herbal Pharmacopoeia. The AHP monograph on St. John's wort was also published in *HerbalGram*, volume 40 (summer 1997) and is available as a reprint. AHP plans

---

The Canadian Pharmacists Association (CPhA), founded in 1907, is the national voluntary organization of pharmacists committed to providing leadership for the profession of pharmacy. Its vision is to establish the pharmacist as the health professional whose practice, based on unique knowledge and skills, ensures optimal patient outcomes. CPhA achieves its vision by serving its members through advocacy, facilitation, provision of knowledge, participation in partnerships, research, and innovation, education, and health promotion.

The Canadian Medical Association (CMA) is the national voice of Canadian physicians. Founded in 1867, CMA's mission is to provide leadership for physicians and to promote the highest standard of health and health care for Canadians. On behalf of its members and the Canadian public, CMA performs a wide variety of functions, such as advocating for access to quality health care, facilitating change within the medical profession, and providing leadership and guidance to physicians to help them influence, manage, and adapt to changes in health care delivery. The CMA is a voluntary professional organization representing the majority of Canada's physicians and comprising 12 provincial and territorial divisions and 42 affiliated medical organizations.

Excerpt from "Finding Accurate and Reliable Information on Herbal Medicines, Appendix I: Selected References for Researching Herbal Medicines." In: *Herbs: Everyday Reference for Health Professionals.* Ottawa, Ontario, Canada: Canadian Pharmacists Association and Canadian Medical Association, 2000. Reprinted with permission of the publishers.

to publish a new monograph every 2 months, starting in the year 2000. Monographs may be ordered through the AHP Web site (www.herbal-ahp.org) or from the American Botanical Council.

Bisset NG, editor. *Herbal Drugs and Phytopharmaceuticals*. Boca Raton (FL): CRC Press; 1994.

Blumenthal M, senior editor. *The Complete German Commission E Monographs: Therapeutic Guide to Herbal Medicines*. Klein S, Rister RS, translators. Austin (TX): American Botanical Council; 1998.

Brinker F. *Herb Contraindications and Drug Interactions*. 2nd ed. Sandy (OR): Eclectic Medical Publications; 1998.

De Smet PAGM, Keller K, Hänsel R, et al, editors. *Adverse Effects of Herbal Drugs*. Vol 1–3. New York: Springer-Verlag; 1992, 1993, 1997.

European Scientific Cooperative on Phytotherapy (ESCOP). *ESCOP monographs on the medicinal uses of plant drugs*. Fascicules 1–5. Exeter, UK: ESCOP; 1996–1997.

McGuffin M, Hobbs C, Upton R, et al, editors. *American Herbal Products Association's Botanical Safety Handbook*. Boca Raton (FL): CRC Press; 1997.

Newall CA, Anderson LA, Phillipson JD. *Herbal Medicines—A Guide for Health-Care Professionals*. London: Pharmaceutical Press; 1996.

Tisserand R, Balacs T. *Essential Oil Safety: A Guide for Health Care Professionals*. London: Churchill Livingstone; 1995.

United States Pharmacopeial Convention. *Botanical monograph series. Drug Information for the Health Care Professional*. Rockville (MD): United States Pharmacopeial Convention; 1998. (Web site: www.usp.org.)

Wagner H, Bauer R. *Chinese Drug Monographs and Analysis*. Geneva: World Health Organization; 1997–1998.

World Health Organization. *WHO Monographs on Selected Medicinal Plants*. Vol 1. Geneva: The Organization; 1999.

Peer-Reviewed Herbal Medicine Journals

Fitoterapia. New York: Elsevier Science Inc.

Pharmaceutical Biology (formerly *International Journal of Pharmacognosy*). Lisse, Netherlands: Swets & Zeitlinger B.V.

Phytomedicine. Stuttgart: Gustav Fischer Verlag.

Phytotherapie. Paris: Masson.

Phytotherapy Research. West Sussex, UK: John Wiley & Sons.

Planta Medica. Stuttgart: Springer-Verlag.

Peer-Reviewed Journals Publishing Phytomedicine and Related Herbal Research

Alternative Therapies in Health and Medicine. Alijo Viejo (CA): Innovision Communications.

Economic Botany. Bronx (NY): New York Botanical Garden Press.

Journal of Alternative and Complementary Medicine: Research on Paradigm, Practice and Policy. Larchmont (NY): Mary Ann Liebert, Inc.

Journal of Ethnopharmacology. New York: Elsevier Science.

Journal of Herbs, Spices and Medicinal Plants. New York: Haworth Herbal Press.

Journal of Natural Products (predominantly chemical constituent data). Cincinnati (OH): American Society of Pharmacognosy.

Phytochemistry (predominantly chemical constituent data). Oxford and New York: Pergamon Press.

Review and Herb News Journals

FACT (Focus on Alternative and Complementary Therapies): An Evidence-Based Approach. London: Pharmaceutical Press.

Healthnotes Review of Complementary and Integrative Medicine (formerly *Quarterly Review of Natural Medicine*). Portland (OR): Healthnotes Inc.

HerbalGram. Austin (TX): American Botanical Council and Herb Research Foundation.

Other Professional Journals

Alternative and Complementary Therapies. Larchmont (NY): Mary Ann Liebert, Inc.

Canadian Journal of Herbalism. Toronto: Ontario Herbalists Association.

Canadian Pharmaceutical Journal. Mississauga: Clifford K. Goodman, Inc.

European Journal of Herbal Medicine. Exeter, UK: National Institute of Medical Herbalists.

Nutrition Research. New York: Elsevier Science.

DATABASES (UP TO DATE AS OF JANUARY 2000)

Agricola. Beltsville (MD): National Agricultural Library. gopher://probe.nalusda.gov:7020/77/agricola/agidx

Biological Abstracts. Philadelphia: BIOSIS. www.biosis.org/home_static.html

Chemical Abstracts. Columbus (OH): Chemical Abstracts Service. www.cas.org/prod.html

The Cochrane Library. The Cochrane Collaboration. hiru.mcmaster.ca/cochrane or www.cochrane.org/cochrane/cdsr.htm

Excerpta Medica database, through *EMBASE.* New York: Elsevier Science. www.bids.ac.uk/embase.html

International Bibliographic Information on Dietary Supplements. Bethesda (MD): Office of Dietary Supplements, National Institutes of Health. odp.od.nih.gov/ods/databases/databases.html

MEDLINE. Bethesda (MD): National Library of Medicine. medline.cos.com

NAPRALERT (natural products alert) database. Chicago: Program for Collaborative Research in the Pharmaceutical Sciences, Department of Medical Chemistry and Pharmacognosy, College of Pharmacy, University of Illinois at Chicago. Access through Bitnet, Internet, Compuserve, Prodigy, EARN or STN International (www.cas.org)

Netting the Evidence: A ScHARR Introduction to Evidence-Based Practice on the Internet. Sheffield, UK: School of Health and Related Research (ScHARR). www.shef.ac.uk/~scharr/ir/netting.html

INTERNET SITES (UP TO DATE AS OF JANUARY 2000)

Algy's Herb Page. www.algy.com/herb/index.html

American Botanical Council Online and *HerbalGram.* Austin (TX): American Botanical Council. www.herbalgram.org

American Herbal Products Association Web site. Silver Spring (MD): The Association. www.ahpa.org

Association of Natural Medicine Pharmacists Web site. San Rafael (CA): The Association. www.anmp.org

Canadian Herb Society Web site. Vancouver: The Society. www.herbsociety.ca

Dr. Duke's Phytochemical and Ethnobotanical Databases. Beltsville (MD): Agricultural Research Service, US Department of Agriculture. www.ars-grin.gov/duke

European Phytojournal (the official newsletter of ESCOP). Exeter: European Scientific Cooperative on Phytotherapy. www.ex.ac.uk/phytonet/phytojournal/contents.htm

Grateful Med. Bethesda (MD): National Library of Medicine. igm.nlm.nih.gov/

Herbal Hall. www.herb.com

HerbCraft Herbal Network (Elizabeth Burch). www.herbcraft.com/monographs.html

HerbMed. Bethesda (MD): Alternative Medicine Foundation. www.amfoundation.org/herbmed.htm

Herb Research Foundation Web site. Boulder (CO): The Foundation. www.herbs.org

MedHerb.com, from *Medical Herbalism.* Boulder (CO): Bergner Communications. www.medherb.com

Medical Herbalism—A Journal for the Clinical Practitioner. Boulder (CO): Bergner Communications. www.medherb.com/DB.HTM

Medicinal Plant Databases (Michael C. Tims). www.wam.umd.edu/~mct/Plants/medicinal.html

National Center for Complementary and Alternative Medicine Web site. Bethesda (MD): The Center. nccam.nih.gov/

National Institute of Medical Herbalists Web site. Exeter, UK: The Institute. www.btinternet.com/~nimh/frameacc.html

Natural Medicines Comprehensive Database. Stockton (CA): Therapeutic Research Center, Inc. www.naturaldatabase.com/

Office of Dietary Supplements Web site. Bethesda (MD): National Institutes of Health. odp.od.nih.gov/ods/

Phytonet. Exeter, UK: Centre for Complementary Health Studies, University of Exeter. www.ex.ac.uk/phytonet/

Planet Herbs Online (Michael Tierra). www.planetherbs.com

PubMed. Bethesda (MD): National Library of Medicine. www.ncbi.nlm.nih.gov/PubMed/

Special Nutritionals Adverse Event Monitoring System. Washington, DC: Office of Special Nutritionals, Center for Food Safety and Applied Nutrition, US Food and Drug Administration. vm.cfsan.fda.gov/~dms/aems.html

Warnings. Ottawa: Health Canada. www.hc-sc.gc.ca/english/news-arc.htm#warn

CHAPTER 63

Interactions of Pharmaceuticals and Botanical Medicines

Francis J. Brinker

INTRODUCTION

As the medicinal use of herbs becomes more common, an understandable concern is the possible interference with prescription drugs. For doctors and pharmacists unfamiliar with the activities and effects of botanical products and their extracted components, a reluctance to recommend these agents to patients or customers may be attributed to a "fear of the unknown." Their concerns are multiple. Will components of botanical remedies interfere with the kinetics of their prescriptions, such as absorption, metabolism, and/or excretion, rendering them less available or more so? Or will the effects of the herbs alter the effect of the drug through metabolic changes, antagonism, or additive effects? Naturopathic physicians and others who use herbal products medicinally often face these same quandaries in prescribing for patients on drug maintenance therapies who wish to explore other approaches for the same or different conditions. This chapter addresses some of the concerns shared by those who administer or pro-

vide pharmaceutical and/or botanical medicines and discusses certain benefits of using botanical remedies and drugs together.

In herbs with primary active constituents, whose pharmacology has been elucidated, a fairly straightforward assessment of potential interactions can be made by those with standard medical/pharmacological training (for example, *Ephedra sinica* with its alkaloids ephedrine and pseudoephedrine). However, the case is not as simple with many herbs. Medicinal plants that have not attracted the attention of research scientists, as well as herbal remedies whose study has revealed a complexity that defies simplistic mechanistic explanations, can baffle even those clinicians who demonstrate an active interest in understanding the interplay of synthetic and natural medicinal agents. In an attempt to help bridge these gaps in knowledge, it is appropriate to address some general considerations and offer a variety of specific examples illustrating how botanical medicines may influence and modify the effects of common pharmaceuticals. Since the vast array of specific concerns cannot be addressed in a limited venue such as this, a practical reference source is needed. To supply this larger need, the author has compiled a more complete reference text from the scientific and medical literature (Brinker, 1997).

Francis J. Brinker, ND, received his doctorate and postgraduate certification in botanical medicine from the National College of Naturopathic Medicine in Portland, Oregon. He is the author of several books on botanical medicine, including *Herb Contraindications and Drug Interactions*. He currently serves as co-facilitator in botanical medicine for the Program in Integrative Medicine at the University of Arizona College of Medicine.

Source: Adapted with permission from F. Brinker, ND, Interaction of Pharmaceuticals and Botanical Medicines, *Journal of Naturopathic Medicine*, Vol. 7, No. 2, pp. 14–22, © 1997, American Association of Naturopathic Physicians.

COMPLEMENTARY COMBINATIONS

In some circumstances, the addition of botanical remedies to other medicines can improve the response or help protect from deleterious side effects of the pharmaceuticals.

This adjunctive approach to prescribing blends the best of both systems in cases in which the prescription drugs are deemed necessary for the patient's recovery or long-term maintenance. While the possibilities in this regard are many and varied, a few examples of how common medical prescriptions can be enhanced by the addition of botanical agents should suffice to illustrate such concomitant treatments.

Immune-Enhancing Botanicals

The standard medical approach to treating infections that led to the dominant success of pharmaceuticals in this field is the administration of antibiotics. The extensive use of these agents has led to a growing crisis in requiring the treatment of new forms of medication that overcome the increasing bacterial resistance to such compounds. The naturopathic approach, meanwhile, has relied heavily on strengthening the body's resistance to infections by employing natural means and substances that enhance the immune response.

Among immune-enhancing botanicals, the American herb *Echinacea* (purple cornflower) is considered foremost. European research on *Echinacea* species has identified a variety of nontoxic active constituents, among them high-molecular-weight polysaccharides, glycoproteins, isobutylamides, polyacetylenes, and caffeic acid derivatives, that together enhance replication, phagocytosis, and cytokine production by various white blood cells. In addition, individual components have shown some antibacterial, antimycotic, and antiviral activities (Brinker, 1995a). In a clinical study on recurrent vaginal candidiasis, the recurrence rate after 6 months when using the topical antimycotic econazole nitrate alone for 6 days was 60.5% in 43 patients. Compared to the recurrence rate of 15.0% in 20 patients using both econazole and *Echinacea purpurea* herb pressed juice topically and 16.7% in 60 patients using econazole topically and *E. purpurea* juice orally, the econazole treatment alone was markedly less effective (Coeugniet and Kuhnast, 1986).

Other botanical remedies are known for immunomodulating benefits that enhance antimicrobial effects in treating infections.

Siberian ginseng (the root of *Eleutherococcus senticosus*) also contains high-molecular-weight heteroglycan polysaccharides that enhance phagocytosis in vitro and in vivo (Wagner et al, 1985). In addition, in a placebo-controlled study the alcoholic extract of *Eleutherococcus* root given in 10-mL doses three times daily to 36 healthy humans for 4 weeks drastically increased the number of immunocompetent cells, especially T-cells (helper/inducer, cytotoxic, and natural killer cells), and generally enhanced the activation of T-lymphocytes with no side effects (Bohn et al, 1987). A study of children ages 0 to 14 years suffering from dysentery caused by *Shigella* species and enterocolitis of *Proteus* etiology compared the use of monomycin and kanamycin together with *Eleutherococcus* and related *Echinopanax elatum* in 157 patients, while using antibiotics alone in 101 patients. The periods of disease decreased for children using the herbs together with the antibiotics (Vereshchagin et al, 1982).

Multiple Complementary Effects: Treatment of Benign Prostatic Hyperplasia

Benign prostatic hyperplasia (BPH) is a condition that involves a number of different processes that seem amenable to treatment with complementary pharmaceutical approaches. Therefore, the smooth muscle relaxing α-adrenergic inhibitor terazosin (Hytrin), proven effective in relieving BPH symptoms, was combined with the 5α-reductase inhibitor finasteride (Proscar) in a clinical study. Though finasteride blocks conversion of testosterone to the more potent prostatic growth stimulator dihydrotestosterone, finasteride combined with terazosin proved no better than terazosin alone in treating BPH as documented by symptom scores in this study (Lepor et al, 1996).

Several botanical remedies have been shown in clinical studies to be effective in treating early stages of BPH. Of greatest benefit are three whose concentrated solid and liquid extracts are commonly used phytomedicinals in Europe: *Serenoa repens* (saw palmetto) fruit, *Pygeum africanum* (African prune) bark, and *Urtica dioica* (stinging nettle) root (Brinker, 1995b). While their extracts have only a mild 5α-reductase inhibitory activity compared to finasteride (Rhodes et al, 1993), they impact the prostate by other means. *Serenoa* has shown some anti-androgenic effects (Brinker, 1995b), but it may be most useful due to its reduction of estrogen and androgen receptors in the nuclei of prostate cells (DiSilverio et al, 1992). In addition to mild 5α-reductase inhibition, *Pygeum* and *Urtica* extracts both demonstrated in vitro aromatase inhibition that reduces the conversion of androgens to estradiol, a contributing factor in BPH. While *Pygeum* was the more potent of the two when used alone, together these extracts had a significantly stronger, synergistic aromatase-inhibiting effect (Hartmann, 1996). It is possible that the combined outcomes of these effective plant remedies together with terazosin would produce better clinical effects than when terazosin is taken alone, based upon their different mechanisms of action from each other and from finasteride.

BOTANICAL PROPERTIES THAT ARE PROTECTIVE AGAINST DRUG SIDE EFFECTS

Botanical medicines can offer protection from some of the undesirable side effects associated with liver compromise due to toxins or the use of pharmaceuticals.

Silybum marianum (milk thistle) fruit flavonolignans have been found protective against liver damage in rodents after exposure to a wide variety of xenobiotic hepatotoxins, including deoxycholate, acetaminophen, halothane, and ethanol due to their antioxidant and lipoxygenase-inhibiting activities (Brinker, 1995a). Clinical studies showed that using the flavonolignan extract called silymarin with patients suffering

from alcoholic cirrhosis decreased mortality and helped normalize serum enzymes indicative of liver damage (Brinker, 1995a; Fintelmann, 1986). Silymarin improves the metabolism of aspirin in cirrhotic rats and may thereby help prevent or reduce side effects from other medications metabolized in the liver of patients with liver disease. In a woman with dilantin-induced hepatitis who required dilantin as a maintenance therapy, the liver enzyme changes normalized after silymarin was given (Fintelmann, 1986). In a double-blind, placebo-controlled study involving 60 patients chronically receiving the psychotropic drugs butyrophenones or phenothiazines, silymarin reduced lipoperoxidative hepatic damage (Palsasciano et al, 1994).

A number of botanically derived compounds have already been used in conventional medicine to enhance the medicinal effects of drugs.

Allantoin has been found to increase the healing of psoriasis when compared to coal tar alone. The cell-proliferant allantoin is found in yields of 1% to 2% in the leaves and roots of *Symphytum officinale* (comfrey); the clinical research used allantoin in 2% concentration topically in a lotion or cream base (Brinker, 1995a).

The immune-stimulant polysaccharide lentinan from the *Lentinus edodes* (shitake) mushroom when given by injection increased the mean survival times in 77 patients over 100% compared to 68 patients given placebo in advanced recurrent stomach cancer patients receiving chemotherapy (Brinker, 1995a). The combination of isolated components from herbs with other pharmaceuticals is an established practice going back to the discovery of alkaloids. Using a more complex extract from a plant increases the number of interactive factors involved in combinations, but this type of botanical medicine is just as capable of increasing the therapeutic potential of other proven remedies.

BOTANICALS THAT REDUCE DRUG AVAILABILITY

There are several general categories of botanical medicines that need to be restricted when vital pharmaceutical drugs are being administered.

It is fairly obvious that if medicines, whatever their source, have antagonistic activities and are prescribed together, they will tend to hinder the effects desired from each one to a greater or lesser extent. The simultaneous prescription of antagonistic agents defies common sense and would be expected to occur only due to a lack of knowledge of the other medication being used. However, interference with medicinal effects not only occurs when two agents are directly antagonistic, but is more common when the absorption, metabolism, or excretion of a drug is compromised.

A delay in absorption of orally administered drugs and nutrients can be caused by certain herbs that delay gastric emptying. This is particularly true of those that are high in water-soluble, hydrocolloidal fiber. Their high viscosity can also produce a semipermeable barrier over the gastrointestinal mucosa, another mechanism that may inhibit absorption.

This mechanism can cause positive or negative consequences, depending on the medical condition and the drug(s) and nutrient(s) involved. Since fiber commonly referred to as gum or mucilage is insoluble in alcohol, this effect is of greatest concern when certain powdered herbs, teas, juices, or dried aqueous extracts are taken orally in large quantities along with medications such as lithium salts, digoxin, or penicillin. Examples of these different types of hydrocolloidal preparations include powdered *Althaea officinalis* (marshmallow) root, cold infusion of *Ulmus fulva* (slippery elm) bark, *Aloe vera* (aloe) leaf gel, and alginate powder from brown algae. Many hydrocolloidal substances can be found in food items like okra and oats or as food additives such as carrageenan, guar gum, locust bean gum, and pectin that are known to absorb cholesterol. Bulk laxative herbs that can also interfere with cholesterol and drug absorption include *Linum usitatissimum* (flax) seed, *Trigonella foenum-graecum* (fenugreek) seed, and *Plantago psyllium* or *P. ovata* (psyllium) seed (Brinker, 1997).

Certain compounds found in botanical medicines can hinder absorption if they bind with alkaloidal medications such as atropine, codeine, ephedrine, and theophylline, which are susceptible to precipitation.

Tannins are the most common cause of this problem though salicylates will also cause alkaloids to precipitate. Since tannins are present in some herbal powders, are extracted in hot water, and are soluble in alcohol, herbs that contain significant quantities of tannins should be avoided in all forms administered orally while taking alkaloid-containing medicines by mouth simultaneously. Tannins can also precipitate proteins and minerals such as iron or copper that may be important factors or cofactors in drug or nutritional therapies. Because the most commonly consumed plant high in tannins is *Camellia sinensis* (black, green, or oolong tea), a case history pertaining to the use of this recreational (and medicinal) beverage is important. Other common beverage and/or medicinal teas that contain high amounts (over 10%) of tannins include *Arctostaphylos uva-ursi* (bearberry) leaves; *Juglans nigra* (black walnut) leaves, bark, and rinds; *Geranium maculatum* (cranesbill) rhizome; *Rubus* species (raspberry) leaves; *Quercus* species (oak) bark; and *Hamamelis virginiana* (witch hazel) leaves and bark. Common salicylate-containing herbs that may precipitate alkaloids include *Filipendula ulmaria* (meadowsweet) flowers, *Populus* species (popular) bark and buds, *Salix* species (willow) bark, and *Gaultheria procumbems* (wintergreen) leaves (Brinker, 1997; Wagner et al, 1985). In summary, two mechanisms by which botanicals can reduce absorption are by reducing mucosal permeability and precipitating alkaloids.

Botanical medicines can also reduce absorption of medicinal agents through their rapid elimination.

High doses of laxatives can lower absorption of orally administered medicinal compounds by increasing peristalsis and reducing the bowel transit time. Although naturopathic physicians tend to avoid the recommendation of herbs known for their excessive cathartic effects, it is still important to be aware of this mechanism. They effectively lower absorption by diminishing the amount of available time and mucosal contact necessary for diffusion or transport to occur across the intestinal mucosa. Prolonged maintenance of such bowel stimulation would be termed abuse and is mostly encountered with self-administration of over-the-counter laxatives by bulimic patients. In cases of anthranoid-containing botanicals, chronic overuse is evidenced by a black discoloration of the rectal mucosa. The more common laxative herbs yielding anthroquinones are *Aloe* species (aloe) leave exudate, *Rheum* species (rhubarb) root, *Rhamnus purshiana* (cascara sagrada) bark, and *Cassia* species (senna) leaves and pods (Brinker, 1997; Brinker, 1996).

The half-life of beneficial medications can also be decreased through the activity of herbs and botanicals that increase liver detoxification.

Many prescribed drugs are metabolized in liver microsomes. The rate of hepatic detoxification of environmental toxins (xenobiotics) can be increased. Herbs such as *Medicago sativa* (alfalfa) have been shown to increase metabolizing enzymes such as mixed-function oxidase in rodents (Brinker, 1997; Brinker 1995). Indoles produced enzymatically after consumption of glucosinolates found in various cruciferous vegetables and plants have a similar effect and enhance the glutathione S-transferase activity (Sparnins et al, 1984). For example, indoles from *Brassica* species crucifers (cabbage, broccoli, etc) increase the liver's metabolism of estradiol. Although increasing microsomal enzyme activity is useful as a means of detoxifying carcinogenic substances, the half-life of beneficial medications can also be decreased (Brinker, 1995a). In addition, the high vitamin K intake from regular consumption of cruciferous vegetables can produce resistance to effects of warfarin (Coumadin) (Walker, 1984).

Specific botanicals and nutrients are known to increase drug metabolism.

Drug metabolism in rats and humans has been shown to increase through the use of the aromatic compound eucalyptol, found in cough drops and in the essential oil of *Eucalyptus* species used in volatile inhalant preparations for steam humidifiers. Eucalyptol decreased plasma and/or brain levels of amphetamine, zoxazolamine, pentobarbital, and aminopyrine in rats exposed to eucalyptol aerosol for 2 to 10 minutes per day for 4 days. In humans exposed to the aerosol for 10 minutes per day for 10 days, the rates of disappearance of plasma aminopyrine and of urinary excretion of 4-aminoantipyrine (its metabolite) were increased (Jori et al, 1970). Eucalyptol was also shown to increase liver metabolism of π-nitro-anisol and aniline. Given as an aerosol to rats for 4 days for either 5 to 10 or 15 to 30 minutes daily, eucalyptol significantly decreased pentobarbital levels in the brain and lowered the induced sleeping time when pentobarbital was given 18 hours after the last eucalyptol exposure (Jori et al, 1969). On the other hand, consumption of *Eucalyptus globulus* leaves increased the toxicity of pyrrolizidine alkaloid-containing *Senecio* species due to the increased metabolic activation of these toxic alkaloids by microsomal enzymes (White et al, 1983).

Not all aromatic oils or terpenes induce microsomal enzyme activity. *Pinus pumilio* oil, guaiacol, menthol, α-pinene, and β-pinene were shown to be without effect (Jori et al, 1969). Aromatic substances that increase microsomal metabolism of drugs include those found in cedarwood *(Juniperus virginiana* and *J. ashei)* oil such as cedrol and cedrene. The inhaled aromatic oil with these components reduced hypnotic effects of hexobarbitone in mice and enhanced the removal of bishydroxycoumarin (Dicourmarol) from the blood in rats. The enzymes enhanced by the cedarwood volatiles were aniline hydroxylase, sulfanilamide acetylase, neoprontosil azoreductase, heptachlor epoxidase, and zoxazolamine hydroxylase (Corrigan, 1993).

POTENTIALLY HAZARDOUS ADDITIVE EFFECTS

Increasing the activity of a pharmaceutical drug is a significant risk due to the side effects or toxicities normally associated with many of these potent synthetic medicines. One means by which this can occur is by increasing the half-life of a drug by slowing its breakdown or excretion.

For example, the suppressive effect of the glycyrrhetinic acid component of *Glycyrrhiza glabra* (licorice) on 5β-reductase effectively delays the clearance of corticosteroids by the liver (Tamura et al, 1979). As far as is known, this type of interference is fairly atypical.

The most common way that mixing medicines accentuates their effects is by combining two agents with similar activities.

There are a number of general categories of drugs for which this holds true. In many cases, botanical medicines with the same or similar effects as botanicals can be used to reduce the dosage of a toxic drug or in some cases to replace a medicine that is not well tolerated. In either of these instances the gradual substitution of a botanical remedy for a prescription drug should only be done under a physician's close supervision and monitoring. Following are examples of serious overmedication resulting from combinations of medicines with comparable effects.

A number of cardiotonic botanical medicines were traditionally used in combination with, or in place of, *Digitalis* species (foxglove) and their extracts. Since *Digitalis* cardiac glycosides and their derivatives have become the standard agents for chronic treatment of cardiac insufficiency, the other botanical heart tonics, with the exception of *Strophanthus* species, have been mostly confined to naturopathic and herbal practice. Most of these remedies share with *Digitalis* structurally similar steroidal glycoside components with comparable activity. Botanicals containing the types of compounds that strengthen the heart's contractions include *Convallaria majalis* (lily-of-the-valley), *Adonis vernalis* (pheasant's eye), *Helleborus niger* (Christmas rose), and *Urginea maritima* (squill) (Brinker, 1997). *Selenicereus grandiflorus* (night-blooming cereus) lacks the steroidal glycoside components typical of this class of drug but acts as a cardiotonic agent nonetheless (Brinker, 1997; Brinker, 1995). Excessive amounts of these cardio-active medications alone or combined with digitalis could result in fatal arrhythmias or cardiac arrest (Brinker, 1996).

Some botanical remedies contain natural compounds that can result in a hemorrhagic diathesis with excessive consumption. These herbs can accentuate the effects of the prescription drug warfarin or other common anticoagulants enough to be of concern with regular consumption.

Plants known to contribute to clotting problems in the past include *Melilotus officinalis* (sweet clover), *Asperula odorata* (woodruff), and *Dipteryx odorata* (tonka beans). Bromelain, the proteolytic enzyme from pineapple (*Ananus comosus*) is also believed to potentiate anticoagulant activity (Hogan, 1983). Other botanicals that may enhance the effects of warfarin include *Aesculus hippocastinum* (horse chestnut) bark, due to the antithrombin activity of its esculetin component, and *Cinchona* species (Peruvian bark) (Brinker, 1997). Garlic (*Allium sativum*) has been shown to inhibit platelet aggregation (Brinker, 1995a), and excessive consumption of garlic has resulted in spontaneous (Rose et al, 1990) and postoperative bleeding episodes (Burnham, 1995).

Anti-anxiety, sedative, and central nervous system depressant medications are prescribed with the warning that they should not be mixed with alcohol due to the deleterious combined effects. A number of botanical medicines have also been shown through research to increase the effects of pharmacological sedatives as demonstrated by increasing the sleeping time in animals induced by the drugs pentobarbital or hexobarbital.

These herbs and their extracts include *Melissa officinalis* (lemon balm), *Eschscholtzia californica* (California poppy), *Humulus lupulus* (hops), *Passiflora incarnata* (passion flower), and *Valeriana officinalis* (valerian) (Brinker, 1997; Brinker, 1995a). Excessive sedation could result from the combination of these herbs with standard depressant drugs.

Monoamine oxidase (MAO) inhibitors given mostly as antidepressant agents have long been known to interact with some drugs and foods that can result in a hypertensive crisis. This is most common with adrenergic agents.

Adrenergic agents include the plant alkaloids ephedrine and pseudoephedrine obtained from *Ephedra* species (ephedra). Another familiar cause of this dangerous interaction are foods high in tyramine such as wine and cheese. The herb *Cytisus scoparius* (Scotch broom) also has a high tyramine content and can additionally aggravate high blood pressure due to the cardiac stimulant activity of its alkaloid sparteine. MAO inhibitors combined with excessive caffeine consumption from such sources as coffee (*Caffea* species), tea (*Camella sinensis*), cola (*Cola nitida*), and chocolate (*Theobroma cacao*) can also result in hypertensive episodes (Brinker, 1997).

Medicinal plants such as *Myristica fragrans* (nutmeg) and *Hypericum perforatum* (St. John's wort) act as MAO inhibitors in vitro (Brinker, 1997). *Hypericum* extract (from St. John's wort) is used effectively as an antidepressant in its own right (Brinker, 1995a). It not only performs as well as the standard tricyclic agents amitriptyline (Bergmann et al, 1993) and imipramine and the tetracyclic antidepressant maprotiline, but was actually shown to be safer than the latter two drugs (Vorbach et al, 1994; Harrer et al, 1994). Due to its impressive clinical effects, it would be prudent to also avoid combining *Hypericum* with other antidepressants, especially MAO inhibitors and those such as fluoxetine (Prozac) that act as selective serotonin reuptake inhibitors.

Certain botanicals known to decrease blood sugar should be monitored to avoid hypoglycemic episodes in individuals with diabetes.

Insulin-dependent diabetics must monitor their blood sugar carefully to avoid hypoglycemic episodes. The combined effect of exogenous hypoglycemic agents with insulin treatment can disrupt the means by which diabetics maintain suitable blood sugar levels and avoid insulin shock. While plant remedies are used to help control Type II diabetes mellitus, those under medication for Type I disease must be concerned about ingesting herbs that can have a significant impact on serum glucose. Certain plants have a well-documented ability to lower blood sugar levels through a variety of mechanisms. Since many hypoglycemic plants are also used as remedies for conditions unrelated to diabetes, their concomitant additive effect with insulin therapy would likely be inadvertent. Foremost among these plants is *Momordica charantia* (bitter melon), which contains a number of hypoglycemic constituents including the steroidal glycoside charantin, proteins p- and v-insulin, alkaloids, and others (Brinker, 1997; Raman and Lau, 1996; Bever and Zahnd, 1979).

Plants whose oral hypoglycemic activity has been confirmed and their active constituents identified include *Allium sativum* (garlic) cloves, *Trigonella foenum-graecum* (fenugreek) seeds, *Vaccinium myrtillus* (bilberry) leaves (Bever and Zahnd, 1979), *Tecoma stans* (tronadora) leaves (Bever and Zahnd, 1979; Perez et al, 1980), and *Olea europaea* (olive) leaves (Gonzalez et al, 1992). Other botanical remedies whose activity has been more or less confirmed without identifying the specific active constituents include *Arctium lappa* (burdock) roots, *Fatsia horrida* (devil's club) root bark, *Gymnema sylvestre* leaves, *Opuntia ficus-indica* (prickly pear) stems, *Syzygium jambolanum* (jambul) seeds, *Bidens pilosa* (aceitilla) plants, and *Turnera diffusa* (damiana) leaves (Bever and Zahnd, 1979; Perez et al, 1980). Hydrocoloidal fiber sources such as guar gum and psyllium taken in large quantities can delay gastric emptying and reduce the rate of absorption of dietary carbohydrates (Brinker, 1997).

Certain botanicals have the capacity to act as phototoxic agents by increasing the skin's sensitivity to ultraviolet radiation.

Plants in the Apiaceae (carrot or parsnip) family typically contain components chemically categorized as furanocoumarins. These psoralen compounds can act as phototoxic agents by increasing the skin's sensitivity to ultraviolet radiation. While occasionally problematic when used alone, the results are much more dramatic and damaging when these plants are taken simultaneously with 8-methoxypsoralen, prescribed to enhance UV therapy for hyperkeratotic conditions such as atopic eczema. Severe burns with swelling and blistering may occur. Those plants containing natural psoralens include *Angelica* species (angelica), *Apium graveolens* (celery), *Ammi visnaga* (khella), *Heracleum* species (hogweed), *Lomatium* species (wild parsnip), and *Daucus carota* (Queen Anne's lace). Plants outside of the Apiaceae family with components known to act as photosensitizers include *Ranunculus* species (buttercups), *Ruta graveolens* (rue), and *Hypericum perforatum* (Brinker, 1997).

Herbs that lower blood pressure may have an additive effect with pharmaceuticals used for this purpose.

Herbal diuretics that reduce fluid volume will also subsequently decrease cardiac output and blood pressure. Diuretic herbs include *Daucus carota*, *Agropyrum repens* (couch grass), *Galium aparine* (cleavers), and *Taraxacum officinale* (dandelion). Herbs used primarily for their hypotensive effects include *Crataegus oxycantha* (hawthorn), *Viscum album* (mistletoe), *Veratrum viride* (green hellebore), and *Rauwolfia serpentina* (snakewood). In an obvious example of avoiding antagonistic herbs, *Glycyrrhiza glabra* root (licorice) and its extracts, unless they are deglycyrrhizinated, should not be used by patients on hypotensive medication due to its potential hypertensive effects (D'Arcy, 1993).

A number of potent alkaloidal drugs are obtained from plant sources. The interactions of the mother plant should be taken as equivalent to those of the isolated alkaloids. Therefore, plants that contain anticholinergic tropane alkaloids such as atropine can potentiate synthetic drugs having sedative, antihistaminic, or antispasmodic activities, and these combinations should be avoided.

Atropine-containing plants include *Atropa belladonna* (deadly nightshade), *Datura stramonium* (Jimson weed), and *Hyoscyamus niger* (henbane) (D'Arcy, 1993). The α_2-adrenergic antagonism of yohimbine and extracts of the bark would be toxic combined with tricyclic antidepressants and phenothiazides and could reverse the effects of antihypertensive drugs (DeSmet and Smeets, 1994). The adverse interactions that may occur with *Rauwolfia serpentina* are the same as for its biogenic amine-depleting alkaloid reserpine. In addition to enhancing antihypertensives as mentioned above, *Rauwolfia* can have a detrimental effect if used with depressants, MAO inhibitors, sympathomimetics, tricyclic antidepressants, or *Digitalis* glycosides (Barnhart, 1991).

Digitalis Combinations with Dissimilar Botanicals

Besides the cardiotonic herbs already mentioned (such as *Strophanthus, Convallaria, Adonis, Helleborus, Urginea,* and *Selenicereus*) that can have an additive effect with digitaloid cardiac glycosides, other herbal remedies can also affect the activity of *Digitalis* constituents or their derivatives. Digitaloids are much-prescribed drugs for atrial tachyrhythmia and congestive heart failure in our ever-aging population. Influencing the activity of these plant-derived medicines can have a profound impact on the life and health of the patient. *Digitalis* glycosides provide a useful example to illustrate the different types of interactions that may occur in conjunction with the use of herbs to the benefit and the detriment of those being medicated.

Besides cardiotonic effects, advantages that can be derived from phytotherapeutic agents in heart disease revolve mainly around the use of coronary vasodilators that improve the perfusion of the cardiac musculature and thereby enhance nutrient availability and metabolic waste removal. *Crataegus* species leaves, flowers, and berries and their extracts have been shown to act therapeutically as vasodilators in relieving anginal pectoris, cardiac arrhythmias, and mild hypertension. A variety of active constituents including triterpene acids, procyanidins, and flavonoids help account for these benefits.

The cardiotonic activity of *Digitalis* was increased by *Crataegus* as well as *Convallaria* and *Adonis* in tests on guinea pigs. In cardiac failure, *Crataegus* functions well in conjunction with *Digitalis* and digoxin. The *Crataegus* extracts increase the response and reduce the toxicity to the cardiac glycosides digoxin and digitoxin, as well as g-strophanthin, allowing a reduction of their doses. *Ammi visnaga* is another botanical with coronary vasodilating components. The constituents khellin, visnadin, samidin, and dihydrosamidin obtained from khella have all shown this activity, with visnadin also producing positive inotropic effects. Visnadin given orally decreases the acute and chronic toxicity of digitoxin in mice by preventing bradycardia and reversing cardiac arrhythmias (Brinker, 1995a).

The absorption of digoxin is slowed by simultaneous consumption of guar gum, which reduces the plasma level temporarily. However, a more threatening interaction with digitaloids involves the use of botanical products that reduce blood potassium levels. Low serum potassium potentiates *Digitalis* effects. The *Glycyrrhiza glabra* root component glycyrrhizin induces potassium excretion in conjunction with sodium and water reabsorption in the kidneys, resulting in hypokalemia and hypertension, if used in large amounts for prolonged periods (Brinker, 1997). However, licorice extracts are safer than consuming an equivalent amount of pure glycyrrhizin, due to modified intestinal absorption and bioavailability of the glycyrrhizin when it is combined with other licorice components (Cantelli-Fort, 1994).

Overuse of laxatives (such as the botanicals *Aloe, Rheum, Rhamnus,* or *Cassica*) can also diminish blood levels of potassium, particularly when combined with potassium-depleting diuretics (Brinker, 1997; Barnhart, 1991). Although some herbal diuretics such as *Equisetum* species (horsetail) lead to significant potassium excretion (Perez Gutierrez et al, 1985), *Taraxacum officinale* leaves compensate for this excretory loss because of their own high potassium content (Racz-Kotilla et al, 1994).

Since one of the uses of *Digitalis* is to slow the contractile rate of the heart, plants with components that affect the autonomic control of this function can disrupt the digitaloid medication's influence. Anticholinergic atropine-containing botanicals (such as *Atropa, Datura,* and *Hyoscyamus*) counteract the bradycardia, an effect that can be utilized in cases of *Digitalis* toxicity (Brinker, 1996). *Ephedra* species containing the sympathomimetic ephedrine can induce tachyrhythmia in patients on digoxin due to enhanced ectopic pacemaker activity. The reserpine in *Rauwolfia* depletes sympathetic neurotransmitters, which may result in bradycardic arrhythmias for patients on digoxin (Barnhart, 1991). Consequently, it is important to monitor botanicals taken in conjunction with *Digitalis* to avoid altering the intended effects of the medication.

CONCLUSION

Whether botanical medicines are additive, are complementary, reduce bioavailability, or alter cofactors, their potential to modify the action of medication suggests the importance of identifying and monitoring herbal products taken in conjunction with pharmaceuticals. To safely prescribe botanicals for patients who are already taking other medicines not only requires a knowledge of the physiologic and pharmacologic effects of the herbal product, but also familiarity with the action of the pharmaceutical as well. All possible interactions cannot be addressed in an article of this scope. The considerations covered do suggest mechanisms of action and general tendencies for combinations of drugs from particular categories. However, each medicine, botanical or otherwise, needs to be studied for its own distinctive patterns of activity and interplay. In any case, an informed, careful approach must be the rule in prescribing all medicines, but most especially when the patient is already taking other medication.

REFERENCES

Barnhart ER, pub. *Physician's Desk Reference.* 45th ed. Oradell, NJ: Medical Economics Data; 1991.

Bergmann R, Nubner J, Demling J. Simple treatment of moderately serious depressions. *Therapie Neurol Psychitrie.* 1993;7:235–240.

Bever VO, Zahnd GR. Plants with oral hypoglycemic action. *Q J Crude Drug Res.* 1979;17:139–196.

Bohn B, Nebe CT, Birr C. Flow-cytometric studies with *Eleutherococcus senticosus* extract as an immunomodulatory agent. *Arzneim-Forsch.* 1987;37:1193–1196.

Brinker F. Botanical medicine research summaries. In: *Eclectic Dispensatory of Botanical Therapeutics.* Vol 2. Sandy, OR: Eclectic Medical Publications; 1995a.

Brinker F. An overview of conventional, experimental and botanical treatments of nonmalignant prostate conditions. In: *Eclectic Dispensatory of Botanical Therapeutics.* Vol 2. Sandy, OR: Eclectic Medical Publications; 1995b.

Brinker F. *Toxicology of Botanical Medicines.* 2nd ed. Portland, OR: Eclectic Medical Publications; 1996.

Brinker F. *Herb Contraindications and Drug Interactions.* Sandy, OR: Eclectic Institute, Inc; 1997.

Burnham BE. Garlic as a possible risk for postoperative bleeding. *Plast Reconstr Surg.* 1995;95:213.

Cantelli-Fort G, Maffei F, Hrelia P, et al. Interaction of licorice on glycyrrhizin pharmacokinetics. *Environ Health Pers.* 1994;102(suppl 9):65–68.

Coeugniet EG, Kuhnast R. Recurrent candidiasis: adjuvant immunotherapy with different formations of Echinacin. *Therapiewoche.* 1986;36:3352–3358.

Corrigan D. *Juniperus* species. In: DeSmet PAGM, et al, eds. *Adverse Effects of Herbal Drugs 2.* Berlin, Germany: Springer Verlag; 1993.

D'Arcy PF. Adverse reactions and interactions with herbal medicines. Part 2—drug interactions. *Adverse Drug React Toxicol Rev.* 1993;12:147–162.

DeSmet PAGM, Smeets OSNM. Potential risks of health food products containing yohimbe extracts. *BMJ.* 1994;309:958.

DiSilverio F, D'Eramo G, Lubrano C, et al. Evidence that *Serenoa repens* extract displays an antiestrogenic activity in prostatic tissue of benign prostatic hypertrophy patients. *Eur Urol.* 1992;21:309–314.

Fintelmann V. Toxic metabolic liver damage and its treatment. *Zeit Phytother.* 1986;(3):65–74.

Gonzalez M, Zarzuelo A, Gamez MJ, Utrilla MP, Jimenez J, Osuna L. Hypoglycemic activity of olive leaf. *Planta Med.* 1992;8:513–515.

Harrer G, Hubner WD, Podzuweit H. Effectiveness and tolerance of the *Hypericum* extract LI 160 compared to maprotiline: a multicenter, double-blind study. *J Geriatr Psychiatr Neurol.* 1994;7(suppl 1):S24–S28.

Hartmann RW, Mark M, Soldati F. Inhibition of 5α-reductase and aromatase by PHL-0080I (Prostatonin), a combination of PY 102 (*Pygeum africanum*) and UR 102 (*Urtica dioica*) extracts. *Phytomedicine.* 1996;3:121–128.

Hogan RP III. Hemorrhagic diathesis caused by drinking an herbal tea. *JAMA.* 1983;249:2679–2680.

Jori A, Bianchetti A, Prestini PE. Effect of essential oils on drug metabolism. *Biochem Pharmacol.* 1969; 18:2081–2085.

Jori A, Bianchetti A, Prestini PE, Garattini S. Effect of eucalyptol (I, 8-cineole) on the metabolism of other drugs in rats and in man. *Eur J Pharmacol.* 1970;9:362–366.

Lepor H, Willford WO, Barry MJ, et al. The efficacy of terazosin, finasteride, or both in benign prostatic hyperplasia. *N Engl J Med.* 1996;335:533–539.

Palsasciano G, Portincasa P, Palmieri V, Ciani D, Vendemiale G, Altomare E. The effect of silymarin on plasma levels of malon-dialdehyde on patients receiving long-term treatment with psychotropic drugs. *Curr Ther Res.* 1994;55:537–545.

Perez GRM, Ocegueda ZA, Munoz LJL, Avila AJG, Morrow WW. A study of the hypoglucemic (sic) effect of some Mexican plants. *J Ethnopharmacol.* 1980;12:253–262.

Perez Gutierrez RM, Yesca Laguna G, Walkowski A. Diuretic activity of Mexican *Equisetum. J. Ethnopharmacol.* 1985;14:269–272.

Racz-Kotilla E, Racz G, Solomon A. The action of *Taraxacum officinale* extracts on the body weight of laboratory animals. *Planta Med.* 1994;26:212–217.

Raman A, Lau C. Anti-diabetic properties and phytochemistry of *Momordica charantia* L. (Cucurbitaceae). *Phytomed.* 1996;2:349–362.

Rhodes L, Primka RL, Berman C, et al. Comparison of finasteride (Proscar), a 5α-reducatase inhibitor, and various commercial plant extracts in in vitro and in vivo 5α-reductase inhibition. *Prostate.* 1993;55:43–51.

Rose KD, Coisant PD, Parliament CF, Levin MB. Spontaneous spinal epidural hematoma with associated platelet dysfunction from excessive garlic ingestion: a case report. *Neurosurg.* 1990;26:880–882.

Sparnins VL, Venegas PL, Wattenberg LW. Gluthathione S-transferase activity: enhancement by compounds inhibiting chemical carcinogenesis and by dietary constituents. *J Natl Cancer Inst.* 1984;68(3):373–376.

Tamura Y, Nichikawa T, Yamada K, Yamamoto M, Kumagai A. Effects of glycyrrhetinic acid and its derivatives on Δ4-5α- and 5β-reductase in rat liver. *Arzneim-Forsch.* 1979;29:647–669.

Vereshchagin IA, Geskina OD, Bukhteeva RR. Increasing of antibiotic therapy efficacy with adaptogens in children suffering from dysentery and *Poteus* infections. *Antibiotiki.* 1982;27:65–69 (BA 75:32108).

Vorbach EU, Hubner WD, Arnold KH. Effectiveness and tolerance of the *Hypericum* extract LI 160 in comparison with imipramine: randomized, double-blind study with 135 outpatients. *J Geriatr Psychiatr Neurol.* 1994;7(suppl I):S19–S23.

Wagner H, Proksch A, Riess-Maurer I, et al. Immunostimulating polysaccharides (heteroglycans) of higher plants. *Arzneim-Forsch.* 1985;35:1069–1075.

Walker FB. Myocardial infarction FTER diet induces warfarin resistance. *Arch Intern Med.* 1984;144:2089–2090.

White RD, Swick RA, Cheeke PR. Effects of microsomal enzyme induction on the toxicity of pyrrolizidine (Senecio) alkaloids. *J Toxicol Environ Health.* 1983;12(4-6):633–640.

CHAPTER 64

Assessing the Effectiveness of Naturopathic Medicine

Carlo Calabrese

In current discussion surrounding the integration of complementary and alternative medicine (CAM) in health care institutions, the first and most frequent question is: Does the treatment alleviate symptoms and cure disease? Naturopathic medicine is one of the practices under consideration. An analysis of the effectiveness of this discipline illustrates some of the difficulties in answering this question for consumers, third-party payers, and policy makers. The intent of this brief discussion is to offer an approach for estimating the potential efficacy of naturopathic medicine (hypothesis generating) and provide additional methodology for its successful investigation (hypothesis testing).

OVERVIEW OF THE PRACTICE

Naturopathy is a primary health care profession that includes the promotion of health, and the prevention, diagnosis, and treatment of disease. The practice is licensed in 11 states and 3 Canadian provinces. In Arizona and British Columbia, acupuncture is a part of the regulated practice; elsewhere, naturopathic physi-

cians must obtain an additional license to practice acupuncture. The license typically is broad, allowing naturopathic doctors (NDs) to diagnose any disease and treat it using any natural means. There are perhaps 2,000 licensed naturopathic physicians in the United States who have been trained in accredited 4-year postbaccalaureate institutions. There may be several thousand more unlicensable naturopaths whose training is highly variable. Licensed naturopaths are considered by many to be the most broadly trained in CAM practices and to be the best prepared for integration into the mainstream health care system due to their preparation in the basic and diagnostic sciences of biomedicine and their broad range of practice.

Basic Principles

The practice is guided by its own principles, articulated by the American Association of Naturopathic Physicians in 1989:

- *First, do no harm;* utilize methods and substances that minimize harm; apply the least force for diagnosis and treatment.
- *Remember "nature heals"* (vis *medicatrix naturae*). Organisms are inherently self-organizing. It is the physician's role to support this process by removing obstacles to health and contributing to the creation of a healthy internal and external environment.
- *Identify and treat the cause.* Symptoms may represent the body's attempt to defend

Carlo Calabrese, ND, MPH, is currently Product Development Manager for Rexall Sundown, Inc. He has served as Co-director of the Research Institute at Bastyr University, where he remains a Senior Scientist. Dr. Calabrese's professional focus includes the development of research methodologies for the investigation of complementary and alternative therapies. He is a graduate of the National College of Naturopathic Medicine and also holds a master's degree in public health from the University of Washington.

itself and to adapt and recover. The physician's optimal approach is to seek and treat the causes of disease rather than suppress the symptoms.

- *Be a teacher.* The physician's role is to educate the patient and emphasize self-responsibility.
- *Treat the whole person.* The multifactorial nature of health and disease requires attention to the physical, mental, emotional, spiritual, social, and ecological aspects of our nature.
- *Prevent disease.* The prevention of disease by the attainment of optimal health is a primary objective.

Clinical Practice

Treatment modalities include among others: botanical medicines; diet; nutritional supplements; homeopathy; physical medicine (physiotherapy, hydrotherapy, and manipulation); counseling; and psychotherapy. A naturopathic physician may arrive at a functional and constitutional assessment as well as a disease diagnosis. Treatment is individualized for the particular patient's condition rather than for a disease entity. Frequently, a combination of treatments is applied and is continuously adjusted over time as the patient's condition changes.

Current State of Research

There is a lack of research on practices that encompass whole systems such as naturopathy, Oriental medicine, and Ayurveda. All three of these approaches are characterized by treatment through multiple modalities with a global approach to individuals and their unique constellation of physical and mental constitutions, stressors, and symptoms. This can be contrasted to conventional practice, which has more tendency to focus on a particular disease or on symptomatic treatment.

Although the intention is to determine whether naturopathic medicine is effective, the body of evidence on the whole practice of naturopathic medicine is as scarce as it is for other nondominant whole systems of practice. Research in whole practices is only recently gaining interest at the National Institutes of Health. New tools for research are also beginning to be accepted with the development of methodologies in practice-based research and outcomes research and health services research.

Biomedical research methods that are considered a gold standard by the scientific community have been typically developed to provide reliable data on a single therapeutic intervention for a specific Western disease. The requirements of these research methods distort naturopathic practice, perhaps rendering it apparently less effective than it may actually be. The measures do not typically take into account the residual benefits to other health problems of the patient nor on more distal effects, such as future health status and health care utilization.

Comparison trials between different systems of practice are needed for holistic practices such as naturopathic medicine. Outcome measures should be not only disease-specific, but both broad and long term, including health status, well-being, utilization, and cost. Only then can the relative utility of the different ways of addressing health care be determined.

Compounding the methodological difficulties of research in this practice, there are structural obstacles as well. There is only a decade of history on the research infrastructure at the academic centers of this profession. Practitioners expert in naturopathic medicine and the individualization of treatment are typically not trained in rigorous comparative trials. Even if the infrastructure and training were in place, sources of funding remain few, and most funding agencies make their decisions on the basis of biomedical theories of a very different nature than those of naturopathy. In the actual research of naturopathic treatment, most studies are focused on substances rather than procedures or lifestyle changes. Without the economic incentives that favor the in-depth study of patentable drugs, trials in naturopathic therapeutics tend to be smaller and with fewer replications. In addition, many practices present special methodological or ethical problems for control, randomization, or blinding, thereby making it more difficult to perform studies as rigorously as desired.

Despite all these hindrances, there are numerous studies and clinical trials that have yielded positive results in evaluating the effect of individual treatments. A pattern of such positive results across the naturopathic treatment modalities in some conditions is very promising. Since comparative trials have not yet been done to assess the whole practice of naturopathic medicine, evidence that suggests the efficacy of naturopathy as a systemic approach is presented in the review below.

EVALUATING EFFECTIVENESS

Since the large trials needed have not yet been done to assess naturopathic medicine, a matrix of clinical trial evidence that may suggest the possibility of marked efficacy in naturopathic medicine as a system is presented here. System variations in development of their respective clinical knowledge bases distinguish naturopathic and conventional medicine and should be considered before going on to the trial evidence:

- *It is not an accurate reflection of naturopathic practice philosophy to address only disease entities.* In a naturopathic approach, the aim is to support healthy function.
- *Consonant with the principle of seeking the cause, the treatment is individualized in a more subtle fashion than just by disease.* Many interventions are used by naturopathic physicians only in a carefully selected subset of patients displaying particular symptoms. For example, about half of depressed women on birth control pills show vitamin B6 (pyroxidine) deficiency, and most of these will improve with pyroxidine supplementation (Adams et al, 1974). Concomitantly, evidence of beneficial effects from pyroxidine supplementation on undifferentiated depression is mixed.
- *Frequently, naturopathic interventions have benefit in more than one disease simultaneously.* It is common for practitioners to choose among therapeutic options that will yield an efficient outcome as well as an effective response, maximizing the cost-benefit ratio.
- *Experimental evidence is not the only form of evidence, and sometimes not the best evidence for particular interventions or therapeutic questions.* Validation for pharmaceutical science is now based on double-blind, controlled clinical trials. However, the literature on this type of research has not served as the primary repository for the practice wisdom of a discipline that has developed empirically by more informal than formal (that is, academic and regulated) epistemological processes.
- *Many naturopathic treatments are based on a long history of human use and comprise the body of expertise of many generations of healers.* These treatments are less likely than patentable drugs to be formally tested in comparison trials. However, because of the relatively benign nature of the agents used, therapeutic trials are very common in naturopathic practice and lead to rapidly accumulated clinical experience.
- *Naturopathic physicians combine many of these relatively nontoxic treatments but, with few exceptions, trials in combination treatment are infrequent.* It may be that even when the right criteria are specified, the benign single agents used do not demonstrate a statistically significant therapeutic difference if used alone. The bioactivity of most nutrients and botanicals is mild and diffuse compared to that of molecularly identified pharmaceutical agents. However, used in combination, they may have additive effects, particularly when the individual remedies work synergistically via differing mechanisms. An example is the treatment

of back pain using an herbal muscle relaxant combined with manipulation. With a well-chosen strategy, the beneficial effects may be amplified. This type of potential benefit is missed in the literature of controlled trials.

- *There are similarities and differences between naturopathy and conventional medicine.* Certain interventions within the naturopathic repertoire are much more frequently used among NDs than among medical doctors. In other cases, the treatment approach may be similar. For example, the management of diabetic nephropathy by protein restriction or of atherosclerosis with a low-saturated fat diet may be just as common among allopathic physicians as among naturopathic ones (though naturopaths may be more aggressive in their application).

- *In naturopathic practice, prevention and health promotion constitute primary treatment strategies.* Review of the literature here focuses on the treatment of disease states. Some of the treatments cited below for osteoarthritis and migraine in fact have side effects that are positive rather than negative. Still, the critical prevention and health promotion goals of ordinary naturopathic practice are not addressed in the evidence below.

Having listed these issues, it may be clear that randomized controlled clinical trials and the extant literature will not tell the whole story of efficacy in naturopathic medicine. In the absence of studies looking at the whole practice, the literature on controlled clinical trials can, however, provide a good suggestion of the potential benefit. One may look at the range of treatments used in naturopathic clinical practice that are tested in randomized, controlled clinical trials for a given health problem. These can be reviewed in the context of an orthodox disease classification. Such an analysis would involve reviewing the medical literature of randomized

trials for all of the naturopathic modalities for a given condition, primarily diet therapy, nutritional supplementation, botanical medicine, homeopathy, physical medicine (physical therapy, hydrotherapy, and manipulation), and counseling/psychotherapy. The criterion for selection of the treatments here is whether there have been clinical trials of acceptable design for which there is no significant evidence controverting the hypothesized effect at the time this chapter was written.

To offer an overall sense of the generalized efficacy of naturopathic medicine, different diseases that span the range of age, gender, chronicity, severity, and mortality could be chosen for review. However, due to space limitations, only two conditions, osteoarthritis and migraine, are reviewed here. The relative benignity of the interventions acting via different mechanisms lends them to polytreatment with the agents. Most conditions are similarly available to treatment with multiple therapeutic approaches. The treatments here would by no means represent complete, or even actual, treatment regimens, but rather possible interventions that have fairly strong experimental evidence in treating the particular disease within the treatment options of naturopathic physicians.

Identifying treatments for which evidence is strongly positive and which are likely to be used in conjunction with each other would give a sense of the possible magnitude of benefit with naturopathic medicine if it were practiced under a treatment selection criterion of randomized trial evidence. It would seem self-evident that coordinated combination therapy with several interventions, each of which is supported by good evidence and works via different pathways, is likelier to work than a single agent.

REVIEW OF CONTROLLED CLINICAL TRIALS

The therapeutic approaches include diet, nutritional supplements, botanical medicine, homeopathy, physical medicine, and counseling/psychology.

Osteoarthritis

Nutritional Supplements

Caruso I, Pietrogrande V. Italian double-blind multicenter study comparing S-adenosyme-thionine (SAMe), naproxen, and placebo in the treatment of degenerative joint disease. *Am J Med.* 1987;83:(5A):66–71. Seven hundred forty-three patients received 1,200 mg SAMe, 750 mg naproxen, or placebo daily. SAMe exerted the same analgesic activity as naproxen; both were more effective than placebo ($p < .01$). SAMe tolerability was better than that of naproxen.

Machtey I, Ouaknine L. Tocopherol in arthritis: a controlled pilot study. *J Am Geriatr Soc.* 1978;26:328. A double-blind, crossover study in which 29 subjects received 600 mg tocopherol or placebo for 10 days in random order. Fifty-two percent had "marked improvement" in pain while on tocopherol versus 4% during placebo ($p < .01$).

Rovat LC. Clinical research in osteoarthritis design and results of short-term and long-term trials with disease modifying drugs. *Int J Tissue Reactions.* 1992;14(5):243–251. Report of three double-blind, randomized trials of oral glucosamine sulfate compared to placebo and ibuprofen. Glucosamine was more effective than placebo (N = 252, $p < .025$) and as effective as ibuprofen (N = 200, $p = .77$). It was as well tolerated as placebo with fewer adverse reactions than ibuprofen ($p < .001$).

Botanicals and Specific Foods

Deal CL, Schnitzer TJ, Lipstein E, Seibold JR, Stevens RM, Levy MD, Albert D, Renold F. Treatment of arthritis with topical capsaicin: a double-blind trial. *Clin Ther.* 1991;13(3):383–395. A study of a constituent of cayenne in 70 patients versus placebo showed a reduction in subjective pain ($p < .003$).

Kulkarni RR, Patki PS, Jog VP, Gandage SG, Patwardhan B. Treatment of osteoarthritis with a combination herbomineral formulation: a double-blind, placebo-controlled, crossover study. *J Ethnopharmacol.* 1991;33(1–2):91–95. Trial of a combination of *Boswellian serrata*, *Curcuma longa*, *Withania somnifera*, and zinc in 42 patients showed a reduction in pain severity ($p < .001$) and disability ($p < .05$).

Rejholec V. Long-term studies of antiosteoarthritic drugs: an assessment. *Semin Arthritis Rheum.* 1987;17(2, suppl 1):35–53. One hundred forty-seven patients received either cartilage extracts or placebo. Placebo patients were permitted to use nonsteroidal anti-inflammatory drugs (NSAIDs) during exacerbations. After 5 years, pain scores in the cartilage patients dropped 85% versus 5% in controls. With cartilage, joint deterioration was 37% less, and less time was lost from work.

Physical Medicine

Trock D, Bollet AJ, Dyer RH Jr, Fielding LP, Miner WK, Markoll R. A double-blind trial of the clinical effects of pulsed electromagnetic fields (PEMF) in osteoarthritis. *J Rheumatol.* 1993;20(3):456–460. Twenty-seven patients were randomized to PEMF or sham treatment; 23–61% improvement in clinical outcome variables was observed in PEMF patients versus 2–18% improvement with sham treatment.

Migraine Headache

Diet

Egger J, Carter CM, Wilson J, Turner MW, Soothill JF. Is migraine food allergy? A double-blind, controlled trial of oligoantigenic diet treatment. *Lancet.* 1983;344:865–869. Of 88 children with severe frequent migraine, 93% recovered on an oligoantigenic diet. Of the 82 who improved, all but 8 relapsed on reintroduction of one or more foods. Of the 82, 40 completed a follow-up with test foods disguised in an oligoantigenic base. There were highly significant relations between the active material and symptoms.

Nutritional Supplements

Schoenen J, Jacquy J, Lenaerts M. Effectiveness of high-dose riboflavin in migraine prophylaxis. A randomized controlled trial. *Neurology*. 1998;50(2):466–470. In a 3 months trial of 400 mg vs placebo in 55 migraineurs, riboflavin was superior in reducing attack frequency ($p = 0.005$) and headache days ($p = 0.012$). The proportion of patients who improved by at least 50%, ie, "responders," was 15% for placebo and 59% for riboflavin ($p = 0.002$). Other studies show the safety profile of riboflavin to be wide.

Faccinetti F, Sances G, Borella P, Genazzani AR, Nappi G. Magnesium prophylaxis of menstrual migraine: effects on intracellular magnesium. *Headache*. 1991;31:298–301. In 20 patients, duration and intensity of migraines were significantly lower in subjects given 360 mg of elemental magnesium daily for 2 months than in the placebo group.

Kangasniemi P, Falck B, Langvik VA, Hyppa MT. Levotryptophan treatment in migraine. *Headache*. 1978;18:161–166. In four of the eight subjects in this double-blind, crossover trial, tryptophan significantly reduced the number and intensity of attacks.

Botanicals and Specific Foods

Murphy JJ, Heptinstall S, Mitchell JRA. Randomized double-blind placebo-controlled trial of feverfew in migraine prevention. *Lancet*.1988;2:189–192. Symptoms were significantly reduced in the group receiving herbal treatment compared to those receiving placebo (N = 72; $p < .005$).

Homeopathy

Brigo B, Serpelloni G. Homeopathic treatment of migraines: a randomized double-blind study of sixty cases (homeopathic remedy versus placebo). *Berlin J Res Homeopathy*. 1991;1(2):98–106. Over 4 months, 80% of patients improved with homeopathy versus 13% on placebo with mean decrease in 10 cm VAS (visual analog scale) of symptom score of 6.2 versus 0.6 cm.

Physical Medicine

Solomon S, Guglielmo KM. Treatment of headache by transcutaneous electrical stimulation. *Headache*. 1985;25:12–15. Subjects treated with transcutaneous electrical stimulation had significantly greater improvement than those receiving placebo.

Robbins LD. Cryotherapy for headache. *Headache*. 1989;29:598–600. In an uncontrolled trial in 45 patients with migraine or migraine plus chronic daily headache, the effectiveness of a cold wrap for relief was evaluated; 64.5% evaluated it as a least mildly effective; 9% judged it as completely effective.

Counseling/Psychology

Fentress DW, Maske BJ, Mehegan JE, Benson H. Biofeedback and relaxation-response training in the treatment of pediatric migraine. *Med Child Neurol*. 1986;28(2):139–146. In 18 children assigned to one of three treatment groups, those receiving electromyography (EMG) biofeedback or relaxation-response training experienced a significant reduction in headache symptoms compared to controls, a difference that was sustained after 1 year.

REFERENCE

Adams PW, Wynn V, Seed M, Folkand. Vitamin B6, depression, and oral contraception. [Letter]. *Lancet*. 1974;2:516–517.

PART XVII

Resources for Continuing Education in Integrative Medicine

CHAPTER 65

Continuing Education in Integrative Medicine

65.1   Approaches to Continuing Medical Education

Andrew Weil and Tracy W. Gaudet with Nancy Faass

INTRODUCTION

Continuing medical education can provide the foundation for a rational working knowledge of complementary therapies and mind-body medi-

cine. Currently, most physicians have patients who make requests for information on complementary and alternative medicine (CAM). At present, the majority of physicians have had little or no formal medical education in alternative therapies or mind-body medicine. Since the practice of medicine is based on the thorough understanding of clinical options, it is important that medical education be available to provide doctors with accurate, meaningful information on complementary therapies. Administrators can facilitate continuing education in integrative medicine in a number of ways:

- *Making information resources available* by perhaps setting aside space on a bookshelf or bookcase where other types of resource material are kept for staff. A wealth of information is currently available on CAM through books, journals, newsletters, audiotapes, and videotapes.
- *Providing in-services or retreats*, or facilitating staff attendance at video conferences, workshops, or conferences.

Andrew Weil, MD, is founder and Director of the Program in Integrative Medicine at the University of Arizona School of Medicine. He is a graduate of Harvard Medical School, has worked for the National Institute of Mental Health, and served as a researcher in ethnopharmacology with the Institute of Current World Affairs and the Harvard Botanical Museum. Dr. Weil is author of numerous highly successful books on health and medicine.

Tracy W. Gaudet, MD, is Associate Director of The Duke Center for Integrative Medicine and has served as executive director and medical director of the University of Arizona, Program in Integrative Medicine. She received her BA cum laude in psychology and sociology and earned her MD degree with honors at Duke University. As Assistant Professor, she has taught Obstetrics and Gynecology at Duke University and the University of Arizona, and at the University of Texas in the Maternal-Fetal Medical Division.

Source: Portions of this chapter have been adapted from Andrew Weil, MD, and Tracy Gaudet, MD.

- *Making CAM services available to staff at no cost or a very low cost.* At the Program in Integrative Medicine, all of the doctors have the opportunity to be treated by CAM practitioners. Everyone is seen by a homeopathic physician and also a Chinese medicine practitioner so that he or she can experience these therapies. Classes on therapies are provided so that the physicians can apply these approaches in their own lives, such as yoga or Qigong.
- *Infusing a philosophy of health into the day-to-day operations of the program.* It is important to model the message throughout the program. For example, many hospitals have fitness facilities that are available to staff as well as the community. The Program in Integrative Medicine encourages staff not only to promote health and prevention to others, but also to evaluate themselves and their own health and well-being. As an organization, the administration consciously supports those efforts.

Life As a Living Laboratory

In medical school, young doctors are expected to stay up all night, eat meals from vending machines, and spend all their free time catching up on sleep or studies. If physicians live that kind of lifestyle, it is more difficult for them to convincingly advise patients to give up smoking, get more exercise, or change their eating habits. Some physicians are looking for an alternative way to practice medicine and still lead a balanced life, rather than one that requires them to forgo sleep, exercise, proper nutrition, and a spiritual life. The Program in Integrative Medicine encourages staff to eat wisely and well, exercise for health and joy, and make time for thinking and reflection. There is value in viewing one's own life as a living laboratory and in being a role model for patients.

THE PROGRAM IN INTEGRATIVE MEDICINE AT THE UNIVERSITY OF ARIZONA

The postdoctoral programs at the University of Arizona include continuing education for physicians through a variety of activities for professional development. These programs are designed to address some of the needs of the large numbers of physicians and other clinicians who wish to incorporate integrative medicine, while remaining in their communities. In 1997, the program's continuing medical education activities reached more than 1,450 health care professionals. To continue the discourse in integrative medicine with a national audience, the program has sponsored:

- a quarterly miniconference series on integrative medicine, broadcast via satellite to sites across the country
- one-day intensive sessions that provide hands-on exposure to specific therapies
- week-long comprehensive conferences for practicing physicians
- in-depth conferences on select topics, such as botanical medicine, and their application in clinical care.

There is a great need for rigorous, in-depth education in a range of specific applications of integrative medicine. The program at the University of Arizona is developing a series of 3- to 5-day courses focusing on integrative practice in given specialties such as cardiology, oncology, and psychiatry. Each of these courses will be co-sponsored with other academic institutions and will alternate locations with these universities. Programs in long-distance learning are being paired with on-site education, supported by both local and remote communities of learning. The goal of the continuing education component is to begin to create a national community of integrative medicine practitioners.

Clinical Education in Integrative Medicine

The Integrative Fellowship Program at the University of Arizona includes medical practice in an integrative clinic. This model is based on the continuum of care, providing services that range from health promotion to acute care. The integrative clinic encourages discourse on alternative therapies and new approaches to practice. Emphasis is also placed on a holistic model of practice that includes mind-body medicine and the expanded context of mind, body, spirit, and community.

Patient care is provided in the integrative clinic by physicians participating in the fellowship program and also by the multidisciplinary team. Physicians see patients for an initial 1-hour interview, which involves case taking and an examination. The patient history is presented in an interdisciplinary case conference, which includes the program director, the medical director, and clinicians representing various systems of medicine, specifically traditional Chinese medicine, homeopathy, mind-body medicine, osteopathy, botanical therapy, nutrition, and spirituality. In this forum, the fellowship students develop a deep appreciation for different systems of medicine and their application, as well the creation of an integrative treatment plan. These plans are individualized, and typically include a combination of alternative and conventional treatments. The patient then returns for a discussion of the treatment options with the physician. The patient may also be scheduled for an evaluation in the clinic by an alternative practitioner together with his or her doctor.

Conference Curriculum in Integrative Medicine

The educational model of the postgraduate program includes a core curriculum of 12 subject areas and clinical training. *These areas reflect our perspective on integrative medicine.*

1. *Healing-Oriented Medicine* focuses on the nature of immunity and the body's healing system; the placebo response as a therapeutic ally; lifestyle medicine; the role of mind-body medicine in healing; and strategies for protecting, enhancing, and activating the immune system and healing responses.

2. *The Philosophy of Science* explores what science is and is not; how quantum theory and chaos theory supersede old Newtonian/Cartesian models; the relationship between medicine and science; and the scientific basis of various treatment modalities.

3. *The Art of Medicine* reflects on the doctor as teacher; effective communication and the art of suggestion; developing the therapeutic relationship; the role of intuition; techniques for motivating behavioral change; and matching therapeutic approaches with individual patients.

4. *Medicine and Culture* reviews the history of medicine; the origins and development of major alternative systems such as Ayurveda, traditional Chinese medicine, homeopathy, osteopathy, and naturopathy; cultural definitions of health, illness, and treatment; and cultural influences on medical thinking.

5. *Research Education* looks at how to design and ask questions; how to design quality studies; how to interpret research findings; and how to identify research methodologies appropriate for integrative medicine.

6. *Nutritional Medicine* teaches the contributions of diet to health and disease; specific information on the benefits and risks of common foods and dietary patterns; the therapeutic role of vitamins, minerals, and other nutritional supplements; and nutritional therapies for specific diseases.

7. *Botanical Medicine* examines the preparations, uses, benefits, and risks of medicinal plants; possible interactions with pharmaceutical medications; and the knowledge of a basic repertory of botanical remedies with known safety and efficacy.

8. *Mind-Body Medicine* addresses the scientific basis of mind-body interactions; a

critical review of existing therapies; the role of the mind in health and illness; the identification of diseases with prominent mind-body components; and how to assess the moods and belief systems of patients.

9. *Spirituality and Medicine* focuses on the spiritual dimension of human life and its relevance to health and illness and healing; the distinction between spirituality and religion; how to take a spiritual history; the relationship between spirituality and medical outcomes; and spiritual healing techniques.

10. *Energy Medicine* provides an overview of dynamic energy systems theory and research; the scientific and clinical basis for informational/energy modalities such as acupuncture, homeopathy, therapeutic touch, and Qigong; bioenergy measurement and treatment devices; and the health benefits and risks of various forms of energy therapy.

11. *Lifestyle Medicine* examines the effect of lifestyle choices, including smoking, vitamins, exercise, alcohol, and food; techniques for motivating behavior change; the physician as a role model of healthy living; and health and the environment.

12. *Leadership in Medicine and Society* focuses on physicians as leaders and as agents of social change; practical skills including public speaking, business planning, and management; political aspects of integrative medicine; medicine and law; and related ethical issues.

Workshops in CAM

The workshops explore the distinction between alternative and integrative medicine; the history of CAM; the history, underlying philosophies, scientific basis, and practical applications of various systems of medicine; and the scientific evidence as it pertains to these systems. The therapies addressed in the workshops and in the fellowship program include acupuncture and Chinese medicine, homeopathy, and osteopathic manipulative therapy, as well as a variety of other systems of healing.

1. *Basics of Chinese Medicine* looks at Eastern traditions with Western sensibilities to explore the foundation concepts, diagnostic techniques, and clinical applications of acupuncture and Chinese herbal medicine. The workshop looks at the Chinese medicine perspective on the patient in the context of its relevance for American patients today. Hands-on experience with pulse and tongue diagnosis and acupuncture first-aid points are demonstrated. A review of current research on the topic is also included.

2. *Basics of Homeopathic Medicine* considers the conceptual challenges of homeopathy and the practical contributions clinicians report. This overview reviews the scientific evidence for the effectiveness of homeopathy and introduces practitioners to acute prescribing for several conditions commonly encountered in primary care practice.

3. *Basics of Osteopathic Manual Medicine* is an intensive overview of the fundamentals course as an introduction for community practitioners, which introduces them to several basic techniques of manual medicine in the clinical setting.

The curriculum is developed as a whole rather than a set of distinct pieces. Consequently, there is significant interplay between the 12 core areas and the themes of the workshops. These programs provide forums in which integrative medicine can continue to be defined.

Associate Fellowship in Integrative Medicine
Malcolm Riley, Director

The most recent continuing education program is the Associate Fellowship in Integrative Medicine. This is a two-year distributed learning program designed to teach integrative medicine to physicians and other health care providers.

The Associate Fellowship Will Prepare Physicians to:
- describe and discuss the philosophical basis of integrative medicine
- incorporate the philosophy and concepts into their personal and professional lives
- discuss integrative medicine with patients
- choose and integrate the most appropriate treatment modalities for patients
- make informed referrals

The Learning Experiences of the Associate Fellowship Include:

Web-based reference and didactic materials. Information resources in Integrative Medicine are sparse and often of dubious quality, we have designed an interactive, trustworthy database of content that Associate Fellows will use initially for learning, but frequently return to for review and reference.

Web-based interactive patient scenarios. The scenarios give the Associate Fellows practice applying an integrative approach to patient care, by focusing on the treatment and prevention of specific diseases and conditions. Each scenario incorporates expertise from many treatment modalities, while giving the Associate Fellows control over what they learn, in what order, and how they choose to apply their new knowledge.

Online collaborative discussions and projects. Integrative medicine is not a field of black and white answers. Therefore, collaboration, teamwork, and communication are essential in the effective application of integrative medicine techniques. Rather than merely teaching facts, we use Web-based discussions including expert integrative medicine practitioners to help Associate Fellows acquire ways of thinking and problem solving. Additionally, these discussions will build a virtual community of physicians working toward the same purpose.

Real-world assignments. Media such as books, articles, audiotapes and videotapes are used when they are the most appropriate to the learning experience. Additionally, we assign "outreach" activities to the Fellows, where they venture into their community and explore the scope and quality of available integrative medicine modalities.

Patient information materials. Studies have shown that continuing medical education is more likely to effect change in the clinic if it includes informational resources for patients. We will couple the learning materials for physicians with patient information materials–ranging from printed patient handouts to recommended medical Web sites.

The Benefits of a Distributed Learning Program Designed in This Way Are:
To the medical education community:
- To create a Web-based, medical education program that maximizes learning and appropriately uses emerging technologies as well as established media, such as video and audio, that can be accessed any where in the world where there is an Internet connection and can serve as a model in other areas of medical education.

To the patient:
- To bring integrative medicine to the most important people—our patients, particularly children and the elderly.
- To increase use of more natural and affordable therapies whenever possible.

- To support healthier lifestyle practices, resulting in lower medical costs and improved quality of life.
- To increase accessibility to informed physicians trained in therapies sought by the public.
- To create of a focus on preventive and healing practices in childhood ensuring lifelong healthy practices that will reap benefit later in life.

To the Physician and Health Professional:

- To provide opportunities for physicians and health professionals to learn and practice integrative medicine.
- To incorporate healthy lifestyle practices into their own lives to benefit themselves, their families, and their patients.
- To increase knowledge of integrative medicine in order to meet the needs of patients for less invasive treatment options.
- To establish a worldwide network, or "virtual community," of fellows and experts in integrative medicine to share information and resources.

Information about the Associate Fellowship is available at: http://integrativemedicine.arizona.edu/af/

65.2 Profile: Three Levels of Integrative Practice

Martin L. Rossman

Integrative medicine is a systems-based medicine that acknowledges the importance of not only physical, but emotional, psychological, social, and spiritual dimensions in health, and seeks to support the patient in exploring these dimensions. It combines the best of conventional medicine with the best of complementary or traditional practices in a rigorously considered way. An integrative approach encourages patient self-care through personal growth and the development of health awareness.

Martin L. Rossman, MD, is a highly recognized leader in the fields of complementary medicine and health psychology. He and David E. Bresler, PhD, are the cofounders and directors of the Academy for Guided Imagery, an accredited postgraduate institute. Over the past 7 years, the academy has provided training and workshops to more than 10,000 psychologists, physicians, social workers, nurses, and other health professionals. The program has certified over 500 professionals in interactive guided imagery, a sophisticated, patient-centered approach to mind-body medicine.

Courtesy of Martin Rossman, MD, San Francisco, California.

There is a growing need for physicians knowledgeable in complementary medicine and skilled in the psychological and emotional aspects of patient care. Physician acceptance of such practices seems to be relatively high although the knowledge level has not kept pace. Several studies in the United States, Canada, and Israel demonstrate that almost 60% of primary care physicians refer to alternative practitioners, and that many use their services for themselves and their families. Yet the same studies suggest that only 8% of these physicians have in-depth knowledge about these alternative practices.

Training in integrative medicine could expand the cadre of physicians who can intelligently guide their patients through a sophisticated understanding of complementary practices. Training would ideally provide insight into the most relevant applications of complementary therapies and effective coordination with biomedicine. There is a need for programs that will allow practicing physicians to upgrade their skills and attain certification without taking time away from their ongoing practices.

Expanding the Continuum of Care

In ancient China, there were five levels of physicians, ranked accorded to their healing skills. The first was the veterinarian, next the acupuncturist, the surgeon, and then the equivalent of an internist, a doctor who used nutrition and herbal medicine. Yet none of these physicians were believed to be able to cure illness. The only doctor who could potentially effect a cure was the highest level physician, whose role was to teach the people how to live in order to sustain health.

This tradition is part of Western culture as well. The word *physician* stems from the root *educare*, which literally means "to draw out," Physicians in our time are still considered the ultimate authorities in health. However, the advent of technology, surgery, and pharmacology has to some degree shifted the focus away from health enhancement and healthy lifestyles. Most medical school curricula have limited course offerings in wellness, nutrition, and psychology. Yet never has physician support and involvement in wellness education been more important. In spite of wondrous advances in medical technology, 19 of the 21 leading causes of death in America are lifestyle related and preventable.

Integrative medicine training could, to some degree, fill this rapidly emerging need. Comprehensive training is most ideally provided through lectures, discussions, case histories, research, group support, personal explorations, sophisticated feedback, and on-line technology to help physicians understand and incorporate integrative medicine principles into their practices.

The Essence of Integrative Practice

Physicians who practice integrative medicine ideally

- Possess knowledge of integrative health principles.
- Encourage patients in effective self-care.
- Are familiar with the major complementary healing practices through clinical observation and personal experience.
- Have access to current information on psychoneuroimmunology.
- Practice a range of approaches to healing based on various scientific, epidemiological, and historical perspectives.
- Possess knowledge and skill in therapeutic listening and communication to maximize the practitioner-patient interface.
- Cultivate personal awareness and development as important aspects of professional development.
- Maintain access to resources to stay abreast of the latest health and medical information.

Three Levels of Practice

Level One

A physician functioning at the initial level of integrative practice reflects a broad, yet thorough understanding of integrative medicine, with insight into the model of integrative health, the principles of integrative medicine, its practices (including alternative practices), and resources for further development. Physicians at this level can intelligently discuss, evaluate, and refer to alternative practices and practitioners, and institute an integrative health model in their practice. The major understandings incorporated at this level include:

- principles and scope of integrative practice
- nutritional factors in illness, treatment, and prevention
- complementary systems of healing, including acupuncture and traditional Chinese medicine, Ayurvedic medicine, herbal medicine, and homeopathy
- bodywork such as chiropractic and osteopathic manipulation, craniosacral therapy, Feldenkrais, yoga, and forms of massage therapy that address both body and emotions
- mind, body, and spirit in medicine; the role of belief systems; meditation; relaxation; stress reduction; imagery; and visualization
- practical and economic aspects of integrative practice, including an inventory of

the physician's practice and the community context in which that practice occurs—available services, community attitudes, needs, resources, and potential barriers to integrative practice.

Level Two

At this stage, physicians begin to deepen their understanding of the integrative approach. Ongoing training consists of workshops, practicums, preceptorships, and home study, ideally combined with expert tutelage in holistic or integrative medicine, practical hands-on experience, and networking. The topics considered at the initial level are revisited in greater depth.

With this foundation, physicians will have a good range of basic information and enough knowledge to skillfully incorporate integrative medicine practices. They have sufficient skills in nutrition and mind-body medicine to have an impact on their practices. The second level of practice also entails a certain amount of self-focus to apply these principles to one's own health patterns. This heightened awareness of the effects of lifestyle also helps when working with patients. The integration of this information on a more subtle level involves not only didactic learning, but experiential exercises and explorations in personal growth. Ongoing home-work is focused in both cognitive and emotional spheres.

Level Three

At this level, education consists of training in one specific complementary clinical discipline compatible with integrative medicine. An appropriate specialization would include one of the following:

- acupuncture
- nutrition
- botanical medicine
- homeopathy
- manual therapy
- mind-body medicine.

This type of training can be obtained through an existing organization such as the American Academy of Medical Acupuncture, Bastyr University, the International Homeopathy Association, or the Academy for Guided Imagery. Training on this level ideally includes in-depth consideration of case history analysis, clinical conferencing, and review with role play and live-patient evaluations. Training is reinforced through ongoing resources for continued learning and the development of a personal network of integrative professionals (see Table 65.2–1).

Table 65.2–1 Experiential Aspects of Integrative Medicine Training

Class	Topics
Personal inventory	Beliefs about medicine and healing, purpose, vision, hopes, intention, resistance, and resources
Practice inventory	Patient's beliefs and needs, partner's beliefs, staff beliefs, resources, and barriers
Community inventory	Available services, community attitudes, community needs, community resources, and community barriers
Personal explorations	Bodywork, acupuncture, homeopathy, herbal exploration, T'ai chi, yoga, cognitive therapy, and interactive imagery
Personal practices	Imagery and visualization, the relaxation response, mindfulness meditation, prayer, and exercise

Courtesy of Martin Rossman, MD, San Francisco, California.

65.3   Continuing Medical Education Resources in Integrative Medicine

Deborah Grandinetti

It is becoming easier to find good information on integrative medicine. The number of relevant resources continues to grow, including professional training programs, conferences, publications, Internet sites, and CD-ROMs. Those looking for information on how to integrate complementary medicine into their practice or introduce it to a hospital or medical group should investigate various specialized conferences, newsletters, and other resources.

BOTANICAL AND NUTRITIONAL MEDICINE

Botanical Medicine in Modern Clinical Practice. Columbia University sponsors an annual 5-day continuing medical education course focused exclusively on botanical medicine. The program provides attendees a scientific framework for understanding the efficacy, benefits, and risks of herbs. It also reviews drug-herb and herb-herb interactions and provides the opportunity to question pharmacologists and physician experts who use herbs in their practices. The conference is cosponsored by Andrew Weil, MD, and the Program in Integrative Medicine at the University of Arizona College of Medicine. Information can be obtained from:
Columbia University
Phone: (212) 543-9550
Web site:
    http://cpmcnet.columbia.edu/dept/rosenthal
    (The site includes a multitude of other useful resources, including scientific databases on herbs.)

Fleming, T, chief ed. *PDR for Herbal Medicines.* Montvale, NJ: Medical Economics;

Source: Adapted with permission from D. Grandinetti, Continuing Medical Education Resources in Integrative Medicine, *Medical Economics Magazine*, February 22, 1999, pp. 153–167, © 2000.

2000–2001. This reference covers more than 600 botanical remedies. Information can be obtained from:
Medical Economics
Phone: (888) 859-8053
Web site: www.pdr.net

HerbalGram. One of the most respected journals on herbs, *HerbalGram* is a quarterly publication cosponsored by the American Botanical Council and the Herb Research Foundation. *HerbalGram* contains feature articles, research, conference reports, and book reviews. Information can be obtained from:
American Botanical Council
Phone: (800) 373-7105
Web site:
    http://www.herbalgram.org/herbalgram

COMPLEMENTARY THERAPIES

Conference. Alternative Medicine: Implications for Clinical Practice. Harvard Medical School provides a comprehensive overview of the disciplines in its annual conference. Information is available at:
Department of Continuing Education
Phone: (617) 432-1525

Books. Micozzi MS, ed. *Fundamentals of Complementary and Alternative Medicine.* New York: Churchill Livingstone; 1996. The book is illustrated, and a CD-ROM package is also available. It is approximately 300 pages and draws on the expertise of 21 contributing authors. Editor Mark Micozzi is a forensic pathologist and executive director of the College of Physicians of Philadelphia.

Fugh-Berman A. *Alternative Medicine: What Works.* Philadelphia: Lippincott, Williams & Wilkins; 1997. Adriane Fugh-Berman, MD, is assistant clinical professor at George Washington University School of Medicine. She coordinated the field investigations program for the Office of Alternative Medicine. This work is 256 pages and covers more than 20 of the most familiar CAM therapies in short chapters that include citations from the scientific literature.

Alternative Medicine: Expanding Medical Horizons: A Report to the National Institutes of Health on Alternative Medical Systems and Practices in the United States. Workshop on Alternative Medicine (1994: Chantilly, VA). Prepared under the auspices of the Workshop on Alternative Medicine. Washington, DC: U.S. Government Printing Office, 1994. NIH Publication No. 94-066. This 372-page resource covers various types of alternative practice and how to conduct and disseminate research. Useful appendices include World Health Organization guidelines for the assessment of herbal medicines; the 20 most popular Asian patent medicines that contain toxic ingredients; and plant sources of modern drugs.

Journals. *Alternative Therapies in Health and Medicine.* This is a bimonthly, peer-reviewed journal that offers original research and papers. The journal is published by InnoVision Communications:
Phone: (800) 899-1712
Web site: http://www.alternative-therapies.com

Integrative Medicine: Integrating Conventional and Alternative Medicine. Andrew Weil's quarterly, peer-reviewed journal includes original studies, critical reviews, major scientific reports, and debates relevant to the field of integrative medicine. The journal is published quarterly by Elsevier Science. A free sample can be requested at the Web site below.
Phone: (888) 437-4636
Web site: http://www-east.elsevier.com/intmed/ order.html

The Journal of Alternative and Complementary Medicine: Research on Paradigm, Practice, and Policy. This is a quarterly, peer-reviewed

journal that includes original research papers, literature reviews, and personal commentary. Included in *Index Medicus* and MEDLINE, it is published by Mary Ann Liebert, Inc. Information can be obtained from:
Phone: (914) 834-3100
Web site: http://www.liebertpub.com

INTEGRATING CAM INTO A MEDICAL PRACTICE

Conference. *The Journal of Alternative Therapies in Health and Medicine* holds an annual alternative-therapies symposium. The conference typically includes a focus on spirituality and healing, reflecting the interests of the executive editor, author Larry Dossey, MD, an internist by training and former chief of staff of Medical City Dallas Hospital. Some of the conferences are cosponsored with other organizations such as the State University of New York. Information can be obtained from:
Phone: (800) 899-1712
Web site: http://www.alternative-therapies.com

Books. Milton D, Benjamin S. *Complementary and Alternative Therapies: An Implementation Guide to Integrative Healthcare.* American Hospital Association and Jossey-Bass Publishers; 1999. This book is a good overview by Doris Milton and Samuel Benjamin, MD, director of the program in Complementary and Alternative Medicine at the State University of New York at Stony Brook. Copies are available from:
Phone: (800) 242-2626

Available in bookstores, the following books are authored by physicians who have developed their own approach to integrative practice:

Gordon J. *Manifesto for a New Medicine: Your Guide to Healing Partnerships and the Wise Use of Alternative Therapies.* Cambridge, MA: Perseus Press; 1996. The author is a Washington, DC-based psychiatrist, founder and director of the Center for Mind-Body Medicine in Washington, DC.

Mehl-Madrona L. *Coyote Medicine*. New York: Scribner; 1997. The author is a Pittsburgh psychiatrist and director of the Center for Complementary Medicine at the University of Pittsburgh.

Galland L. *The Four Pillars of Healing*. New York: Random House; 1999. The author is a New York internist and former medical director of the Gesell Institute at Yale.

POSTGRADUATE PROGRAMS IN INTEGRATIVE MEDICINE

In-depth training in integrating conventional and alternative medicine is available through Andrew Weil's fellowship program. Initiated in 1997, the 2-year fellowship is open to MDs and DOs who have completed residencies. There is also a distance learning course paralleling the fellowship that is designed for clinicians in practice. For more information, see the Web site of the Program in Integrative Medicine: http://integrativemedicine.arizona.edu

At least a dozen other medical schools also provide some form of postgraduate training in integrative medicine, including Harvard and Columbia.

ECONOMIC DEVELOPMENTS

The Integrator for the Business of Alternative Medicine. This periodical is a 12-page monthly newsletter focusing on the challenges and business opportunities inherent in CAM integration, from hospital/health system-based integrated clinics to HMO benefit trends and venture capital initiatives. Information is available from:
Phone: (877) 426-6633

Physicians who accept capitated patients should be especially attuned to scientific literature on CAM therapies. Thousands of studies can be accessed online on PubMed.
Web site: http://www.ncbi.nlm.nih.gov

A good source of information on ongoing studies is the National Center for Complementary and Alternative Medicine (NCCAM), which conducts and supports biomedical research in this area. The center is under the auspices of the National Institutes of Health.
Web site: http://nccam.nih.gov
NCCAM Clearinghouse
Phone: (888) 644-6226

65.4   Internet Resources

William Mac Beckner

EVALUATING WEB SITES

The same set of quality standards that aid users of medical information navigate print should apply in the digital world. These core standards should apply when assessing information "published" on CAM Web sites and Internet discussion forums. Through the utilization of standards, consumers and professionals alike can reasonably judge whether what they

William Mac Beckner coordinates the Cochrane Collaboration registry of randomized controlled trials in the Complementary Medicine Field, as well as the NIH NCCAM databases on CAM in Pain and Arthritis. In conjunction with his role at the Complementary Medicine Program, he is an instructor in CAM research evaluation at the University of Maryland, School of Medicine. He has also served as project manager for the NIH Office of Alternative Medicine's research database on complementary and alternative medicine.

are reading is credible, reasonable, or useful. Core standards that help in evaluating digital material include:

1. **Authorship:** Authors and contributors, their affiliations and relevant credentials should be provided.
2. **Attribution:** References and sources for all content should be listed clearly, and all relevant copyright information noted.
3. **Disclosure:** Web site "ownership" should be prominently and fully disclosed, as should any sponsorship, advertising, underwriting, commercial funding arrangements or support, or potential conflicts of interest. This includes arrangements in which links to other sites are posted as a result of financial considerations. Similar standards should hold in discussion forums.
4. **Currency:** Dates that content was posted and updated should be indicted.

Web sites and other Internet-based sources of CAM information that fail to meet these basic standards should be considered suspect.

NEWSLETTERS

The Cochrane Collaboration Complementary Medicine Field Newsletter: Karen Soeken, editor. Covers the activities of the Cochrane Complementary Medicine Field.
www.compmed.ummc.umaryland.edu/
Compmed/Cochrane/Cochrane.htm

Bandolier: Andrew Moore, executive editor, NHS R&D Directorate. It contains bullet points (hence Bandolier) of evidence-based medicine and covers CAM topics.
www.jr2.ox.ac.uk/Bandolier/

Natures Herbs: Jim Duke: editor. A Detailed description of herbs used in the U.S.
www.naturesherbs.com/nh/index14.html

HerbClip: Herb Research Foundation.
www.herbs.org/green aper.html

Integrative Medicine Consult: Leonard Wisneski, editor. This site provides impartial, up-

to-date, science-based information about alternative therapies and botanical medicines.
www.onemedicine.com

Herbal Gram: The American Botanical Council.
www.herbalgram.org/herbalgram/index.html

The Integrator: John Weeks, editor and publisher. "For the Business of Alternative Medicine."
www.onemedicine.com

Alternative Medicine Business News: Atlantic Information Services, Elaine Zablocki, editor

Alternative Health News Online:
www.altmedicine.com/

Queensland Herb Society: Newsletter: Australian newsletter with herb resources.
www.powerup.com.au/~sage/

Townsend Letter for Doctors and Patients:
http://tldp.com

Alternative Therapies in Women's Health:
www.ahcpub.com/ahc_root_html/products/
newsletters/atwh.html

Alternative Medicine Alert:
www.ahcpub.com/ahc_root_html/products/
newsletters/ama.html

SPECIAL REPORTS

Five-Year Strategic Plan: National Center for Complementary and Alternative Medicine.
http://nccam.nih.gov/nccam/strategic/

Milk Thistle: Effects on Liver Disease and Cirrhosis and Clinical Adverse Effects.
www.ahrq.gov/clinic/milktsum.htm

Garlic: Effects on Cardiovascular Risks and Disease, Protective Effects Against Cancer, and Clinical Adverse Effects.
www.ahrq.gov/clinic/garlicsum.htm

Integrated Healthcare: A Way Forward for the Next Five Years? Published by the Foundation for Integrated Medicine, 1997.
www.fimed.org/

Alternative Medicine: Expanding Medical Horizons.
https://orders.access.gpo.gov/

Enhancing the Accountability of Alternative Medicine. New York: Milbank Memorial Fund, NY, 1998. Patient protection and the communication of scientific information. www.milbank.org/mraltmed.html

National HMO Survey of Alternative Care: Landmark Healthcare, Inc., 1999. www.landmarkhealthcare.com/99tlrII.htm

Complementary and Alternative Health Practices and Therapies: York University Centre for Health Studies. www.yorku.ca/research/ychs/html/ publications.html

AMERICAN MEDICAL ASSOCIATION— PUBLISHED SPECIAL REPORTS

JAMA, November 11, 1998
http://jama.amaassn.org/issues/v283n10/ toc.html

Archives of Internal Medicine, November 9, 1998
http://archinte.amaassn.org/issues/v158n20/ toc.html

Archives of Neurology, November 1998
http://archneur.amaassn.org/issues/v55n11/ toc.html

Archives of General Psychiatry, November 1998
http://archpsyc.amaassn.org/issues/v55n11/ toc.html

Archives of Pediatrics & Adolescent Medicine, November 1998
http://archpedi.amaassn.org/issues/v152n11/ toc.html

Archives of Surgery, November 1998
http://archsurg.amaassn.org/issues/v133n12/ toc.html

American Medical Association: Report of the Council on Scientific Affairs. Alternative Medicine. Summary. CSA Report 12-A-97 www.ama-assn.org/med-sci/csa/1997/ rep12a97.htm

BRITISH MEDICAL ASSOCIATION

BMJ Collected Resources in Complementary Medicine.
www.bmj.com/cgi/collection/ complementary_medicine

BOOKS

Zollman R, Vickers, A. *ABC of Complementary Medicine.* London: BMJ Books, 2000

Blumenthal M, Golberg A, Brinckmann J. *Herbal Medicine, Expanded Commission E Monographs.* Newton: Integrative Medicine Communications, 2000.

Pelletier, Kenneth R. *The Best Alternative Medicine: What Works? What Does Not?* (Hardcover - February 2000)

Cross, John R., Oschman James L. *Acupressure: Clinical Applications in Musculo-Skeletal Conditions*

Stux, G. *Clinical Acupuncture: Scientific Basis.* Berlin. Springer- Verlag.2000

Helms JM. *Acupuncture energetics: a clinical approach for physicians.* Berkeley: Medical Acupuncture Publishers, 1995

Horstman, Judith, William J. Arnold. *The Arthritis Foundation's Guide to Alternative Therapies*: 1999

Jonas, & Levin. *Essentials of Complementary and Alternative Medicine:* Lippincott Williams & Wilkins, 1999

Lewith, George T. and David Aldridge (ed.) *Clinical Research: Methodology for Complementary Therapies.* London: Hodder & Stroughton, 1987

Cassileth, Barry R., Ph.D., *The Alternative Medicine Handbook:* W.W. Norton & Company, 1998.

Fugh-Berman, Adraine, *Alternative Medicine: What Works:* William & Wilkins, 1997.

Fulder, Stephen, *The Handbook of Alternative and Complementary Medicine:* Oxford University Press, 1996.

Werbach, Melvyn R. and Murray, Michael T.-*Botanical Influences on Illness:* Oxford University Press, 1994.

Werbach, Melvyn R. *Foundations of Nutritional Medicine: A Sourcebook of Clinical Research*, Third Line Press, 1997

Cohen, Micheal H., *Complementary and alternative medicine: legal boundaries and regulatory perspectives.* Johns Hopkins University Press, 1998.

Lewith, George, Kenyon, Julian, *Complementary Medicine An Integrated Approach;* Oxford University Press, 1997

Micozzi, Marc S. *Fundamentals of Complementary and Alternative Medicine:* Churchill Livingston, 1998

Cassileth, Barrie R., *The Alternative Medicine Handbook: The Complete Reference Guide to Alternative and Complementary Therapies* WW Norton & Co, 1998

Fetrow, Charles W. and Juan R. Avila, *Professional's Handbook of Complementary and Alternative Medicines* Springhouse, Pa, Springhouse Corp, 1999.

Goldstein, Michael S., *Alternative Health Care: Medicine, Miracle, or Mirage?,* Philadelphia, Pa, Temple University Press, 1999.

Torkelson, Anthony R., *The Cross Name Index to Medicinal Plants (Plants in Indian Medicine A-Z,* vol 4) Boca Raton, Fla, CRC Press, 1999.

Turchaninov, Ross and Cox, Connie A., *Medical Massage,* with illus, paper, 02-X, Scottsdale, Ariz, Stress Less Publishing, Phoenix, Ariz, Aesculapius Books, 1998.

Novey, Donald., *Clinician's Complete Reference to Complementary & Alternative Medicine,* Mosby 2000

FEDERAL AND STATE RESOURCES IN CAM

National Center for Complementary and Alternative Medicine.
http://nccam.nih.gov/

The Office of Cancer Complementary and Alternative Medicine.
http://occam.nci.nih.gov/

Clinical Trials.gov. 10 clinical trials are now recruiting patients, use "Alternative Medicine" as the search term.
http://clinicaltrials.gov/

The US Government Healthfinder
www.healthfinder.gov

FDA guide to dietary supplements
www.fda.gov/fdac/features/1998/598_guid.html

Current Bibliographies in Medicine 97-6, 1/70 through 10/97. 2302 Citations. Prepared by Lori J. Klein, M.A.L.S., National Library of Medicine, Alan I. Trachtenberg, M.D., M.P.H., National Institute on Drug Abuse 1997 October
www.nlm.nih.gov/pubs/cbm/acupuncture.html

Consensus Development Statement, National Institutes of Health, November 3-5, 1997, Revised Draft 11/5/97
http://odp.od.nih.gov/consensus/cons/107/107_intro.htm

Alternative Medicines from the Federal Trade Commission
www.ftc.gov/bcp/conline/pubs/health/whocares/altmeds.htm

Commission on Dietary Supplement Labels
http://web.health.gov/dietsupp/

FDA Guide to Choosing Medical Treatments by Isadora B. Stehlin appeared in FDA Consumer June 1995, United States Food and Drug Administration
www.fda.gov//oashi/aids/fdaguide.html

Health Information, National Institutes of Health: publications, consumer health information, clearinghouses, health hotlines, consensus statements, rare diseases, and clinical alerts.
www.nih.gov/health/

Health Protection Branch, Canada regulation and control of medical devices, product safety, drugs, etc.
www.hc-sc.gc.ca/hpb/

Federation of State Medical Boards of the United States, Inc. Report of the Special Committee on Health Care Fraud
www.hc-sc.gc.ca/hpb/

Latest State News: State of the State Health Freedom Movement
www.healthlobby.com/news.html

Legislation, from Natural Health Village contains congressional information, federal legislation, and special reports includes:

Access Medical Bill and H.R.1055, the
National Center for Integral Medicine
Establishment Act
www.naturalhealthvillage.com/

Natural Products Branch, National Cancer
Institute: "responsible for coordinating
programs directed at the discovery and
development of novel naturally-derived
agents to treat cancer and AIDS."
http://dtp.nci.nih.gov/

United States Food and Drug Administration
www.fda.gov/

Dietary supplements information
http://vm.cfsan.fda.gov/~dms/supplmnt.html

NCCAM FUNDED SPECIALIZED RESEARCH CENTERS

NCCAM Research Funding Breakdown
http://nccam.nih.gov/nccam/research/grants/
rfb/fy99.html

University of Maryland Complementary
Medicine Program Center for Alternative
Medicine Research on Arthritis.
www.compmed.ummc.umaryland.edu

Minneapolis Medical Research Foundation
Center for Addiction and Alternative
Medicine Research (CAAMR)
www.mmrfweb.org/caamrpages/caamrcover.
html

Consortial Center for Chiropractic Research/
Palmer Center for Chiropractic Research
www.palmer.edu

Columbia University Center for CAM Research
in Aging and Women's Health
http://cpmcnet.columbia.edu/dept/rosenthal/

University of Arizona Health Sciences Center
Pediatric Center for Complementary and
Alternative Medicine (No Link)

Maharishi University Center for Natural
Medicine and Prevention, (No Link)

Center for Health Research Center for
Complementary and Alternative Medicine
Research in Craniofacial Disorders (No Link)

Oregon Health Sciences University Center for
Complementary and Alternative Medicine in
Neurological Disorders (No Link)

The Purdue Center for Dietary Supplement
Research on Botanicals (No Link)

University of Arizona Center on Botanicals (No
Link)

The Johns Hopkins Center for Cancer
Complementary Medicine (No Link)

The University of Michigan CAM Research
Center for Cardiovascular Diseases (No
Link)

University of Pennsylvania Specialized Center
of Research in Hyperbaric Oxygen Therapy.
(No Link)

USEFUL EVIDENCE-BASED MEDICINE SITES FOR CAM RESEARCHERS

The Cochrane Collaboration Complementary
Medicine Field Registry of Controlled Trials
search under "Compmed"
www.update-software.com/clibhome/
clib.htm

Compmed Trials
www.mailbase.ac.uk/lists-a-e/comp-med-
trials

Bandolier Evidence-based healthcare. A
website and newsletter about evidence-based
health care; generally considered one of the
top sources for such information on the net
(has information on CAM therapies)
www.jr2.ox.ac.uk/Bandolier/

Organizing Medical Networked Information
(search under Alternative Medicine)
http://omni.ac.uk/

FREE ONLINE SEARCHABLE DATABASES IN CAM RESEARCH

The Cochrane Collaboration Complementary
Medicine Field Registry of Randomized
Controlled Trials.
www.compmed.ummc.umaryland.edu/ris/
risweb.isa

The Complementary Medicine Program
CAMPAIN database and Complementary
Medicine Program Arthritis database
www.compmed.ummc.umaryland.edu/ris/
risweb.isa

NCCAM Citation Index
http://altmed.od.nih.gov/nccam/resources/
cam-ci/search.cgi
The International Bibliographic Information
on Dietary Supplements (IBIDS) is a
database IBIDS database
http://odp.od.nih.gov/ods/databases/ibids.
html
The Combined Health Information Database
(CHID)
http://chid.nih.gov/
Medline/PubMed
www.nlm.nih.gov
HerbMed® is a project of the Alternative
Medicine Foundation, Inc,
www.herbmed.org/

RESEARCH ORGANIZATIONS, INSTITUTIONS, AND ASSOCIATIONS

McMaster University Health Information
Research Unit
http://hiru.mcmaster.ca/default.htm
Research Council for Complementary Medicine
(RCCM)
www.gn.apc.org/rccm
Münchener Modell
www.lrz-muenchen.de/~
ZentrumfuerNaturheilkunde/muemo.html
Exeter University
www.ex.ac.uk/
Glasgow Homeopathic Hospital
www.homeoint.org/morrell/glasgow/
index.htm
Royal London Homeopathic Hospital NHS
Trust.
http://194.70.69.3/tagish/health/a4f6_
17e.htm
American Botanical Council:
www.herbalgram.org/
The American Herbal Pharmacopoeia
www.herbal-ahp.org/

Herb Research Foundation
www.herbs.org/
American Association of Naturopathic
Physicians: directories to licensed
naturopathic physicians, school and
information use their media web site
www.naturopathic.org/
American Chiropractic Association
www.amerchiro.org/
American Herbal Pharmacopoeia herbal
monographs.
www.herbal-ahp.org
American Holistic Medical Association
http://holisticmedicine.org/
American Massage Therapy Association
www.amtamassage.org/
HealthInform: "providing access to reliable,
research-based information on alternative
and complementary health for consumers
and healthcare professionals through its
publications and customized research
services"
www.healthinform.com/
Homœopathic Pharmacopœia Convention of
the United States (HPCUS)
www.hpus.com/
OncoLink is the University of Pennsylvania's
comprehensive cancer education resource.
http://cancer.med.upenn.edu/
Ask NOAH About: Alternative
(Complementary) Medicine
www.noah-health.org/
Landmark Healthcare, Inc: nationwide
alternative managed care company
specializing in the provision of clinically
supported alternative care therapies
www.landmarkhealthcare.com/
National Center for Homeopathy
www.healthy.net/nch/
Touch For Health Association:
www.tfh.org/

CAM JOURNALS

Journal	Web Site	Indexed in MEDLINE
Advances	www.harcourt-international.com/journals/ambm/	✓
Alternative and Complementary Therapies	www.liebertpub.com/pubs1.htm	✓
Alternative Therapies in Health and Medicine	www.alternative-therapies.com/	✓
American Journal of Acupuncture	www.read-aja.com/	✓
American Journal of Chinese Medicine	www.ajcm.org/editorial0198.html	
American Journal of Clinical Nutrition	www.ajcn.org/	✓
British Homeopathic Journal	www.stockton-press.co.uk/0007-0785/News/ Hel89377...	
British Journal of Clinical Pharmacology	www.blackwell-science.com/~cgilib/jnlpage. bin?Journal=BJCP&File=BJCP&Page=aims	✓
Chinese Journal of Integrated Traditional and Western Medicine	www.chinainfo.gov.cn/periodical/zgzxyjh-E/	✓
Chiropractic Research Journal	www.life-research.edu/crj/crj.html	✓
Complementary Therapies in Medicine	www.healthworks.co.uk/hw/publisher/ churchill/church4.html	✓
European Journal of Herbal Medicine	www.btinternet.com/~nimh/journal.html	
Fact Focus on Complementary Therapies	www.ex.ac.uk/FACT/ - 7k	
Forschende Komplementarmedizin	www.karger.com/journals/fkm/fkm_jh.htm 4	
Journal of Alternative and Complementary Medicine	www.liebertpub.com/acm/default.htm	✓
Journal of Complementary and Alternative Medicine	www.liebertpub.com/acm/default.htm	
Journal of Ethnopharmacology	http://sciserv.ub.uni-bielefeld.de/elsevier/03788741/	✓
Journal of Manipulative and Physiological Therapeutics	http://national.chiropractic.edu/jmpt/	✓
Medical Hypothesis	www.harcourt-international.com/journals/ mehy/default.cfm?jhome.html	✓
Phytomedicine	www.urbanfischer.de/journals/phytomed/ frame_template.htm?/journals/phytomed/phytmed.htm	✓
Planta Medica	www.thieme.com/onGILGJAIJMKF/display/772	✓

THE FUTURE

PART **XVIII**   Future Perspectives

Future Perspectives

CHAPTER 66

Envisioning the Future

66.1   Evolving Paradigms

Clement Bezold

The paradigms that defined U.S. health care for most of the twentieth century are vanishing. During that period, medicine assumed a new identity, evolving from the sphere of the sole practitioner to a system of medical complexes and tertiary care centers, research campuses, and international biotechnical consortiums, in just 100 years. Now another phase of rapid change is occurring as a result of influences ranging from new technologies to new paradigms.

In the evolving health care system, it is probable that:

- Disease and risk will be defined much more broadly.

- The placebo effect will be applied as a therapeutic strategy.
- Medicine will encompass a broader range of paradigms.
- Outcomes research will increasingly focus on clinical utility.
- Health systems will focus on earlier intervention—"Forecast, Prevent, and Manage."
- Consumers will play a greater role in managing their own care.
- Increased customization will occur in both conventional and complementary medicine.
- Expanded applications of epidemiology will leverage broader health gains.

BROADER INTERPRETATIONS OF HEALTH AND ILLNESS

In the future, health care providers will not only treat the direct, localized, physical, or biochemical effects of a disease, they will increasingly take into account the effects of a disease on the patient's other body systems and mental

---

Clement Bezold, PhD, is founder and President of the Institute for Alternative Futures, a nonprofit research and educational organization that assists organizations and individuals in creating their preferred futures. IAF provides environmental scanning and prepares presentations and workshops on trends, visioning, alternative futures, and foresight.

Source: Adapted with permission from C. Bezold, PhD, *Institute for Alternative Futures (IAF) Report on the Future of Complementary and Alternative Approaches in U.S. Health Care,* © 1998, NCMIC Group, Inc.

state. Recent research, for example, shows that psychological traits correlate with health status and mortality (Weiss, 1997). Increasingly, providers will view disease as a dynamic element affecting and being affected by a series of concentric systems—from genetic to cellular to organ to body to mind-body-spirit to individual-family to family-community-health system to global systems. In the future, such systems view will constitute the overarching paradigm for addressing health and disease.

Many complementary and alternative medicine (CAM) practitioners already operate within some form of this systems perspective. James Gordon, director of the Center for Mind-Body Medicine and a physician who uses alternative therapies in his practice, believes we can look at illness as an opportunity to examine and improve our lives (Gordon, 1996). Disease can be a catalyst to explore what it means to be truly healthy and in harmony with our surroundings.

Emerging Perspectives

Placebo Effect and Remembered Wellness

As we consider the future of outcome measures and outcomes for health care, it is relevant to consider our capacity for self-healing—the placebo effect—and its potential role as a therapeutic tool.

In research studies, the placebo response is the healing response demonstrated in patients who believe they have been given appropriate medication when, in actuality, they may have been given an inactive substance. The placebo response and its role in healing are well documented in the scientific literature. In double-blind-controlled studies that use placebos, such as pharmaceutical research, placebo response rates of 30% are common. Some researchers argue that 40–70% of the success of all patient care can be attributed to the placebo response and, therefore, that the patient's belief should be harnessed as a therapeutic tool (Brown and Avram, 1997). Herbert Benson, a Harvard University professor and physician, supports the higher end of the range, suggesting that the placebo response is twice as common as previously believed. Benson also proposes that we rename the placebo effect "remembered wellness," and that practitioners use it consciously and concertedly to augment treatment. Benson estimates that evoking remembered wellness through relaxation and cognitive-behavioral techniques could result in savings of over $50 billion a year (Benson, 1996).

If this projection is correct, the application of the placebo response in the context of *all* modalities, mainstream and alternative, could be significant. In addition, there are other mind-body phenomena, involving prayer, personality, or belief systems, which could be put to use for clinical benefit. Ultimately, any safe and effective approach that stimulates a person's innate healing capacity and engages the immune system may come to be considered as a potential tool for healing.

Clinical Utility

As a broad range of models are factored into outcomes research, the resulting knowledge base will become increasingly focused on utility—on what works to improve health. Both genomics and CAM will have significant impact on diagnostic categories over the next decade. Genomics will enable us to determine individual proclivities to disease and comorbidity factors. Cancers will no longer be defined only by organ or site—breast cancer or lung cancer—but will also be described by the genotypes and phenotypes that have been associated with the deterioration or remediation of these conditions.

Genotype and Phenotype

A genotype implies having a particular gene sequence. Phenotype focuses on physical, biochemical, or behavioral characteristics, as determined genetically and environmentally. Thus, genotype describes whether an individual or group has a specific gene or set of genes, whereas phenotype describes the expression of genes through the process of interaction with the environment.

Diagnostic categories from complementary medicine that reflect phenotypic differences will be added to the universal nomenclature. Constitutional homeopathy, for instance, finds relevance in behavioral and morphologic characteristics. Oriental medicine incorporates information from differences in pulse diagnosis. Constitutional categories in Ayurveda are based on body type—endomorph, ectomorph, and mesomorph. Factors of this type will be integrated into diagnostic categories, as they prove useful. Clinical utility will become a component of health care outcomes, particularly in the absence of a transparadigm science that would define clinical outcomes in terms of multidisciplinary categories. The definition of utility itself will become more complex as it is modulated by patient preferences.

Early Intervention: Forecast, Prevent, and Manage

A paradigm focused on early intervention reflects a fundamental shift in the perspective underlying health care—a move from treating disease after the fact to greater emphasis on preventing the disease process before it begins or escalates. This paradigm moves practitioners away from treating symptoms of disease to anticipating changes in health status, preventing morbidity wherever possible, and proactively managing morbidity when it does occur (Goldsmith, 1996).

This shift in the focus of treatment will entail a concurrent paradigm shift in institutional practice and investment. The entire health care community, from practitioners to policy makers, will likely expand the prevailing focus to encompass all aspects of lifestyle. This shift will be supported by the development of informational systems that emphasize prevention and self-care; the development of approaches designed to prevent potential health problems; the use of new biomonitoring techniques; and a new generation of DNA vaccines.

Together, these tactics will allow:

- The application of outcomes from both CAM and advanced biomedical research
- Early detection of illness and abnormal functioning
- More accurate diagnosis and treatment of genetically defined subtypes of disease
- Gene therapy, which designs out disease and addresses subtle malfunctions in the physiology
- A dramatic increase in available interventions—new generations of antibiotics and vaccines
- Customized care in which therapeutics are more precisely tailored to individual biochemistry
- Minimization of disease by targeting the social and environmental risk factors in communities
- New forms of immunotherapy, including CAM treatments that enlist and bolster immunity
- Disease management using a wide range of therapeutic tools, including lifestyle change.

Managed Self-Care

More and more, consumers are becoming involved in their own care. The largest proportion of health care has always been self-care, but with the proliferation of knowledge and knowledge tools, consumers are gaining greater understanding of health and self-management. Within the provider community, expertise is also expanding, from specialist physicians to general practitioners, nurses, and other health care providers.

The category of people who were called patients in the past will be recognized in the future as sophisticated health care consumers. The culmination of this model is the concept of patient as healer, in which the patient actively participates in his or her own care, in tandem with health care professionals.

At least three trends are converging in favor of self-care:

- Consumers' willingness to take charge of their health
- Growing desire among providers to encourage self-care and to practice demand management
- Insurers, self-funded employers, and capitated providers who now have greater incentives to promote self-care.

For consumers interested in taking an active role in their care, one of the highest value-added services provided by many professionals will be their capacity to motivate and guide their patients to manifest healthier behavior. This health coach role will grow in importance, and schools must enable future practitioners to become effective health coaches.

CUSTOMIZATION OF HEALTH CARE

The growing interest in customization by conventional medicine stems in part from its own tradition as a primarily empirical science, focusing on specific and measurable dimensions of the human body and its reactions to internal and external stimuli. This focus has led to, among other things, the discovery of DNA and the rise of genomics, with its implications for increased capacity to treat the individual.

The capacity of genomics for customization has been a long-term systemic focus of certain complementary and alternative approaches. In fact, some of the alternative disciplines have incorporated and tracked the diagnostic and therapeutic significance of phenotypic differences—not for centuries, but for millennia! Most leading complementary approaches have developed elaborate "phenotypic" systems for differentiating among individuals. These represent evidence-based observations over long periods of time: in Oriental medicine, for example, the knowledge base has been accrued over as much as 2,500 years.

Ayurvedic approaches, most common in India, use the "dosha" system to characterize individuals. Doshas can be thought of as beginning with body types (ectomorph, endomorph, and meso-

morph) and adding layers of information about emotional tendencies, intellectual styles, and spiritual inclinations (Gottlieb, 1995). Likewise, Oriental medicine and homeopathy have complex approaches to subgrouping individuals phenotypically, apart from their specific disease diagnosis. Homeopathy considers persons having similar syndromes, such as migraine headaches, for example, not as having the same disease but as having similar symptoms pointing to deeper conditions that may be radically different. These deeper conditions cannot usually be addressed by suppressing the symptoms. Homeopathy incorporates individualization of care by tailoring the remedy to various phenotypic characteristics of the individual being treated (Ullman, 1995).

Insights from mind-body approaches will also contribute to customization. One of the most popular phenotypic groupings, the Myers-Briggs Type Indicator (MBTI) is based on Carl Jung's observation that we all have different "gifts" in the way we process information and come to decisions (Briggs-Myers, 1995). For example, some people focus on facts and details, others on concepts and larger patterns; some operate analytically, whereas others are more influenced by their values and beliefs. The resulting differences have been shown to be important in how individuals operate at work and in their relationships. It is possible that personality type has clinical relevance in a range of diseases and health conditions.

Redefining Health Care through Customization

Implications for Research and Regulatory Approaches

Conventional health care will increasingly "customize" or personalize preventive methods and treatment to achieve the greatest benefit and cause the least harm. Genotype and phenotype will provide the basis for this approach. Some of the research on clinically relevant customization is likely to focus on complementary medicine and wellness. This will increase the complexity and sophistication of our understanding and will challenge current regulatory approaches. For example, how should clinical trials, drug regulation, and formulary development change if we can identify various factors that consistently predict whether a medication will be successful? What if these pheonotypes are derived from observations drawn from Oriental medicine? Health care will face interesting challenges.

A related challenge for the development of new pharmaceutical therapies relates to the conduct of clinical trials. If drugs become customized and focused on specific genotypes, the population for which the drugs would be used might be relatively small. Likewise, outcome measures might become more complex as genotype differences lead to different definitions of outcomes.

Integrated and Customized Therapies

Customized and integrative therapeutics are being applied in expanded applications. Nutritional expert Jeffrey Bland, PhD, founder and CEO of HealthComm International (Gig Harbor, Washington), has developed several products for nutritional modulation of liver detoxification. The customized products are selected on the basis of the user's diagnosis and biochemical profile, reflected in laboratory testing. The products are typically used as a component of a customized nutritional protocol to provide macro-, micro-, and accessory nutrients that support the restoration of functional detoxification capabilities (Bland, 1999; HealthComm International, 2000).

In the field of cancer treatment, Keith Block, MD, a Chicago-area physician, has created a program that enables him to better individualize treatment protocols for his patients. Before developing a treatment regimen, he creates biomedical, biochemical, and biomechanical profiles, as well as a psychosocial profile (including patient needs, attitudinal tendencies, and stress level). Based on the outcomes of these detailed studies of each patient, Block individualizes the nutritional program, including diet change and nutritional supplements. According to Michael Lerner, PhD, an expert on complementary

cancer approaches at Commonweal, Block's approach is a "model that could fit easily into the mainstream practice of hematology-oncology" (Lerner, 1994). By 2010, we will be much farther along in understanding how to integrate complementary and alternative approaches with conventional medicine and to customize and personalize the resulting mix of therapeutics to the individual.

LEVERAGING BROADER HEALTH GAINS THROUGH EPIDEMIOLOGY

Most health care professionals make their contribution one patient at a time. This is appropriate but no longer sufficient. Health professions should enable their members to make greater contributions by leveraging health gains for broader groups in the population.

One approach is to apply the professions' unique tools to populations in which epidemiology suggests that the greatest health gains can be achieved. This matrix of linkages will include not only mainstream medical specialties, but also the range of CAM therapies. For example, chiropractors could determine which populations have high morbidity from back problems and provide preventive strategies to these groups—such as retail sales personnel who spend most of the work day standing.

Once this commitment is established, creativity will be required to discover and design appropriate roles for each of the health professions. If the professions recognize and make a commitment to address these problems in ways appropriate to their disciplines, the health professions and society will have the opportunity to leverage broader health gains.

THE EVOLVING FUTURE

In 1998, the *Institute for Alternative Futures (IAF) Report on the Future of Complementary and Alternative Approaches in U.S. Health Care* presented a range of forecasts. Five key issues were explored through expert opinion, a consensus process, focus groups, and a review of the literature.

Typically, forecasts are developed based on patterns of experience, established and newly emerging trends, and expert judgment. Trends are monitored in science and technology, health care delivery, and in clinical therapeutics. Experts are interviewed for their insights, their forecasts, and their response to potential scenarios. For this report, a range of opinion was also sought through focus groups ranging from managed care executives to consumers. An extensive search of the medical literature was performed.

The five key forecasts that evolved from the 1998 study are as follows:

1. CAM therapies will become major tools for health promotion and prevention.
2. CAM will be integrated into conventional medical protocols.
3. Some CAM providers will become recognized as primary care providers.
4. Conventional and automated providers will increase the use of alternative therapies.
5. Providers that take a role in creating healthy communities will gain a competitive advantage.

Hypothesis #1: Complementary and alternative approaches will become major tools for health promotion and prevention

Trends in Health Enhancement

Broader Use of Health Promotion. In the future, we will engage an expanded range of approaches to health—physical, nutritional, psychological, and spiritual—that will tend to make people healthier and provide higher quality of life. These approaches will come to be seen as meaningful strategies, even for patients with potentially fatal conditions, such as late-stage cancer. In some cases, health promotion interventions may be all that is needed to restore health, as in the Ornish program; in other cases, they will be focused on prevention, risk reduc-

tion, or helping individuals with terminal illness to have quality of life.

Greater Routine Use of Core Complementary Modalities. CAM disciplines such as Oriental medicine, chiropractic, and Ayurveda are all based on philosophies that encourage holistic health practices on the part of the individual. These and many other CAM therapies conceptually reinforce health promotion. The same can be said for biomedical care, at its philosophical best. In practice, both types of providers can become overly focused on the immediate complaint at hand, using a limited bag of tools. In the future, complementary medicine is likely to be applied more frequently in health promotion, based on feedback from long-term outcomes research and consumer satisfaction. The lifestyle components of CAM will see their greatest application in prevention and wellness.

Health Promotion through Routine Wellness Visits. Leading providers in certain CAM disciplines firmly believe that periodic visits are beneficial in maintaining patients' health. Some chiropractors recommend quarterly or monthly checkups. Some physicians using integrated practices recommend quarterly visits for rebalancing through acupuncture or a review of diet, supplements, and lifestyle. The services of a health coach are also based on the idea of periodic monitoring and reinforcement. Visits for care can vary widely in terms of time and cost. An office visit involving only spinal manipulation might involve patient-chiropractor contact of as few as 7–10 minutes, whereas a wellness visit incorporating a range of approaches, including acupuncture, might consist of 45–60 minutes of the consumer's time and 30–45 minutes for the practitioner. Additional outcomes data will be required to determine the cost/benefit ratio of these periodic visits.

Until we have more data, the question of wellness visits is likely to remain unresolved. For example, in chiropractic care, an estimated 14–35% of services provided in this country consist of these wellness visits (Institute for

Alternative Futures, 1998). Their popularity has been driven by consumer demand, and many consumers are willing to pay for them out of pocket. Some experts suggest that such visits reduce the need for more costly diagnostic or treatment approaches, including hospital utilization. The utilization of wellness visits will probably continue to increase, paid for by consumers as noncovered services.

Hypothesis #2: CAM will be integrated into conventional medical protocols

This trend has already begun to occur. In the next decade, CAM therapies will be integrated into the protocols of conventional medicine. The extent to which they will be integrated will vary according to the particular complementary discipline, the type of health system and its organizational culture, the availability of coverage, demographics, and the health care needs of the target population.

The degree of integration will also depend on:

- The development of a substantial evidence basis for CAM
- The nature of customization of care
- Whether conventional medicine absorbs various CAM disciplines into its practices
- Whether medicine also includes CAM providers in mainstream practice
- Whether, alternatively, mainstream providers refer patients outside the system to CAM providers

New Protocol Development

A Shift toward Integrative Therapeutics, Including CAM Therapies. Biomedicine is moving away from an intensive focus on disease treatment toward integrative therapeutics that emphasize treating the whole person (mind and body), enhancing the immune system, and supporting self-healing capacity. A ground-breaking example of this are the programs of Dean Ornish for the treatment of heart disease, using a combination of diet, exercise, group support,

and mental and attitudinal approaches, including spiritual orientation. Each participant's regimen is individualized to some degree, so they receive medication as necessary. The program has been documented to successfully reverse advanced heart disease for many participants (Ornish et al, 1998). This integrated approach, customized to the needs of the individual, could become a major form of disease management in the United States.

A Search for Definitive Treatments for Chronic Conditions. In the treatment of chronic illness, most approaches used in biomedicine tend to be palliative, rather than curative. Medical scientist Lewis Thomas (1977) suggests that, in this new century, we will find definitive treatments for these disorders. Traditionally, health care has sought definitive treatments, sometimes conceived of as "magic bullets" that target the problem or disease but require little behavioral change on the part of the patient. Highly successful examples include antibiotics and many other types of drug therapy, as well as surgery. Some CAM therapies provide magic bullets, such as herbal or homeopathic remedies for various conditions or chiropractic manipulation for certain back problems. Yet a profound lesson is now being absorbed by the health care system from integrated approaches. Ornish's program (Ornish et al, 1998) can reverse heart disease by reducing plaque buildup in the arteries. Ornish has proposed that this approach can also be used to reverse cancer and will be researching this premise in a sizable clinical trial. This represents a more holistic approach to combating disease but one that clearly requires significant participation from patients (particularly in the areas of diet, exercise, stress reduction, spiritual and personal growth, and psychosocial involvement).

There will also continue to be interest in and support for quick fixes, by both consumers and health care providers. There will be more powerful magic bullets in the classic pharmacological sense, for example, of drugs that effectively melt plaque in the arteries. We are likely to develop new definitive treatments, which will be preventive in nature. The paradigm of being healthier rather than relying on a crisis orientation will become the overriding characteristic of health care. Complementary and alternative approaches will be a growing component of these healthier approaches.

Increased Use of Cost-Effective Supportive Approaches. Complementary and alternative medicine offers great promise for enhancing the quality of life for those with chronic conditions and for those undergoing therapy that is physically taxing, such as cancer chemotherapy. Complementary therapies are already widely used by consumers in these areas. As evidence makes it clear that CAM is highly relevant in supportive and adjunctive therapeutics, health care providers will incorporate more alternative approaches into their practices. Providers will prescribe some CAM therapies in the same way that they now prescribe over-the-counter remedies. There will continue to be some financial tension as long as consumers must pay for these remedies out of pocket. As more CAM therapies are proven to be effective, some will be covered by health plans, but others will remain nonreimbursable items. In both cases, CAM will continue to be used as supportive therapy.

Hypothesis #3: Some CAM providers will become recognized as primary care providers and will be funded by the dominant health care systems

Trends in Integration

Some CAM Practitioners Will Function as Primary Care Providers. The definition of a primary care provider is shifting from "primary contact" to imply the practitioner who assumes overall responsibility for effectively managing the patient's problems, including referrals to other health care professionals. Increasingly, the role also involves prevention—acting as a consultant on health promotion. As evidence from outcomes research becomes more available and as CAM practitioners prove themselves able

to work within health care delivery systems, their role as primary care providers will grow, particularly if they offer less expensive or more highly effective care (which is ultimately less expensive).

Expanded Reimbursement by Health Systems. Increasingly, health care providers are including CAM, both therapeutics and providers, in their coverage. As noted, many leading health care providers are opening CAM centers in their systems and incorporating CAM into standard practice. Given the high degree of consumer interest and presumably growing evidence for cost-effectiveness, complementary therapeutics and services will be funded with greater frequency by the dominant health systems.

Hypothesis #4: The use of alternative therapies by conventional providers and automated providers will increase

New Patterns of Utilization

Use by Conventional Providers. In the coming decade, U.S. health care will become more effective and cost-effective. The integration of new technology, wellness initiatives, and appropriate CAM therapies will be part of this enhancement. These trends will be supported by the development of integrated protocols, best practices, and expert systems. Among health care providers, as job competition increases, professionals are likely to diversify the services they offer to increase their competitiveness in the market. The expanded use of integrative medicine will create demand for practitioners with dual training and expertise in various fields of biomedicine and CAM.

Extensive outcomes data will enable health care professionals to incorporate wellness and CAM programming that has been shown to be cost-effective. Increasingly, health systems will advertise their complementary services and holistic approaches. Report cards are likely to assess providers and health systems in terms of the complementary approaches they use and, ultimately, how successful they are in applying various complementary therapeutics for prevention and the treatment of specific conditions.

Some aspects of the knowledge base of CAM may be easily incorporated into clinical protocols. However, there are CAM disciplines that require significant training and can take years to fully master—for example, comprehensive training in Oriental medicine includes pulse diagnosis; acupuncture; herbal medicine; treatments such as moxibustion, principles of diet; therapeutic exercise such as Qigong and T'ai chi; and the understanding of the body from the perspective of Chinese medicine. Effective chiropractic manipulation is an advanced skill related to sophisticated diagnostic requirements and clinical therapeutic technique. However, certain aspects of CAM modalities may be seamlessly incorporated into biomedical treatment—for example, the use of some nutritional supplements and herbal remedies—if the relevant expertise has been incorporated into the training, protocols, and expert systems used by the health care organization.

An interesting question for the integration of these best practices is whether not only the practices themselves, but also their accompanying diagnostic systems, will be incorporated. Customization of care on the basis of genotype and phenotype will be integrated to a greater degree into mainstream medicine over the next decade. In diagnosis and screening, some of the CAM therapies use typologies and patterns of individual characteristics that are essentially systems of phenotypic characteristics. This approach is particularly true of Oriental medicine, Ayurvedic medicine, and homeopathy. Some of these phenotypic schematics will prove to be clinically useful and will be incorporated into mainstream diagnostic and treatment protocols.

Use by Automated Providers. Many aspects of health care will be provided by expert systems and/or intelligent devices. This will be true of health care in general and of preventive strategies and CAM specifically. Understandably, most physicians and providers dislike the notion of being partially or wholly displaced by equipment or software. Most argue that these devices will interfere with the doctor–patient relationship. Some are frank about the economic threat they represent. Bank tellers undoubtedly had a similar response to automated teller machines (ATMs) when they were being proposed 20 years ago. However, there is much more to the doctor–patient interaction than the teller–customer interaction—and the subtle effects of the therapeutic relationship on healing are only just beginning to be understood. Yet even if we honor the provider–patient relationship more fully, the decentralizing capacity of expert systems will give consumers far greater capacity for self-care, enabling the provider to focus on higher-value aspects of the relationship, including coaching and counseling.

Availability of Therapeutic Devices. In terms of equipment, will there be machines for taking a pulse diagnosis or providing acupuncture? This is feasible. For example, one can currently purchase enhanced versions of the acupressure chair and also equipment that facilitates spinal stretching. Many small hand-held acupuncture devices are now on the market that can be used to identify and treat sensitive points with very low-level electromagnetic stimulation. (In Hong Kong, these devices are ubiquitous.) Another likely innovation will be computer-based expert systems.

Expansion of Self-Care. In the next decade, much health care that is currently provided by professionals will be supplanted by sophisticated self-care; individuals and families will conceivably handle far more of their own health care needs at home than they do now. These efforts are likely to be aided by automated and electronic information tools and fee-for-service care, perhaps reinforced by medical savings accounts and other incentives to make the best use of health care, and with the protection of catastrophic health insurance against excessive expenditures.

Proliferation of Expert Systems. The role of complementary and alternative approaches in this self-care environment will grow most quickly for therapies that are amenable to inclusion in the protocols of expert systems. Self-help guides to conventional and complementary care are being transformed into sophisticated software. Homeopathy, for example, has spawned high-end expert systems for use by homeopaths. Software like this will become more consumer-friendly and accessible, built into expert systems for integrative self-care. In the next decade, expert systems will be able to customize their recommendations to the user, based on the appropriate phenotypes drawn from alternative medical systems such as acupuncture, Ayurveda, and homeopathy. Simultaneously, software that acts as a personal coach via individualized intelligent agents will become common.

Hypothesis #5: CAM and mainstream providers who assume a significant role in creating healthy communities have the potential to gain a competitive advantage

This hypothesis is based on observation of developments in health care in the United States and other regions of the world. Health care providers will not only become responsible for health outcomes, but may also share greater responsibility for the health of the communities they serve. To the extent that they can help to create healthy communities, they will gain competitive advantage. This forecast is made with less certainty than the others. It is as much an aspiration or statement of hope as a plausible forecast. To date, community health has not been a primary focus for either alternative or mainstream providers. Yet leveraging true gains in health requires moving upstream to the causes of ill health, many of which can be dealt with only by focusing on the community and the environment. Complementary and alternative approaches offer unique opportunities for contribution in this area. Shared vision—both within and across therapeutic communities—is essential to identify and achieve long-term goals for improved community health.

CONCLUSION

By 2010, at least two-thirds of the U.S. population will be using one or more of the approaches we now consider alternative. Complementary and alternative therapies and preventive programs will be integral to many of the future changes in health care. Consequently, all stakeholders—allopathic providers, complementary medicine practitioners, insurers, payers, the pharmaceutical industry, consumers, and policy makers—need to explore how health care can evolve in order to yield the greatest health gains. Whether future trends are more or less healthy will be a matter of our choices and commitments.

REFERENCES

Benson H. *Timeless Healing.* New York: Scribner; 1996.

Bland J. *Genetic Nutritioneering.* Chicago: NTC Publishing; 1999.

Briggs-Myers I, Myers P. *Gifts Differing.* Menlo Park: Consulting Psychologists Press; 1995.

Brown D, Goldstein A. Long and short of life. *The Washington Post.* December 4, 1997: A1.

Goldsmith J. Managed care comes of age. In: *Future Care: Responding to the Demand for Change*, eds. C Bezold and E Mayer. New York: Faulkner & Gray; 1996.

Gordon J. *Manifesto for a New Medicine.* New York: Addison-Wesley; 1996.

Gottlieb W. *New Choices in Natural Healing.* Emmaus, PA: Rodale Press; 1995:5.

HealthComm International, Web site www.healthcomm.com. Accessed March 2000.

Institute for Alternative Futures. *The Future of Complementary and Alternative Approaches (CAAs) in U.S. Health Care.* Alexandria, VA: NCMIC Insurance Company; 1998:4–14.

Lerner M. *Choices in Healing.* Boston: MIT Press; 1996.

Thomas L. 1977. Biomedical science and human health: The long-range prospect. *Daedalus.* 1997(Summer):168.

Ornish D, Scherwitz LW, Billings JH, et al. Intensive life-style changes for reversal of coronary heart disease. *JAMA.* 1998;280(23):2001–2007.

Ullman D. *The Consumer's Guide to Homeopathy.* New York: GP Putnam's Sons; 1995:8.

Weiss R. Your personality may be killing you. *The Washington Post.* July 22, 1997; Health Section:16.

66.2   Vantage Point: Managing Demand

Christopher Foley

Health care shares characteristics with three other major institutions: the police and fire departments, and the military. These are all institutions that ideally should make efforts to manage demand down, rather than up. They should all be essentially trying to put themselves out of a job. The problem in health care is that we make our living when demand is up, and we are affiliated with vendors who also benefit from high demand.

Our economic partners include four major industries: the pharmaceutical industry, hospitals, the diagnostic imaging industry, and surgical instrument manufacture. We make more money if we manage demand up, but, ethically, we should be trying to manage demand down. The primary tools that physicians have been given to manage demand in a capitated system are surgery and pharmaceuticals. These methods are appropriate for acute conditions but are not always effective in addressing chronic conditions. With the development of new paradigms and new tools,

we approach the dawn of an era in which we are beginning to manage upstream—which ultimately means reducing demand downstream.

For each of the four sectors, there is an integrative and upstream adaptation that can be made in response to the changing economic and technologic environment.

The key is to retool gradually in every sector in order to adapt to new requirements (Table 66.2–1).

- *The pharmaceutical industry* will continue to thrive as the paradigm shift occurs because it also owns nutraceutical and botanical manufacturing. In those dual roles, the industry will retain market share as a portion of consumer demand shifts to another sector of the industry.
- *The hospital sector*, in the future, will expand beyond the provision of acute care to the community. Clearly, we will always need the acute care services, but the demand will decrease over time. As our capabilities in the provision of acute and trauma care continue to be refined, patient market share will be reduced. This is a phenomenon that can be observed in other sectors, as well. In response, hospital services will become diversified to include health management services and facilities such as fitness clubs and community health centers.
- *The use of diagnostic technology* will potentially be applied to a greater range of

Christopher Foley, MD, completed his medical education at the University of Minnesota and practiced internal medicine in St. Paul for 18 years. In 1995 he left his private practice to direct the HealthEast Healing Center in the St. Paul/Minneapolis area—one of the first clinics in the country designed to provide alternative therapies in conjunction with mainstream medicine. HealthEast's integrative health initiatives have been relocated to HealthEast's new twenty-first century hospital, Woodwinds, in Woodbury, a suburb of St. Paul. Dr. Foley is also a clinical assistant professor at the University of Minnesota.

Table 66.2–1 Managing Down Demand: New Applications of Technology and Information

Institution	New Applications
Pharmaceutical industry	Continued development of the pharmaceutical industry; the creation of new antibiotics and vaccines; and extensive expansion into nutrients (nutraceuticals) and botanicals (phytomedicine)
Hospitals	Continued function as a medical resource to the community through an expanded continuum of services that includes fitness centers, community health facilities and outpatient centers, risk reduction, and disease management.
Diagnostic imaging and therapeutic radiology	Expanded use of energy medicine and electromagnetic fields to treat depression; facilitate bone regeneration and wound healing; and heal degenerative diseases. Expanded applications in functional testing and diagnosis
Surgical instrument industry	Continued market to expand to new applications in orthopedic surgery and organ transplants, as well as elective cosmetic surgery for an aging population

evaluative capabilities. For example, positron emission tomography (PET) technology, currently utilized to diagnose acute conditions such as brain tumors, will be applied in more subtle diagnostic evaluations, such as malfunctions related to the gut–brain axis, which manifest in behavioral disorders. Magnetic resonance imaging (MRI) technology will be expanded into the field of energetic medicine—the use of low-level electromagnetic fields in healing. For example, molecular magnetic energizing (MME) units, which are comparable to the MRI, are now being used in bone regeneration and wound healing. Many additional applications will be developed. Pioneers in this field will become widely recognized, such as Norman Sheeley, who treats depression with low-level electromagnetic stimulation.

- *The surgical instrument industry* will be adapted to the needs of an aging population. We are likely to see increases the number of surgical procedures for aging knees, organs, and faces.

This situation is in some ways comparable to the auto industry. As consumers have become

more knowledgeable about the market and as competition has increased, manufacturers have responded by developing higher-quality cars. Manufacturers now offer good-quality, long-lasting products. If one is considering the automobile simply as a mode of transportation, it is possible to buy a very good car quite inexpensively. Consequently, other aspects of the products must be emphasized in order to differentiate them, so the marketing of style and power becomes more important.

The corollary to health care is that we are moving toward a system that teaches people how to manage their health quite inexpensively, with an emphasis on how to live a long time and remain highly functional by managing genetic expression. At the same time, because of the need to change the system incrementally, earlier services will be recast in order to continue to use the capacity of the system to the fullest. Luxury services, such as organ replacements and face-lifts, are the equivalent in health care of expensive automobiles.

Corporations in the auto industry now market themselves as providers of all types of transportation rather limiting themselves to any one product. Whether consumers want an economy car or a luxury car, the goal of the manufacturer is to meet the need by providing a range of options. The companies that accommodate that range of consumer need will be the survivors.

In the pharmaceutical industry, for example, if a manufacturer wants to be the provider of choice for treating depression, it is most likely to be successful if it is the company that helps people to manage their condition successfully. A company is most likely to capture market share by offering the physician a product line that includes a range of choices for patients, such as medication, botanicals, and nutrients. Physicians will choose the company that provides a truly integrative approach in order to offer their patients effective options. Manufacturers have not yet conceptualized their separate service lines from an integrative perspective, but this is clearly the wave of the future.

The successful business plan of the large drug conglomerate of tomorrow will be highly integrative and will reflect the breadth of consumer demand and interest. Those that are not integrative may lose market share, unless the industry is restructured or unless vendors become fully involved with service provision linked to the new paradigms, as well.

CHAPTER 67

The Total Customer Relationship in Health Care: Broadening the Bandwidth

Donald M. Berwick

The health care system is in the midst of a market revolution, driven by cost containment but also fully charged by the idea that competition among providers will lead to reforms that neither the government nor the professions have been able to achieve by themselves. An agenda of "reports to consumers" has been advanced as a new hope for improving the health care system. An alternative to this notion of consumerism is far broader—the concept of total relationship.

THE BANDWIDTH OF TOTAL RELATIONSHIP

In the hands of masters outside the health care domain, the total customer relationship *embraces several elements that can be imported into health care:*

- customers as assistants in decreasing waste
- mass customization and stratification of need
- shaping demand
- immediate recovery
- delight as the objective
- customer knowledge and innovation.

A useful model can be found in modern, globally competitive companies. The idea of customer-mindedness is a vast and expansive notion of *customer relationship* and how powerful the totality of that relationship can be in ensuring the success of organizations. Applied in the fields of health care, this becomes the notion of *total relationship* with those who depend on health care for their safety, security, and comfort. Understanding the breadth of the bandwidth of total relationship is a key to the next phase of maturation of our industry's ability to give people what they need and deserve from us. Following are some elements of a total customer relationship in the hands of masters.

Customer As Assistants in Decreasing Waste

General Motors defines *waste* as "anything the customer would not willingly pay for." That is an extremely demanding definition. It broadens the concept of waste and, therefore, the opportunities for efficiency far beyond the obvious forms of scrapped materials and lost time. For a modern company, motion of people or supplies is waste, inventory is waste, and inspection is

Donald M. Berwick, MD, MPP, President and CEO of the Institute for Healthcare Improvement, is a practicing pediatrician who teaches regularly at both Harvard Medical School and the Harvard School of Public Health. He is current Chair of the National Advisory Council of the Agency for Healthcare Research and Quality, as well as an elected member of the Institute of Medicine of the National Academy of Sciences. He has published over 80 scientific articles in numerous professional journals and is co-author of the books, *Curing Health Care* and *New Rules: Regulation, Markets and the Quality of American Health Care*.

The Institute for Healthcare Improvement (IHI) is a non-profit organization designed to be a major force for integrative and collaborative efforts to accelerate improvement in health care systems. The Institute provides bridges connecting people and organizations who are committed to real reforms, and who believe they can accomplish more together than they can separately.

Courtesy of Donald Berwick, MD, Boston, Massachusetts.

waste. So are unused space, idle equipment, and most documents. At the world-class level, the search for and removal of waste (what the Japanese call *muda*) can itself become the heart of a business strategy (Womack and Jones, 1996). "The more waste is removed," said Taiichi Ohno, the genius behind the Toyota production process, "the more every customer can appear as an individual" (Ohno, 1988).

If waste is defined in terms of the customer viewpoint, then inquiry about customer viewpoint is an essential step in its discovery. The Cadillac Division of General Motors studied the question, How many different Cadillacs can we make? This meant adding up all possible combinations of color, style, equipment, and so on. The answer was more than 4 billion, an immense latent capability, but of what use? How many different Cadillacs were ever actually ordered by a customer? The answer: More than 99% of all orders could be accounted for by 8,000 different Cadillacs. The rest of the latent capacity was pure waste—a capability no customer ever cared about.

In designing health care systems of the future, it will be as important to understand what our patients and families do not want as what they do want. Like Cadillac, our capacities in many functions far outstrip any plausible need.

Mass Customization and Stratification of Need

The best service companies in the world feel to the consumer as though the work were individualized. When it counts, it is. However, a good deal of the efficiency and effectiveness of those companies comes not from knowing each customer as an individual but rather from their deep understanding of the stratification of people in their own market. They do not necessarily know you as an individual, but they can find out quickly where, among several general types of customers, you fit most closely.

These companies are mass-customizing their work. They have abandoned a policy of "one size fits all" in favor of a much more powerful

set of market strata—something like "five sizes fit 75% of our customers." Airlines treat frequent travelers differently from the rest, and they treat platinum-level frequent travelers differently again.

Yet in many emergency departments you can find a sign prominently posted that says something like "Only one visitor may accompany the patient to the examination room." What about the child with two parents or the elderly person with three attendants, or the out-of-towner brought in by the couple hosting him? The sign is out of place in a world of customer-mindedness. Rules, like products, can be customized.

In evaluating need, some advocates of "leveling the playing field" would eliminate variables such as race, income, and prior health status in order to promote a greater fairness within the system. However, this strategy does not bring us closer to understanding the needs of customers. Rather, it factors them out.

Shaping Demand

Powerful companies in the world market do not just meet customer expectations, they actively shape them. Health care managers sometimes characterize the expectations of the consumer public as "excessive" or "unrealistic," but remarkably few maintain and improve active processes for causing those expectations to change over time.

Yet the opportunities for shaping demand are extraordinary in health care. Consider the recommendations of the second edition of the *Guide to Clinical Preventive Services* from the U.S. Preventive Services Task Force (USPSTF) of the Department of Health and Human Services (1996). Five years of work on that edition included the review of more than 6,000 scientific articles bearing on more than 200 current or proposed clinical preventive services, such as screening tests, immunizations, and behavioral counseling. For most of the services reviewed, including many in common use today, the USPSTF found little or no scientific evidence of efficacy, and even some evidence of active harm. Excessive use of fetal monitoring, for example, can raise the Caesarean section rate unnecessarily. Routine screening with chest X-rays for lung cancer or with ultrasonography for ovarian cancer adds to costs without any evidence of benefit in reduced morbidity or mortality. A preventive services package for a group practice or a managed care system modeled on the recommendations of the USPSTF would be both more effective and less expensive overall than the informal packages that abound today. To accomplish such a change, however, would require a highly coordinated effort to change, using processes of public relations, clinician education, media, and many others in a managed, coordinated organizational effort.

John Scott, an internist in Kaiser-Permanente's Colorado Region, has taken customer-mindedness seriously in a new design that illustrates how powerful shaping demand can be to improve service. Noticing that he was repeating the same instructions over and over again for his hypertensive patients, he offered several a chance to visit him as a group, then to have personal sessions if they needed them. He applied the same thinking to his diabetic patients and to other subgroups. The groups were successful, so much so that when he informed one set of patients that a forthcoming meeting had to be canceled because he was going to be away, they told him that they would still like to meet anyway.

Supporting Self-Care

The most exciting applications of customer focus in health care today engage patients and families in learning to perform tasks in diagnosis and care that were formerly reserved for doctors and nurses (Greenfield et al, 1988). Asthma patients today measure their own peak flow rates, adjust their own medications, and administer their own nebulizer treatments at home with machines that, a decade ago, were found only in hospitals (Lahdensuo et al, 1996).

Larry Staker, an internist at Intermountain Health Care's LDS Hospital in Salt Lake City, is teaching diabetic patients how to keep statistical control charts of their glucose levels and how to adjust their insulin on their own. He is doing similar work with patients who have hypertension, who learn to adjust their own blood pressure medications, and with people on anticoagulation, who learn to adjust their own coumadin. His case series suggests that when patients are taught to make their own decisions, they can often be effective participants in their own care.

In the pursuit of total customer relationship, the health care organization of the future will be continually searching for ways to transfer care into the hands of patients and families when it is wise, humane, and logistically successful to do so. Organizations will not preserve prerogatives that they do not need. Alaska Airlines lets me issue myself my own boarding pass, and today I am effectively my own bank teller.

Immediate Recovery

In great organizations, when a customer gets abraded, recovery rebuilds loyalty. In fact, a great company's most loyal customers include those who have suffered some damage, then experienced immediate and thorough redress. The classiest organizations do not just replace the service or product, they use a concept called "replace plus one," under which customers receive more than they lost, out of respect for the misuse of their time and as a form of additional apology.

This approach, called "immediate recovery" in service industries, requires a sense of guarantee, a commitment to promises. Standing behind a product or service is most effective when there are no excuses allowed. ("Guaranteed, period" is the promise of the mail order company Lands' End.) Only a few health care systems have grappled with guarantee as a strategy. To do so places the relationship with the customer at the highest level of priority. A strong recovery strategy speaks volumes to a work force if people are well supported to deliver on the guarantee. The best immediate recovery programs place great authority in local, low-level personnel to offer and deliver whatever it takes to restore the faith and loyalty of the customer. Immediate-recovery events, when carefully documented, constitute a source of ongoing information on patterns of both defect and need, providing grist for longer-term improvements and for new product and service designs.

Total relationship with patients and families as customers requires an answer to the question, What do we promise, and how do we back up that promise when we fail? Few report card systems raise questions at this level of discipline and commitment, and few patients completing a rating questionnaire will think to report on a "failed promise," because that is not the current vocabulary in health care scoring.

Becoming a Customer Yourself

The surest way to experience care as a patient does is to become a patient oneself. In fact, clinicians and others in health care often have the chance to do so, either personally or through the eyes of a relative—such as a child or an aging parent. Ask almost any audience of health care professionals to report on their own experiences as patients. They tend to be just as frustrated as patients by long waits, unanswered questions, poor designs, and wrong treatments (Berwick, 1996).

Equally disturbing, however, is the schizophrenic separation between the frustration of doctors and nurses as patients on the one hand and their rationale as caregivers on the other. The explanation for this disconnection lies, of course, not in blindness but in a sense of powerlessness: Clinicians feel helpless to change the systems that they know full well are inadequate to meet needs. No one likes long waits, but those waits seem inescapable. No one favors errors, but mistakes happen.

World-class health care systems, focused on customers, will not avoid the experiences of patienthood but rather will amplify them. The best way to do so for many executives and clinical leaders would be to reconnect personal experiences with public priorities. This can begin with

simulation. A few courageous health care leaders are arranging to have themselves admitted to their own hospital or examined in their own clinic, usually with the full knowledge of the staff involved in their simulated care, then to document and debrief carefully what they notice. Wisely done, this exercise leads not, as some fear, to impulse on anecdote but to renewed understanding of what may be salient to study more and to correct in general (see Chapter 44 on the Griffin Hospital experience).

Continual Innovation

In the long run, the biggest problem with report cards as drivers of improvement is their limited view of what is possible. Great companies and great health care systems will seek to produce the unexpected, to cause patients and families to boast about their care, not merely to be satisfied with it. Delight in those we serve must come from much deeper understandings of the lives, needs, and sensibilities of our patients and families, rather than from rating scales.

The ability to produce customer delight depends on continual innovation. Knowledge for invention is not generally quantitative; it is narrative. The stories, not the rating scores, contain the possibilities. To learn what we can do for people that is absolutely unprecedented in their experience will require that we meet them, know them, and create with them.

Score cards to date neither study nor reward the inventiveness that will define the future of our industry. They focus on known processes and familiar services, and they divert energy from the task of creation in many organizations. Excellent organizations will not yield to the temptation of short-run numerical gains at the expense of basic redesign of care. In that redesign process, the customer is a partner, a co-architect of the future, and welcome at our table.

CONCLUSION: A CUSTOMER FOCUS CREDO

The bandwidth of total customer relationship for health care is broad. My list of elements is only partial. The justification for these elements and ideas for others lie in several tenets about the wisdom of those we serve and the nature of our purpose. Taken together, those tenets provide a credo for the next phase of the development of our industry:

1. *In a helping profession, the ultimate judge of performance is the person helped.* In the last analysis, we have nowhere else to turn for the true compass directions to excellence. In the quest for total relationship with customers, a world-class health care system, like the best health care providers, will ask continually, "What do you need?" and "How did I do at meeting that need?"

2. *Most people, including sick people, are reasonable most of the time.* An uncompromising intention to meet needs invites fears that those needs may be insatiable. It is also true that some patients are unreasonable some of the time. However, the more important question is about the majority of patients and their expectations most of the time. Commitment to customers begins with trust in customers. They are, after all, not just like us, they *are* us.

3. *Different people have different, legitimate needs.* What customers need most is our understanding and agile systems that respect their diversity. A world-class

health system exhibits flexibility and makes the effort to discover what it must and can do for patients, one by one. I once saw a hospital that had engraved above its door the words "Every patient is the only patient."

4. *Pain and fear produce anxiety in both the patient and the caregiver.* The impact of constantly dealing with emergent situations makes it tempting to take certain liberties. This is a centuries-old precedent in health care. However, the context of emergency should not provide a reason for removing the focus from the customer. Clinicians earn their high status best by remaining mindful at all times of the needs of those who depend on them.

5. *Meeting needs without waste is a strategic and moral imperative.* "Customer focus" is neither the motto of marketing nor a sideline to the true work of medicine. It is at the very heart of health care. It is its *raison d'être*. Without pursuit of the social need, for which the term *customer focus* is only shorthand, health care has no legitimate claim to its trillion dollars in spending. When the patient enters our gates, all our encounters must begin with a single question, How can I help you? All the investments of our time, our energies, and our dollars must move ever in the direction of the answers to that question.

REFERENCES

Berwick DM. Quality comes home. *Ann Intern Med.* 1996;125:839–843.

Greenfield S, Kaplan SH, Ware JE Jr, Yano EM, Frank HJ. Patients' participation in medical care. Effects on blood sugar control and quality of life in diabetes. *J Gen Intern Med.* 1988;3(5):448–457.

Lahdensuo A, et al. Randomised comparison of guided self management and traditional treatment of asthma over one year. *BMJ.* 1996;312:748–752.

Ohno T. *The Toyota Production System: Beyond Large-Scale Production.* Portland, OR: Productivity Press; 1988.

U.S. Preventive Services Task Force. *Guide to Clinical Preventive Services*, 2nd Edition. Baltimore: Williams & Wilkins; 1996.

Womack JP, Jones DT. *Lean Thinking: Banish Waste and Create Wealth in Your Corporation.* New York: Simon & Schuster; 1996.

Index

Page numbers in *italics* denote figures and exhibits; those followed by "t" denote tables; those followed by "n" denote footnotes.